Treatments in Hepatology

Treatments in Hepatology

Vicente Arroyo

Professor of Medicine and Chief of Section, Liver Unit and Department of Medicine,
Hospital Clínic i Provincial, University of Barcelona, Barcelona, Spain

Jaume Bosch

Associate Professor of Medicine and Chief of Section, Liver Unit and Department of Medicine,
Hospital Clínic i Provincial, University of Barcelona, Barcelona, Spain

Juan Rodés

Professor of Medicine and Director of the Liver Unit, Department of Medicine,
Hospital Clínic i Provincial, University of Barcelona, Barcelona, Spain

MASSON, S.A.

Barcelona - Madrid - Paris - Milano - Asunción - Bogotá - Buenos Aires - Caracas - Lima - Lisboa - México
Montevideo - Rio de Janeiro - San Juan de Puerto Rico - Santiago de Chile

MASSON, S.A.
Avda. Príncipe de Asturias, 20 - 08012 Barcelone

MASSON, S.A.
120, Bd. Saint-Germain - 75280 Paris Cedex 06

MASSON S.P.A.
Via Statuto, 2 - 20121 Milano

ISBN 84-458-0341-7
Depósito Legal: B. 10.516 - 1995
Cover Designer: Angel García
Compositor: A. Parras - Avda. Meridiana, 93-95 - Barcelone (1995)
Printer: Gràfiques 92, S.A. - Torrassa, 108 E - Sant Adrià de Besòs (Barcelone) (1995)
Printed in Spain

Contributors

Luis Álvarez
Instituto de Investigaciones Biomédicas, Consejo Superior de Investigaciones Científicas, Madrid, Spain.

Francis E. Andre
Medical and Scientific Services SmithKline Beecham Biologicals, Rixensart, Belgium.

Adrian M. Bisceglie
Department of Internal Medicine, Saint Louis University Health, Sciences Center, Saint Louis, USA.

Henri Bismuth
Hepatobiliary Center, Paris South University, Hôpital Paul Brousse, Villejuif, France.

Andres T. Blei
Section of Gastroenterology and Hepatology, Lakeside VA Medical Center and Northwestern University, Chicago, USA.

Loreto Boix
Liver Unit, Hospital Clínic i Provincial, University of Barcelona, Barcelona, Spain.

Jaume Bosch
Liver Unit, Hospital Clínic i Provincial, University of Barcelona, Barcelona, Spain.

Concepció Brú
Liver Unit, Hospital Clínic i Provincial, University of Barcelona, Barcelona, Spain.

Miguel Bruguera
Liver Unit, Hospital Clínic i Provincial, University of Barcelona, Barcelona, Spain.

Jordi Bruix
Liver Unit, Hospital Clínic i Provincial, University of Barcelona, Barcelona, Spain.

A. K. Burroughs
Liver Transplantation and Hepato Biliary Medicine, Royal Free Hospital, London, UK.

David L. Carr-Locke
Endoscopy Service, Brigham and Women's Hospital, Harvard Medical School, Boston, USA.

Antoni Castells
Liver Unit, Hospital Clínic i Provincial, University of Barcelona, Barcelona, Spain.

Marielle Cohard
Service d'Hépato-Gastroentérologie, Clinique d'Hépato-Gastroentérologie, CHRU, Grenoble, France.

Antonio Craxi
Instituto di Medicina Generale e Pneumologia, University of Palermo, Italy.

David L. Cutler
Director Division of Clinical Pharmacology, Schering-Plough Research Institute, Kenilworth, USA.

Gennaro D'Amico
Clinica Medica R, Divisione di Medicina, Ospedale V. Cervello, Palermo, Italy.

Gary L. Davis
Section of Hepatobiliary Diseases, University of Florida, College of Medicine, Gainesville, USA.

Geoffrey M. Dusheiko
Department of Medicine, Royal Free Hospital and School of Medicine, London, UK.

Juan I. Esteban
Liver Unit, Hospital Universitari Vall d'Hebron, Universitat Autònoma, Barcelona, Spain.

Olivier Farges
Hepatobiliary Center, Paris South University, Hôpital Paul Brousse, Villejuif, France.

Cyrille Feray
Hepatobiliary Center, Paris South University, Hôpital Paul Brousse, Villejuif, France.

Faust Feu
Liver Unit, Hospital Clínic i Provincial, University of Barcelona, Barcelona, Spain.

Joan C. García-Pagán
Liver Unit, Hospital Clínic i Provincial, University of Barcelona, Barcelona, Spain.

Jane M. Geders
Section of Gastroenterology and Hepatology, Tulane University and Veterans Administration Medical Center, New Orleans, USA.

Angels Ginès
Liver Unit, Hospital Clínic i Provincial, University of Barcelona, Barcelona, Spain.

Pere Ginès
Liver Unit, Hospital Clínic i Provincial, University of Barcelona, Barcelona, Spain.

Antonio González
Liver Unit, Hospital Universitari Vall d'Hebron, Universitat Autònoma, Barcelona, Spain.

Norman D. Grace
Department of Gastroenterology, Tufts University School of Medicine, Faulkner Hospital, Boston, USA.

Roberto J. Groszmann
Digestive Disease Section, Yale University School of Medicine, Veterans Affairs Medical Center, West Haven, USA.

Carlos Guarner
Gastroenterology Service, Hospital de la Santa Creu i Sant Pau, Universitat Autònoma, Barcelona, Spain.

M. Hoyumpa
Department of Medicine, Division of Gastroenterology and Nutrition, The University of Texas Health Science Center at San Antonio and Audie L. Murphy Memorial Veterans' Hospital, San Antonio, USA.

A. M. Lacy
Department of Surgery, Hospital Clínic i Provincial, University of Barcelona, Barcelona, Spain.

Vincent Leroy
Service d'Hépato-Gastroentérologie, Clinique d'Hepato-Gastroentérologie, CHRU, Grenoble, France.

Charles S. Lieber
Mt. Sinai School of Medicine (CUNY); Alcohol Research and Treatment Center and GI/Liver & Nutrition Program, Bronx VA Medical Center, New York, USA.

Cristina Linea
Instituto di Medicina Generale e Pneumologia, University of Palermo, Italy.

Anna S. F. Lok
Section of Gastroenterology and Hepatology, Tulane University and Veterans Administration Medical Center, New Orleans, USA.

Silvio Magrin
Divisione di Medicine Interna, Ospedale V. Cervello, Palermo, Italy.

Masatoshi Makuuchi
Second Department of Surgery, Faculty of Medicine, University of Tokyo, Tokyo, Japan.

Michael Peter Manns
Department of Gastroenterology and Hepatology, Center of Internal Medicine, Medizinische Hochschule Hannover, Hannover, Germany.

Philippe Mathurin
Service d'Hépato-Gastroentérologie, Groupe Hospitalier Pitié-Salpêtrière, Paris, France.

José M. Mato
Instituto de Investigaciones Biomédicas, Consejo Superior de Investigaciones Científicas, Madrid, Spain.

David Multimer
Liver and Hepatobiliary Unit, Birmingham, UK.

Miquel Navasa
Liver Unit, Hospital Clínic i Provincial, University of Barcelona, Barcelona, Spain.

Andreas Ochs
Medizinische Universitätsklinik, Freiburg, Germany.

Pierre Opolon
Service d'Hépato-Gastroentérologie, Groupe Hospitalier Pitié-Salpêtrière, Paris, France.

Pablo Ortiz
Laboratorio Europharma, Grupo Boehringer, Madrid, Spain.

J. B. Otte
Department of Surgery, Cliniques Universitaires St. Luc, Brussels, Belgium.

María A. Pajares
Instituto de Investigaciones Biomédicas, Consejo Superior de Investigaciones Científicas, Madrid, Spain.

D. Patch
Liver Transplantation and Hepato Biliary Medicine, Royal Free Hospital, London, UK.

Robert P. Perrillo
Section of Gastroenterology and Hepatology, Ochsner Clinic, New Orleans, USA.

Ramón Planas
Gastroenterology Department, Hospital Universitari Germans Trias i Pujol, Badalona, Spain.

Gudrun Pöschl
Salem Medical Center, University of Heidelberg, Heidelberg, Germany.

Raoul Poupon
Unité d'Hépato-Gastroentérologie, Hôpital Saint-Antoine, Paris, France.

Renée E. Poupon
INSERM Unit 21, Villejuif, France.

Thierry Poynard
Service d'Hépato-Gastroentérologie, Groupe Hospitalier Pitié-Salpêtrière, Paris, France.

M. J. Ramond
Service d'Hépatologie, Hôpital Beaujon, Clichy, France.

Jürg Reichen
Department of Clinical Pharmacology, University of Berne, Berne, Switzerland.

Jennifer A. Roberts
Department of Public Health and Policy, London School of Hygiene and Tropical Medicine, London, UK.

Simon C. Robson
Department of Surgery, New England Deaconess Hospital, Boston and MRC UCT Liver Center, Groote Schuur Hospital, Cape Town, USA.

Nancy Rolando
Institute of Liver Studies, King's College Hospital and King's College School of Medicine & Dentistry, London, UK.

Martin Rössle
Medizinische Universitätsklinik, Freiburg, Germany.

B. Rueff
STAMA, Hôpital Beaujon, Clichy, France.

Bruce A. Runyon
Department of Medicine, University of Louisville, Louisville, USA.

Mikko Salaspuro
Research Unit of Alcohol Diseases, University of Helsinki, Helsinki, Finland.

Luis Salleras
Department of Preventive Medicine, Hospital Clínic i Provincial, University of Barcelona, Barcelona, Spain.

Joan Saló
Liver Unit, Hospital Clínic i Provincial, University of Barcelona, Barcelona, Spain.

Didier Samuel
Hepatobiliary Center, Paris South University, Hôpital Paul Brousse, Villejuif, France.

Steven Schenker
Department of Medicine, Division of Gastroenterology and Nutrition, The University of Texas Health Science Center at San Antonio and Audie L. Murphy Memorial Veterans' Hospital, San Antonio, USA.

Andreas Schüler
Department of Gastroenterology and Hepatology, Center of Internal Medicine, Medizinische Hochschule Hannover, Hannover, Germany.

Helmut K. Seitz
Department of Medicine and Laboratory of Alcohol Research, Liver Disease and Nutrition, Salem Medical Center, University of Heidelberg, Heidelberg, Germany.

Greg Van Stiegmann
Surgical Endoscopy Service, University of Colorado and Denver, Veterans Affairs Hospitals, Denver, USA.

Gregorio Varela
Instituto de Investigaciones Biomédicas, Consejo Superior de Investigaciones Científicas, Madrid, Spain.

Roger Williams
Institute of Liver Studies, King's College Hospital and King's College School of Medicine & Dentistry, London, UK.

Catherine H. Wu
University of Connecticut School of Medicine, Farmington, USA.

George Y. Wu
Division of Gastroenterology-Hepatology, Herman Lopata Chair in Hepatitis Research, University of Connecticut School of Medicine, Farmington, USA.

Jean Pierre Zarski
Service d'Hépato-Gastroentérologie, Clinique d'Hépato-Gastroentérologie, Grenoble, France.

Introduction

J. Rodés

Treatment in liver diseases has experienced great progress over the last few years, largely enhancing the possibility of improving survival and quality of life for patients with both acute and chronic liver diseases. This book includes the contributions to a meeting held in Barcelona in March 1995 aimed at updating, most, albeit not all, therapies in hepatology.

The spectrums covered in the book have been selected to include new procedures and management, and the topics which are, today, of greatest interest in Hepatology. The book is divided into 9 sections devoted to Pharmacological Treatment of Portal Hypertension, Treatment of Complications of Cirrhosis, Treatment of Bacterial Infections in Liver Diseases, Treatment of Chronic Viral Hepatitis, Prophylaxis of Hepatitis Virus Infection, Advances in Liver Transplantation, Treatment of Alcoholic Liver Disease, Treatment of Biliary Diseases and Hepatocellular Carcinoma, and, finally, a miscellaneous section dedicated to Other Treatments in Liver Diseases.

In the section on Pharmacological Treatment of Portal Hypertension, the mechanisms of this frequent complication, particularly collateral formation and rupture of esophageal varices, drug therapy in acute bleeding episodes, pharmacological prevention of variceal hemorrhage and evaluation and indication of pharmacological treatment of patients with portal hypertension are discussed. The section on Treatment of Complications of Cirrhosis analyzes the new technical developments in the management of patients bleeding from esophageal varices such as endoscopic variceal ligation and the transjugular intrahepatic portosystemic shunt. In addition, the treatment of ascites, renal dysfunction and hepatic encephalopathy are also discussed indicating the most rational approaches to these complications. The incidence of bacterial infections, especially spontaneous bacterial peritonitis, is very high. At present, antibiotic regimes have been widely investigated achieving good results in controlling these infections. Furthermore, the prevention of bacterial infections in both, fulminant hepatic failure and cirrhosis, has also been developed and is discussed in section 3. Without a doubt interferon, as an antiviral therapy in chronic hepatitis B and C infection, is the only treatment that has been demonstrated to be effective in these clinical conditions. However, more clinical research is required to further improve the results of this therapy. Section 4 also looks at several other possible mechanisms of action, new treatments and new therapeutic schedules in these patients. The discovery of hepatitis A and B vaccines has been one of the most important events to occur in modern Hepatology. At present, however, we still do not have a vaccine against hepatitis C. This is the future challenge. All these aspects are widely discussed in section 5 of this book. Liver transplantation has changed Hepatology. It is probably the most important advance in the treatment of severe acute liver failure and end-stage chronic liver disease. The survival of patients submitted to liver transplantation is excellent. However, a lot of problems remain to be solved. In section 6, all these aspects, particulary immunosuppression and new surgical techniques, including xenotransplantation, are discussed in depth. Alcoholic liver disease remains one of the most frequent clinical problems in Hepatology. It has been well established that abstinence is the best treatment. It is, however, quite difficult to achieve this objective, and now there are relatively well established therapies and the arrival of new and old drugs is discussed in section 7.

Section 8 includes the treatment of biliary diseases such as gallstones and malignant strictures by laparoscopic surgery and endoscopic procedures. These two new techniques clearly have changed the management of these frequent disorders. In the same section the surgical and medical treatment of hepatocellular carcinoma are reported. Finally, section 9 is devoted to updating the treatment of acute hepatic failure, autoimmune hepatitis and chronic cholestasis. There are two other very interesting topics. The first, gene therapy, will be of great interest in the near future and, the second, prescribing in liver disease, is very useful and practical, and in turn, very little known by most physicians.

All these topics are covered by 50 internationally distinguished speakers considered as leaders and experts in each topic. I am very grateful that these people have accepted our invitation to participate in this book.

In closing, I would like to express my gratitude to all the patronage and sponsors: University of Barcelona, Hospital Clínic i Provincial of Barcelona, International Association for the Study of the Liver, European Association for the Study of the Liver, Spanish Association for the Study of the Liver, Schering Plough, Europharma, Ferring Pharmaceuticals, Hoechst, Knoll-Basf-Pharma, Sandoz Pharma SAE, Smith Kline French, Dr. Falk Pharma GMbh, Madaus Cerafarm, Medical Europa and Pfizer. Without their cooperation this meeting could not have been held and consequently this book could never have been published.

Index

Section 3

TREATMENT OF BACTERIAL INFECTIONS IN LIVER DISEASES

Section 4

TREATMENT OF CHRONIC VIRAL HEPATITIS

Section 7

TREATMENT OF ALCOHOLIC LIVER DISEASE

Section 8

TREATMENT OF BILIARY DISEASES AND HEPATOCELLULAR CARCINOMA

Section 9

OTHER TREATMENTS IN LIVER DISEASES

Treatments in Hepatology

Section 1

Pharmacological Treatment of Portal Hypertension

Mechanisms of Portal Hypertension: Collateral Formation and Rupture

R. J. Groszmann

INTRODUCTION

Portal hypertension is the main consequence of cirrhosis and is responsible for the majority of its complications. Varices and variceal hemorrhage are a direct consequence of portal hypertension and account to a large extent for the high morbidity, the high mortality and the high care costs associated with cirrhosis (1).

Practically all patients with cirrhosis, irrespective of etiology, will develop portal hypertension. Initially, portal pressure increases as a consequence of an increased resistance to portal flow du to scarring, compression and narrowing of hepatic sinusoids. Later on, in addition to this elevated resistante to blood flow, there is an increase in portal blood inflow (2). When *both* resistance and flow are elevated, portal pressure increases even further and when a minimal pressure threshold is reached, the clinical complications of portal hypertension appear (3).

Studies from our and other laboratories support the contention that a minimal portal pressure gradient of around 12 mmHg is necessary for the development of varices and variceal bleeding (3). In this context, we have recently demonstrated that a reduction in portal pressure gradient below 12 mmHg protects patients from variceal bleeding (4). Reducing pressure below the bleeding threshold not only protects patients from variceal hemorrhage but also increases survival (fig. 1) (4).

Portal pressure is the result of the interrelationship between portal blood flow and the resistance developed by the obstructed portal system to that flow. In order to understand this relationship, it is necessary to apply the concepts of fluid dynamics that govern all living and nonliving systems. Ohm's law applied to the vascular system states that the pressure gradient between

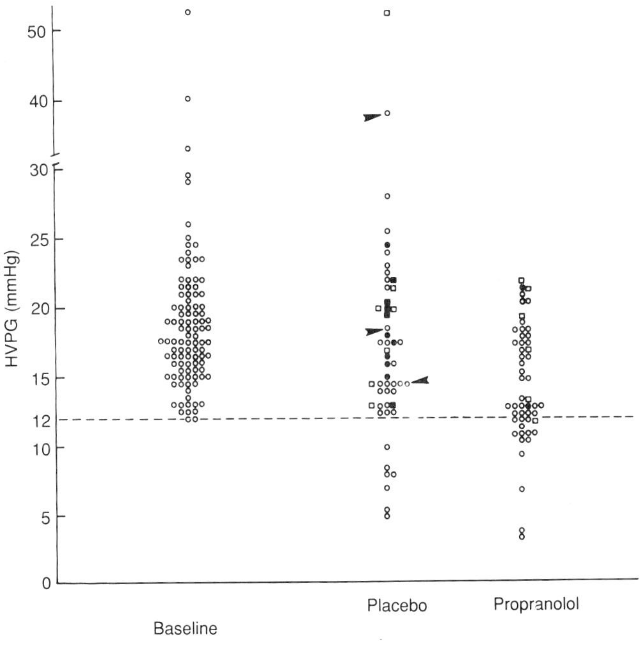

Fig. 1. Effects on portal pressure of long-term treatment with propranolol or placebo. Patients that have bled from portal hypertensive gastropathy are depicted with or → or ↙ and patients that have bled from gastro-esophageal varices are depicted with ● or ■. Patients that have one measurement of HVPG are depicted ■ ❑ and patients that have more than one measurement of HVPG are depicted ●○. None of the patients that have a reduction in the hepatic venous pressure gradient (HVPG) below 12 mmHg bled from varices (4).

two ends of a vascular circuit depends on the relationship between flow (Q) in the circuit and the resistance (R) to that flow: $P_1 - P_2 = Q \times R$. Resistance is expressed by Poiseuille's formula $R = nl/\pi r^4$ where n is the viscosity of blood, r is the vessel radius and l is the length of the system. Under physiologic conditions, n and l are constants hence pressure is directly related to flow and inversely related to changes in vessel size. Since resistance changes in proportion to the fourth power of the radius, small changes in vessel size produce large changes in pressure. In portal hypertensive states, in experimental animal models and man, portal pressure is elevated due to an increase in both resistance and portal venous flow (5).

INTRAHEPATIC VASCULAR RESISTANCE

Increased resistance to portal venous flow may be localized at prehepatic, intrahepatic, or posthepatic sites. In prehepatic and posthepatic portal hypertension, this is secondary to obstruction of portal venous inflow or hepatic venous outflow, respectively. Intrahepatic portal hypertension is more complex and is usually a consequence of anatomic derangements of the hepatic lobule and liver microcirculation.

While structural alterations in the hepatic microcirculation due to fibrosis and nodular regeneration is the most important factor, a primary increase in vascular tone similar to that observed in arterial hypertension may also contribute to the increased intrahepatic resistance observed in chronic liver disease. Hepatic lipocytes have been shown to play a role in hepatic fibrogenesis. In addition, there is evidence suggesting that they may act as liver specific pericytes, a type of cell that has been shown to regulate blood flow in other organs (6). In acute and chronic liver injury, hepatic lipocytes acquire contractile characteristics and may contribute to the dynamic modulation of intrahepatic resistance (7). These cells, which may also be the predominant source of collagen synthesis in chronic liver disease, may contribute to the regulation of hepatic blood flow at the microcirculatory level. Lipocytes are strategically located in the sinusoids with perisinusoidal and interhepatocellular branching processes containing actin-like filaments. They also express the alpha smooth muscle actin gene which is characteristic of vascular smooth muscle cells. This feature is similar to that observed in myofibroblasts which may be derived from lipocytes. Myofibroblasts are intermediate in structure between smooth muscle cells and fibroblasts. Bundles of actin microfilaments are demonstrated within their cytoplasm and these cells are thought to be responsible for the contraction of maturing scar tissue. Myofibroblast-like cells have been shown to exist in fibrous septa around sinusoids and terminal hepatic venules in cirrhotic livers where their density may correlate with vascular resistance. These cells are postulated to have a role in the regulation of vascular resistance in the isolated perfused cirrhotic rat liver (8). Normal lipocytes, when activated in culture, acquire contractile properties with an enhanced response to endothelial derived vasoconstrictors such as endothelins (9). Recently, the vascular endothelium has been shown to play an important role in regulating vascular tone by synthesizing potent vasoconstrictors (endothelins) and vasodilators (prostacyclin and nitric oxide) (10). Nitric oxide has been shown to regulate intrahepatic resistance in normal and cirrhotic rat livers (11, 12). Nitric oxide (NO), being a vasodilator that exerts its action locally is considered a major «fine tuner» of vascular tone. In fact, one of the most important vascular roles of NO is to balance the effect of humoral and local vasoconstrictors. Vascular beds with a defective NO synthesis demonstrate an abnormally increased vascular resistance. There are several different processes that impair endothelial cell function and the local synthesis of NO. These include trauma, arteriosclerosis, and arterial hypertension (13, 14). In fact, we have observed that rats with spontaneous arterial hypertension have a high portal pressure and an increased intrahepatic vascular resistance (15). We have recently demonstrated that NO contributes to the regulation of intrahepatic resistance in the normal rat liver (11). Mechanisms that regulate the production of NO in the hepatic microcirculation and the role NO plays in pathological states such as cirrhosis remain to be determined. Preliminary studies from our laboratory performed in the isolated perfused cirrhotic liver, suggest that NO plays a major role in the modulation of intrahepatic vascular resistance (16). Our preliminary data suggest that NO production is deficient in the hepatic microcirculation of the cirrhotic liver.

SPLANCHNIC AND SYSTEMIC CIRCULATION

A hyperdynamic splanchnic and systemic circulation is observed in all forms of portal hypertension and is associated with extensive portosystemic shunting and/or hepatic failure. The pathophysiologic basis of this hyperdynamic circulation is still controversial though it is probably due to an increase in activity of endothelial independent and endothelial dependent vasodilators. The resultant vasodilatation leads to sodium retention and increased intravascular volume. This combination of vasodilatation and an expanded intravascular volume is necessary for the full expression of the hyperdynamic state (5, 17).

Vasodilatation

Elevated levels of circulating endogenous vasodilators may account for the hyperdinamic circulation in portal hypertensive states. Cross-perfusion studies between portal hypertensive and normal rats demonstrated an increase in flow and decrease in vascular resistance in the splanchnic and systemic circulation of the normal animal (18). The failure of a parabiotic model to confirm these findings may be the result of rapid metabolism of the circulating vasodilator(s) by the liver of the normal animal of the parabiotic pair (19).

A variety of gut peptides have been proposed as the circulating vasodilatory substance which mediates the hyperdynamic circulation with glucagon being the most likely candidate (20). Glucagon levels are elevated in a rat model of prehepatic portal hypertension and in patients with portal hypertension and portosystemic shunting (21, 22). Infusion of glucagon in normal animals to achieve levels observed in portal hypertensive controls was associated with a significant reduction in splanchnic vascular resistance (23). Although infusion of a glucagon-specific antiserum resulted in a significant reduction in portal venous inflow, this was not accompanied by a modulation of the systemic hyperdynamic circulation nor by a significant reduction in portal pressure (24). Thus, the significance of glucagon as a mediator of the hyperdynamic circulation remains unclear.

A variety of circulating vasodilators have been evaluated including bile acids, histamine, adenosine, and others without a clear demonstration that they contribute to the hyperdynamic state.

Vascular hyporeactivity to endogenous vasoconstrictors has been demonstrated in animal models of portal hypertension and cirrhotic patients (25, 26). A postreceptor defect induced by circulating vasodilators can explain the impairment in vascular contractility observed in portal hypertension.

Recent studies have emphasized the role of endotelial dependent mechanisms in the regulation of vascular tone. Endothelial cells synthesize vasoconstrictors (endothelins) and vasodilators (prostacyclins and nitric oxide). In rabbits with pre-hepatic portal hypertension, mesenteric blood flow, decreased vascular resistance, and increased portal pressure are associated with a significant increase (27%) in the systemic arterial concentration of prostacyclin (26). While cyclooxygenase blockade results in a decrease in prostacyclin levels and diminution in the hyperdinamic circulation, these agents also cause deleterious effects on renal function in cirrhotic patients (27).

Nitric oxide (NO) is a potent endotelial-derived vasodilator that is formed from L-arginine. Recent studies suggest that NO may play an important role in the hyperdynamic circulation of portal hypertension. *In vitro* studies, using perfused mesenteric artery preparations from normal and portal hypertensive rats, demonstrated that vessels from portal hypertensive animals exhibited significant hyporeactivity to norepinephrine, vasopressin, potassium chloride and methoxamine (28, 29). Since this preparation is free of circulating vasodilators, this hyporesponsiveness may be mediated by an endothelial-dependent mechanism. Incubation of this system with the stereospecific NO biosynthesis inhibitor N^{ω}-nitro-L-arginine (NNA) reversed the blunted response to these pressors in vessels of rats with prehepatic portal hypertension induced by partial ligation of the portal vein (PVL) to a greater extent than that observed in normal vessels, suggesting that enhanced NO secretion may contribute significantly to the vascular hyporeactivity to endogenous vasoconstrictors observed in portal hypertension. This conclusion is supported by *in vivo* studies en PVL and cirrhotic rats, which show that blockade of NO formation significantly decreases the systemic hyperdynamic circulation and splanchnic hyperemia and reverses the hyporeactivity to methoxamine in PVL rat (30, 32). Thus, alterations in systemic and splanchnic hemodynamics seen in portal hypertension may be mediated in part by excess formation of NO.

Intravascular Volume

Development of a hyperdynamic circulation requires both vasodilation and intravascular volume expansion. In normal animals and humans, vasodilators alone either have no effect or actually diminish cardiac output rather than produce a hyperdynamic circulatory state. In PVL rats, volume expansion is preceded by vasodilation and in turn leads to the full expression of the hyperdinamic circulation (33, 34). In this same rat model, dietary sodium restriction ameliorates the development of the hyperdinamic circulation and institution of a sodium restricted diet in rats with established portal hypertension, decreases the hyperdynamic circulatory state (35).

Octreotide and nitric oxide blockade decrease renal sodium retention and plasma volume expansion by diminishing vasodilatation thereby, preventing the full expression of the hyperdynamic circulation (36, 37). Plasma volume expansion has been demonstrated in cirrhotic patients (38). An increased splanchnic blood flow, which is part of the hyperdynamic syndrome, is an important contributing factor to the severity of portal hypertension (5).

COLLATERAL CIRCULATION

Porto-systemic collaterals develop as a result of portal hypertension. Although they partially decompress the portal circulation, they also lead to important complications. The most lethal is the development of gastroesophageal varices and variceal hemorrhage. Also, in advanced disease, splanchnic blood flow is diverted through the collateral system bypassing the liver, depriving it of blood flow and providing a conduit through which toxins escape hepatic metabolism. This diversion of portal blood flow leads to hepatic failure and encephalopathy.

The vascular resistance of the collateral bed, although lower than that of the obstructed portal system, is nevertheless higher than normal portal resistance (5). Hence, the development of portosystemic collaterals does not lead to complete portal decompression. Portal hypertension persists even when the entire portal flow escapes through collaterals. Although collaterals develop as a consequence of an increased portal pressure, they then contribute importantly to the circulatory derangements characteristics of portal hypertension. Factors that modulate the development of the collateral system and that regulate collateral blood flow are not yet completely understood. However, since portosystemic collaterals receive much of the splanchnic blood in portal hypertension, it is clear that factors affecting collateral circulation will have a great impact on portal hemodynamics. *In situ* perfusion of this vascular bed has been performed demonstrating that collateral vessels are rich in alpha & beta-adrenergic receptors as well as 5-hydroxytryptamine receptors most likely of the $5HT_2$ subtype (39). In addition, the collateral vascular tone is markedly influenced by endothelial dependent (i.e. nitric oxide) factors though it is unclear whether this is a primary pathway responsible for vasodilatation of this system or a secondary consequence of hemodynamic alterations observed in this and other models of portal hypertension.

VARICEAL RUPTURE

Approximately 20-30% of patients with varices will develop variceal hemorrhage within a two-year period. However, no single risk factor has been shown to accurately identify this subset of patients. Variceal wall tension, a concept that integrates local factors, variceal or portal pressure and varix size may be the decisive factor that determines rupture (40). Expressed as a modification of Laplace's law: $T = TP \times r/w$ where T = tension, TP = transmural pressure, r = vessel radius and w = wall thickness. TP is the gradient between intravariceal pressure and esophageal luminal pressure. Tension (T), a property of the vessel wall, is an inwardly directed force that opposes an outwardly directed expanding force ($TP \times r/w$). When the elastic limit of the vessel is reached, further increments in expanding force cannot be balanced by a compensatory increase in T and rupture occurs (fig. 2).

Experimental studies have shown that the expanding force and the opposing T required to prevent vessel rupture increase out of proportion to increases in TP, due to the influence of an increase in vessel radius and decrease in wall thickness that accompany increments in TP (40). Likewise, small reductions in TP induced by pharmacologic agents may result in a significant decrease in the expanding force and the wall tension required to prevent rupture due to an associated reduction in vessel radius and increase in wall thickness. In this way, modest decreases in portal and variceal pressure induced by pharmacologic therapy may significantly decrease the risk of variceal rupture.

After variceal rupture occurs, the factors that modulate the severity of bleeding can be expressed by the equation:

$$\text{Severity of bleed} \therefore TP \times \text{area of rent/viscosity}$$

At this point, the size of the varix rent or tear is the major determinant of the severity of the hemorrhage. Pharmacologic agents probably have little effect on the size of the rent may limit efficacy of pharmacologic therapy in this situation.

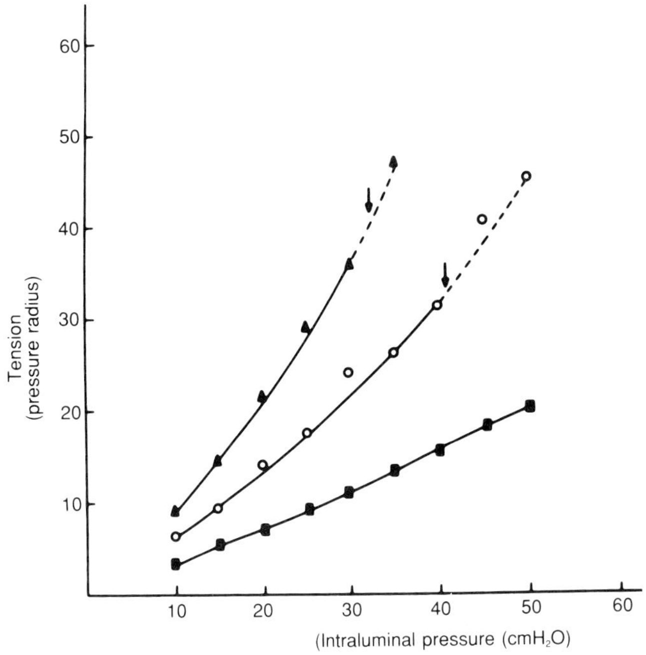

Fig. 2. Importance of varix wall thickness on the relationship between intraluminal pressure and tension. Initial varix radius is constant (6.25 mm) and wall thickness is variable (▲ = 75 μ; ■ = 150 μ; ○ = 225 μ). Each point represents the mean of 15 determinations in five identical models of each varix. The rupture zone (---) is the range of pressures at which rupture occurred. The mean rupture pressure (↓) is illustrated. Tension was greater in the thin-walled (▲) varix compared with the moderate (■) and thick-walled (○) varices. Rupture occurred only in the thin-walled (▲) varix accompanied by increases in varix radius (40, with permission).

REFERENCES

1. Schlichting P, Christensen E, Faurholdt L, Poulsen H, Juhl E, Tygstrup N. Main causes of death in cirrhosis. Scand J Gastroenterol 1983; 18:881-888.
2. Vorobioff J, Bredfeldt JE, Groszmann RJ. Increased blood flow through the portal system in cirrhotic rats. Gastroenterology 1984; 87:1120-1126.
3. Garcia-Tsao G, Groszmann RJ, Fisher R, Conn HO, Atterbury CE, Glickmann M. Portal pressure, presence of gastroesophageal varices and variceal bleeding. Hepatology 1985; 5:419-424.
4. Groszmann RJ, Bosch J, Grace N, Conn HO, Garcia-Tsao G, Navasa M, Albert J, Rodes J, Fischer R, Bermann M, Rofe S, Patrick M, Lerner E. Hemodynamic events in a prospective randomized trial of propranolol vs placebo in the prevention of the first variceal hemorrhage. Gastroenterology 1990; 99:1401-1407.
5. Genecin P, Groszmann RJ. Biology of Portal Hypertension. In: Arias I, Boyer J, Fausto N, Jakoby W, Schachter D, Shafritz D, eds. The Liver: Biology and Pathobiology. 3rd ed. New York: Raven Press, 1994; 1327-1341.
6. Pinzani M, Failli P, Ruocco C, Casini A, Milani S, Baldi E, Giotti A, Gentilini P. Fat-storing cells as liver-specific pericytes-spatial dynamics of agonist-stimulated intracellular calcium transients. J Clin Invest 1992; 90:642-646.
7. Rudolph R, McClure WJ, Woodward M. Contractile fibroblasts in chronic alcoholic cirrhosis. Gastroenterology 1979; 76:704-709.
8. Bhathal PS, Grossman HJ. Reduction of the increased portal vascular resistance of the isolated perfused cirrhotic rat liver by vasodilators. J Hepatol 1985; 1:325.
9. Rockey DC, Housset CN, Friedman SL. Contractility of Hepatic Lipocytes: Implications for the pathogenesis of portal hypertension. Hepatology 1992; 16:316 (Abstr).

10. Rubanyi GM. Endothelium-derived relaxing and contracting factors. J Cell Biochem 1991; 46:27-36.
11. Mittal MK, Gupta T, Lee FY, Sieber CC, Groszmann RJ. Nitric oxide modulates vascular tone in normal rat liver. Am J Physiol 1994; 267:G416-G422.
12. Gupta TK, Groszmann RJ. Administration of L-arginine, the physiological precursor of nitric oxide, reduces portal perfusion pressure and ameliorates hepatic vascular hyperreactivity in experimental cirrhosis. Hepatology 1994; 20:200A (Abstr).
13. Mayhan WG. Impairment of endothelium-dependent dilatation of basilar artery during chronic hypertension. Am J Physiol 1990; 259:H1455-1462.
14. Raij L. Hypertension, endothelium, and cardiovascular risk factors. Am J Med 1991; 90:13S-18S.
15. Polio J, Groszmann RJ. Increased intrahepatic resistance in a genetic rat model of arterial hypertension: studies in isolated perfused rat liver. Gastroenterology 1988; 94:A357 (Abstr).
16. Mittal MK, Lee FY, Groszmann RJ. Role of nitric oxide in the intrahepatic portal circulation of cirrhotic rats. Gastroenterology 1993; 104:A956(Abstr).
17. Genecin P, Groszmann RJ. Portal Hypertension. In: Schiff E and Schiff L, eds. Diseases of the Liver. 7th ed. Philadelphia: J B Lippincott, 1993; vol. 2; 935-973.
18. Benoit JN, Barrowman JA, Harper SL, Kvietys PR, Granger DN. Role of humoral factors in the intestinal hyperemia associated with chronic portal hypertension. Am J Physiol 1984; 247:G486-G493.
19. Sikuler E, Groszmann RJ. Hemodynamic studies in a parabiotic model of portal hypertension. Experientia 1985; 41:1323-1324.
20. Benoit JN, Granger DN. Splanchnic hemodynamics in chronic portal hypertension. Sem Liver Dis 1986; 6:287-298.
21. Sherman R, Joshi P, Hendler R, Felig P, Conn HO. Hyperglucagonemia in Laennecs cirrhosis: the role of portal-systemic shunting. N Engl J Med 1974; 290:239-242.
22. Silva G, Navasa M, Bosch J, Chesta J, Pizcueta PM, Casamitjana R, Rivera F, Rodes J. Hemodynamic effects of glucagon in portal hypertension. Hepatology 1990; 11:668-673.
23. Benoit JN, Zimmerman B, Premen AJ, Go VL, Granger DN. Role of glucagon in splanchnic hyperemia of chronic portal hypertension. Am J Physiol 1986; 251:G674-G677.
24. Sikuler E, Groszmann RJ. Hemodynamic studies in long and short term portal hypertensive rats: the relation of systemic glucagon levels. Hepatology 1986; 414-418.
25. Polio J, Sieber CC, Lerner E, Groszmann RJ. Cardiovascular hyporesponsiveness to norepinephrine, propranolol and nitroglycerin in portal hypertensive and aged rats. Hepatology 1993; 18:128-136.
26. Sitzmann JV, Bulkley GB, Michael MC, Campbell K. Role of prostacyclin in the splanchnic hyperemia contributing to portal hypertension. Ann Surg 1989; 209:322-327.
27. Wong F, Massie D, Hsu P, Dudley F. Indomethacin-induced renal dysfunction in patients with well-compensated cirrhosis. Gastroenterology 1993; 104:869-876.
28. Sieber CC, Groszmann RJ. In vitro hyporeactivity to methoxamine in portal hypertensive rats: reversal by nitric oxide blockade. Am J Physiol 1992; 262:G996-G1001.
29. Sieber CC, Groszmann RJ. Nitric oxide mediates hyporeactivity to vasopressors in mesenteric vessels of portal hypertensive rats. Gastroenterology 1992; 103:235-239.
30. Pizcueta MP, Pique JM, Fernández M et al: Modulation of the hyperdynamic circulation of cirrhotic rats by nitric oxide inhibition. Gastroenterology 1992; 103:1909-1915.
31. Pizcueta MP, Pique JM, Bosch J, Whittle BJ, Moncada S. Effects of inhibiting nitric oxide biosynthesis on the systemic and splanchnic circulation of rats with portal hypertension. Br J Pharmacology 1992; 105:184-190.
32. Lee FY, Albillos A, Colombato LA, Groszmann RJ. The role of nitric oxide in the vascular hyporesponsiveness to methoxamine in portal hypertensive rats. Hepatology 1992; 16:1043-1048.
33. Albillos A, Colombato LA, Groszmann RJ. Vasodilatation and sodium retention in prehepatic portal hypertension. Gastroenterology 1992; 102:931-935.
34. Colombato LA, Albillos A, Groszmann RJ. Temporal relationship of peripheral vasodilatation, plasma volumen expansion and the hyperdynamic circulatory state in portal hypertensive rats. Hepatology 1992; 15:323-328.
35. Genecin P, Polio J, Groszmann RJ. Na restriction blunts expansion of plasma volume and ameliorates hyperdynamic circulation in portal hypertension. Am J Physiol 1990; 259:G498-G509.
36. Albillos A, Colombato LA, Lee FY, Groszmann RJ. Octreotide ameliorates vasodilation and Na^+ retention in portal hypertensive rats. Gastroenterology 1993; 104:575-579.
37. Lee FY, Colombato LA, Albillos A, Groszmann RJ. N^{ω}-nitro-L-arginine administration corrects peripheral vasodilation and systemic capillary hypotension and ameliorates plasma volume expansion and sodium retention in portal hypertensive rats. Hepatology 1993; 17:84-90.
38. Murray JF, Dawson AM, Sherlock S. Circulatory changes in chronic liver disease. Am J Med 1958; 24:358-367.
39. Mosca P, Lee FT, Kaumann AJ, Groszmann RJ. Pharmacology of portal-systemic collaterals in portal hypertensive rats: role of endothelium. Am J Physiol 1992; 263:G544-G550.
40. Polio J, Groszmann RJ. Hemodynamic factors involved in the development and rupture of esophageal varices: a pathophysiologic approach to treatment. Sem Liver Dis 1986; 6:318-331.

The Acute Bleeding Episode: Advances in Drug Therapy

F. Feu, G. D'Amico, J. Bosch

INTRODUCTION

Variceal bleeding is a frequent and severe complication of patients with cirrhosis and portal hypertension. In spite of recent therapeutic advances, the mortality associated with each bleeding episode is still very high, averaging 35% (1-6).

The prognosis of variceal hemorrhage is mainly influenced by the magnitude of blood loss, severity of liver failure and occurrence of complications (infections, multiorgan failure, encephalopathy) (1-6). A distinct characteristic of variceal bleeding is that it is very frequently associated with early rebleeding in the first days following admission. This occurs in 30-50% of patients within 7 to 10 days after admission (1-6), specially in those with advanced liver failure (2). Therefore, a correct therapeutic approach should be aimed not only at controlling the acute variceal bleeding episode, but also preventing early rebleeding during the period in which patients are at high risk.

The initial management of cirrhotic patients with acute variceal bleeding is very important to reduce the mortality. This general management includes adequate blood volume replacement, support of vital organ function and prevention of complications due to hypovolemic shock and worsening of liver function. Overtransfusion should be avoided to prevent a further increase in portal pressure that may reactivate variceal bleeding. Treatment of these patients should be performed under intensive care facilities, preferably in units dealing with gastrointestinal bleeding patients.

Specific therapy to stop bleeding is usually started following diagnostic endoscopy. Different techniques have been used to control variceal hemorrhage, including drugs, esophageal tamponade, endoscopic sclerotherapy, banding ligation, TIPS and emergency surgery (7). As a consequence of the marked progress in the understanding of the pathophysiology of portal hypertension, the pharmacological therapy has experienced an important development, and the use of drugs in the treatment of acute variceal bleeding has gained wide acceptance. It is important to remark that pharmacological therapy offers the unique advantage of not requiring sophisticated equipment or specialized personnel, thus allowing to deliver specific therapy for bleeding not only immediately after admission, but also while the patient is being transferred to hospital (7). However, as no therapy is effective in 100% of the cases, hospitals dealing with the treatment of variceal hemorrhage should have expertise in more than one therapeutic option to be used when the initial one fails. Decision making is often difficult, and physicians have to choose the appropriate therapy among different treatments, most of them incompletely or poorly evaluated.

Acknowledgements. Supported in part by grants from the Fondo de Investigaciones Sanitarias 94/0734 and 94/0757. The authors are indebted to Drs. JC García-Pagán, A Escorsell and A Luca for their cooperation, and to Ms. D Bird for secretarial support.

Many randomized clinical trials comparing pharmacological agents with placebo, non-active treatments or other therapeutic options for variceal bleeding have been performed. Interpretation of the results of these studies is sometimes difficult because of differences in prognostic variables and criteria to define success or failure. These issues have been extensively discussed in a recent international consensus conference (8), from which guidelines for designing future randomized controlled trials have emerged.

In this review the randomized controlled trials using pharmacological agents for variceal bleeding are summarized using meta-analysis when possible. Meta-analysis provides a more reliable estimate of the effect of therapy and overcomes problems of low power in trials including a small number of patients. Pooled estimates of the effects of therapy are presented as pooled odds ratios (POR) according to the Mantel-Haenszel-Peto method (7,9). For control of bleeding, values of POR greater than 1.00 indicate a favorable effect of treatment under investigation as compared to control therapy. This effect is statistically significant when the 95% confidence interval does not include values equal or lower than 1.00. For mortality and complications, values of POR lower than 1.00 indicate a favorable effect of the experimental treatment. This effect is statistically significant when the 95% confidence interval does not include values equal or higher than 1.00. Before reviewing the most commonly used drugs in the treatment of variceal bleeding, the rational basis for the use of pharmacological agents is discussed.

RATIONAL BASIS FOR PHARMACOLOGICAL THERAPY

As in any hydrodynamic system, the portal pressure gradient is the result of the product of blood flow (Q) and vascular resistance (R) within the portal-collateral system. These factors are mathematically related by Ohms' law:

$$\Delta P = Q \times R$$

Increased portal pressure in cirrhosis is promoted by a combination of both factors; an increase in vascular resistance is the initiating event, and in advanced stages, when collaterals have already developed, increased portal blood inflow significantly contributes to the maintenance and aggravation of portal hypertension (10). Therefore, it is possible to reduce portal pressure by decreasing portal-collateral blood flow (using vasoconstrictors), by decreasing vascular resistance of the intrahepatic and portal-collateral circulation (using vasodilators), or by a combination of both.

VASOPRESSIN

For many years vasopressin has been the most frequently used pharmacological agent for the therapy of acute variceal bleeding, though its efficacy in the treatment of this complication has not been proved unequivocally (7). Vasopressin is a very powerful vasoconstrictor (11). At pharmacological doses, it reduces blood flow to all splanchnic organs, and thereby decreases portal blood flow and portal pressure (12). Vasopressin is also effective in reducing collateral blood flow (13) and variceal pressure (14). However, vasopressin administration is associated with adverse effects on systemic hemodynamics owing to its marked vasoconstrictor effect on systemic circulation, with increased peripheral vascular resistance and reduced cardiac output, heart rate and coronary blood flow. These effects may result in serious complications such as myocardial ischemia or infarction, arrythmias, mesenteric ischemia, ischemia of lower extremities and cerebrovascular accidents. Because of that, vasopressin administration has to be stopped in about 25% of cases (15-26). Infusions of low doses of vasopressin in the superior mesenteric artery have been used in an attempt to decrease the systemic toxicity of the drug; however, comparative studies have shown similar effects as intravenous vasopressin administration (20-22). As a result, vasopressin is administered as continuous i.v. infusion, starting at 0.4 U/min, which may be increased up to 0.6 and 0.8 U/min. Therapy is usually maintained until bleeding has been controlled for 12-24 hours. If more than 0.4 U/min are required, the rate of infusion is decreased stepwise prior to discontinuation of therapy.

Table 1. Summary and meta-analysis of randomized controlled trials comparing vasopressin with placebo or non-active treatments for acute variceal bleeding

Author	N of patients (C/VP)	Dose of VP	Duration of infusion	Control of bleeding C/VP (%)	Mortality C/VP (%)
Merigan et al. (1962) (15)	24/29	20 U	20 min	0/55	80/93
Conn et al. (1975) (16)*	16/17	0.05-0.4 U/min	28 hours	25/71	62/53
Mallory et al. (1980) (17)*	20/18	0.2-0.4 U/min	46 hours	15/45	45/44
Fogel et al. (1982) (18)	19/14	0.6-6.2 U/min	24 hours	37/29	42/50
POR (95% CI)				4.54 (2.32-8.33)	1.11 (0.54-2.28)

C: placebo or non-active treatment; VP: vasopressin; POR: pooled odds ratio; CI: confidence interval.
* Intra-arterial vasopressin.

The efficacy of vasopressin in the control of acute variceal bleeding has been compared with placebo or non-active treatments in four randomized controlled trials (RCTs) (15-18) (table 1). In three of these studies vasopressin was more effective than non-active treatment. However, in the first study (15) the treatment outcome was assessed just 1 hour after starting a 20-minute vasopressin infusion. Using meta-analysis, the pooled estimate of these trials shows a significant beneficial effect of vasopressin in the control of bleeding [pooled odds ratio (POR): 4.54; 95% confidence interval (CI): 2.32-8.33] (fig. 1); no significant effect on mortality is observed (fig. 2). Complications appeared in 32% to 64% of patients receiving vasopressin. Three out of 78 vasopressin-treated patients died because of complications related to therapy.

Table 2 summarizes the results of 5 randomized controlled trials comparing vasopressin and emergency sclerotherapy in the treatment of acute variceal bleeding (27-31). The only trial showing a favorable effect of sclerotherapy (30) had a possible bias in the assessment of treatment outcome. Success of therapy was evaluated by repeated endoscopy at 12 hours only in the vasopressin group, whereas in the sclerotherapy group endoscopy was repeated only if bleeding was suspected. Meta-analysis of these trials shows that in patients treated with sclerotherapy there is a strong trend towards a reduction in the rebleeding rate during hospital admission (POR: 0.66; 95% CI: 0.44 to 1.0) and mortality (POR: 0.65; 95% CI: 0.42 to 1.01) (fig. 3). Finally, vasopressin alone (32) or in association with nitroglycerin (33) showed similar efficacy in controlling bleeding and mortality than balloon tamponade (table 2 and fig. 3).

VASOPRESSIN ASSOCIATED WITH NITROGLYCERIN

Hemodynamic studies have shown that the association of nitroglycerin to vasopressin administration causes a further reduction in portal pressure and reduces the adverse systemic effects associated with vasopressin (19). This is achieved because nitroglycerin, which is a powerful venous dilator, reduces the increase in portal vascular resistance induced by vasopressin and improves myocardial performance.

This combined therapy has been compared to vasopressin alone in 3 RCTs (23-25). In these studies nitroglycerin was given sublingually (23), intravenously (24), or transdermally (25) using continuous release preparations. All three investigations showed that the association of vasopressin plus nitroglycerin was more effective in controlling bleeding than vasopressin alone (table 3). In 2 of these trials the side effects were significantly reduced in the group treated with combined therapy (23, 24). The only trial performed in a double-blind fashion (25) further showed that the association of transdermal nitroglycerin to i.v. vasopressin significantly reduced the transfusion requirements, the need of balloon tamponade, and the number of pa-

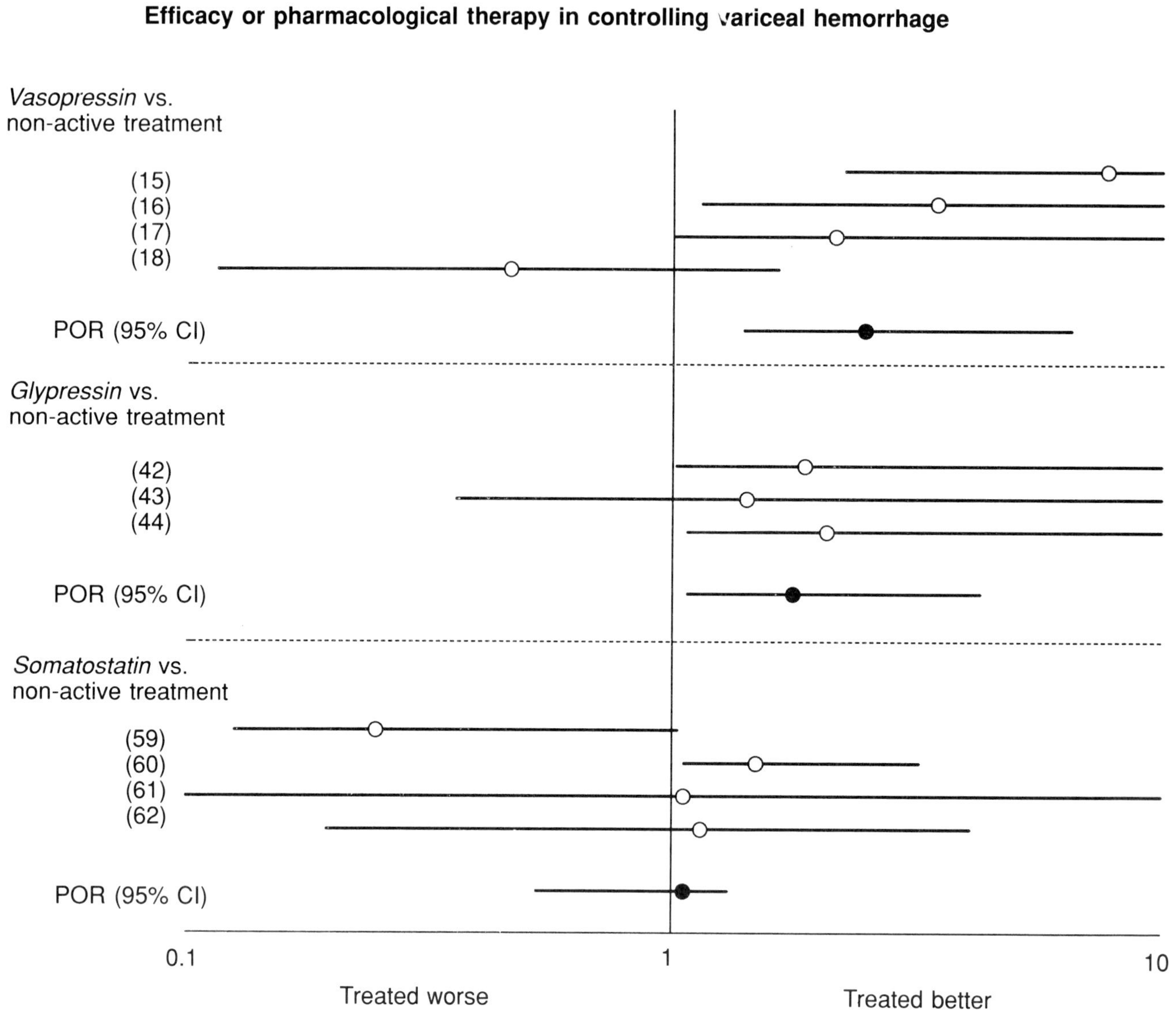

Fig. 1. Control of variceal bleeding in randomized controlled trials comparing pharmacological agents with placebo or non-active treatments. Results of individual studies are expressed as odds ratios with 95% confidence intervals (–○–). Using meta-analysis the pooled estimates of treatment effects are presented as pooled odds ratios (POR) with 95% confidence intervals (–●–). Values of POR > 1.00 indicate a favorable effect of drug therapy, and this effect is statistically significant when the 95% CI does not include values ≤ 1.00. Figures between brackets indicate reference number.

tients requiring emergency surgery. The pooled estimate of the treatment effect shows a significant increase in the success to control bleeding with the combination therapy (POR: 2.56; 95% CI: 1.39-4.54) (fig. 3). This was associated with a significantly lower incidence of complications (POR: 0.29; 95% CI: 0.12-0.73) (fig. 3), but mortality was not significantly different (POR: 0.94; 95% CI: 0.50-1.79). These studies suggest that if vasopressin is still used, it should always be associated with nitroglycerin.

GLYPRESSIN (TERLIPRESSIN)

This synthetic vasopressin analogue (triglycyl-lysine-vasopressin or terlipressin) is slowly converted in vivo into lysine-vasopressin by enzymatic cleavage of the glycyl residues. Glypressin, unlike vasopressin, does not enhance fibrinolysis and has a longer biological activity, which makes continuous i.v. infusion unnecesary (26). The preferred schedule of administration is as i.v. injections of 2 mg/4h. The slow

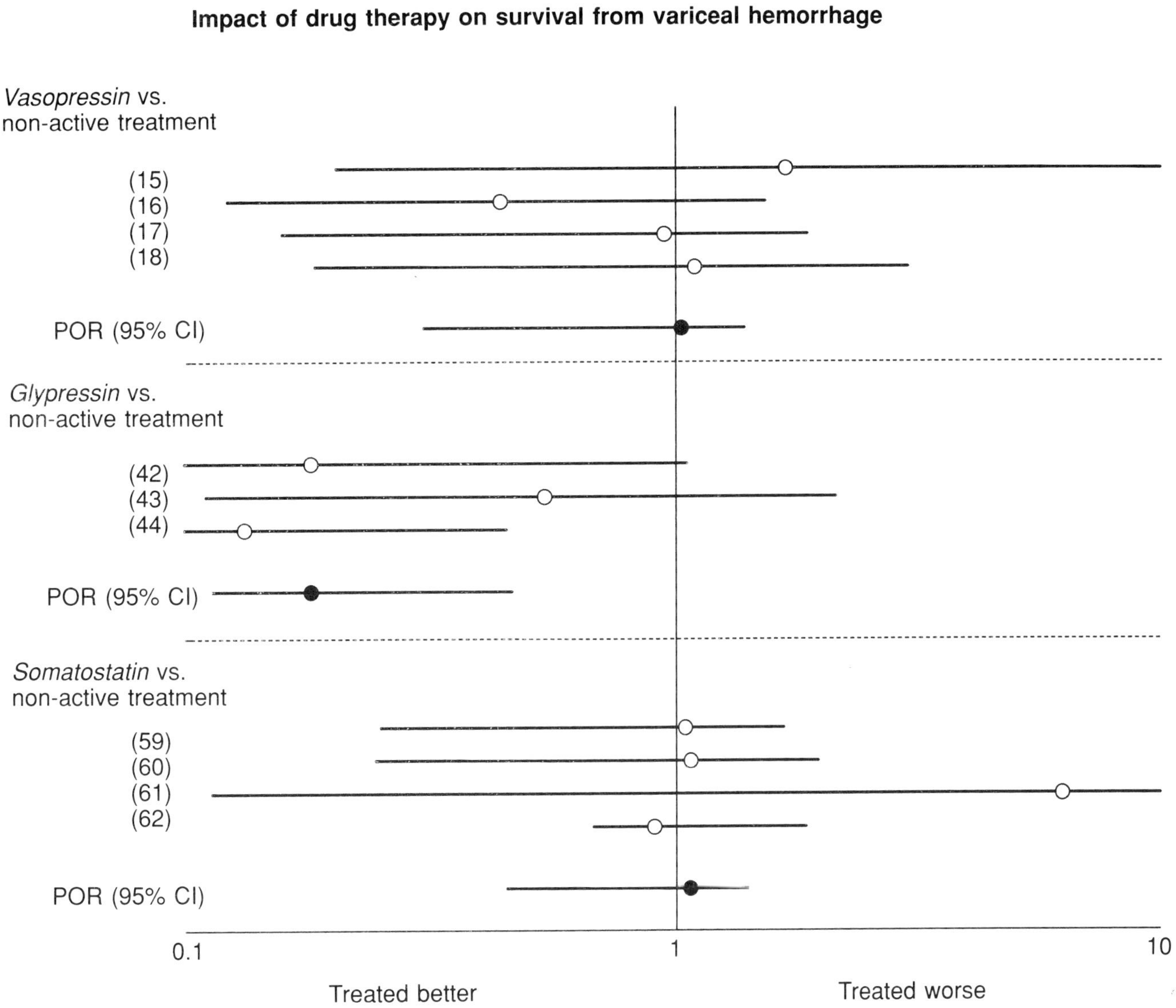

Fig. 2. Mortality associated with variceal bleeding in randomized controlled trials comparing pharmacological agents with placebo or non-active treatments. Results of individual studies are expressed as odds ratios with 95% confidence intervals (–○–). Using meta-analysis the pooled estimates of treatment effects are presented as pooled odds ratios (POR) with 95% confidence intervals (–●–). Values of POR < 1.00 indicate a favorable effect of drug therapy, and this effect is statistically significant when the 95% CI does not include values ≥ 1.00. This analysis showed that glypressin was the only drug that significantly decreased mortality from variceal bleeding. Figures between brackets indicate reference number.

transformation of glypressin into vasopressin in the tissues allows the achievement of high local concentrations with low circulating levels, which results in reduced systemic toxicity.

Confirming previous results in experimental models (34), hemodynamic studies performed in patients with cirrhosis and portal hypertension have shown that intravenous injections of 1 to 2 mg of glypressin cause marked reductions in portal pressure (ranging from 16% to 35%) (35-38) and azygos blood flow (by an average of 32%) (35, 38). These effects are still present up to 3-4 hours after glypressin administration (38). In addition, Cestari et al. (39) have shown a 28% reduction in esophageal variceal pressure after i.v. injection of 2 mg of glypressin. In association with these changes, glypressin significantly increases mean arterial pressure and decreases heart rate and cardiac output (35-38). The systemic hemodynamic effects of

Table 2. Summary of randomized controlled trials comparing vasopressin with sclerotherapy (including meta-analysis) and balloon tamponade in the treatment of acute variceal bleeding

Author	N of patients (C/VP)	Control of bleeding C/VP (%)	Mortality C/VP (%)	Complications C/VP (%)
Vasopressin compared with sclerotherapy				
Soderlund et al. (1985) (27)	57/50	95/84	28/36	30/10
Larson et al. (1986) (28)	44/38	NR/NR	5/13	25/63
El-Zayadi et al. (1988) (29)	63/55	NR/NR	11/20	30/0
Westaby et al. (1989) (30)*	33/31	88/65	27/39	9/10
Alexandrino et al. (1990) (31)	41/42	71/71	29/41	–/–
POR (95% CI)		0.52 (0.28-0.98)	1.54 (0.99-2.38)	0.66 (0.39-1.09)
Vasopressin compared with tamponade				
Pinto Correia et al. (1984) (32)	20/17	70/65	20/12	10/12
Terés et al.(1990) (33)*	52/56	87/66	31/30	8/9
POR (95% CI)		0.43 (0.20-0.89)	0.89 (0.43-1.88)	1.18 (0.38-3.67)

C: control treatment; VP: vasopressin; POR: pooled odds ratio; CI: confidence interval; NR: not reported.
* Vasopressin plus nitroglycerin.

glypressin may be attenuated by the association of nitroglycerin (40, 41), although the decrease in portal pressure is not significantly enhanced.

Three placebo controlled trials have been published assessing the efficacy of glypressin in controlling variceal bleeding (42-44) (table 4). Two trials (42, 44) showed that glypressin was significantly better than placebo. The pooled estimates showed a highly significant increase in success to control bleeding (POR: 3.23; 95% CI: 1.64-6.67) (fig. 1). The mean success rate with

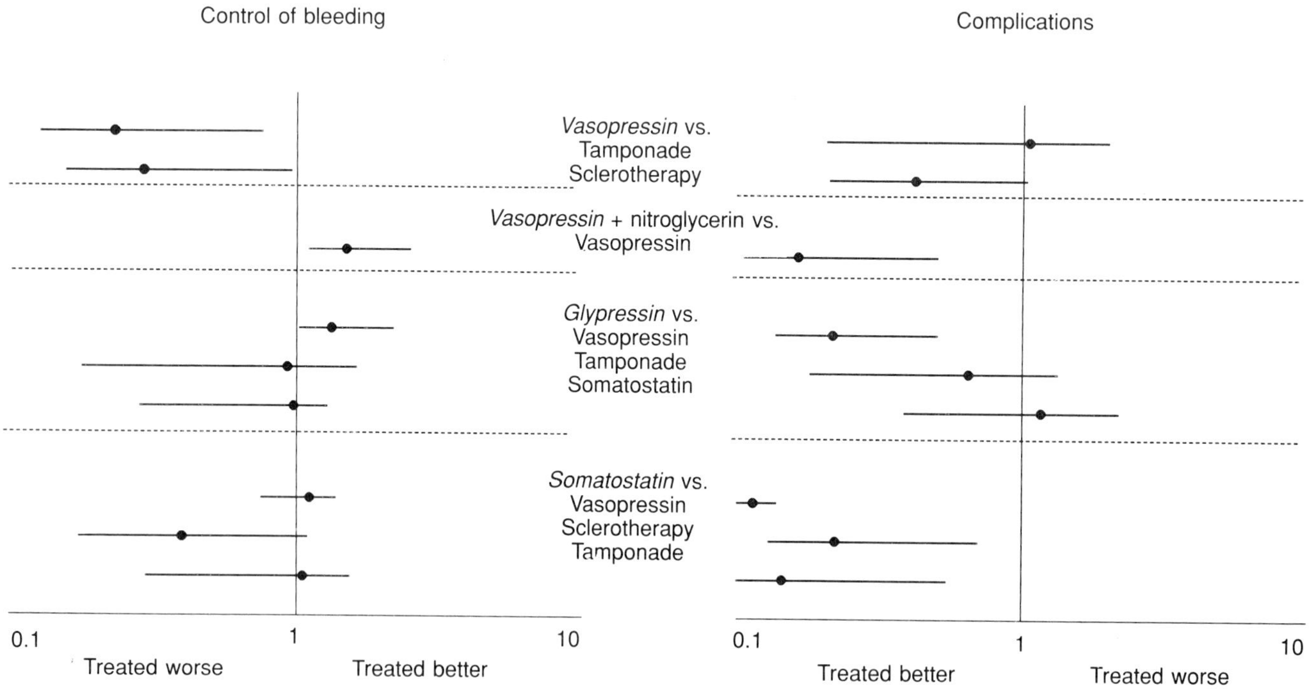

Fig. 3. Summary of the meta-analysis of efficacy and complications of different pharmacological treatments as compared with other therapeutic options. Data are presented as pooled odds ratios (POR) with the 95% confidence intervals (CI). For the efficacy of therapy values of POR > 1.00 indicate a favorable effect of experimental treatment, and this difference is statistically significant when the 95% CI does not include values ≤ 1.00. For complications the experimental treatment has a favorable effect when values of POR are lower than 1.00, being the difference significant if the 95% CI does not include values ≥ 1.00.

Table 3. Results and meta-analysis of the randomized controlled trials comparing vasopressin alone versus vasopressin plus nitroglycerin in the treatment of variceal bleeding

Author	Route of NTG	N of patients VP/VP + NTG	Control of bleeding VP/VP + NTG (%)	Mortality VP/VP + NTG (%)	Complications VP/VP + NTG (%)
Tsai et al. (1986) (23)	Sublingual	19/20	21/45	58/55	32/10
Gimson et al. (1986) (24)	i.v.	34/38	44/68	26/24	21/3
Bosch et al. (1989) (25)	Transdermal	35/30	54/73	29/30	9/7
POR (95% CI)			2.56 (1.39-4.54)	0.94 (0.50-1.79)	0.29 (0.12-0.73)

VP: vasopressin; NTG: nitroglycerin; POR: pooled odds ratio; CI: confidence interval.

glypressin was 75%. A remarkable effect associated with glypressin therapy was a clear reduction of mortality associated with bleeding episodes (42, 44). The pooled estimates show a significant decrease in mortality (POR: 0.32; 95% CI: 0.15-0.70) (table 4). As illustrated in figure 2, glypressin is the only pharmacological treatment that has been shown to reduce the mortality associated with variceal bleeding. A recent double-blind ambulance study evaluated the efficacy of glypressin vs. placebo administered prior to admission (at patients' home and during transferral). This trial again showed a significant reduction of mortality associated with variceal hemorrhage in patients who received glypressin (45). Glypressin therapy was associated with a higher incidence of side-effects than placebo (table 4). These side effects, however, were usually mild and rarely required discontinuation of therapy.

Table 4. Results and meta-analysis of randomized controlled trials comparing glypressin with placebo and other active treatments for acute variceal bleeding

Author	N of patients C/GLY	Control of bleeding C/GLY (%)	Mortality C/GLY (%)	Complications C/GLY (%)
Glypressin compared with placebo				
Walker et al. (1986) (42)	25/25	52/80	32/12	0/20
Freeman et al. (1989) (43)	16/15	38/60	25/20	0/7
Soderlund et al. (1990) (44)	29/31	55/84	38/10	14/48
POR (95% CI)		3.23 (1.64-6.67)	0.32 (0.15-0.70)	5.75 (2.34-14.2)
Glypressin compared with vasopressin				
Freeman et al. (1982) (46)	11/10	9/70	27/20	–/–
Desaint et al. (1987) (47)	6/10	83/80	33/30	17/0
Chiu et al. (1990) (48)	28/26	54/50	36/46	–/–
D'Amico et al. (1994) (49)	55/56	76/91	16/25	60/38
POR (95% CI)		2.09 (1.09-4.01)	1.40 (0.75-2.64)	0.40 (0.22-0.73)
Glypressin compared with somatostatin				
Walker et al. (1992) (50)	25/25	80/68	16/24	8/0
VBSG (1993) (51)	81/80	84/80	14/16	6/14
POR (95% CI)		0.99 (0.51-1.93)	1.01 (0.49-2.09)	1.58 (0.63-4.01)
Glypressin compared with tamponade				
Colin et al. (1987) (52)	27/27	88/88	22/15	15/11
Fort et al. (1990) (53)	24/23	79/78	8/13	46/43
POR (95% CI)		0.97 (0.33-2.86)	0.87 (0.29-2.59)	0.83 (0.33-2.09)

C: control treatment; GLY: glypressin; POR: pooled odds ratio; CI: confidence interval.

Other studies have shown that glypressin is more effective than vasopressin, alone (46-48) or associated with nitroglycerin (49), in the control of bleeding (table 4 and fig. 3). It is important to note that these studies found a significantly lower complication rate with glypressin, even when vasopressin was associated with nitroglycerin (49) (fig. 3). Two recent trials have compared glypressin with somatostatin (50, 51); these studies showed that the two drugs were highly effective in arresting variceal bleeding, with no differences either in the control of bleeding, mortality or complications (table 4 and fig. 3). Finally, glypressin was found to be as effective as balloon tamponade in controlling variceal hemorrhage in two trials (52, 53).

Thus, available data indicate that glypressin is highly effective in the control of variceal bleeding and reduces mortality. It is simpler, more effective and safer than vasopressin (even when associated with nitroglycerin), and is as effective as somatostatin or balloon tamponade. Glypressin is safe enough to be given for longer periods to prevent early rebleeding (54).

SOMATOSTATIN

Somatostatin has been widely used in the treatment of acute variceal bleeding because it decreases portal pressure and portal-collateral blood flow without the adverse systemic effects of vasopressin (55). Somatostatin causes a selective splanchnic vasoconstriction which leads to a decrease in portal and collateral blood flow resulting in a reduction of portal pressure (55). This is probably due to the inhibition of the release of splanchnic vasodilatory peptides, such as glucagon, caused by somatostatin (56). Bolus injections of somatostatin cause a marked vasoconstriction in cirrhotic patients, which leads a rapid and intense reduction in portal pressure and azygos blood flow (55). These changes are much greater than those caused by continuous infusions; this suggests that repeated bolus injections during the first hours of therapy may be useful to improve the efficacy of therapy. Somatostatin is usually given as a continuous i.v. infusion at a dose of 250 µg/h after a bolus injection of 250 µg. When successful, therapy is maintained for 2-5 days (57).

Since the first report of Tyden et al in 1978 (58) using somatostatin in the treatment of acute variceal bleeding, several studies have been performed comparing the efficacy of somatostatin with other treatments for variceal bleeding. Somatostatin was compared with placebo in two randomized placebo controlled trials (59, 60) and with non-active treatments in 2 trials (61, 62). The results of these studies are summarized in table 5. Valenzuela et al. (59) failed to show any beneficial effect of treatment, which was mainly due to an unexpectedly high spontaneous rate of cessation of bleeding in the placebo group (75%). This study may thus represent an example of a false-negative investigation, probably due to some inadvertent bias. In a second large study Burroughs et al. (60) reported a significantly higher efficacy of somatostatin as compared to placebo in controlling variceal bleeding. The two trials differed in the duration of treatment, 30 hours in the first study (59) and 5 days in the second (60), and probably more important, in the definition of treatment success: achivement of a bleeding-free period of 4 hours and 5 days, res-

Table 5. Summary and meta-analysis of randomized controlled trials comparing somatostatin with placebo and non-active treatment for acute variceal bleeding

Author	N of patients C/SMT	Control of bleeding C/SMT (%)	Mortality C/SMT (%)
Valenzuela et al. (1989) (59)*	36/48	75/56	28/31
Burroughs et al. (1990) (60)*	59/61	41/64	11/15
Testoni et al. (1986) (61)	14/15	93/93	0/7
Loperfido et al. (1987) (62)	25/22	16/23	28/27
POR (95% CI)		1.22 (0.75-2.04)	1.27 (0.69-2.34)

C: placebo or non-active treatment; SMT: somatostatin; POR: pooled odds ratio; CI: confidence interval.
* Placebo.

Table 6. Summary and meta-analysis of randomized controlled trials comparing somatostatin with vasopressin in the treatment of acute variceal bleeding

Author	N of patients VP/SMT	Control of bleeding VP/SMT (%)	Mortality VP/SMT (%)	Complications VP/SMT (%)
Kravetz et al. (1984) (63)	31/30	58/53	45/47	26/0
Jenkins et al. (1985) (64)	12/10	33/70	33/20	17/0
Bagarani et al. (1987) (65)	25/24	32/67	40/25	13/6
Cardona et al. (1989) (66)	18/20	56/40	17/30	33/0
Hsia et al. (1990) (67)	24/22	37/55	62/63	46/18
Saari et al. (1990) (68)	22/32	52/65	36/34	52/3
Rodriguez-Moreno et al. (1991) (69)	16/15	63/40	19/20	63/0
POR (95% CI)		1.40 (0.89-2.20)	0.93 (0.58-1.51)	0.12 (0.07-0.22)

VP: vasopressin; SMT: somatostatin; POR: pooled odds ratio; CI: confidence interval.

pectively. In two studies comparing somatostatin with non-active treatment (H_2-blockers), this drug was as effective as H_2-blockers (61, 62). When these four trials comparing somatostatin with placebo or H_2-blockers were grouped in a meta-analysis, the pooled estimates showed a non-significant trend for a beneficial effect of somatostatin increasing the success to control bleeding (POR: 1.22; 95% CI: 0.75-2.04) (fig. 1). Mortality was unaffected (fig. 2).

Seven trials compared somatostatin with vasopressin (table 6) (63-69), and showed a slightly higher efficacy of somatostatin than vasopressin in controlling variceal bleeding, but the difference was not statistically significant (POR: 1.40; 95% CI: 0.89-2.20). It is important to remark that in all trials complications were virtually absent with somatostatin (mean 3.9%, range 0-18%), whereas the mean complication rate was 36% (13-63%) with vasopressin (fig. 3).

Somatostatin has also been compared with more invasive therapies, such as balloon tamponade (70, 71) and emergency sclerotherapy (72-74) (fig. 3). These studies showed that somatostatin was as effective as tamponade and sclerotherapy, with no significant differences in mortality, but with a significantly lower incidence of complications (table 7).

The lack of complications of somatostatin administration suggested that this drug could be used for longer periods to prevent early rebleeding. This was investigated in a multicenter RCT performed in 6 hospitals in Spain (75). The study included 170 cirrhotic patients who had achieved a 24 hour bleeding-free period by means of medical therapy. Patients were randomized to receive a single course of sclerotherapy or a continuous i.v. infusion of somatostatin for 5 days. There were no differences between the two treatments in the incidence of early

Table 7. Summary and meta-analysis of randomized controlled trials comparing somatostatin with sclerotherapy and balloon tamponade in the treatment of acute variceal bleeding

Author	N of patients C/SMT	Control of bleeding C/SMT (%)	Mortality C/SMT (%)	Complications C/SMT (%)
Somatostatin compared with sclerotherapy				
Di Febo et al. (1990) (72)	24/23	92/78	21/26	8/4
Shields et al. (1992) (73)	41/39	83/77	19/31	29/13
Planas et al. (1994) (74)	35/35	83/80	23/28	28/14
POR (95% CI)		0.64 (0.32-1.31)	1.52 (0.80-2.89)	0.41 (0.20-0.86)
Somatostatin compared with tamponade				
Jaramillo et al. (1991) (70)	20/19	50/58	25/26	5/0
Avgerinos et al. (1991) (71)	30/31	67/68	33/23	33/9
POR (95% CI)		1.18 (0.53-2.66)	0.74 (0.31-1.77)	0.24 (0.07-0.76)

C: control treatment; SMT: somatostatin; POR: pooled odds ratio; CI: confidence interval.

variceal rebleeding (17% with sclerotherapy and 19% with somatostatin) or mortality at 6 weeks (9% vs. 11%, respectively). However, the incidence of severe complications was significantly higher in patients treated with sclerotherapy than in those receiving somatostatin (10% vs. 0%).

Therefore RCTs comparing somatostatin with placebo or non-active treatment and other therapeutic options support that somatostatin is effective in the treatment of variceal hemorrhage. Moreover, somatostatin is certainly a very safe therapy, which makes it possible to start treatment immediately after admission or even while the patient is transferred to hospital, and maintain treatment for several days to prevent early rebleeding.

OCTREOTIDE

The role of octreotide, a synthetic somatostatin derivative with longer biological half life (76) in the treatment of variceal bleeding is still under investigation. Although studies in animals have shown that octreotide causes a reduction in portal pressure (77, 78), this effect is uncertain in patients with cirrhosis (76, 79-81). The reduction in portal pressure observed by McKee et al. (79) has not been confirmed by other authors. Octreotide infusion caused a transient reduction in azygos blood flow (80). The effect of octreotide on variceal pressure is unpredictable (82). It has been suggested that octreotide may prevent the increase of portal pressure induced by the volume replacement following hemorrhagic shock (83) or by a meal (84). However, the clinical relevance of these effects is not known.

There are still few trials comparing octreotide with other therapies in the treatment of acute variceal bleeding. Octreotide has been compared with vasopressin (85), glypressin (86), balloon tamponade (79) and emergency sclerotherapy (87, 88). In all these studies the success and mortality rates in patients receiving octreotide were similar to control treatments. However, the small sample sizes, different schedules of octreotide treatment, and unclear end-points of these trials indicate that there is not enough data to support the use of octreotide in the treatment of acute variceal bleeding out of the context of controlled trials (table 8).

OTHER AGENTS

A different approach in the therapy of variceal bleeding may be the use of drugs that increase the pressure of the lower esophageal sphincter, such as metoclopramide and domperidone. This suggestion was raised by portographic studies showing that these drugs may reduce blood flow through esophageal varices by increasing the lower esophageal sphincter pressure (89, 90). Moreover, hemodynamic studies performed in patients with cirrhosis and portal hypertension have shown that metoclopramide and domperidone cause a significant decrease in azygos blood flow (91) and esophageal variceal pressure (92). Nevertheless, the utility of these drugs either in arresting or preventing variceal bleeding is still uncertain (93, 94).

SUMMARY

Acute variceal hemorrhage is one of the most severe complications of patients with cirrhosis and portal hypertension, and represents an important cause of death in these patients. After a

Table 8. Results of clinical studies comparing the efficacy of octreotide with other therapies for variceal bleeding

Author	Control treatment	N of patients C/OCT	Control of bleeding C/OCT (%)	Mortality C/OCT (%)
Hwang et al. (1992) (85)	Vasopressin	24/24	46/63	50/46
Silvain et al. (1993) (86)	Glypressin + NTG	41/46	46/57	27/22
Mc Kee et al. (1990) (79)	Balloon tamponade	20/20	70/50	25/0
Jenkins et al. (1992) (87)	Sclerotherapy	20/20	90/90	NR/NR
Sung et al. (1993) (88)	Sclerotherapy	49/49	74/69	41/29

C: control treatment; OCT: octreotide; NTG: nitroglycerin; NR: not reported.

correct resuscitation, a specific therapy to arrest bleeding should be started. Pharmacological treatment has gained wide acceptance in recent years because of its unique advantages: no specialized personnel or sophisticated equipment are required, may be given immediately after admission or even when patients are transferred to hospital.

Vasopressin infusion should not longer be used because its efficacy has not been clearly established and the high incidence of severe side-effects. Whenever used, it should be associated with nitroglycerin. Glypressin is better than vasopressin alone or associated with nitroglycerin, is as effective as somatostatin and balloon tamponade, and more important, is the only pharmacological agent that improves survival in patients with variceal bleeding. Somatostatin injections, followed by a continuous intravenous infusion, have similar efficacy as other treatments. An important advantage of somatostatin is the lack of severe side-effects. Octreotide shares some of the properties of somatostatin, but its utility in the treatment of variceal bleeding is still under investigation.

REFERENCES

1. D'Amico G, Morabito A, Pagliaro L, Marubini E. Liver Study Group of V Cervello Hospital. Survival and prognostic indicators in compensated and decompensated cirhhosis. Dig Dis Sci 1986; 31:468-475.
2. García-Pagán JC, Terés J, Calvet X, Bosch J, Rodés J. Factors which influence the prognosis of the first episode of variceal hemorrhage in patients with cirrhosis. Recent advances in the pathophysiology and therapy of portal hypertension. Serono Simposia Review 1989; 287-302.
3. de Dombal FT, Clarke JR, Clamp SE, Malizia G, Kotwal MR, Morgan AG. Prognostic factors in upper G.I. bleeding. Endoscopy 1986; 18:6-10.
4. Cardin F, Gori G, Mc Cormick PA, Burroughs AK. A predictive model for very early rebleeding from varices. Gut 1990; 31:A1204.
5. Graham DY, Smith JL. The course of patients after variceal hemorrhage. Gastroenterology 1981; 80:800-809.
6. D'Amico G, Morabito A, Pagliaro L, Traina M, Montalbano L. Six-week prognostic indicators in upper gastrointestinal hemorrhage in cirrhosis. Frontiers of gastrointestinal research 1986; 9:247.5.
7. D'Amico G, Pagliaro L, Bosch J. The treatment of portal hypertension. A meta-analytic review. Hepatology 1995 (in press).
8. De Franchis R, Pascal JP, Ancona E Burroughs AK, Henderson M Fleig W, Groszmann R, Bosch J, Sauerbruch T Soederlund C, Lebrec D, Soerensen TIA, Pagliaro L. Consensus Report. Definitions, methodology and therapeutic strategies in portal hypertension: a consensus development workshop. Baveno, April 1990. J Hepatol 1992; 15: 256-261.
9. Collins R, Yusuf S, Peto R. Overview of randomised trials of diuretics in pregnancy. Br Med J 1985; 290:17-23.
10. Bosch J, Pizcueta P, Feu F, Fernández M, García-Pagán JC. Pathophysiology of Portal Hypertension. Gastroenterol Clin North Am 1992; 21:1-14.
11. Altura BM, Altura BT. Vascular smooth muscle and neurohypophyseal hormones. Fed Proc 1977; 36:1853-1860.
12. Bosch J. Effect of pharmacological agents on portal hypertension: a hemodynamic appraisal. Clin Gastroenterol 1985; 14:169-183.
13. Bosch J, Mastai R, Kravetz D, Bruix J, Rigau J, Rodés J. Measurement of azygos venous blood flow in the evaluation of portal hypertension in patients with cirrhosis. Clinical and haemodynamic correlations in 100 patients. J Hepatol 1985; 1:125-139.
14. Bosch J, Bordas JM, Mastai R, Kravetz D, Navasa M, Chesta J, Pizcueta P, García-Pagán JC, Rodés J. Effects of vasopressin on the intravariceal pressure in patients with cirrhosis: Comparison with the effects on portal pressure. Hepatology 1988; 8:861-865.
15. Merigan TC, Plotkin GR, Davidson CS. Effect of intravenously administered posterior pituitary extract on hemorrhage from bleeding esophageal varices. N Engl J Med 1962; 266:134-135.
16. Conn HO, Ramsby GR, Storer EH, Mutchnick MG, Joshi PH, Phillips MM, Cohen GA, Fields GN, Petroski D. Intraarterial vasopressin in the treatment of upper gastrointestinal hemorrhage: a prospective controlled clinical trial. Gastroenterology 1975; 68:211-221.
17. Mallory A, Schaefer JW, Cohen JR, Holt AS, Norton LW. Selective intra-arterial vasopressin infusion for upper gastrointestinal tract hemorrhage. A controlled trial. Arch Surg 1980; 115:30-32.
18. Fogel RM, Knauer MC, Andres LL, Mahal AS, Stein D, Kemeny JM, Rinki MM, Walker JE, Siegmund D, Gregory PB. Continuous intravenous vasopressin in active upper gastrointestinal bleeding. A placebo-controlled trial. Ann Int Med 1982; 96:565-569.
19. Groszmann RJ, Kravetz D, Bosch J, Glickman M, Bruix J, Bredfelt J, Conn HO Rodés J, Storer EH. Nitroglycerin improves the hemodynamic response to vasopressin in portal hypertension. Hepatology 1982; 2:757-762.
20. Johnson WC, Widrich WC, Ansell JE, Robbins AH, Nabseth DC. Control of bleeding varices by vasopressin: a prospective randomized study. Ann Surg 1977; 186:369-376.
21. Clanet J, Tournet R, Fourtanier G, Joncquiert F, Pascal JP. Traitement pour la pitressin des hemorragies pou rupture de varices oesophagiennes chez le cirrhotique. Etude controlleé. Acta Gastroenterol Belg 1978; 41:539-543.

22. Chojkier M, Groszmann RJ, Atterbury CE, Bar-Meir S, Blei AT, Frankel J, Glickman MG, Kniaz JL, Schade R, Taggart GJ, Conn HO. A controlled comparison of continuous intraarterial and intravenous infusion of vasopressin in hemorrhage from esophageal varices. Gastroenterology 1979; 77:540-546.
23. Tsai YT, Lay CS, Lai KH, Ng WW, Yeh YS, Wang JY, Chiang TT, Lee SD, Chiang BN, Lo KJ. Controlled trial of vasopressin plus nitroglycerin vs vasopressin alone in the treatment of bleeding esophageal varices. Hepatology 1986; 6:406-409.
24. Gimson AES, Westaby D, Hegarty J, Alastair W, Williams R. A randomized trial of vasopressin plus nitroglycerin in the control of acute variceal hemorrhage. Hepatology 1986; 6:410-413.
25. Bosch J, Groszman RJ, García-Pagán JC, Terés J, García-Tsao G, Navasa M, Mas A, Rodés J. Association of transdermal nitroglycerin to vasopressin infusion in the treatment of variceal hemorrhage: a placebo-controlled clinical trial. Hepatology 1989; 10:962-968.
26. Blei AT. Vasopressin analogs in portal hypertension: different molecules but similar questions. Hepatology 1986; 6:146-147.
27. Soderlund C, Ihre T. Endoscopic sclerotherapy vs. conservative management of bleeding esophageal varices. Acta Chir Scand 1985; 151:449-456.
28. Larson AW, Cohen H, Zwieiban B, Chapman D, Gourdji M, Korula J, Weiner D. Acute esophageal variceal sclerotherapy. JAMA 1986; 255: 497-500.
29. El-Zayadi A, El-Din S, Kabil M. Endoscopic sclerotherapy versus medical treatment for bleeding esophageal varices in patients with schistosomal liver disease. Gastrointest Endosc 1988; 34:314-317.
30. Westaby D, Hayes P, Gimson AES, Polson R, Williams R. Controlled clinical trial of injection sclerotherapy for active variceal bleeding. Hepatology 1989; 9:274-277.
31. Alexandrino P, Alves MM, Fidalgo P, Matos L, Esteves AV, Veloso J, Olivera AG, Moura MC. Is sclerotherapy the first choice treatment for active oesophageal variceal bleeding in cirrhotic patients? Final report of a randomized clinical trial. J Hepatol 1990; 11(Suppl):S1.
32. Pinto Correia J, Martins Alves M, Alexandrino P, Silveira J. Controlled trial of vasopressin and balloon tamponade in bleeding esophageal varices. Hepatology 1984; 4:885-888.
33. Terés J, Planas R, Panés J, Salmerón JM, Mas A, Bosch J, Llorente C, Viver J, Feu F, Rodés J. Vasopressin/nitroglycerin infusion vs esophageal tamponade in the treatment of acute variceal bleeding: a randomized controlled trial. Hepatology 1990; 11:964-968.
34. Blei AT, Groszmann RJ, Gusberg R, Conn HO. Comparison of vasopressin and triglycyl-lysine vasopressin on splanchnic and systemic hemodynamics in dogs. Dig Dis Sci 1980; 25:688-694.
35. Valla D, Lee SS, Moreau R, Hadengue A, Sayegh R, Lebrec D. Effets de la glypressine sur les circulations splanchnique et systémique des malades atteints de cirrhose. Gastroenterol Clin Biol 1985; 9:877-880.
36. Lebrec D. Hemodynamic effects of terlipressin (glypressin) in patients with cirrhosis. In: Lebrec D, Blei AT, eds. Vasopressin analogs and portal hypertension. Paris: John Libbey Eurotext, 1987; 105-112.
37. Merkel C, Gatta A, Bolognesi M, Finucci G, Battaglia G, Angeli P, Zuin R. Hemodynamic changes of systemic, hepatic, and splenic circulation following triglycyl-lysin-vasopressin administration in alcoholic cirrhosis. Dig Dis Sci 1988; 33:1103-1109.
38. Escorsell A, Feu F, García-Pagán JC, Luca A, Trejo R, Bosch J, Rodés J. Long-term reduction of portal pressure and collateral blood flow after single IV injection of 1 and 2 mg of glypressin in patients with cirrhosis. A double-blind controlled study. J Hepatol 1994; 21:S134.
39. Cestari R, Braga M, Missale G, Ravelli P, Burroughs AK. Haemodynamic effect of triglycyl-lysine-vasopressin (glypressin) on intravascular oesophageal variceal pressure in patients with cirrhosis. A randomized placebo controlled trial. J Hepatol 1990; 10:205-210.
40. Lin HC, Tsai YT, Lee FY, Chang TT, Wang SS, Lay CS, Lee SD, Lo KJ. Systemic and portal haemodynamic changes following triglycyllysine vasopressin plus nitrglycerin administration in patients with hepatitis B-related cirrhosis. J Hepatol 1990; 10:370-374.
41. Moreau R, Soubrane O, Hadengue A, Sogni P, Gaudin C. Effets hémodynamiques de l'administration de terlipressine seule ou associé à la nitroglycérine chez les malades atteints de cirrhose. Gastroenterol Clin Biol 1992; 16:680-686.
42. Walker S, Stiehl A, Raedsch R, Kommerell B. Terlipressin in bleeding esophageal varices. A placebo controlled double-blind study. Hepatology 1986; 6:112-115.
43. Freeman JG, Cobden MD, Record CO. Placebo-controlled trial of terlipressin (glypressin) in the management of acute variceal bleeding. J Clin Gastroenterol 1989; 11:58-60.
44. Soderlund C, Magnusson I, Torngren S, Lundell L. Terlipressin (triglycyl-lysine vasopressin) controls acute bleeding oesophageal varices. A double-blind, randomized, placebo-controlled trial. Scand J Gastroenterol 1990; 25:622-630.
45. Levacher S, Blaise M, Pateron D, Letoumelin Ph, Lapandry C, Pourriat JL. Early administration of terlipressin plus transdermal nitroglycerin of active upper gastrointestinal hemorrhage in cirrhotic patients. J Hepatol 1994; 21:S46.
46. Freeman JG, Cobden I, Lishman AH, Record CO. Controlled trial of terlipressin ("glypressin") versus vasopressin in the early treatment of esophageal varices. Lancet 1982; 2:66-68.
47. Desaint B, Florent C, Levy VG. A randomized trial of triglycyl-lysine vasopressin versus lysine vasopressin in active cirrhotic variceal hemorrhage. In: Lebrec D, Blei AT, eds. Vasopressin analogs and portal hypertension. Paris: John Libbey Eurotext, 1987; 155-157.
48. Chiu WK, Sheen IS, Liaw YF. A controlled study of glypressin versus vasopressin in the control of blee-

ding from esophageal varices. J Gastroenterol Hepatol 1990; 5:549-553.
49. D'Amico G, Traina M, Vizzini G, Tinè F, Politi F, Montalbano L, Pasta L, Pagliaro L, Morabito A and The Liver Study Group of V. Cervello Hospital. Terlipressin or vasopressin plus transdermal nitroglycerin in a treatment strategy for digestive bleeding in cirrhosis. A randomized clinical trial. J Hepatol 1994; 20:206-212.
50. Walker S, Kreichgauer HP, Bode JC. Terlipressin vs somatostatin in bleeding esophageal varices: a controlled double blind study. Hepatology 1992; 15:1023-1030.
51. Variceal Bleeding Study Group. Glypressin vs somatostatin in the treatment of acute variceal bleeding in patients with cirrhosis. A double-blind randomized controlled trial. Hepatology 1994; 19:136I (Abstr).
52. Colin R, Giuli N, Czernichow P, Ducrotte P, Lerebours E. Prospective comparison of glypressin, tamponade and their associacion in the treatment of bleeding esophageal varices. In: Lebrec D, Blei AT, eds. Vasopressin analogs and portal hypertension. Paris: John Libbey Eurotext, 1987; 149-153.
53. Fort E, Sautereau D, Silvaine C, Ingrand P, Pillegand B, Beauchant M. A randomized trial of terlipressin plus nitroglycerin vs balloon tamponade in the control of acute variceal hemorrhage. Hepatology 1990; 11:678-681.
54. Fiaccadori F, Pedreti G, Biraghi M, Arcidiacono R. Terlypressin and endoscopic sclerotherapy control variceal bleeding and prevent early rebleeding in cirrhotic patients. Current Therap Research 1993; 54:1-10.
55. Bosch J, Kravetz D, Rodés J. Effects of somatostatin on hepatic and systemic hemodynamics in patients with cirrhosis of the liver: comparison with vasopressin. Gastroenterology 1981; 80:518-525.
56. Kravetz D, Bosch J, Arderiu MT, Pizcueta MP, Casamitjana R, Rivera F, Rodés J. Effects of somatostatin on splanchnic hemodynamics and plasma glucagon in portal hypertensive rats. Am J Physiol 1988; 254:G322-G328.
57. Kravetz D, Bosch J, Terés J, Bruix J, Rimola A, Rodés J. Comparison of intravenous somatostatin and vasopressin infusions in treatment of acute variceal hemorrhage. Hepatology 1984; 4:442-446.
58. Tyden G, Samnegard H, Thulin L, Friman L, Efendic S. Treatment of bleeding esophageal varices with somatostatin. N Engl J Med 1978; 299:1466-1467.
59. Valenzuela JE, Schubert T, Fogel MR, Strong RM, Levine J, Mills PR, Fabry TL, Taylor LW, Conn HO, Posillico JT, and a Multicentre Study Group. A multicentre, randomised, double-blind trial of somatostatin in the management of acute hemorrhage from esophageal varices. Hepatology 1989; 10:958-961.
60. Burroughs AK, McCormick PA, Hughes MD, Sprengers D, D'Heygere F, McIntyre N. Randomized, double-blind, placebo- controlled trial of somatostatin for variceal bleeding. Emergency control and prevention of early variceal rebleeding. Gastroenterology 1990; 99:1388-1395.
61. Testoni PA, Masci E, Passaretti S, Malesci A, Tittobello A, Comin U, Ballarin E. Comparison of somatostatin and cimetidine in the treatment of acute esophageal variceal bleeding. Curr Ther Res 1986; 39:759-766.
62. Loperfido S, Godena F, Tosolini G, De Matte P, Burei F, Gasparini G, Sartori C, Valbusa A, Bulfoni A, Buttola Q. La somatostatina nel trattamento dell'emorragia da varici esofago-gastriche. Recenti Prog Med 1987; 78:82-86.
63. Kravetz D, Bosch J, Terés J, Bruix J, Rimola A, Rodés J. Comparison of intravenous somatostatin and vasopressin infusion in treatment of acute variceal hemorrhage. Hepatology 1984; 4:442-446.
64. Jenkins SA, Baxter JN, Corbett WA, Devitt P, Ware J, Shields R. A prospective randomized controlled clinical trial comparing somatostatin and vasopressin in controlling acute variceal haemorrhage. Br Med J 1985; 290:275-278.
65. Bagarani M, Albertini V, Anza M, Barlattani, Bracci F, Cucchiara G, Gizzonio D, Grassini G, Mari T, Procacciante F. Effect of somatostatin in controlling bleeding from esophageal varices. Ital J Surg Sci 1987; 17:21-26.
66. Cardona C, Vida F, Balanzo J, Cusso X, Farre A, Guarner C. Eficacia terapeutica de la somatostatina versus vasopressina mas nitroglicerina en la hemorragia activa por varices esofagogástricas. Gastroenterol Hepatol 1989; 12:30-34.
67. Hsia HC, Lee FY, Tsai YT, Lee SD, Lai HK, Lin WJ, Lay CS, Wang SS, Lo KJ. Comparison of somatostatin and vasopressin in the control of acute esophageal variceal hemorrhage. A randomized, controlled study. Chinese J Gastroenterol 1990; 7:71-78.
68. Saari A, Klvilaakso E, Inberg M, Paakkonen M, Lahtinem J, Hockerstedt K, Schroder T. Comparison of somatostatin and vasopressin in bleeding esophageal varices. Am J Gastroenterol 1990; 85:804-807.
69. Rodríguez-Moreno F, Santolaria F, Glez-Reimers E, Gómez JL, Batista N, Conde A, Martínez A, Rodríguez E. A randomized trial of somatostatin vs vasopressin plus nitroglycerin in the treatment of acute variceal bleeding. J Hepatol 1991; 13:S162.
70. Jaramillo JL, de la Mata M, Mino G, Costàn G, Gòmez-Camacho F. Somatostatin versus Sengstaken balloon tamponade for primary haemostasia of bleeding esophageal varices. J Hepatol 1991; 12:100-105.
71. Avgerinos A, Klonis C, Rekoumis G, Gouma P, Papedimitriou N. Controlled trial of somatostatin and balloon tamponade in bleeding esophageal varices. J Hepatol 1991; 13:78-83.
72. Di Febo G, Siringo S, Vacirca M, Santoro P, Merighi S, Mustafà A, Barbara L. Somatostatin and urgent sclerotherapy in active esophageal variceal bleeding. Gastroenterology 1990; 98:A583.
73. Shields R, Jenkins SA, Baxter JN, Kingsnorth AN, Ellenbogen S, Makin CA, Gilmore I, Morris AI, Ashby D, West CR. A prospective randomised controlled trial comparing the efficacy of somatostatin with injection sclerotherapy in the control of oesophageal varices. J Hepatol 1992; 16:128-137.
74. Planas R, Quer JC, Boix J, Canet J, Armengol M, Cabrè

E, Pintanel T, Humbert P, Oller B, Broggi MA, Gassull MA. A prospective randomized trial comparing somatostatin and sclerotherapy in the treatment of acute variceal bleeding. Hepatology 1994; 20:370-375.

75. Variceal bleeding study group. Randomized controlled trial of sclerotherapy vs somatostatin infusion in the prevention of early rebleeding following variceal hemorrhage in patients with cirrhosis. J Hepatol 1994; 21:S7.
76. Eriksson LS, Brundin T, Söderlund C, Wahren J. Hemodynamic effects of a long-acting somatostatin analogue in patients with liver cirrhosis. Scand J Gastroenterol 1987; 22:919-925.
77. Jenkins SA, Baxter JN, Corbett WA, Shields R. Effects of a somatostatin analogue SMS 201-995 on hepatic hemodynamics in the pig and on intravariceal pressure in man. Br J Surg 1985; 72:1009-1012.
78. Cerini R, Lee SS, Hadengue A, Koshy A, Girod C, Lebrec D. Circulatory effects of somatostatin analogue in two conscious rat models of portal hypertension. Gastroenterology 1988; 94:703-708.
79. McKee R. A study of octreotide in oesophageal varices. Digestion 1990; 45:60-65.
80. MacCormick PA, Dick R, Siringo S, Wagstaff D, Chesta J, McIntyre N, Burroughs AK. Octreotide reduces azygos blood flow in cirrhotic patients with portal hypertension. Eur J Gastroenterol Hepatol 1990; 2:489-492.
81. Lin HC, Tsai YT, Lee FY, Lee SD, Hsia HC Lin WJ, Lo KJ. Hemodynamic evaluation of octrotide in patients with hepatitis B-related cirrhosis. Gastroenterology 1992; 103:229-234.
82. Primignani M, Nolte A, Vazzoler MC, Hall de Lima MC, Carpinelli L, Marcelli R, de Franchis R. The effect of octreotide on intraesophageal variceal pressure in liver cirrhosis is unpredictable. Hepatology 1990; 12:989 (Abstr).
83. Greig JD, Carter DC. Effect of SMS 201-995 on portal pressure and porta-systemic shunting following haemorrhagic shock and blood volume restitution in portal hypertension. Gut 1990; 31:A1183 (Abstr).
84. MacCormick PA, Biagino MR, Dick R, Greenslade L, Chin J, Cardinn F, Wagstaff D, McIntyre N, Burroughs AK. Octreotide inhibits the meal-induced increases in portal venous pressure in cirrhotic patients with portal hypertension. A double blind placebo controlled study. Hepatology 1992; 16:1180-1186.
85. Hwang JS, Lin CH, Chang CF, Lee FY, Lu WC, Hsia HC, Wang SS, Wang SS, Lee SD, Tsai YT, Lo KJ. A randomized controlled trial comparing octreotide and vasopressin in the control of acute esophageal variceal bleeding. J Hepatol 1992; 16:320-325.
86. Silvain C, Carpentier S, Sautereau D. Czernichow B, Métreau JM, Fort E, Ingrand P, Boyer J, Pillegand B, Doffël M, Dhumeaux D, Beauchant M. Terlipressin plus transdermal nitroglycerin vs. octreotide in the control of acute bleeding from esophageal varices: a multicenter randomized trial. Hepatology 1993; 18:61-65.
87. Jenkins SA, Copeland G, Kingsworth A, Shields R. A prospective randomized controlled clinical trial comparing Sandostatin and injection sclerotherapy in the control of acute variceal haemorrhage: an interine report. Gut 1992; 33:F221. (Abstr).
88. Sung JJ, Chung SCS, Lai CW, Chan FKL, Leung JWC, Yung MY. Octreotide infusion of emergency sclerotherapy for variceal hemorrhage. Lancet 1993; 342:637-641.
89. Miskowik J, Burcharth F, Jensen L. Effect of lower oesophageal sphincter on oesophageal varices. A portographic study. Scand J Gastroenterol 1981; 16:957-960.
90. Owman T, Lunderquist A. Pharmacologic manipulation of lower esophageal sphincter pressure. A possible means of treatment of variceal bleeding. Radiology 1983; 23:139-142.
91. Mastai R, Grande L, Bosch J, Bruix J, Rigau J, Kravetz D, Navasa M, Pera C, Rodés J. Effects of metoclopramide and domperidone on azygos venous blood flow in patients with cirrhosis and portal hypertension. Hepatology 1986; 6:1244-1247.
92. Kleber G, Sauerbruch T, Fisher G, Geigenberger G, Paumgartner G. Reduction of transmural oesophageal variceal pressure by metoclopramide. J Hepatol 1991; 12:362-366.
93. Feu F, Mas A, Bosch J, Salmeron JM, Garcia Pagan JC, Terés J, Rodés J. Domperidone or metoclopramide vs placebo in the prevention of early variceal rebleeding in cirrhosis. A prospective, randomized trial. J Hepatol 1988; 7 (Suppl 1):S31.
94. Hosking SW, Doss W, El-Zeiny H, Robinson P, Barsoum MS, Johnson AG. Pharmacological constriction of the lower esophageal sphincter: a simple method of arresting variceal hemorrhage. Gut 1988, 29:1098-1102.

Pharmacological Prevention of Variceal Hemorrhage

N. D. Grace

INTRODUCTION

Long-term epidemiologic studies have shown that up to 90% of patients with cirrhosis will eventually develop esophageal varices as a complication of portal hypertension (1). Based on data from prospective endoscopic studies of patients with esophageal varices and from the medical control groups of randomized controlled trials for the prevention of first variceal hemorrhage (2-4), 25 to 30% of these patients will experience an episode of variceal bleeding. Most bleeding episodes occur within a year of the initial diagnosis of varices, with the risk of bleeding decreasing significantly in patients with varices of longer duration (2). However, once a patient has experienced an episode of variceal bleeding and has been successfully treated for the acute event, the risk of recurrent variceal bleeding approaches 70%, with most episodes occurring within 6 months of the index bleed (5). The mortality for each bleeding episode is 30 to 50% depending on the clinical status of the patient. Variceal hemorrhage remains a major cause of death in patients with cirrhosis with 10-15% of untreated patients expiring from a variceal bleed within one year of the diagnosis of esophageal varices. Therefore, effective therapy for the prevention of variceal hemorrhage might be expected to favorably influence the mortality rate in patients with cirrhosis.

RISK FACTORS

Since the majority of patients with esophagogastric varices will not have bleeding as a complication, it is important to determine risk factors that will identify patients more likely to experience a variceal bleed. Prospective studies have shown that the size of varices (large varices), the presence of endoscopic red color signs and advanced liver disease as determined by Child's classification, especially the presence of ascites, are predictive of a variceal bleed (2, 6-8). In patients with alcoholic cirrhosis, continued consumption of alcohol is also associated with a high risk of bleeding (8). A number of classifications have been proposed, using various combinations of these risk factors (2, 7, 8). Although these classifications have been successful in identifying a group of patients with an increased risk of variceal hemorrhage, a number of patients who do not meet the high risk criteria will nevertheless have an esophageal variceal bleed (6, 9). Until better criteria are established, a reasonable argument can be made for placing all patients with endoscopically proven esophageal varices, especially patients with large varices, on prophylactic therapy to prevent first variceal hemorrhage.

BASIS FOR PHARMACOLOGIC THERAPY

The pathophysiology of portal hypertension has been discussed in a previous chapter. As portal pressure is a function of portal venous blood flow and intrahepatic and portocollateral resistance, drugs that will either decrease portal venous blood flow (vasoconstrictors) or alter intrahepatic and/or portocollateral resistance (vasodilators) have the potential for decreasing portal pressure. A number of potential drugs have been studied in animal models of portal hypertension but only the vasoconstrictive non-selective beta adrenergic blockers (propranolol, nadolol) and the vasodilatory long-acting nitrates (isosorbide-5-mononitrate) have been evaluated in long-term randomized controlled trials. There is limited data to determine how much of a decrease in portal pressure is necessary to prevent a bleeding episode. However, Feu et al. reported that patients in whom the HVPG decreased by greater than 20% in response to propranolol or the combination of propranolol and isosorbide-5-mononitrate after 3 months of treatment had significantly fewer episodes of recurrent variceal bleeding than patients with less than a 20% decrease (11% vs. 54%) (10). Using a combination of nadolol and isosorbide-5-mononitrate, Villanueva et al. found significantly less recurrent variceal bleeding in patients in whom there was a decrease of greater than 10% in the HVPG at 3 months compared to baseline than in patients without a significant decrease in HVPG (17% vs. 67%) (11). In patients with an initial hepatic venous pressure gradient greater than 12 mmHg, a decrease to less than 12 mmHg will essentially eliminate the risk of bleeding (12).

PREVENTION OF FIRST VARICEAL BLEEDING

There are 9 RCT's (7 published (13-19), 2 in abstract only (20, 21) that have compared non-selective beta adrenergic blockers (7 propranolol, 2 nadolol) to a placebo control group for the prevention of first variceal hemorrhage. A meta-analysis of the published studies (9) shows a significant benefit for beta adrenergic blockers in the prevention of initial variceal hemorrhage ($p < 0.01$) (fig. 1) and a trend for prevention of mortality ($p = 0.112$) (fig. 2). Although one of the studies published in abstract only (20) reported more bleeding episodes in patients treated with propranolol, inclusion of this abstract in a meta-analysis does not alter the favorable outcome for the use of beta adrenergic blockers (22).

Of the seven published trials, four report a significant benefit for prevention of variceal bleeding (14-16, 19), one found a significant advantage for the subgroup of patients who were compliant in taking their medication (17), one found patients who did not have ascites at the time of randomization had a lower incidence of variceal bleeding when treated with propranolol (18) and one found no difference between propranolol and control group (13). Combining data from these trials, 16.3% of patients randomized to non-selective beta adrenergic blockers experienced an episode of upper gastrointestinal hemorrhage compared to 27.2% of the control patients, a reduction of 40% in the risk of first variceal hemorrhage (9). Only Pascal et al. reported a statistically significant improvement in survival (15). Using a 3 way randomization, Andreani et al. (14) showed propranolol to be superior to both sclerotherapy and a control group for prevention of first variceal hemorrhage, with no difference found between the latter groups. There was also a trend toward improved survival in the propranolol-treated patients. The Prova study (13) used a 4 way randomization between propranolol, sclerotherapy, propranolol plus sclerotherapy, and a control group. This trial was terminated prematurely after 3 years because of an unexpected high mortality associated with sclerotherapy treatment. The propranolol and control groups had similar survival curves, which were both slightly better than the survival curves for patients receiving sclerotherapy.

Although an improvement in survival associated with beta adrenergic blocker therapy was not statistically significant, analysis of data from four of the trials (23) revealed a significant decrease in death due to gastrointestinal hemorrhage. In the six trials where data is available, gastrointestinal bleeding was the cause of death in 26.0% of patients receiving beta adrenergic blockers compared to 36.2% in the control population. Although the majority of deaths in both beta adrenergic blocker treated patients and control groups were due to non-bleeding events, there was no significant difference between the treatment groups for death due to liver failure (24).

Using nine criteria for judging the quality of design Pagliaro et al. (22) gave all of these trials excellent ratings with a mean score that was 76% of the maximal obtainable score. This is in contrast to the trials evaluating sclerotherapy

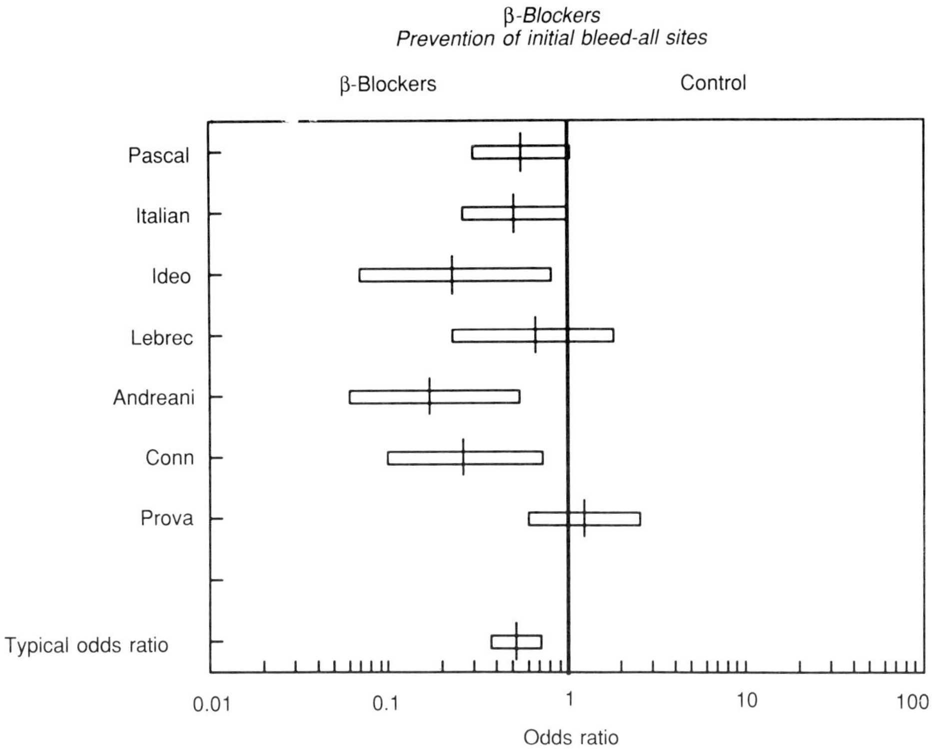

Fig. 1. Randomidez, controlled trials of β-blockers (propranolol, nadolol) versus placebo for prevention of first variceal hemorrhage. Bleeding refers to the number of patients experiencing bleeding from all sources, not just esophageal varices. Odds ratio is 0.52; 95% CI, 0.38 to 0.71 ($p < 0.01$).

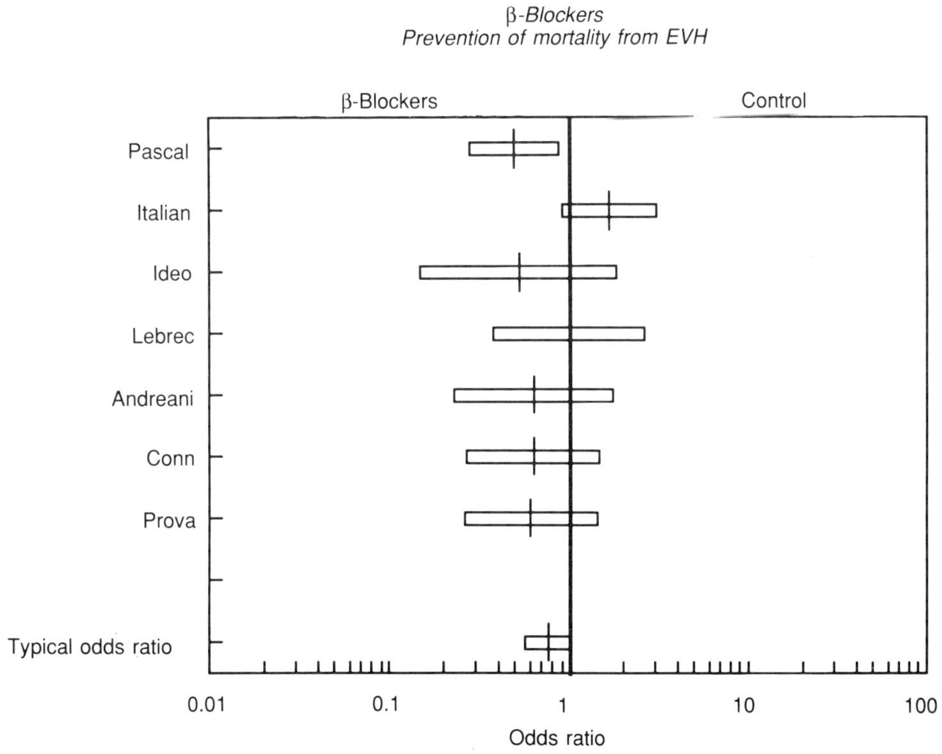

Fig. 2. Randomidez, controlled trials of β-blockers (propranolol, nadolol) versus placebo for prevention of first variceal hemorrhage. Prevention of mortality. Odds ratio is 0.75; 95% CI, 0.57 to 1.03 ($p = 0.112$).

for prevention of initial variceal hemorrhage where there was marked heterogeneity in the quality of design scores and an inverse relationship between the quality of design and the enthusiasm for the use of sclerotherapy.

SUBGROUP ANALYSIS

Variceal Size

Since only 25-30% of patients with esophageal varices will experience an episode of variceal bleeding, should all patients with varices be placed on prophylactic beta adrenergic blocker therapy? There is uniform agreement that large varices are a risk factor for variceal bleeding, prompting 4 of the 7 published controlled trials to include only patients with varices of moderate to large size. Combining data from three trials that included patients with small varices (13, 14, 19), 2 of 41 patients with small varices randomized to a beta adrenergic blocker had an episode of variceal bleeding compared to 4 of 46 randomized to placebo (fig. 3). Although beta adrenergic therapy was highly effective for the prevention of first variceal hemorrhage in patients with large varices, the number of patients with small varices included in these trials is inadequate to draw any conclusions about recommending beta adrenergic therapy for this group of patients.

Severity of Liver Disease

Six of the seven published trials provide data relating the severity of liver disease as judged by Child's criteria to the risk of gastrointestinal bleeding. While the seventh study (13) did not give data on Child's classification, a multivariate analysis found only sex, bilirubin and albumin to have significant, independent prognostic value. In four studies (14-16, 19), patients classified as Child's B appear to derive the greatest benefit from beta adrenergic blocker therapy, whereas one study (18) reports a significant benefit only for patients classified as Child's A and one study (17) found no difference in bleeding events between Child's A and B patients when compared to the corresponding control groups. In the five studies that presented data on Child's status at the time of randomization, only 61 patients with Child's Class C were included, a sample size that is inadequate to draw conclusions about the use of beta adrenergic blockers for this subgroup of patients.

Ascites

Concern about the efficacy of beta adrenergic blocker therapy in patients with ascites has been raised, based on a retrospective analysis of data from the Italian Multicenter trial in which propranolol was found to be most effective in the prevention of first variceal hemorrhage in patients without ascites at the time of randomization (18). In contrast, Conn et al. (19) found a benefit for propranolol only in the group of patients with ascites at entry as only one patient without ascites experienced a bleeding event. In an analysis of individual patient data combining four of the European trials, Poynard et al. (23) found nonselective beta adrenergic blocker therapy effective for both patients with and wit-

	Total patients	Large varices	Small varices
β-Blockers	458	377 (82,3 %)	81 (17,7 %)
Placebo	462	377 (81,6 %)	85 (18,4 %)

	Large varices			Small varices		
	N	EVH	%	N	EVH	%
β-Blockers	317	42	(13,2 %) *	41	2	(4,9 %)
Placebo	316	84	(26,6 %)	46	4	(8,7 %)

Fig. 3. Comparison of incidence of variceal hemorrhage in patients with large versus small varices as judged by endoscopy at the time of randomization. (Data from controlled trials by Conn et al. [19], Andreani et al. [14] and the Prova Study Group [13].) *, Statistically significant.

hout ascites at the time of randomization. Since ascites is an independent risk factor for variceal bleeding, patients with mild to moderate ascites and esophageal varices should be placed on prophylactic beta adrenergic blocker therapy.

TOLERANCE TO BETA ADRENERGIC BLOCKER TREATMENT

Not all patients are candidates for beta adrenergic blocker therapy. Congestive heart failure, severe chronic obstructive pulmonary disease, asthma and insulin dependent diabetes mellitus are considered relative contraindications to the use of beta adrenergic blockers. In the study by Conn et al. (19), a screening log revealed that 20% of patients with cirrhosis considered for the study had contraindications to beta adrenergic blockers or were already receiving them. In addition, side effects requiring cessation of propranolol therapy were found in 14% of patients by Conn et al. (19), 11% by Pascal et al. (15), 27% by the Italian Multicenter Project (18), 7% by Andreani et al. (14) and 17% in the Prova Study (13) compared to 4% by Lebrec et al. (17) and 3% by Ideo et al. (16) for patients treated with nadolol. Although there are no controlled trials directly comparing propranolol and nadolol, the implication of this data is that nadolol may be better tolerated. This may reflect the fact that nadolol is not metabolized by the liver and does not penetrate the blood brain barrier although the difference in side effects between the beta adrenergic blockers is not primarily a reflection of CNS side effects.

UNSETTLED ISSUES

Duration of Beta Adrenergic Blocker Therapy

Is the reduction in portal pressure achieved over 1-2 years sustained over a longer period of treatment? In a hemodynamic study by Groszmann et al. (12), there was a significant reduction in the hepatic venous pressure gradient (HVPG) at 3 months in patients treated with propranolol when compared to baseline values (18.1 ± 4.2 to 15.7 ± 3.4 mmHg; $p < 0.05$) but no significant change was observed in the placebo group (19.6 ± 6.8 to 17.5 ± 5.3 mmHg, NS). At one year, there was a significant reduction in the HVPG in both groups but this may be a consequence of more patients in the placebo group leaving the study because of terminating events. There are no published data on the effect of beta adrenergic blocker treatment on the HVPG when patients have been on treatment for greater than 2 years. In a study designed to evaluate the prognostic value of sequential hemodynamic measurements in patients with alcoholic cirrhosis and esophageal varices and no prior history of portal hypertensive related bleeding Vorobioff et al. (25) demonstrated that, without the institution of prophylactic treatment, a reduction in the HVPG >15% was associated with significantly greater probability of remaining free of bleeding and surviving. They noted a greater decrease in HVPG in patients who abstained from alcohol. A multivariate analysis demonstrated that the HVPG had independent prognostic value for both bleeding and survival at 10 months, a trend that was also evident with measurements at 25 months and 45 months. Although this study does not address the effect of beta adrenergic blocker therapy, the implication is that a sustained reduction in HVPG of >15% and, especially a reduction to less than 12 mmHg, may be associated with a continuing decrease in the risk of variceal hemorrhage.

Is the initiation of beta adrenergic blocker therapy a life long commitment? The mean follow-up period for the published RCT's ranged from 12 to 28 months. The Barcelona-Boston-New Haven study (19) was designed to taper patients not meeting a study end point off propranolol at the completion of the study. Approximately half of the patients in each arm of the study were tapered and followed prospectively. Six of twenty-five patients who had been treated with propranolol subsequently bled compared to three of twenty-four who had been on placebo (26). Variceal hemorrhage was the cause of death in four patients from the group that had been on propranolol compared to none in the placebo group. The earliest bleeding episode occurred 2 months after discontinuation of medication so that bleeding was unlikely to represent a rebound phenomena. These findings suggest that beta adrenergic blocker therapy needs to be continued indefinitely, a hypothesis requiring verification by a long-term controlled trial.

Alternative Pharmacologic Therapy

For patients who either have contraindications to the use of beta adrenergic blockers or who are unable to tolerate the drugs because of side effects, long acting nitrates may be a reasonable alternative. García-Pagán et al. (27) demonstrated a sustained reduction in the HVPG over a 3 month follow-up on patients with cirrhosis receiving isosorbide-5-mononitrate when compared to a group given a placebo. These investigators further showed that the combination of propranolol and isosorbide-5-mononitrate produced a greater reduction in the HVPG than propranolol alone (28, 29). This additional effect of isosorbide-5-mononitrate was especially evident in patients who did not sustain a significant decrease in HVPG when treated with propranolol alone (28). Vorobioff et al. (30) demonstrated a similar enhanced reduction in HVPG for the combination of propranolol and isosorbide dinitrate compared to propranolol given alone.

In a controlled trial comparing propranolol and isosorbide-5-mononitrate for the prevention of first variceal hemorrhage, Angelico et al. (31) found the drugs comparable for the prevention of variceal hemorrhage with no difference in side effects requiring cessation of therapy or in survival between the 2 groups. Potential concerns about isosorbide-5-mononitrate causing a deterioration in renal function in patients with ascites (30) were not substantiated in this trial. A second study comparing nadolol plus isosorbide-5-mononitrate versus nadolol alone for the prevention of initial variceal hemorrhage reported very few bleeding episodes in either group in a mean follow-up period of 19 months (32).

CONCLUSIONS

Non-selective beta adrenergic blockers (propranolol, nadolol) are effective in the prevention of first variceal hemorrhage in patients with cirrhosis and large esophageal varices, with a reduction in risk of approximately 40%. They are especially effective in patients classified as Child's B and are effective for both patients with and without ascites. Selecting patients who will be compliant in taking their medication is a necessity. Isosorbide-5-mononitrate is a reasonable alternative for patients who are either intolerant of or have contraindications to the use of beta adrenergic blockers. Although improvement in survival does not quite reach statistical significance in the published RCT's, a significant reduction in variceal hemorrhage as a cause of death is achieved.

PREVENTION OF RECURRENT VARICEAL HEMORRHAGE

There are 11 randomized controlled trials comparing non-selective beta adrenergic blockers (propranolol 10, nadolol 1) to a placebo for the prevention of recurrent variceal hemorrhage (20, 33-42). A recent meta-analysis of these trials shows a significant reduction in rebleeding with a pooled relative risk of 0.38, 95% CI, 0.29-0.52 (43). The non-selective beta adrenergic blocker was either superior to or equivalent to the placebo in all of these studies, with no study showing beta adrenergic blocker therapy less effective than placebo. Combining the data from these trials, the risk of recurrent bleeding is reduced from 65.9% in the control groups to 44.7% in the beta adrenergic blocker treated patients, a reduction of 32% ($p < 0.0001$) (44). Patients with good liver function (Child's A or B) were especially benefited by beta adrenergic therapy. Although this was not quite statistically significant there was a trend toward improved survival (RR, 0.7; 95% CI, 0.44-1.05) (43). Comparison of these trials is complicated by differences in the etiology and severity of liver disease and especially differences in the time interval between the index bleed and the initiation of therapy which ranged from a mean of 12 hours to 21 days (43). Graham et al. (5) have shown that the highest risk period for rebleeding is within the first 2 weeks after index bleed so a delay in initiation of treatment could miss high risk patients and therefore influence long term morbidity and mortality. Although the mean dose of propranolol varied in these trials, this did not seem to account for the differences in rebleeding rates. A multivariate analysis showed that the occurrence of hepatocellular carcinoma, lack of compliance, lack of persistent decrease in resting heart rate and lack of abstinence from alcohol were associated with a higher risk of rebleeding (45). In general, the beta adrenergic blocker therapy was well tolerated; the most common side effects reported were loss of energy, dyspnea, depression, cold extremities, impotence and headache (43). Only a relatively small number of patients had side effects severe enough to prompt discontinuation of therapy. Hepatic encephalopathy or renal failure were not a significant problem in patients receiving beta adrenergic blocker therapy.

Propranolol has also been shown to be superior to a placebo for the prevention of recurrent bleeding form portal hypertension gastropathy, an entity in which endoscopic therapy has no role (46). In a trial with an 18 month follow-up period, Pérez-Ayuso et al. (46) demonstrated a trend toward improved survival as well as reduction in recurrent bleeding in patients receiving propranolol.

A number of controlled trials have compared propranolol to sclerotherapy or the combination of propranolol and sclerotherapy to either sclerotherapy or propranolol alone for the prevention of recurrent variceal bleeding. Results of these studies are discussed in chapter: «Drug therapy: comparison with other therapies for portal hypertension».

CONCLUSION

Non-selective beta adrenergic blocker therapy is a reasonable choice as initial therapy for the prevention of recurrent bleeding both from esophageal varices and from portal hypertensive gastropathy. However, since 45% of patients will experience recurrent bleeding despite beta adrenergic blocker therapy, there is a need for more effective therapy. Measurements of hemodynamic response to beta adrenergic blocker therapy may help select patients more likely to respond to treatment. Future research should evaluate the effect of combinations of pharmacologic agents and the combination of pharmacologic and endoscopic therapy.

REFERENCES

1. Christensen E, Fauerholdt L, Schlichting P, Juhl E, Poulsen H, Tygstrup N. Aspects of the natural history of gastrointestinal bleeding in cirrhosis and the effects of prednisone. Gastroenterology 1981; 81:944-952.
2. The North Italian Endoscopic Club for the Study and Treatment of Esophageal Varices. Prediction of the first variceal hemorrhage in patients with cirrhosis of the liver and esophageal varices: a prospective multicenter study. N Engl J Med 1988; 319:983-989.
3. Gores GJ, Wiesner RH, Dickson ER, Zinmeister AR, Jorgensen AR, Langworthy A. Prospective evaluation of esophageal varices in primary biliary cirrhosis: development, natural history and influence in survival. Gastroenterology 1989; 96:1552-1559.
4. Grace ND. Prevention of initial variceal hemorrhage. In: Groszmann RJ, Grace ND, eds. Gastroenterology Clinics of North America: Complications of portal hypertension: Esophagogastric varices and ascites. Philadelphia: WB Saunders, 1992; 149-161.
5. Graham D, Smith JL. The course of patients after variceal hemorrhage. Gastroenterology 1981; 80:800-809.
6. Rigo GP, Merighi A, Chalen NJ, Mastronardi M, Codeluppi PL, Ferrari A. A prospective study of the ability of three endoscopic classifications to predict hemorrhage from esophageal varices. Gastrointest Endosc 1992; 38:425-429.
7. Beppu K, Inokuchi K, Koyanagi N, Nakayama S, Sakata H, Kitarro S, Kobayaski M. Prediction of variceal hemorrhage by esophageal endoscopy. Gastrointest Endosc 1981; 27:213-218.
8. Dagradi AE. The natural history of esophageal varices in patients with alcoholic liver cirrhosis: an endoscopic and clinical study. Am J Med 1972; 57:520-540.
9. Grace ND. Management of Portal Hypertension. The Gastroenterologist 1993; 1:39-58.
10. Feu F, García-Pagán JC, Luca A, Teres J et al. Clinical-hemodynamic correlations during pharmaceutical prevention of variceal rebleeding in cirrhosis. Hepatology 1992; 16:123A.
11. Villanueva C, Balanzo J, Novella MT, Torras X et al. A prospective and randomized trial of endoscopic sclerotherapy vs. nadolol plus isosorbide-5-mononitrate for the prevention of variceal rebleeding. Hepatology 1994; 20:268A.
12. Groszmann RJ, Bosch J, Grace ND, Conn HO, García-Tsao G, Navasa M. Hemodynamic events in a prospective randomized trial of propranolol versus placebo in the prevention of a first variceal hemorrhage. Gastroenterology 1990; 99:1401-1407.
13. The Prova Study Group. Prophylaxis of first hemorrhage from oesophageal varices by sclerotherapy, propranolol or both in cirrhotic patients. A randomized multicenter trial. Hepatology 1991; 14:1016-1024.
14. Andreani T, Poupon RE, Balkau B, Trinchet JC, Grnage JD, Peigney N. Preventive therapy of first gas-

trointestinal bleeding in patients with cirrhosis: results of a controlled trial comparing propranolol, endoscopic sclerotherapy and placebo. Hepatology 1990; 12:1413-1419.
15. Pascal JP, Cales P, A Multicenter Study Group. Propranolol in the prevention of first upper gastrointestinal tract hemorrhage in patients with cirrhosis of the liver and esophageal varices. N Engl J Med 1987; 317:856-861.
16. Ideo G, Bellati G, Fesce E, Grimoldi D. Nadolol can prevent the first gastrointestinal bleeding in cirrhosis: a prospective, randomized study. Hepatology 1988; 8:6-9.
17. Lebrec D, Poynard T, Capron JP, Hillon P, Geoffroy P, Roulot D. Nadolol for prophylaxis of gastrointestinal bleeding in patients with cirrhosis. A randomized trial. J Hepatology 1988; 7:118-125.
18. The Italian Multicenter Project for Propranolol in Prevention of Bleeding. Propranolol prevents first gastrointestinal bleeding in nonascitic cirrhotic patients. Final report of a multicenter randomized trial. J Hepatology 1989; 9:75-83.
19. Conn HO, Grace ND, Bosch J, Groszmann RJ, Rodés J, Wright SC. Propranolol in the prevention of the first hemorrhage from esophageal varices: results of a randomized double blind cooperative clinical trial. Hepatology 1991; 13:902-912.
20. Colman J, Jones P, Finch C, Dudley F. Propranolol in the prevention of variceal hemorrhage in alcoholic cirrhotic patients. Hepatology 1990; 12:851.
21. Strauss E, Desa MFG, Albano A, Lacet CMC, Leite MO, Maffei RA, Jr. A randomized controlled trial for the prevention of the first upper gastrointestinal bleeding due to portal hypertension in cirrhosis: sclerotherapy or propranolol versus control groups. Hepatology 1988; 8:1395.
22. Pagliaro L, D'Amico G, Sorensen TIA, Lebrec D, Burroughs AK, Morabito A. Prevention of first bleeding in cirrhosis: A meta-analysis of randomized trials of nonsurgical treatment. Ann Intern Med 1992; 117:59-70.
23. Poynard T, Cales P, Pasta L, Ideo G, Pascal JP, Pagliaro L, Lebrec D. Beta-adrenergic-antagonist drugs in the prevention of gastrointestinal bleeding in patients with cirrhosis and esophageal varices: An analysis of data and prognostic factors in 589 patients from four randomized clinical trials. N Engl J Med 1991; 324:1532-1538.
24. Grace ND. Prevention of initial variceal hemorrhage. Progress in Hepatic, Biliary and Pancreatic Surgery. In: Najarian JS, Delaney JP, eds. Chicago: Year Book, 1990; 409-418.
25. Vorobioff J, Groszmann RJ, Picabea E, Villavicencio R, Passamonti M, Lerner E, Tanno H, Gamen M, Audano M. Prognostic value of sequential measurement of portal pressure in alcoholic cirrhotic patients. Hepatology 1994; 20:103A.
26. Grace ND, Conn HO, Groszmann RJ, Richardson CR, Matloff DS, García-Tsao G. Propranolol for prevention of first esophageal variceal hemorrhage: a lifetime commitment? Hepatology 1990; 12:407(A).
27. García-Pagán JC, Feu F, Navasa M, Bru C, Del Árbol LR, Bosch J, Rodés J. Long-term haemodynamic effects of isosorbide-5-mononitrate in patients with cirrhosis and portal hypertension. J Hepatol 1990; 11:189-195.
28. García-Pagán JC, Navasa M, Bosch J, Bru C, Pizcueta P, Rodés J. Enhancement of portal pressure reduction by the association of isosorbide-5-mononitrate to propranolol administration in patients with cirrhosis. Hepatology 1990; 11:230-238.
29. García-Pagán JC, Feu F, Bosch J, Rodés J. Propranolol compared with propranolol plus isosorbide-5-mononitrate for portal hypertension: a randomized controlled study. Ann Int Med 1991; 114:869-873.
30. Vorobioff J, Picabea E, Gamen M, Villavicencio R, et al. Propranolol compared with propranolol plus isosorbide dinitrate in portal-hypertensive patients: Long-term hemodynamics and renal effects. Hepatology 1993; 18:477-484.
31. Angelico M, Carli R, Piat C, Gentile S, Rinaldi V, Bologna E, Capocaccia L. Isosorbide-5-mononitrate versus propranolol in the prevention of first bleeding in cirrhosis. Gastroenterology 1993; 104:1460-1465.
32. Merkel C, Gatta A, Amodio P et al. Nadolol or nadolol plus isosorbide-5-mononitrate in the prophylaxis of first variceal bleeding in patients with cirrhosis. Interim analysis of a multicenter study. J Hepatol 1993; 8:1:s147-148.
33. Burroughs AK, Jenkins WJ, Sherlock S, Dunk A, Walt RP, Osuafor TOK et al. Controlled trial of propranolol for the prevention of recurrent variceal hemorrhage in patients with cirrhosis. N Engl J Med 1983; 309:1539-1542.
34. Lebrec D, Poynard T, Bernuau J, Berkoff E, Nouel O, Capron JP et al. A randomized controlled study of propranolol for prevention of recurrent gastrointestinal bleeding in patients with cirrhosis: A final report. Hepatology 1984; 4:355-358.
35. Villeneuve JP, Pomier-Layrargues G, Infante-Rivard C, Willems B, Huet PM, Marleau D, Viallet A. Propranolol for the prevention of recurrent variceal hemorrhage: A controlled trial. Hepatology 1986; 6:1239-1243.
36. Queuniet AM, Czernichow P, Lerebours E, Ducrotte P, Tranvouez JL, Colin R. Etude controllée du propranolol dans la prevention des recidives hemorragiques chez les patients cirrhotiques. Gastroenterol Clin Biol 1987; 11:41-47.
37. Gatta A, Merkel C, Sacerdoti D, Bolognesi M, Caregaro L, Zuin R et al. Nadolol for prevention of variceal rebleeding in cirrhosis: A controlled clinical trial. Digestion 1987; 37:22-28.
38. Colombo M, Defranchis R, Tommasini M, Sangiovanni A, Dioguardi N. Beta blockade prevents recurrent gastrointestinal bleeding in well-compensated patients with alcoholic cirrhosis: A multicenter randomized controlled trial. Hepatology 1989; 9:433-438.
39. Sheen IS, Chen TY, Liaw YF. Randomized controlled study of propranolol for prevention of recurrent esophageal varices bleeding in patients with cirrhosis. Liver 1989; 9:1-5.

40. Garden OJ, Mills PR, Birnie GG, Murray GD, Carter DC. Propranolol in the prevention of recurrent variceal hemorrhage in cirrhotic patients: A controlled trial. Gastroenterology 1990; 98:185-190.
41. Rossi V, Cales P, Burtin P et al. Prevention of recurrent variceal bleeding in alcoholic cirrhotic patients: prospective controlled trial of propranolol and sclerotherapy. J Hepatol 1991; 12:283-289.
42. Cerbelaud P, Cales P, Pascal B, Charneau J et al. Propranolol et prevention des recidives de rupture de varice oesophagienne du cirrhotique. Gastroenterol Clin Biol 1986; 18:A10.
43. Burroughs AK, McCormick PA. Prevention of variceal rebleeding. Groszmann RJ, Grace ND, eds. Gastroenterology Clinics of North America: Complications of portal hypertension: Esophagogastric varices and ascites. Philadelphia: WB Saunders, 1992; 119-147.
44. Grace ND. A hepatologist's view of variceal bleeding. Am J Surg 1990; 160:26-31.
45. Poynard T, Lebrec D, Hillon P, Sayech R et al. Propranolol for prevention of recurrent gastrointestinal bleeding in patients with cirrhosis: A prospective study of factors associated with rebleeding. Hepatology 1987; 7:447-451.
46. Pérez-Ayuso R, Piqué JP, Bosch J, Panés J et al. Propranolol in prevention of recurrent bleeding from severe portal hypertensive gastropathy in cirrhosis. Lancet 1991; 337:1431-1434.

Clinical-Hemodynamic Correlations in the Evaluation and Treatment or Portal Hypertension

J. C. García-Pagán, J. Bosch

INTRODUCTION

Portal hypertension is a frequent clinical syndrome characterized by a pathological increase in portal venous pressure. As discussed before (see chapter: «Mechanisms of portal hypertension: collateral formation and rupture»), the maintenance of an increased portal pressure leads to the formation of portalsystemic collaterals that divert portal blood to the systemic circulation bypassing the liver, including the gastroesophageal varices, that are the most clinically relevant. After their formation, varices can progressively increase in size until their rupture and bled which is one of the most severe complications of cirrhosis (fig. 1). It is well known that, once gastroesophageal varices have bled, the risk of rebleeding is extremely high, if no effective treatment to prevent rebleeding is performed, reaching 70% after one year (1).

The present chapter is aimed at reviewing the natural history of gastroesophageal varices from their formation to their rupture in accordance with the hemodynamic changes observed either spontaneously or by therapeutic intervention (table 1).

Acknowledgements. We are indebted to D. Bird for secretarial help and to Drs. F Feu, A Escorsell and A Luca for their cooperation. These studies have been supported by grants from the Fondo de Investigaciones Sanitarias (94/0068 and 94/0757) and Fundació Catalana per a l'Estudi de les Malalties del Fetge.

FORMATION OF GASTROESOPHAGEAL VARICES

Portal hypertension is defined by the finding of an increased portal pressure gradient (PPG: the difference between free portal or wedged portal venous pressure and free hepatic venous pressure) above the normal value (up to 5 mmHg). Ho-

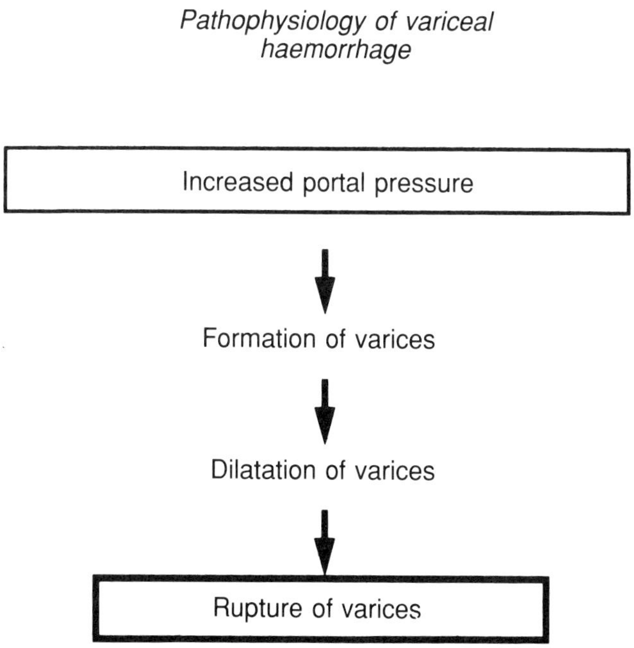

Fig. 1. Natural history of esophageal varices from its formation to its rupture.

Table 1: Clinical hemodynamic correlations and natural history of portal hypertension. Summary of studies

Reference	Type of study	N patients	Hemodynamic threshold	Clinical event
Formation of varices				
2	Crossectional	53	⩾ 10 mmHg	Presence of varices (endoscopy)
3	Crossectional	87	⩾ 12 mmHg	Presence of varices (endoscopy)
First variceal bleeding				
2	Crossectional	27	⩾ 12 mmHg	Bleeding from varices
3	Crossectional	49	⩾ 12 mmHg	Bleeding from varices
4	Crossectional	19	⩾ 12 mmHg	Bleeding from varices
15	Crossectional	70	⩾ 12 mmHg or VP > 10 mmHg	Bleeding from varices
8	Longitudinal	84	Reduction PPG to ⩽ 12 mmHg at 3 months	Protection from bleeding
14	Longitudinal	30	Reduction PPG ⩾ 15% or <12 mmHg at 10 months	Protection from bleeding
Acute bleeding episode				
35	Longitudinal	22	> 16 mmHg at index bleed	High % continued bleeding or early rebleeding
38	Longitudinal	31	Reduction by drugs of VP >10% at index bleed	No early rebleeding
Rebleeding				
42	Longitudinal	69	Reduction PPG ⩾ 20% at 3 months < 12 mmHg at 3 months	Marked reduction rebleeding Protection from rebleeding
43	Longitudinal	62	Reduction PPG ⩾ 20% at 3 months	Marked reduction rebleedin
41	Longitudinal	11	Reduction PPG > 12% at 1 months	No rebleeding
44	Longitudinal	16	Reduction VP > 20% at 3 months	Low variceal rebleeding

PPG, portal pressure gradient; VP, variceal pressure.

wever, clinically significant portal hypertension (associated with the development of complications from portal hypertension) requires that the PPG increases above a threshold value. Several studies have demonstrated that for varices to develop, the PPG shall increase above 10 mmHg (2-4). This observation suggests that it could be possible to prevent the development of gastroesophageal varices by an early pharmacological intervention, preventing a sustained increase of PPG above this threshold value. Furthermore, it is likely that reduction of PPG below this value may cause a gradual disappearance of gastroesophageal varices. Actually, there is experimental evidence indicating that development of portal-systemic collaterals can be prevented by agents that reduce portal pressure (5-7). Moreover, in a recent study we demonstrated that patients with varices in whom the PPG was reduced below a threshold value had a significant reduction in the size of varices (8). However, although all cirrhotic patients with varices have a PPG above 10 mmHg, there are also cirrhotic patients with PPG above this value but without varices. Clinical data from French (9) and Italian studies (10) showed that, in patients with liver cirrhosis and no esophageal varices at endoscopy, the incidence of new varices were 8% and 23% respectively after one year of follow-up. This different incidence could be related to the severity of liver disease and etiology of cirrhosis (10). However, multivariate analysis (9, 10) did not identify any variable with independent predictive value for development of varices. In an ongoing prospective study at our institution we have evaluated 31 consecutive cirrhotic patients without esophageal varices. Ten had a PPG < 10 mmHg, but 21 (68%) had a PPG ≥ 10 mmHg. It is likely that these latter patients are at greater risk of developing varices than those with a PPG < 10 mmHg, but this contention has not been proved yet. This can only be answered by longitudinal hemodynamic and endoscopic investigations in untreated patients.

FIRST VARICEAL BLEEDING EPISODE

Prospective randomized controlled clinical trials for the prevention of first variceal bleeding in patients with cirrhosis and esophageal varices have shown that the incidence of variceal bleeding ranges between 19 to 40% in control groups (11). Esophageal size, presence of red color signs in the variceal wall and degree of liver failure are the main variables correlating with an increased risk of variceal bleeding (12, 13). Hemodynamic studies have shown that a PPG $\geq$ 12 mmHg is necessary for the occurrence of variceal bleeding (2-4). This was first observed in retrospective studies comparing the PPG of patients with or without previous bleeding from esophageal varices (2-4). More recently this has been confirmed in prospective follow-up studies (8, 14). One of them, a prophylactic propranolol-placebo trial (8) clearly showed that the risk of experiencing the first episode of bleeding was abolished when the PPG was decreased to 12 mmHg or below. Furthermore, this selected group of patients also experienced a reduction in variceal size and prolonged actuarial probability of survival in comparison with those patients maintaining a PPG > 12 mmHg. Therefore, 12 mmHg seems to be the threshold gradient necessary for varices to bleed. However, among patients with a PPG above this threshold, the relationship between PPG and variceal bleeding is less evident (2-4, 8), since in some retrospective studies (2, 15-17), PPG was similar in variceal bleeders and non bleeders. However, other studies (3, 18) found higher PPG in patients with previous variceal bleeding. Nevertheless, in these studies there was marked overlap in PPG values between previous bleeders and non-bleeders.

How can we explain the lack of a good relationship between PPG measurements and variceal bleeding? There is new information which clarifies this issue showing that this relationship indeed exists.

On one hand, it has been shown that variceal pressure, measured non-invasively by means of an endoscopic pressure-sensitive gauge device, was significantly higher in variceal bleeders than in non-bleeders, despite similar PPG (15, 19), which was explained on the basis of the finding that variceal pressure was significantly lower than portal pressure (15, 19, 20). In these studies it was also shown that patients with large varices had greater variceal pressure than those with small varices (19). The measurement of variceal pressure with the combined semiquantitative assessment of variceal size allows for a rough estimation of variceal wall tension (as the product of variceal pressure and diameter), that was shown to be much higher in variceal bleeders than in non bleeders (15). In addition, repeated measurements showed that variceal pressure remained higher in patients bleeding on follow-up than in those who did not bleed (21). These observations reinforce the concept that variceal wall tension (determined by the interaction of variceal pressure, variceal size and thickness of the wall of the varices) is the main factor leading to variceal rupture (22). Therefore, despite a similar PPG elevation a higher variceal size or pressure may result in a greater risk of bleeding.

On the other hand, the lack of apparent relationship between PPG and bleeding in some retrospective studies may be due to temporal (chronological) dissociation between measurements of PPG and previous bleeding events (recent or remote). In that regard, Vinel et al. (23) showed that PPG measurements have prognostic value for short-term survival in patients with cirrhosis bleeding from esophageal varices. A delay between the occurrence of bleeding and measurement of PPG may select survivors with lower PPG. In addition, it has been shown that, among survivors, PPG is significantly higher immediately after an episode of variceal bleeding than 10 days later, due to a spontaneous reduction (24).

There is now evidence suggesting that changes in PPG during follow-up may correlate better than baseline PPG with the risk of bleeding. As previously mentioned, the study by Groszmann et al. (8) showed no incidence of bleeding in patients in whom PPG decreased below 12 mmHg in the follow-up. This has been recently confirmed by Vorobioff et al. (14) showing that the actuarial probability of first bleeding was significantly lower in those patients in whom PPG decreased more than 15% than in those who did not despite a similar baseline PPG. The study confirmed that no patient decreasing PPG below 12 mmHg bled. At least two other studies have shown that either PPG (25) or wedged hepatic vein pressure (26) was significantly higher in cirrhotic patients developing the first variceal hemorrhage during follow-up than in those who did not.

It has also been proposed that the finding of a reversal of portal blood flow, evidenced by Doppler ultrasonography or portography, correlates with a low risk of bleeding on follow up (27, 28). This, however, has not been confirmed by others (29-31). Nevertheless, the low prevalence of hepatofugal blood flow, 8.3% in a series of 228 unselected cirrhotic patients (31), makes the possible prognostic value of portal blood flow direction of small clinical impact.

ESOPHAGEAL VARICEAL REBLEEDING

Variceal bleeding is the most severe complication of portal hypertension (32). In addition, rebleeding is exceedingly common among survivors (33). Rebleeding can occur in the first few days after the index-bleed (*early rebleeding*) or later during the follow-up (*late rebleeding*), the incidence of rebleeding remains high during the first 6 weeks and decreases rapidly thereafter, becoming finally almost equal to that before bleeding (1).

FAILURE TO CONTROL BLEEDING OR EARLY REBLEEDING

Identification of patients who will continue to bleed or that will soon rebleed from esophageal varices may help to define the strategy of treatment in patients with variceal bleeding. Early prognostic assessment may be of help in deciding which patients will require rapid aggressive treatment. However, routine clinical and laboratory assessment is of little value; the severity of liver disease is the only factor associated with a high risk of early rebleeding (34). What do we know about possible relationships between hemodynamic parameters and outcome of patients with acute variceal bleeding?. There are recent data suggesting that either measurements of PPG or variceal pressure may correlate with the clinical evolution of these patients (27, 35-38). Early studies performed by Adamson et al. in the 70's (27), measuring portal pressure in patients during acute variceal hemorrhage, suggested that the degree of portal hypertension may be related to the persistence of the bleeding episode. This study showed that the higher the portal pressure, the higher the probability of persistence of variceal bleeding. More recently, Ready et al. (35), in a small group of patients with variceal bleeding who had the PPG measured in the day of the index bleeding episode, found that those with a PPG greater or equal to 16 mmHg had a chance of continued bleeding or early rebleeding greater than 50% (34). This was not observed in patients with lower PPG even in the absence of a specific treatment such as drugs or sclerotherapy (34). It has also been suggested that repeated measurements of variceal pressure, measured by endoscopy during the bleeding episode, may be of value identifying patients with a high risk of rebleeding (37). Thus, the preliminary results of a study by Ruiz del Árbol et al. (37) showed that those patients exhibiting an early (3 days) spontaneous decrease of variceal pressure, greater than 20% from its basal value during the day of the index bled, had a very low risk of rebleding. The same group (38) suggested that the response of variceal pressure to vasoactive drugs may help predict the outcome in these patients. Early rebleeding was only observed in patients with no or less than 10% reduction in variceal pressure after a bolus injection of somatostatin or glypressin (38).

Although provocative, the hemodynamic correlations observed in the context of acute variceal bleeding should be confirmed in larger series of cirrhotic patients. It should be noted, however, that because of the difficulties inherent to these hemodynamic measurements, it is unlikely that adequate studies could be done in patients in unstable hemodynamic conditions, which is the subset in whom it will be more useful to have prognostic indicators that could help in the decision for aggressive intervention (TIPS, surgery).

LATE REBLEEDING

Because of the high risk of rebleeding, it is accepted that patients surviving an acute variceal hemorrhage should receive effective long-term therapy to reduce the risk of recurrent variceal bleeding. Available data suggests that patients in Child-Pugh class B or C have higher rates of both rebleeding and death, and that variceal size and continued alcohol abuse are related to rebleeding risk (2, 10, 17, 29).

In patients with previous variceal bleeding, the PPG (25) or the wedged hepatic vein pressure (26, 39) have been shown to be independent prognostic factors of rebleeding during follow-up in some studies (25, 26, 39) but not in others (40-42). Possible explanations for such a discrepancy include: *a*) different time interval from bleeding to hepatic venous pressure measurements. As it has been shown, patients with high PPG may dye early after hemorrhage (23) and those who survive frequently exhibit a spontaneous reduction in PPG, that may be detected as early as 10 days after the bleeding episode (24), and *b*) the different treatments used to prevent rebleeding that may have influenced the outcome in these different series. Presently, as in predicting the first variceal bleeding, there is evidence suggesting that changes in PPG during follow-up, rather than baseline PPG values, may be a more important prognostic indicator for rebleeding (41-43). Sacerdoti et al. (41), in 11 cirrhotic patients treated with beta-blockers to prevent rebleeding, showed that no patient exhibiting a reduction in PPG greater than 12% after 1 month of beta-blockade rebled. However, these results should be taken with caution because of the small number of patients studied and the small number of events (4 rebleeds). A recent study performed in our unit (42) in a group of 69 cirrhotic patients receiving elective pharmacological therapy following variceal hemorrhage, showed that a fall in the PPG of more than 20% of baseline values or below 12 mmHg (after 3 months treatment) is associated with a very low risk of rebleeding on long-term follow-up: 8% vs. 55% in patients failing to exhibit such a decrease in PPG. In a multivariate analysis using a Cox's model (including demographic, clinical and endoscopic data) only a reduction in PPG greater than 20% had independent prognostic value for rebleeding. These results strongly suggest that repeated measurements of PPG during continued pharmacological therapy provide useful prognostic information on the risk of variceal rebleeding. Our study confirms that decreasing PPG below the 12 mmHg threshold value is associated with a complete protection from the risk of rebleeding (8). Almost the same protective value is associated with marked reductions in PPG (more than 20% of baseline), even if not reaching the 12 mmHg mark.

These findings have been confirmed in a recent study by Villanueva et al. comparing pharmacological treatment vs. sclerotherapy for the prevention of variceal rebleeding (43). This study showed that patients with a reduction in PPG greater or equal to 20% had an actuarial probability of rebleeding significantly lower than patients with lower decrease in PPG (43). The protective effect of a PPG reduction greater than 20% was observed either in patients treated with drugs or with sclerotherapy. Recent data from Ruiz del Árbol et al. (44) also suggests that a decrease in variceal pressure greater than 20% from baseline, after 3 months of propranolol treatment, had an independent prognostic value for rebleeding. Contrary to all these studies, Valla et al. (40) could not find any relationship between changes in PPG after an acute oral dose of 40 mg of propranolol and the probability of rebleeding on follow-up. However, the acute effects of a single fixed dose of propranolol may not be representative of what happens in clinical practice since the dosage of propranolol should be individually titrated. Actually, some studies have documented differences between the acute and chronic response to propranolol (45,46).

The good relationship between marked decrease in PPG (> 20%) and good clinical outcome suggests that this parameter may be used as a guidance for decision-making during therapy. Thus, the results of our study raise the question of whether it is adequate to continue drug therapy in patients with a poor hemodynamic response or it might be convenient to shift to other therapies. This, however, should be confirmed by additional prospective investigations.

SURVIVAL

The main factor predicting survival in all series analyzing this issue is the degree of liver failure usually evaluated as the Child-Pugh score. However, hemodynamic parameters such as arterial pressure (47) or hepatic venous pressures had also been considered to be independent predictors of survival in different series of cirrhotic patients (8, 14, 25, 26) but not in others (39, 48). A study performed in our unit showed that wedged hepatic venous pressure correlated with survival both in cirrhotic patients with or without previous variceal bleeding (26). Changes in PPG observed during follow-up were not only correlated with the incidence of rebleeding but also with survival. Thus, patients without previous variceal bleeding with a reduction in PPG to or below 12 mmHg (8) or more than 15% from its baseline value (14) had a prolonged survival than those who did not fulfill these criteria. In patients with previous variceal bleeding, there was a trend toward a lower actuarial mortality in patients who had a decrease of PPG greater than 20% than in those who had not (4% vs. 29% at 3 years follow-up: NS) but only Child-Pugh score was an independent predictor of mortality. As mentioned before, PPG measurements early in the course of the bleeding episode have prognostic value (23).

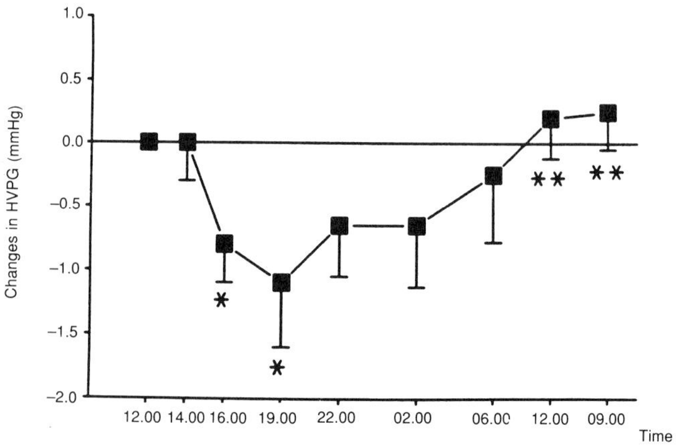

Fig. 2. Circadian changes in portal pressure gradient (HVPG) in patients with cirrhosis and portal hypertension. Data are shown as absolute changes from 12 a.m. (mean ± SEM). *, Significantly different from 12 a.m. ($p < 0.05$). **, Significantly different from 7 p.m. ($p < 0.05$). (Reproduced with permission from García-Pagán et al [49].)

OTHER SITUATIONS: CIRCADIAN CHANGES IN PORTAL PRESSURE

A recent study in our unit, performing serial measurements of portal pressure in patients with cirrhosis, showed that PPG exhibit a circadian variation (49). Thus, PPG progressively declined over the afternoon and evening reaching a nadir at 19.00 hours. Thereafter, PPG increased during the night, returning to baseline values at 09.00 h (fig. 2). In addition, we evaluated the time of occurrence of variceal bleeding in 101 consecutive cirrhotic patients presenting with a hematemesis of fresh blood and in whom the variceal origin of bleeding was confirmed by early endoscopy. The analysis of the time of occurrence of variceal hemorrhage using multiple components rhythmometry test, disclosed two peaks in the prevalence of variceal bleeding, the more pronounced being at 22.44 hours, when PPG started to increase, and the second at 09.12 hours, close to the maximum value of PPG. Furthermore, the lowest prevalence of variceal bleeding was at 15.20 hours, a time when portal pressure was declining in most patients. Such a rhythm in the time of occurrence of variceal bleeding has been confirmed by other authors in other countries (50, 51). The findings of this study suggested that spontaneous variations of PPG may be clinically relevant, since the lower and higher prevalence of bleeding occurred respectively during the periods of spontaneous decrease and increase in PPG.

It has also been shown that PPG can increase after other different physiological stimuli such as meals (52, 53), or physical exercise (54). Thus, PPG measurements in patients with portal hypertension cannot be considered a static but a dynamic parameter. The amplitude of these changes may influence the evolution of portal hypertension. It is likely that repeated bounds in portal pressure may lead to progressive dilatation of the varices. Preventing such increments may slow down the incidence of complications from portal hypertension.

REFERENCES

1. Graham DY, Smith JL. The course of patients following variceal hemorrhage. Gastroenterology 1981; 80:800-809.

2. Lebrec D, DeFleury P, Rueff B, Nahum H, Benhamou JP. Portal hypertension, size of esophageal varices and risk of gastrointestinal bleeding in alcoholic cirrhosis. Gastroenterology 1980; 79:1139-1144.
3. García-Tsao G, Groszmann RJ, Fisher RL, Conn HO, Atterbury CE, Glickman M. Portal pressure presence of gastroesophageal varices and variceal bleeding. Hepatology 1985; 5:419-424.
4. Viallet A, Marleau D, Huet M, Martin F, Farley A, Villeneuve JP, Lavoie P. Hemodynamic evaluation of patients with intrahepatic portal hypertension: relationship between bleeding varices and the portohepatic gradient. Gastroenterology 1975; 69:1297-1300.
5. Sarin SK, Groszmann RJ, Mosca PG, Rojkind M, Stadecker MJ, Bhatanagar R, Reuben A, Dayal Y. Propranolol ameliorates the development of portal-systemic shunting in a chronic murine schistosomiasis model of portal hypertension. J Clin Invest 1991; 87:1032-1036.
6. Lin HC, Soubrane O, Lebrec D. Prevention of portal hypertension and portosystemic shunting by early chronic administration of clonidine in conscious portal vein stenosed rats. Hepatology 1991; 14:325-330.
7. Lin HC, Soubrane O, Cailmail S, Lebrec D. Early chronic administration of propranolol reduces the severity of portal hypertension and portal systemic shunting in conscious portal vein stenosed rats. J Hepatol 1991; 13:213-219.
8. Groszmann RJ, Bosch J, Grace ND, Conn HO, García-Tsao G, Navasa M, Fischer R, Bermann M, Rofe S, Patrick M, Rodés J. Hemodynamic events in a prospective randomized trial of propranolol vs placebo in the prevention of a first variceal hemorrhage. Gastroenterology 1990; 99:1401-1407.
9. Calès P, Desmorat H, Vinel JP, Caucanas JP, Ravaud A, Gerin P, Brouet P, Pascal JP. Incidence of large esophageal varices in patients with cirrhosis: aplication to prophylaxis of first bleeding. Gut 1990; 31:1298-1302.
10. Pagliaro L, D´Amico G, Pasta L, Politi F, Vizzini G, Traina M, Madonia S, Luca A, Guerrera D, Puleo A, D´Antoni A. Portal hypertension in cirrhosis: Natural history. In: Bosch J, Groszmann RJ, eds. Portal Hypertension. Pathophysiology and Treatment. Oxford: Blackwell, 1994; 72-92.
11. Poynard T, Calès P, Pasta L, Ideo G, Pascal JP, Pagliaro L, Lebrec D, et al. Beta-adrenergic-antagonist drugs in the prevention of gastrointestinal bleeding in patients with cirrhosis and esophageal varices. An analysis of data and prognostic factors in 589 patients from four randomized clinical trials. N Engl J Med 1991; 324:1532-1538.
12. The North Italian Endoscopic Club for the study and the treatment of esophageal varices. Prediction of the first variceal hemorrhage in patients with cirrhosis of the liver and esophageal varices. N Engl J Med 1988; 319:983-989.
13. Beppu K, Inokuchi K, Koyanagi N, Nakayama S, Sakata H, Kitano S, Kobayashi M. Prediction of variceal hemorrhage on esophageal endoscopy. Gastrointest Endosc 1981; 27: 213-218 .
14. Vorobioff J, Groszmann RJ, Picabea E, Villavicencio R, Passamonti M, Lemer E, Tanno H, Gamen M, Audano M. Prognostic value of sequential measurement of portal pressure in alcoholic cirrhotic patients. Hepatology 1994; 20:103A.
15. Rigau J, Bosch J, Bordas JM, Navasa M, Mastai R, Kravetz D, Bruix J, Feu F, Rodés J. Endoscopic measurement of variceal pressure in cirrhosis: correlation with portal pressure and variceal hemorrhage. Gastroenterology 1989; 96:873-880.
16. Vinel JP, Cassigneul J, Louis A. Clinical and prognostic significance of portohepatic gradient in patients with cirrhosis. Surg Gynecol Obstet 1982, 155:347-352.
17. Rector WJ Jr, Reynolds TB. Risk factors for hemorrhage from esophageal varices and acute gastric lesions. Clin Gastroenterol 1985; 14:139-153.
18. Butzow GH, Novak D. Clinical value of hepatic vein catheterization. Gastrointest Radiol 1977; 2:153-161.
19. Feu F, Bordas JM, Luca A, García-Pagán JC, Escorsell A, Bosch J, Rodés J. Reduction of variceal pressure by propranolol: Comparison of the effects on portal pressure and azygos blood flow in patients with cirrhosis. Hepatology 1993; 18:1082-1089.
20. Bosch J, Bordas JM, Rigau J, Viola C, Mastai R, Kravetz D, Navasa M, Rodés J. Noninvasive measurement of the pressure of esophageal varices using an endoscopic gauge: comparison with measurement by variceal puncture in patients undergoing endoscopic sclerotherapy. Hepatology 1986; 6:667-672.
21. Feu F, Bordas JM, García-Pagán JC, Bosch J, Rodés J. Endoscopic measurement of variceal pressure in patients with cirrhosis. Correlation with the NIEC index and with the risk of variceal hemorrhage. J Hepatol 1990; 11:S22.
22. Polio J, Groszmann RJ. Hemodynamic factors incolved in the development and rupture of esophageal varices: a pathophysiologic approach to treatment. Semin Liver Dis 1986; 6:318-331.
23. Vinel JP, Cassigneul J, Levade M, Voigt JJ, Pascal JP. Assessment of short-term prognosis after variceal bleeding in patients with alcoholic cirrhosis by early measurement of portohepatic gradient. Hepatology 1986; 6:116-117.
24. Pomier-Layrargues G, Villeneuve J, Willems B, Huet PM, Marleau D. Systemic and hepatic hemodynamics after variceal hemorrhage: effects of propranolol and placebo. Gastroenterology 1987; 93:1218-1224.
25. Merkel C, Bolognesi M, Bellon S, Zuin R, Noventa F, Finucci G, Sacerdoti D, Angeli P, Gatta A. Prognostic usefulness of hepatic vein catheterization in patients with cirrhosis and esophageal varices. Gastroenterology 1992; 102:973-979.
26. Viola C, Bosch J, Mastai R, Terés J, Navasa M, Kravetz D, Grima N, Rodés J. Prognostic value of measurements of portal pressure in patients with cirrhosis. J Hepatol 1987; 5 (S1):S71.
27. Adamson RJ, Butt K, Dennis CR, Kinkhabwala M, Moskowitz H, Gordon D. Prognostic significance of portal pressure in patients with bleeding esophageal varices. Surg Gynecol Obstet 1977; 145:353-356.

28. Lam KC, Juttner HJ, Reynolds TB. Spontaneous portosystemic shunt relationship to spontaneous encephalopathy and gastrointestinal hemorrhage. Dig Dis Sci 1981; 26:346-352.
29. Rouselot LM, Moreno AH, Panke WF. Studies on portal hypertension. The clinical and physiopathological significance of self-established (non surgical) portal systemic venous shunt. Ann Surg 1959; 150: 384-410.
30. Nunez D Jr, Russel E, Yrizarry J, Pereiras R, Viamonte M Jr. Portosystemic communications studied by transhepatic portography. Radiology 1978; 127:75-79.
31. Gaiani S, Bolondi L, Li Bassi S, Zironi G, Siringo S, Barbara L. Prevalence of spontaneous hepatofugal portal flow in liver cirrhosis. Clinical and endoscopic correlation in 228 patients. Gastroenterology 1991; 100:160-167.
32. García-Pagán JC, Terés J, Calvet X, Bosch J, Rodés J. Factors which influence the prognosis of the first episode of variceal hemorrhage in patients with cirrhosis. In: Bosch J, Rodés J, eds. Recent advances in the pathophysiology and therapy of portal hypertension. Serono, Symposia Review n.° 22. 1989; 287-302.
33. De Dombal FT, Clarke JR, Clamp SE, Malizia G, Kotwal MR, Morgan AG. Prognostic factors in upper GI bleeding. Endoscopy 1986; 18(S2):6-10.
34. Burroughs AK, McCormick PA, Hughes MD, Sprengers D, D'Heygere F, McIntyre N. Randomized, double-blind, placebo-controlled trial of somatostatin for variceal bleeding. Emergency control and prevention of early variceal rebleeding. Gastroenterology 1990; 99:1388-1395.
35. Ready JB, Robertson AD, Goff JS, Rector WG. Assessment of the risk of bleeding from esophageal varices by continuous monitoring of portal pressure. Gastroenterology 1991; 100:1403-1410.
36. De Franchis R, Pascal JP, Ancona E, Burroughs AK, Henderson M, Fleig W, Groszmann RJ, Bosch J, Sauerbruch T, Soederlund C, Lebrec D, Soerensen TIA; Pagliaro L. Definitions, methodology and therapeutic strategies in portal hypertension. J Hepatol 1992; 15:256-261.
37. Ruiz del Árbol L, Arocena C, Vázquez M, Defarges V, Maroño E, García-Plaza A, Fresneda V. Endoscopic measurement of variceal pressure during hemorrhage from esophageal varices. J Hepatol 1992; 16:S36.
38. Ruiz del Árbol L, Monescillo A, Arocena C, Gisbert J, Martín de Argila C, Boixeda D. Efectos sobre la presión variceal de glipresina frente a somatostatina en el tratamiento de la hemorragia por varices esofágicas. Gastroenterol Hepatol 1994; 17: 226.
39. Vlavianos P, Gimson AES, Hayllar K, MacMathuna P, Westaby D, Williams R. Prognostic significance of systemic and portal haemodynamic parameters in patients with cirrhosis and previous variceal bleeding. Gut 1990: 31:A592.
40. Valla D, Jiron MI, Poynard T, Braillon A, Lebrec D. Failure of haemodynamic measurements to predict recurrent gastrointestinal bleeding in cirrhotic patients receiving propranolol. J Hepatol 1987; 5:144-148
41. Sacerdoti D, Merkel C, Gatta A. Importance of the 1-month-effect of nadolol on portal pressure in predicting failure of prevention of rebleeding in cirrhosis. J Hepatol 1991; 12:124-125.
42. Feu F, García-Pagán JC, Luca A, Terés J, Bosch J, Rodés J. Clinical hemodynamic correlations during pharmacological prevention of variceal rebleeding in cirrhosis. Hepatology 1992; 16:123A.
43. Villanueva C, Balanzó J, Novella MT, Torras X, Sainz S, Soriano G, Guarner C, Vilardell F. A prospective and randomized trial of endoscopic sclerotherapy vs nadolol plus isosorbide-5-mononitrate for the prevention of variceal rebleeding. Hepatology 1994; 20:688.
44. Ruiz del Árbol L, Monescillo A, LaFuente C, Arocena C, Erdozain JC. Variceal pressure response during propranolol therapy is useful in predicting the risk of variceal rebleeding. J Hepatol 1993; 18:S34.
45. García-Tsao G, Grace ND, Groszmann RJ, Conn HO, Fisher RR, Atterbury CE, Glickman M. Short term effects of propranolol on portal venous pressure. Hepatology 1986; 6:101-106.
46. Vorobioff J, Picabea E, Villavicencio R, Puccini V, Rossi O, Bordato J, Audano M. Acute and chronic hemodynamic effects of propranolol in unselected cirrhotic patients. Hepatology 1987; 7:648-653.
47. Llach J, Ginès P, Arroyo V, Rimola A, Tító Ll, Badalamenti S, Jiménez W, Gaya J, Rivera F, Rodés J. Prognostic value of arterial pressure, endogenous vasoactive systems, and renal function in cirrhotic patients admitted to the hospital for the treatment of ascites. Gastroenterology 1988; 94:482-487.
48. Urbain D, Muls V, Makoul E, Jeghers O, Thys O, Ham HR. Prognostic significance of hepatic venous pressure gradient in medically treated alcoholic cirrhosis: comparison to aminopyrine breath test. Am J Gastroenterol 1993; 88:856-859.
49. García-Pagán JC, Feu F, Luca A, Bosch J, Rodés J. Circadian variation of portal pressure in patients with cirrhosis. Hepatology 1994; 19:595-601.
50. Siringo S, Di Febo G, Bolondi L, Sofia S, Gaiani S, Rigamonti A, Miglioli M, et al. Circadian occurence of variceal bleeding in cirrhotics. Gastroenterology 1992; 102:A890.
51. Sprengers D, D' Heygere F, Cook D, McCormick PA, Mc Intyre N, Burroughs AK. Biphasic diurnal pattern of onset of bleeding from oesophageal varices. J Hepatol 1987; 5(S1):s204.
52. Lee S, Hadengue A, Moreau R, Sayegh R, Hillon P, Lebrec D. Postprandrial hemodynamic response in patients with cirrhosis. Hepatology 1988; 8:647-651.
53. McCormick PA, Dick R, Graffeo M, Wagstaff D, Madden A, McIntyre N, Burroughs AK. The effect of non-protein liquid meals on the hepatic venous pressure gradient in patients with cirrhosis. J Hepatol 1990; 11:221-225.
54. García-Pagán JC, Santos C, Barberá JA, Feu F, Luca A, Roca J, Rodriguez-Roisin R, Bosch J, Rodés J. Physical exercise increases portal pressure in patients with cirrhosis and portal hypertension. J Hepatol 1993; 18 (Suppl 1):S40.

Drug Therapy: Comparison with Other Therapies for Portal Hypertension

A. K. Burroughs, D. Patch

INTRODUCTION

The evaluation of drugs for the treatment of portal hypertension is best considered in the clinical settings of the acute variceal bleeding episode, prevention of rebleeding from varices and portal hypertensive gastropathy, and primary prophylaxis of such bleeding.

ACUTE VARICEAL BLEEDING

Bleeding from oesophageal and particularly gastric varices can be massive, but there is considerable variation in the severity of initial presentation. Mortality is not only related to the severity of bleeding, but also to the severity of the underlying liver disease (1, 2). In some series there is a greater than 50% mortality in Child-Pugh grade C patients. A particular feature of variceal bleeding is the frequency of very early rebleeding which is a prognostic factor for death (as for peptic ulcer bleeding). Emergency treatment follows the same principles as for other types of gastrointestinal bleeding and consists of resuscitation, diagnosis and control of bleeding.

Many therapies are used for acute bleeding, including administration of vasoactive drugs but also balloon tamponade, endoscopic injection therapy or banding ligation, intrahepatic portosystemic stent shunt (TIPS) and surgery. The latter is used less and less because the operative mortality in cirrhotics is high (3).

The aims of managing acute variceal bleeding are to control the haemorrhage, prevent early rebleeding, minimise the deterioration in liver function and treat complications associated with blood loss.

The only specific treatment for bleeding that does not require special skill and is immediately available, is vasoactive drug therapy. Until recently drug have been considered as a stop gap therapy until «definitive» endoscopic therapy could be used. However, some recent studies suggest drugs may be a substitute for endoscopic therapy. Moreover, there is recent evidence that patients who continued to bleed or rebleed early are those with high variceal or portal pressure (4, 5). This suggests that use of vasoactive drugs to lower portal pressure over days, with minimal side effects, is of potential therapeutic benefit and, therefore, might be used in combination with endoscopic methods.

Randomised Trials of Drugs versus Balloon Tamponade (table 1)

There are 8 studies (6-13). Unfortunately, comparison between these treatments is difficult, because of defining end points for efficacy. If tamponade is used properly there is good control of bleeding during inflation of the balloons, but early rebleeding is frequent once tamponade is removed. It is not always clear from the trial reports, when efficacy is being assessed, eg. during therapy when one would expect good control with tamponade, and less with drugs, or

Table 1. Drugs versus balloon tamponade

Author	Year	Drug type	Total number patients (p) or episodes (e)	Child-pugh C patients (%)	Efficacy drug:tamponade (%)	Death drug:tamponade (%)
Pinto-Correia	1984	Vasopressin	37 (e)	13	65:70	12:20
Colin	1987	Terlipressin	54 (e)	22	74:74*	15:22
Teres	1990	Vasopressin + nitroglycerin	108 (p)	–	66:87	30:31
Fort	1990	Terlipressin + nitroglycerin	47 (e)	55	78:79	0:8
McKee	1990	Octreotide	40 (e)	7	0:25*	50:70
Avgerinos	1991	Somatostatin	61 (p)	26	55:33	23:33
Jaramillo	1991	Somatostatin	39 (p)	41	58:50*	26:25
Blanc	1994	Terlipresin	40 (e)	–	70:95	35:35

* No information on blood transfusion requirements.

at the end of an interval of 24 hours after the termination of drug infusion or tamponade. However, there is no significant difference between treatments in mortality, despite any potential differences in describing the end point for efficacy. In fact, there are no statistically significant differences in efficacy either.

A recent meta-analysis performed for the Athens 1992 World Congress of Gastroenterology demonstrated no differences in efficacy or mortality ($p = 0.37$ and $p = 0.15$ respectively) between balloon tamponade and vasoactive therapy, with no particular differences regarding the type of drug used.

Moreover, the complication rates are very poorly documented. It is difficult to differentiate serious side effects from minor ones. One could expect a higher complication rate from balloon tamponade, compared to drugs but as reported in these trials, there is no statistical difference in complication rates.

However, it is clear that as balloon tamponade, has poor patient acceptability, and a potential fatal complication rate, it can never be first line treatment. Comparisons with drugs should be made in a selected group of patients with similar severity of bleeding. The available trials do not address this question. Furthermore, it is difficult to justify starting such studies today, as tamponade is most often used to stem massive variceal bleeding and for transport of the patient. It's use is not a routine first line therapy in any patient with bleeding varices.

Randomised Trials of Drugs versus Endoscopic Sclerotherapy (tables 2 and 3)

All except one (14) of the early studies, compared a vasoactive drug and balloon tamponade versus sclerotherapy (15-18). In addition emergency injection sclerotherapy was used in the drug and balloon group if required. Therefore, the differences between treatments in these studies (table 2) are difficult to evaluate. There were no differences in efficacy or mortality.

Table 2. Drugs and balloon tamponade versus endoscopic sclerotherapy*

Author	Year	Drug type	Total number patients	Child-pugh patients (%)	Efficacy drugs/T:sclerotherapy (%)	Death drugs/T:sclerotherapy (%)
Larson	1986	Vasopressin	82	57	13:5	79:95
Copenhagen	1984	Vasopressin	187	–	–:–	48:48
Soderlund	1985	Vasopressin	107	72	84:95	36:28
Alexandrino	1990	Vasopressin + nitroglycerin	83	49	71:71	40:39

* In these trials sclerotherapy was given if necessary to the group initially treated with drugs and balloon tamponade.

Table 3. Drugs versus endoscopic sclerotherapy

Author	Year	Drug type	Length of treatment	Total number patients (p) or episodes (e)	Child-pugh patients (%)	Efficacy drug:sclerotherapy (%)	Death drug:sclerotherapy (%)
Westaby	1989	Vasopressin + nitroglycerin	12 hrs	64 (e)	34	65:88	39:27
DiFebo	1990	Somatostatin	48 hrs	47 (p)	–	78:92	26:21
Shields	1992	Somatostatin	5 days	80 (p)	54	77:83	31:20
Jenkins	1992	Octreotide	48 hrs	40 (p)	70	90:90	25:25
Sung	1993	Octreotide	48 hrs	98 (p)	45	72:58	29:41
Morillas	1994	Somatostatin	48 hrs	70 (p)	–	80:83	29:23
VSBG	1994*	Somatostatin	5 days	170 (p)	–	81:83	11:9

* Randomized 24 hours after admission.

In the trials in which a simple comparison was made between vasoactive drugs and sclerotherapy (14, 19-24) all but one trial (14), compared either somatostatin or octreotide to sclerotherapy. Surprisingly, there are no statistically significant difference between these treatments in this group of trials. This suggests that the therapies may be equivalent in the management of acute variceal bleeders. However, the varying definitions of success, although consistent between therapies in each single trial are not so between trials. As for the group of trials of drugs versus tamponade, there are some difficulties in interpreting this group as being homogenous.

If both groups of trials are taken together viz the use of sclerotherapy versus the standard therapy of drugs with or without balloon tamponade, then there is a statistically significant difference in favour of sclerotherapy, using meta analysis, for both efficacy ($p < 0.0008$), and mortality ($p < 0.02$). However, when analysed by year of publication the more recent the study, the less difference there is between therapies, or indeed no differences can be found. This may suggest a different definition of end points rather than drug therapy becoming more effective, or sclerotherapy less effective in more recent times.

LONG TERM DRUG THERAPY

Prevention of the First Gastrointestinal Haemorrhage

There are 9 trials comprising 996 patients (25-33), 6 with propranolol and 2 with nadolol (table 4). Most of these patients had large esophageal varices at entry. Two trials also evaluated prophylactic sclerotherapy. A comprehensive meta-analysis (34) and an update (35) show

Table 4. Randomized trials of β-blockers for the primary prevention of variceal bleeding

Trial (author)		Sample size	Mean or median follow-up (months)	Bleeding rate (%)		Death rate (%)	
				Control	β-Blocker	Control	β-Blocker
Pascal	1987	230	16	27	17	36	21
IMPP	1989	174	28	35	21	31	44
Ideo*	1988	79	23	22	3	18	10
Lebrec*	1988	106	12	19	13	19	19
Conn	1991	102	34	22	4	22	16
Strauss	1988	36	16	25	20	44	35
Andreani**	1990	84	c. 20	32	5	41	30
PROVA**	1991	140	15	18	18	22	15
Colman	1990	48	–	8	35	28	26

* Nadolol.
** Also had a prophylactic sclerotherapy group.

that the incidence of first bleeding is significantly reduced without evidence of statistical heterogeneity. The pooled relative risk of bleeding taking β-blockers is almost half that of placebo: 0.48 (95% CI, 0.35-0.66), $p < 0.001$, and including the Australian study: 0.53 (95% CI 0.39-0.74), $p < 0.001$. In this latter analysis there is heterogeneity. The mortality rate is also reduced but not significantly so: pooled relative risk 0.8 (95% CI, 0.6-1.0) (35). Using individual patient data, rather than trial outcomes, a meta-analysis of 4 of the trials comprising 589 patients has shown that after 2 years (taking age and severity of cirrhosis into account, as these affected mortality), the survival rate was only slightly better in the β-blocker group ($p = 0.09$) (36). However, prevention of fatal bleeding by β-blockers was highly significant ($p = 0.004$) —a saving of 8 lives amongst 100 patients followed for 2 years. This was also true for the prevention of bleeding per se: a mean of 78% free of bleeding in the propranolol group versus 65% in the control group ($p = 0.002$). These differences remained after adjustment for the cause and severity of cirrhosis, ascites and size of varices. The former two factors were associated with bleeding and death in both the β-blocker and control groups. The advantage of analysing individual patient data is that censored data and prognostic data can all be taken into account. Secondly, data can be evaluated for the same period of follow-up. Comparison between proportional hazard models and adjusted log-rank tests were made for several subgroups of interest, eg. alcoholics versus non-alcoholics, ascitic versus non-ascitic patients, and nadolol versus propranolol, as was done in this meta-analysis. None of these analyses affected the overall difference between treatment groups.

The data from prophylactic trials suggests that screening for moderate and large varices in cirrhotics should become part of routine clinical practice, and that if these are found, β-blockers should be given to reduce the incidence of bleeding and death from bleeding. Whether the benefit holds true for smaller varices it is not known for certain. If patients are intolerant or have contraindications for β-blockers, nitrovasodilators might be tried, as in a recent trial (37), but the renal side effects may be significant in ascitic cirrhotics (37). This trial has shown equivalent results for isosorbide mononitrate and propranolol.

Prevention of Bleeding from Portal Hypertensive Gastropathy

In the first propranolol trial, patients who had gastric mucosal bleeding were also included. Propranolol was shown to protect from rebleeding from this source but the numbers were too small to establish statistical significance. Portal hypertensive gastropathy is now a well recognized entity, also known as congestive gastropathy. It may lead to chronic anaemia as well as upper gastrointestinal bleeding (38). Whatever the triggering agent for occult or frank blood loss, propranolol has been shown to prevent both acute and chronic bleeding in a single blind randomized study (39). Thus the actuarial percentages of patients free of re-bleeding from portal hypertensive gastropathy at 12 months were 65% versus 38% ($p < 0.05$) and at 30 months 52% versus 7% ($p < 0.05$). There were also fewer episodes of acute re-bleeding (mean episodes/patient/month: 0.01 vs. 0.12).

Prevention of Re-bleeding from Varices: β-blockers Compared to no Treatment

There are 12 trials comprising 803 patients (table 5). Meta-analyses based on the first 9 trials show that the risk of re-bleeding is significantly reduced by β-blockers (34, 35). The pooled relative risk is 0.4 (95% CI, 0.3-0.5), $p < 0.001$ with no statistical heterogeneity. However, there is no significant effect on mortality, the pooled relative risk being 0.7 (95% CI, 0.5-1.04). The difference in mortality is far less than in the primary prevention trials. In another meta-analysis including all 12 studies (40) and excluding re-bleeding or death within one year of follow up, the mean odds ratio for re-bleeding was 2.3 (95% CI, 1.7-3), $p < 0.0001$ with no statistical heterogeneity, in favour of β-blockers. Survival was also improved: mean odds ratio of 1.4 (95% CI, 1-1.9), $p < 0.05$. A cumulative meta-analysis showed this to be significant for mortality in 1990. Clinical factors which might predict the therapeutic response for re-bleeding

Table 5. Randomized trials of β-blockers for the prevention of re-bleeding from varices

Trial (author)		Sample size	Mean or median follow-up (months)	Bleeding rate (%)		Death rate (%)	
				Controls	β-Blocker	Controls	β-Blocker
Lebrec	1994	74	29	64	16	22	8
Burroughs	1993	48	21	59	54	23	15
Villeneuve	1986	79	23	81	76	38	45
Queuniet	1987	99	25	65	57	21	24
Gatta	1987	24	14	67	25	25	8
Colombo	1989	62	12	47	25	23	12
Colombo	1989	62	12	47	31	23	10
Sheen	1989	36	12	56	28	11	0
Garden	1990	81	16	77	47	44	37
Cerebelaud	1986	84	16	66	34	–	–
Von Kobe	1987	54	–	46	38	32	23
Colman	1990	100	–	50	35	4	4

with propranolol are not yet known, but non-compliance, presence of hepatocellular carcinoma and non-reduction of resting heart rate have been suggested as negative predictors by Lebrec's group. Some haemodynamic criteria may be shown to be useful in the future, but their measurement remains invasive and not practical. A partial solution to this problem may be the correlation of intravariceal pressure reduction measured endoscopically and the incidence of re-bleeding.

Prevention of Re-bleeding from Varices: β-Blockers Compared to Sclerotherapy

There are 9 trials comprising 735 patients (table 6) (40-49). Meta-analyses showed that the 2 therapies are equivalent, with a relative risk of 1 (95% CI, 0.7-1.7) for mortality, and 0.7 (95% CI, 0.5-1.1) for re-bleeding (35), p = 0.06. The difference in re-bleeding is very small. Another meta-analysis excluding those with re-bleeding or death within one year showed similar results (50). Thus, on this basis, β-blockers can be considered as the treatment of first choice for the prevention of re-bleeding, bearing less contraindications, as it is less expensive and less invasive than sclerotherapy, and does not increment endoscopy work load. However, many groups still use long-term sclerotherapy as first-line therapy for preventing re-bleeding. In the future, combination drug therapy should make the pharmacological approach even more effective. There are no trials versus banding. There is one study comparing sclerotherapy versus nadolol and isosorbide mononitrate (51). Rebleeding occurred in 11 of 43 (26%) in the drug group versus 24 of 43 (56%) of the sclerotherapy group. There was no difference in mortality.

Table 6. Randomized trials of β-blockers versus sclerotherapy for the prevention variceal bleeding

Trial		Sample size	Mean or median follow-up (months)	Bleeding rate (%)		Death rate (%)	
				β-Blocker	Sclerotherapy	β-Blocker	Sclerotherapy
Alexandrino	1988	65	29	74	55	32	29
Feig	1987	105	26	48	31	32	36
Dollet	1988	51	36	44	64	32	29
Westaby	1990	108	24	52	42	77	64
Teres	1993	72	11	49	21	31	21
Liu	1990	118	?	75	35	41	53
Rossi	1991	53	19	48	50	26	23
Martin	1991	76	36	53	55	23	31
Dasarathy	1992	91	36	67	42	41	22

Table 7. Randomized trials of β-blockers combined with sclerotherapy versus sclerotherapy alone

Trial		Sample size	Mean or median follow-up (months)	Bleeding rate (%)		Death rate (%)	
				β-Blockers and sclerotherapy	Sclerotherapy	β-Blockers and sclerotherapy	Sclerotherapy
Westaby	1986	53	6	27	30	35	26
Vickers	1987	69	24	51	44	37	26
Vinel	1990	65	12	21	38	12	19
Jensen	1989	31	–	20	75	7	6
Gerunda	1990	60	6	20	17	–	–
Lundell	1990	41	–	12 (e)	11 (e)	5	26
Bertoni	1990	28	–	7	29	7	21
Villanueva	1993	40	12	55	39	9	11
Avgerios	1993	85	24	31	52	18	22.5
Acharya	1993	114	24	17	21	9	12.5

e: episodes.

Prevention of Re-bleeding from Varices: Addition of β-Blockers to Sclerotherapy versus Sclerotherapy Alone, or versus β-Blockers Alone

There are 10 trials of sclerotherapy and β-blockers versus sclerotherapy alone comprising 586 patients (table 7) (52-61). Meta-analysis of the first seven trials showed that there is no advantage in combining β-blockers with long term sclerotherapy to prevent re-bleeding: relative risk 0.7 (95% CI, 0.45-1.2) (35). Theoretically the drug might prevent re-bleeding before variceal obliteration. Only one group (55, 62) shows re-bleeding is significantly decreased both before and after eradication and only one other trial shows a significant advantatge of adding a β-blocker (54). Mortality is unchanged: relative risk 0.95 (95% CI, 0.5-1.75) (35).

There are 2 trials of sclerotherapy and β-blockers versus β-blockers alone (63, 64). Both show a significant advantage of adding sclerotherapy to β-blockers in terms of re-bleeding: β-blockers alone versus combination therapy: 65% vs. 45% (63) and 59% vs. 42% (64). There was no difference in mortality. The results of all 12 trials do not justify the routine use of the combination of β-blockers and sclerotherapy.

Drugs versus Surgery or Sclerotherapy, and Drugs and Sclerotherapy versus Tips

There is only one study which has evaluated drug therapy versus shunt surgery (if good liver function) or sclerotherapy (if poor liver function) (65). In this 3 centre study, the applicability of drug therapy was superior to surgery with similar results for re-bleeding at 2 years: 54% propranolol plus isosorbide mononitrate (drugs), 44% sclerotherapy or shunts (invasive therapy), and similar mortality at 2 years 29% drugs and 33% invasive therapy. Assigned treatment was given to 103 of 120 randomized to drug therapy and 96 of 112 invasive treatment —analysis by treatment received did not change the outcome. This study suggests that if no contraindications exist drug therapy should be tried first. Its applicability is good and it is also the cheapest treatment, giving similar results to more invasive treatments.

Another study comparing TIPS to the combination of propranolol and sclerotherapy in 54 patients (66), showed that severe re-bleeding occurred in 26% of the combined group compared to 8% of the TIPS group, without difference in mortality. Follow-up was only for a mean of 8 months.

THE FUTURE OF DRUG THERAPY FOR THE MANAGEMENT OF PORTAL HYPERTENSION

In acute variceal bleeding, drug therapy is the only treatment which can be used immediately and in contrast to endoscopic therapies is not dependent on the availability of skilled staff. Its future role will be in combination with endoscopic therapy to prevent the early re-bleeding seen frequently in such patients. To date the best candidates are glypressin and somatostatin or octreotide.

The future long-term management of portal hypertension will increasingly be based on drug therapy. Drug combinations will be used as in systemic hypertension. It may even be possible to prevent the development, or the extension of the collateral circulation and thus the development of varices. This has already been shown in animal models of portal-hypertension using propranolol. However, the current problem is the lack of a simple «splanchnic sphygmomanometer» which could be used to monitor therapy precisely. HVPG measurement is invasive and not routinely available. In addition, there is no reliable clinical or haemodynamic index which can be measured *prior* to therapy, which will reliaby predict the therapeutic efficacy. However gradient changes in hepatic venous pressure measurement following propranolol administration may predict the therapeutic response. Future studies will be directed at simple ways of establishing individual patient response to portal hypotensive agents in relation to target reduction of pressure levels.

REFERENCES

1. Graham DY, Smith JL. The course of patients after variceal haemorrhage. Gastroenterology 1981; 80:800-809.
2. Burroughs AK, Mezzabitte G, Phillips A et al. Cirrhotic with variceal haemorrhage: The importance of the time interval between admission and the start of analysis for survival and rebleeding rates. Hepatology 1989; 9:801-807.
3. Spence RAJ. Surgical measures for active variceal bleeding. Gastrointest Endosc (Clin North Am) 1992; 2:77-94.
4. Del Árbol R, de Argila M, Vásquez C et al. Endoscopic measurement of variceal pressure (VP) during haemorrhage from oesophageal varices (HEV). Hepatology 1992; 16:81A.
5. Ready JB, Robertson AD, Goff JS, Rector et al. Assessment of the risk of bleeding from esophageal varices by continous monitoring of portal pressure. Gastroenterology 1991; 100:1403-1410.
6. McKee R. A study of octreotide in oesophageal varices. Digestion 1990; 45(Suppl 1):60-65.
7. Avgerinos A, Klonis C, Rekoumis G, Gouma P, Papadimitriou N, Raptis S. A prospective randomized trial comparing somatostatin, balloon tamponade and the combination of both methods in the management of acute variceal hemorrhage. J Hepatol 1991; 13:78-83.
8. Jaramillo JL, De la Mata M, Mino G, Costán G, Gómez-Camacho F. Somatostatin versus Sengstaken balloon tamponade for primary haemostasis of bleeding oesophageal varices. A randomized pilot study. J Hepatol 1991; 12:100-105.
9. Colin R, Giuli N, Czernichow P, Ducrotte P, Lerebours E. Prospective comparison of Glypressin, tamponade and their association in the treatment of bleeding esophageal varices. In: Lebrec D, Blei AT, eds. Vasopressin analogs and portal hypertension. London: John Libbey Eurotext, 1987; 149-153.
10. Pinto Correia J, Martins Alves M, Alexandrino P, Silveira J. Controlled trial of vasopressin and balloon tamponade in bleeding oesophageal varices. Hepatology 1984; 4:885-888.
11. Fort E, Sautereau D, Silvain C, Ingrand P, Pillogand B, Beauchant M. A randomized trial of terlipressin plus nitroglycerin vs balloon tamponade in the control of acute variceal hemorrhage. Hepatology 1990; 11:678-681.
12. Teres J, Planas R, Panés J. Salmerón JM, Mas A, Bosch J, Llorente C, Viver J, Feu F, Rodés J. Vasopressin/nitroglycerin infusion vs oesophageal tamponade in the treatment of acute variceal bleeding: a randomized controlled trial. Hepatology 1990; 11:964-968.
13. Blanc P, Bories J, Desprez D et al. Balloon tamponade with Linton-Michel tube versus terlipressin in the treatment of acute esophageal and gastric variceal bleeding. J Hepatol 1994; 21:S133.
14. Westaby D, Hayes PC, Gimson AES, Polson RJ, Williams R. Controlled clinical trial of injection sclerotherapy for active variceal bleeding. Hepatology 1989; 9:274-277.
15. Alexandrino P, Alves MM, Fidalgo P et al. Is sclerotherapy the first choice treatment for active oesophageal variceal bleeding in cirrhotic patients? J Hepatol 1990; 11:S1.
16. The Copenhagen Esophageal Varices Sclerotherapy Project. Sclerotherapy after first variceal hemorrhage in cirrhosis. A randomized multicenter trial. N Engl J Med 1984; 311:1594-1600.
17. Larson AW, Cohen H, Zweiban B et al. Acute esophageal variceal sclerotherapy. Results of a prospective randomized controlled trial. JAMA 1986; 255:497-500.
18. Soderlund C, Ihre T. Endoscopic sclerotherapy vs conservative management of bleeding oesophageal varices. A 5-year prospective controlled trial of emergency and long-term treatment. Acta Chir Scand 1985; 151:449-456.
19. Shields R, Jenkins SA, Kingsworth AN et al. A prospective randomized controlled trial comparing the efficacy of somatostatin with injection sclerotherapy in the control of bleeding oesophageal varices. J Hepatol 1992; 16:128-137.
20. Jenkins SA, Yates J, Baxter JN et al. A prospective randomized controlled clinical trial comparing sandostatin and injection sclerotherapy in the control of

acute variceal haemorrhage: an interim report. Gut 1992; 23(Suppl 1):F233.
21. Sung JY, Chung S, Lai CW et al. Octreotide infusion or emergency sclerotherapy for variceal haemorrhage. Lancet 1993; 342:657-641.
22. Morillas R, Quer JC, Planas R et al. Somatostatin vs. endoscopic sclerotherapy in the treatment of acute variceal bleeding: final results of a prospective randomized trial. Hepatology 1994; 19:4-1051.
23. Di Febo G, Siringo S, Varia M et al. Somatostatin (SMS) and urgent sclerotherapy in active oesophageal variceal bleeding. Gastroenterology 1990; 99:A583.
24. Variceal Bleeding Study Group. Randomized controlled trial of sclerotherapy versus somatostatin infusion in the prevention of early rebleeding following varical haemorrhage in patients with cirrhosis. Hepatology 1994; 19:1361.
25. Pascal JP, Cales P and Multicenter Study Group. Propranolol in the prevention of first upper gastrointestinal tract hemorrhage in patients with cirrhosis of the liver and esophageal varices. N Engl J Med 1987; 317:856-861.
26. Ideo G, Bellati G, Fesce E, Grimoldi D. Nadolol can prevent the first gastrointestinal bleeding in cirrhotics: a prospective, randomized study. Hepatology 1988; 8:6-9.
27. Lebrec D, Poynard T, Capron JP, Hillon P, Geoffroy P, Roulot E et al. Nadolol for prophylaxis of gastrointestinal bleeding in patients with cirrhosis. A randomized trial. J Hepatology 1988; 7:11-25.
28. The Italian Multicenter Project for Propranolol in Prevention of Bleeding. Propranolol prevents first gastrointestinal bleeding in non ascitic cirrhotic patients. Final report of a multicenter randomized trial. J Hepatol 1989; 9:75-83.
29. Andreani T, Poupon RE, Balkau B, Trinchet JC, Grange JD, Peigney N et al. Preventive therapy of first gastrointestinal bleeding in patients with cirrhosis: results of a controlled trial comparing propranolol, endoscopic sclerotherapy and placebo. Hepatology 1990; 12:1413-1419.
30. Conn HO, Grance N, Bosch J, Groszmann RJ, Rodés J, Weight SC et al. Propranolol in the prevention of the first hemorrhage from oesophageal varices: results of a randomized double-blind cooperative clinical trial. Hepatology 1991; 13:902-912.
31. The PROVA Study Group. Prophylaxis of first hemorrhage from oesophageal varices by sclerotherapy, propranolol or both in cirrhotic patients. A randomized multicenter trial. Hepatology 1991; 14:1016-1024.
32. Strauss E, de Sa MF, Albano A, Lacet CM, Leite MO, Maffei RA Jr. A randomized controlled trial for the prevention of the first upper gastrointestinal bleeding due to portal hypertension in cirrhosis: sclerotherapy or propranolol versus control groups (Abstr). Hepatology 1988; 8:1395.
33. Colman J, Jones P, Finch C, Dudley F. Propranolol in the prevention for variceal hemorrhage in alcoholic cirrhotic patients (Abstr). Hepatology 1990; 12:851.
34. Pagliaro L, Burroughs AK, Sorensen T et al. Therapeutic controversies and randomised controlled trials (RCT's): prevention of bleeding and re-bleeding in cirrhosis. Gastroenterol Int 1989; 2:71-84.
35. Pagliaro L, Burroughs AK, Sorensen TIA et al. β-Blockers for preventing variceal bleeding. Lancet 1990; 336:10012(Correspondence).
36. Poynard T, Cales P, Pasta L et al. Beta-adrenergic antagonist drugs in the prevention of gastro-intestinal bleeding in patients with cirrhosis and esophageal varices. N Engl J Med 1991; 324:1532-1538.
37. Angelico G, Carli L, Piai C et al. Isosorbide-5-mononitrate versus propranolol in the prevention of first bleeding in cirrhosis. Gastroenterology 1993; 104:1460-1465.
38. D'Amico G, Montalbano L, Traina M et al. Natural history of congestive gastropathy in cirrhosis. Gastroenterology 1990; 99:1558-1564.
39. Pérez-Ayuso R, Piqué J, Bosch J et al. Propranolol in prevention of recurrent bleeding from severe portal hypertensive gastropathy in cirrhosis. Lancet 1991; 337:1431-1434.
40. Bernard B, Lebrec D, Mathurin P, Opolon P, Poynard T. Meta-analysis of β-blockers in the prevention of recurrent variceal bleeding in patients with cirrhosis. Hepatology 1994; 20:106A.
41. Alexandrino PT, Alves MM, Pinto Cozzeia J. Propranolol or endoscopic sclerotherapy in the prevention of recurrence of variceal bleeding: a prospective, randomized controlled trial. J Hepatol 1988; 7:175-185.
42. Fleig WE, Stang EF, Huncke R et al. Prevention of recurrent bleeding in cirrhotics with recent variceal haemorrhage: prospective randomized comparison of propranolol and sclerotherapy. Hepatology 1987; 7:355-361.
43. Dollet JM, Champigneulle B, Patris A et al. Endoscopic sclerotherapy versus oral propranolol after variceal haemorrhage in cirrhosis: results of a 4 year prospective randomized trial. Gastroenterol Clin Biol 1988; 12:234-239.
44. Westaby D, Polson RJ, Gimson AE et al. A controlled trial of oral propranolol compared with injection sclerotherapy for the long-term management of variceal bleeding. Hepatology 1990; 11:353-359.
45. Teres J, Bosch J, Bordas JM et al. Propranolol versus sclerotherapy in preventing variceal rebleeding. A randomized controlled trial. Gastroenterology 1993; 105:1508-1514.
46. Liu JD, Yeng YS, Chen PH et al. Endoscopic injection sclerotherapy and propranolol in the prevention of recurrent variceal bleeding. World Congress of Gastroenterology, Sydney 1990; FP118(Abstr).
47. Rossi V, Cales P, Burtin P et al. Prevention of recurrent variceal bleeding in alcoholic patients: prospective controlled trial of propranolol and sclerotherapy. J Hepatol 1991; 12:283-289.
48. Martin T, Taupignon A, Lavignolle A, Perrin D, Le-Bodic L. Prevention des recidives hemorragigues chez des malades atteints de cirrhose. Resultats d'une étude controlée comparant propranolol et sclérose endoscopique. Gastroenterol Clin Biol 1991; 15:833-837.

49. Dasarathy S, Dwivedi M, Bhargava DK et al. A prospective randomized trial comparing repeated endoscopic sclerotherapy and propranolol in decompensated (Child Class B and C) cirrhotic patients. Hepatology 1992; 16:89-94.
50. Bernard B, Lebrec D, Mathurin P, Opolon P, Poynard T. Meta analysis of propranolol and endoscopic sclerotherapy in the preention of gastrointestinal rebleeding in patients with cirrhosis. Hepatology 1994; 20:106A.
51. Villanueva C, Balanzo J, Novella ME et al. A prospective and randomized trial of endoscopic sclerotherapy vs nadolol plus isosorbide 5 mononitrate for the prevention of variceal rebleeding. Hepatology 1994; 20:268A.
52. Westaby D, Melia E, Hegarty J et al. Use of propranolol to reduce the rebleeding rate during injection sclerotherapy prior to variceal obliteration. Hepatology 1986; 6:673-675.
53. Vickers C, Rodes J, Hillenbrand P et al. Prospective controlled trial of propranolol and sclerotherapy for prevention of re-bleeding from esophageal varices. Gut 1987; 28:A1359(Abstrt).
54. Vinel JP, Lamouliliette H, Cales P et al. Propranolol reduced the re-bleeding rate during injection sclerotherapy: results of a randomized study. Gastroenterology 1990; 98:A644(Abstrt).
55. Jensen LS, Krarup N. Propranolol in prevention of re-bleeding from esophageal varices during the course of endoscopic sclerotherapy. Scand J Gastroenterol 1989; 24:339-345.
56. Gerunda GE, Neri D Cangrandi F et al. Nadolol does not reduce early rebleeding in cirrhotics undergoing endoscopic variceal sclerotherapy: a multicenter randomized controlled trial. Hepatology 1990; 12:988(Abstrt).
57. Lundell L, Leth R, Lind T et al. Evaluation of propranolol for prevention of recurrent bleeding from esophageal varices between sclerotherapy sessions. Acta Chir Scand 1990; 156:711-715.
58. Bertoni G, Fornaciari G, Beltrami M et al. Nadolol for prevention of variceal re-bleeding during the course of endoscopic injection sclerotherapy: a randomised pilot study. J Clin Gastroenterol 1990; 12:364-365(Letter).
59. Villanueva C, Balanzo J, Martínez FJ et al. Nadolol does not improve the results of sclerotherapy in prevention of variceal rebleeding. Gut 1993; 34(Suppl):S5.
60. Avgerinos A, Rekoumis G, Klonis C et al. Propranolol in the prevention of recurrent upper gastrointestinal bleeding in patients with cirrosis undergoing endoscopic sclerotherapy. A randomized controlled trial. J Hepatol 1993; 19:301-311.
61. Acharya Sk, Dasarathy S, Sakena S et al. A prospective randomized study to evaluate propranolol in patients undergoing long-term endoscopic sclerotherapy. J Hepatol 1993; 19:291-300.
62. Jensen LS, Krarup N. Propranolol may prevent recurrence of oesophageal varices after obliteration by endoscopic sclerotherapy. Scand J Gastroenterol 1990; 25:352-356.
63. O'Connor KW, Lehman G, Yne H et al. Comparison of three non-surgical treatments for bleeding esophageal varices. Gastroenterology 1989; 96:899-906.
64. Ink O, Martin T, Poynard T et al. Does elective sclerotherapy improve the efficacy of long-term propranolol for prevention of recurrent bleeding in patients with severe cirrhosis? A prospective multicenter randomized trial. Hepatology 1992; 16:912-919.
65. McCormick PA, Feu F, Sabrin C, Planas R and the Anglo-Spanish Variceal Rebleeding Group. Propranolol and isosorbide mononitrate versus sclerotherapy or shunt surgery for the prevention of variceal rebleeding: a randomized trial. Hepatology 1994; 20:106A(Abstrt).
66. Rossle M, Deibert P, Haag K, Ochs A, Siegerste Her V, Langer M. TIPS versus sclerotherapy and β-blockade: preliminary results of a randomized study in patients with recurrent variceal haemorrhage. Hepatology 1994; 20:107A(Abstrt).

Section 2

Treatment of the Complications of Cirrhosis

Endoscopic Ligation of Esophageal Varices

G. Van Stiegmann

INTRODUCTION

In the mid-1980's our group showed that elastic band ligation could be used to treat esophageal and gastric varices (1). We hypothesized, based on results of controlled trials which compared sclerotherapy with elastic band ligation for treatment of hemorrhoids, that this new treatment could be safer and more effective than injection sclerotherapy when used to treat esophagogastric varices. Results of experimental and clinical investigation have supported this hypothesis. The purpose of this chapter is to present the technique of endoscopic ligation, detail effects of this treatment, and highlight results of clinical studies.

ENDOSCOPIC LIGATING DEVICE

The endoscopic ligating device (C. R. Bard, Tewksberry, MA) has been described in detail elsewhere (2). Variations of the original design are currently available outside of the United States. One such modification employs a clear plastic outer and inner cylinder (fig. 1). This does not change the nature of operation of the the device (overtube still necessary) but substantially increases the field of view of the endoscopist. The second modification, available only in prototype form, consists of device which allows endoscopic ligation of up to three targets without need to reload after each firing. Disadvantages of the multiple fire ligator include a relatively narrow field of view and a slightly larger diameter of the ligator itself. It is uncertain at this time if multiple fire capability will benefit treatment of esophageal varices or eliminate the need for use of an endoscopic overtube.

EFFECTS OF ELASTIC BAND LIGATION

Tissue effects resulting from elastic band ligation are consistent and reproducible. Studies in portal hypertensive dogs with esophageal varices showed ligated varices initially blanched and become cyanotic within 3-7 minutes (3). Microscopic examination of treatment sites 24

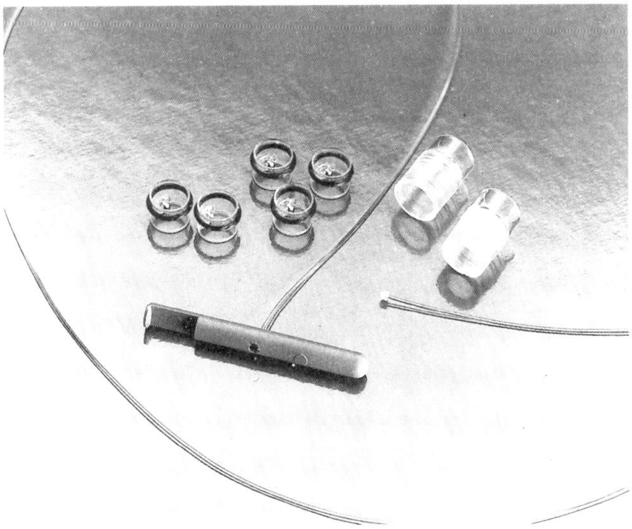

Fig. 1. «See through» endoscopic ligation device. The translucent device results in a wider field of view for the endoscopist. (Photo courtesy of Bard Interventional Products, Inc. Tewksberry, MA.)

hours after ligation showed ischemic necrosis of the mucosa and submucosa. All treatment sites had developed shallow (1-2 mm) ulcerations from 8-12 mm in length by day seven. Microscopic examination showed granulation tissue, sloughing necrotic tissue, and intense inflammatory reaction in the ulcer base. Varices were replaced by 6-10 mm diameter depressions in the esophageal mucosa by day 14 to 21. Microscopy showed replacement of vascular structures in the submucosa with maturing scar tissue. The underlying muscular wall was intact and no animals had complications of treatment.

Studies by Jensen and his colleagues compared endoscopic ligation with sclerotherapy for treatment of bleeding varices in a portal hypertensive canine model (4, 5). Test animals received one form of endoscopic treatment and control animals no therapy. Bleeding from either esophageal or gastric varices was controlled with either treatment. Ulceration was present at all treated sites in the stomach with either ligation or sclerotherapy. Ninety per cent of ligated esophageal sites ulcerated in contrast to only ten per cent of sites treated with sclerotherapy.

A controlled clinical trial by Young et al. compared ulcers resulting from sclerotherapy with those caused by ligation (6). Sclerotherapy ulcers were deeper and ligation-related ulcers were larger in surface area and circular in shape compared to the linear lesions resulting from sclerotherapy. One hundred percent of ligation treatment sites ulcerated in contrast to a 90 percent incidence of ulceration with sclerotherapy. Ligation-induced ulcers healed in a mean of 14 days compared with a mean of 21 days for those resulting from sclerotherapy. Two of 13 sclerotherapy patients developed esophageal stricture. None of the ten ligation treated group had complications. Bleeding from ulcers was not observed in either cohort.

Goff et al. performed esophageal manometric examinations on patients who had undergone endoscopic ligation, on patients who had been treated with sclerotherapy, and on untreated controls who had esophageal varices (7). Sclerotherapy patients had a greater incidence of stricture formation and less ability to relax the lower esophageal sphincter. There were, however, no persistent long-term manometric differences between the three groups.

TECHNIQUE OF ELASTIC BAND LIGATION

Patients with active upper gastrointestinal bleeding are stabilized and prepared as for routine emergent diagnostic endoscopic examination. Most receive intravenous sedation (usually meperidine and midazolam) and topical pharyngeal anesthesia. Complete survey examination of the esophagus, stomach and duodenum is done. If varices are to be treated, an endoscopic overtube is inserted after completion of the survey examination. Overtube insertion is accomplished by using either the endoscope or an appropriately sized esophageal dilator as an obturator (8). The endoscope and attached ligating device is then inserted via the overtube.

The sequence of ligation treatment is predicted on the presence or absence of active bleeding. If a discrete site of active bleeding is identified it should be ligated directly or alternatively, ligation should be done immediately caudad and cephalad to the bleeding site. If active bleeding is present and no discrete bleeding site can be identified treatment is carried out as in the non-bleeding patient. Treatment begins with ligation of the largest most distal varix, usually at or just caudad to the gastroesophageal junction. Subsequent ligations are done at the same level or more cephalad until all variceal channels in the distal five to seven cm of the esophagus are ligated at least once. Patients with bleeding from gastric fundal varices are probably best treated with a combination of ligation and sclerotherapy administered at the same sitting.

Combination treatment is performed by injection of sclerosant immediately following elastic band ligation of varices. Ligation of individual esophageal varices is first done near the gastroesophageal junction. Each variceal channel is ligated once. Intravariceal sclerotherapy is then done using one ml of sclerosant per varix at sites from one to three cm cephalad to the site of ligation. Combination treatment of gastric varices is done by first ligating the fundic varices, a task which usually requires use of a retroflexed position. After ligation has been done, 1 to 5 ml of sclerosant are injected into the varix on the non-luminal side of the elastic band.

Following endoscopic ligation, those treated for bleeding gastric fundal varices are placed on the best available acid suppressing regimen to minimize the risk of autodigestion of the ligated tissue with subsequent early slough and bleeding. Repeat ligation treatments aimed at eradication of esophageal varices are done at seven to 14 day intervals until varices are obliterated. Elective repeat treatments are done on an outpatient basis.

RESULTS OF ENDOSCOPIC LIGATION

Two uncontrolled studies suggest that elastic band ligation is effective for control of hemorrhage in patients who are actively bleeding from varices at the time of treatment. Our group treated 23 actively bleeding patients and achieved 72 hour control of hemorrhage in 96% (9). Rebleeding within 30 days occurred in 18% and overall survival was 61% at nine months. Saeed et al. treated 10 actively bleeding patients who had failed endoscopic sclerotherapy (mean 4.5 prior sclerotherapy sessions) and achieved early control in 90% (10). Rebleeding occurred in six patients by 90 days follow up and was controlled again by ligation in five of the six. Survival was 66% at follow up ranging to 22 months. Four controlled trials which compared conventional sclerotherapy with endoscopic ligation confirmed these findings (11-14). Sclerotherapy controlled acute hemorrhage in from 77 to 92% of those actively bleeding compared with 86 to 94% control for endoscopic ligation. An ongoing prospective randomized study compares endoscopic ligation with the cyanoacrylate glue injections for control of ative variceal bleeding (15). Preliminary data indicates the two methods are equally effective, however, further patient accrual is needed before firm conclusions can be drawn.

Elastic band ligation was used to prevent recurrence of hemorrhage in 146 consecutive cirrhotic patients who had previously bled from esophageal varices (16). Retreatment was done at seven to 14 day intervals until distal esophageal varices were eradicated. One hundred fourteen patients survived initial hospitalization. Sixty-five (57%) had 72 episodes of recurrent bleeding. Overall survival was 73%. Eighty percent of the patients who remained in the study more than 30 days had varices eradicated from the distal esophagus with a mean of 5.5 treatment sessions. During the course of this study, there were four non-bleeding complications which required treatment: two esophageal strictures (single bouginage each); one meat impaction; and one patient with dysphagia which lasted for 36 hours.

Five controlled trials comparing sclerotherapy with elastic band ligation are published or have been presented in abstract form (11-14, 17). Data from these trials is summarized in table 1. Results to date support elastic band ligation as equal or superior to sclerotherapy in all outcome variables. Moreover, the new treatment appears to be associated with signifi-

Table 1. Results from five prospective randomized trials which compared endoscopic ligation with endoscopic sclerotherapy

Study	Patients	Therapy	#Rebled	# Rx to eradicate (mean)	Survival (%)	Compl. (%)
Multicenter	65	ES	48	5	55*	22*
(14)	64	EVL	36	4	72*	02
Laine	39	ES	44	6*	77	54*
(13)	38	EVL	26	4	81	21
Gimson	49	ES	53*	5*	52	NA
(11)	54	EVL	30	3	37	NA
Avgerinos	40	ES	40	6*	79	60*
(17)	37	EVL	27	4	80	32
Lo	59	ES	44*	6*	68	27*
(12)	61	EVL	15	4	84	05

* $p < 0.05$.
ES: endoscopic sclerotherapy; EVL: endoscopic variceal ligation; # Rx to eradicate (mean): mean number of treatments needed to eradicate esophageal varices; Compl: non-bleeding complications requiring active treatment.

cantly fewer non-bleeding complications. The greater incidence of pulmonary complications in sclerotherapy treated patients in the multicenter study suggests a beneficial effect of ligation over sclerotherapy in this regard (14). Alternatively, fewer pulmonary complications in ligation patients may have resulted from prevention of tracheal aspiration by use of the endoscopic overtube which in this trial was employed only in the group treated with ligation. The incidence of pulmonary complications (pneumonias) was similar in both ligation and sclerotherapy arms of the Los Angeles study in which both cohorts were treated using an overtube, thus suggesting use of the overtube may prevent some pulmonary problems (13).

A trend toward fewer episodes of recurrent bleeding in patients treated with ligation has been observed in all of the controlled trials to date. This finding, along with fewer deaths from infection related complications, contributed to improved survival in ligation treated patients in the multicenter trial (14). The lower incidence of recurrent bleeding in ligation treated patients may result from greater efficiency of ligation at eradication of varices. Fewer numbers of treatments (one to two less per patient) were required to eradicate varices in three of the four trials. This advantage of elastic band ligation may provide both outcome and economic advantages over sclerotherapy.

Results: Combined Elastic Band Ligation and Sclerotherapy

Forty six patients were enrolled in a pilot study of combination endoscopic ligation and low volume sclerotherapy administered synchronously (18). Eradication of esophageal varices was accomplished with a mean of approximately two treatment sessions. Ulcerations at the site of ligation and sclerosant injection were seen in most patients within the first few days of treatment but resulted in few adverse effects. The overall rebleeding rate with mean follow up of 8 months was 30% with only one death resulting from hemorrhage. Serious complications associated with combination ligation sclerotherapy in this trial included one proximal esophageal perforation and two cases of spontaneous bacterial peritonitis.

Data from a French prospective randomized trial which compared endoscopic ligation with combined ligation and sclerotherapy confirmed findings in the study above and found eradication of varices could be accomplished with a mean of 1.2 combined ligation and sclerotherapy treatments in contrast to a mean of 4.4 treatments to eradicate using sclerotherapy alone (19). A recent prospective randomized trial which compared combination ligation/sclerotherapy with ligation alone failed to comfirm advantage for the combined method. Saeed et al. (10) found a higher complication rate in patients treated with synchronous sclerotherapy and ligation and no difference in numbers of treatment sessions required to eradicate varices. They concluded the increased costs and higher complication rate associated with combined therapy did not justify its use.

Hashizume et al. described the use of endoscopic ligation as initial treatment followed by subsequent sclerotherapy (20). The design of this trial underscores an observation made by many who have used endoscopic ligation: smaller varices are harder to ligate than larger ones. Patients treated with this metachronous combination therapy were selected randomly and prospectively compared with a group treated by sclerotherapy alone. Most patients had not bled from varices and were treated to prevent a first bleed. The initial ligation treatment was followed at weekly intervals by sclerotherapy to obliterate residual varices. Patients treated with this regimen required less sclerosant to eradicate varices and had fewer complications such as renal and pulmonary insufficiency, fever, pain, and pleural effusion than those treated with sclerotherapy alone. It stands to reason that use of less sclerosant should result in fewer sclerosant-related complications and this group has taken advantage of thrombosis and venous stasis induced by elastic band ligation to enhance the effects and minimize complications of subsequent sclerotherapy. More efficient eradication of varices may be possible with combined ligation and sclerotherapy. Determination of the optimal combination of these methods and the best time sequencing (synchronous vs. metachronous treatment) is needed.

A small number of patients with bleeding gastric fundal varices have been treated with elastic band ligation and with combination ligation sclerotherapy. Our initial attempts to treat gastric varices with ligation alone resulted in early rebleeding as the devitalized ligated tissue was rapidly autodigested in spite of optimal acid suppression. In subsequent cases, the use of sclerotherapy immediately following ligation (as described above) resulted in control of bleeding and eradication of varices in several patients. Chon et al. report using combined endoscopic ligation and sclerotherapy in 32 patients with gastric fundal varices with control of bleeding and no rebleeding or complications during a mean follow up of 10 months (21). The small number of patients treated precludes firm conclusions. I believe that some patients with bleeding fundal varices can be controlled and successfully treated using endoscopic methods. On the other hand, when recurrent hemorrhage from fundal varices does occur it is often torrential. Combined elastic band ligation and sclerotherapy is probably best used as an interim measure to halt acute bleeding while semielective preparations are made for more definitive control by either surgical or radiological shunt insertion.

Complications Associated with Elastic Band Ligation

Complications of elastic band ligation can be classified in two categories: those resulting from elastic band ligation and its subsequent tissue effects and those from use of the overtube. Several published case reports describe mechanical complications caused by introduction of the overtube. These mishaps consisted of partial or complete esophageal perforations or trauma causing bleeding. Berkelhammer et al. and Goldschmeidt et al. (8, 22) concluded that overtube trauma was usually caused by "pinching" of the esophageal wall in the gap between the overtube and the endoscope when the latter was used as an obturator to facilitate introduction. The optimal solution to this problem is use of an esophageal dilator which completely fills the lumen of the overtube as the obturator to facilitate introduction into the esophagus.

Complications directly related to endoscopic ligation, in contrast to those from the overtube, are less common. Saltzmann and Arora report transient obstruction of the esophagus by boluses of ligated tissue (23). We observed one such case and concluded that a combination of the tissue boluses and distal esophageal spasm were to blame. The distal esophagus in our patient was tightly closed and an endoscope could not pass, but symptoms of dysphagia resolved without treatment. Transient distal esophageal spasm at the site of either ligation or sclerosant injection is not uncommon and may contribute to hemostasis in patients treated for active bleeding.

SUMMARY

Endoscopic elastic band ligation for bleeding esophageal varices is a new form of endoscopic treatment based on principles developed for elastic band ligation of internal hemorrhoids. Experimental studies have shown ligation results in replacement of submucosal structures, including varices, with scar tissue resulting in eradication of varices. Clinical studies have shown ligation results in consistent shallow ulceration at each treatment site. Such ulcers appear to have no greater propensity to bleed than ulcers induced by sclerotherapy and cause few esophageal strictures and no measurable effects on esophageal motility and function. Elastic band ligation appears equal in efficacy to sclerotherapy for control of active bleeding from esophageal varices. Ligation appears equal or superior to sclerotherapy for long-term prevention of recurrent variceal bleeding in all outcome variables and results in significantly fewer treatment related complications. The combination of elastic band ligation with sclerotherapy, either synchronously or with metachronous application of the latter, may produce results superior to those obtainable with either treatment used alone.

REFERENCES

1. Stiegmann G, Goff J. Endoscopic esophageal varix ligation: preliminary clinical experience. Gastrointest Endosc 1988; 34:113-117.
2. Stiegmann GV, Cambre T, Sun J. A new endoscopic elastic band ligating device. Gastrointest Endosc 1986; 32:230-233.

3. Stiegmann GV, Sun JH, Hammond WS. Results of experimental endoscopic esophageal varix ligation. Am Surg 1988; 54:105-108.
4. Egan J, Jensen DM, Hirabayashi K, Machicado GA. Randomized controlled study of endoscopic rubber band ligation and high volume sclerotherapy for actively bleeding gastric varices in dogs. Gastrointest Endosc 1991; 37:239 (Abstr).
5. Jensen DM, Weisz N, Hirabayashi K, Machicado GA. Randomized controlled study of rubber band ligation and sclerotherapy for active esophageal varix bleeding in dogs. Gastroenterol 1991; 100:A 92 (Abstract).
6. Young M, Sanowski R, Rasche R. Comparison and characterization of ulcerations induced by endoscopic ligation of esophageal varices versus endoscopic sclerotherapy. Gastrointest Endosc 1993; 39:119-122.
7. Goff JS, Reveille RM, Stiegmann GV. Endoscopic sclerotherapy versus endoscopic variceal ligation: Esophageal symptoms, complications, and motility. Am J Gastroenterol 1988; 83:1240-4.
8. Goldschmiedt M, Haber G, Kandel G et al. A safety maneuver for placing overtubes during endoscopic variceal ligation. Gastrointest Endosc 1992; 38:399-400.
9. Stiegmann GV, Goff JS, Sun JH, Wilborn S. Endoscopic elastic band ligation for active variceal hemorrhage. Am Surg 1989; 55:124-128.
10. Saeed Z, Stiegmann G, Ramirez F, Reveille R, Goff J, Hepps K, Cole R. Endoscopic variceal ligation versus combined ligation and low dose sclerotherapy: a multi-center randomized trial. Am J Gastroenterol 1994; 89:1626.
11. Gimson A, Ramage J, Panos M, Hayllar K, Harrison P, Williams R, Westaby D. Randomised trial of variceal banding ligation versus injection sclerotherapy for bleeding oesophageal varices. Lancet 1993; 342:391-394.
12. Lo G, Lai K, Chang C, Jeng J, Chen S, Lin C, Chiang H. A prospective, randomized trial of injection sclerotherapy vs banding ligation in the management of bleeding esophageal varices. Gastroenterology 1994; 106:A933.
13. Laine L, El-Newihi H, McGinn F. Endoscopic ligation compared with sclerotherapy for treatment of bleeding esophageal varices. Ann Int Med 1993; 119:1-8.
14. Stiegmann G, Goff J, Michaletz-Onody P, Korula J, Lieberman D, Saeed Z, Reveille R, Sun J, Lowenstein S. Endoscopic sclerotherapy as compared with endoscopic ligation for bleeding esophageal varices. N Engl J Med 1992; 326:1527-1532.
15. Khandelwal M, Jones W, Akerman P, Raijman I, Siemens M, Kandel G, Kortan P, Marcon N, Haber G. Preliminary results of a prospective randomized trial of Histoacryl vs endoscopic band ligation (EBL) for acute esophago-gastric variceal hemorrhage. Gastrointest Endosc 1994; 40 (Part 2):P76.
16. Goff JS. Endoscopic variceal ligation. Can J Gastroenterol 1990; 4:639-642.
17. Avgerinos A, Armonis A, Manolakopoulos S, Rekoumis G, Sgourou A, Gouma P, Raptis S. Endoscopic sclerotherapy (ES) versus endoscopic ligation (EVL) for prevention of recurrent oesophageal variceal haemorrhage in cirrhotics. A prospective study. Gastroenterology 1994; 106:A861.
18. Reveille RM, Goff JS, Stiegmann GV, Stauffer JT. Combination endoscopic variceal ligation (EVL) and low volume sclerotherapy (ES) for bleeding esophageal varices: A faster route to variceal eradication? Gastrointest Endosc 1991; 37:243 (Abstr).
19. Koutsomanis D. Endoscopic variceal ligation combined with low volume sclerotherapy: a controlled study. Gastroenterology 1992; (102):A835 (Abstr).
20. Hashizume M, Ohta M, Ueno K, Tanoue K, Kitano S, Sugimachi K. Endoscopic ligation of esophageal varices significantly reduces adverse effects of injection sclerotherapy: a prospective randomized trial. Gastrointest Endosc 1993; 39:123-126.
21. Chon J, Song C, Lee S, Choi J, Kim C, Ryu H, Hyun J. A new method of endoscopic variceal ligation-injection sclerotherapy (EVLIS) for gastric varix. Gastroenterology 1994; 106:A875.
22. Berkelhammer C, Madhav G, Lyon S, Roberts J. "Pinch" injury during overtube placement in upper endoscopy. Gastrointest Endosc 1993; 39:187-189.
23. Saltzman J, Arora S. Complications of esophageal variceal band ligation. Gastrointest Endosc 1993; 39:185-187.

The Transjugular Intrahepatic Portosystemic Shunt (TIPS): Efficiency and Clinical Complications

M. Rössle, A. Ochs

INTRODUCTION

The performance of TIPS involves the puncture of an intrahepatic branch of the portal vein and the implantation of a metallic stent into the parenchymal channel between the hepatic and portal veins. This procedure is probably the most demanding interventional technique and, therefore, its mortality, complications and clinical results are closely related to the expertise of the team. This presentation concentrates on published data regarding response to treatment (lack of rebleeding in patients with variceal bleeding or recurrence of ascites in patients treated for refractory ascites), and long-term complications (i.e., hepatic encephalopathy, liver failure). Results on long-term mortality are not presented, since they are only meaningful in the context with comparable data from randomized controlled studies which are not accomplished at present.

VARICEAL REBLEEDING

Variceal rebleeding is almost always a consequence of shunt insufficiency. This is a frequent event and appears in about 50% of the patients within the first year of follow-up (1-4) (table 1). After the first year of follow-up, primary shunt insufficiency is rare (1). The estenosis/occlusion may be located within the stent-shunt or at the hepatic venous outflow. It may be related to the various stents implanted, the anatomy of the shunt and the use of post-procedural anticoagulation. In our hospital, heparin is given to all patients with prothrombin activity greater than 30% and platelet count over 40.000/µl. After a 1-week continuous intravenous infusion of heparin, low molecular heparin is given subcutaneously for another 4 weeks. To our knowledge, other centers do not give heparin because of the fear of bleeding complications. As shown by platelet labeling, heparin significantly reduces platelet aggregation to the metallic stent within the first 24 hours after its implantation (5). This may reduce primary thrombus formation as well as delay intima proliferation. The latter may be related to a direct inhibitory effect of heparin on factors inducing intima hyperplasia (6). If shunt insufficiency occurs, reestablishment of the shunt can be achieved almost always by balloon dilatation or implantation of additional stents (1-4).

Intimal hyperplasia causing stenosis may also be due to leakage of bile into the lumen of the shunt (7). This complications has been reported to occur in 36% of cases (8) and may be prevented by the use of covered stents which will be available soon.

Variceal rebleeding occurs in 5 to 20% of the patients (1-4) (table 1). However, only 1 of our 300 patients treated for variceal bleeding died from variceal hemorrhage. This may be due to the frequent (3 months) sonographic evaluations, which allowed early redilatation when occlusion was diagnosed. Angiography of the shunt revealed complete occlusion in only one third of the

Table 1. Rates (%) of primary shunt insufficiency and variceal rebleeding in 4 studies on TIPS for variceal bleeding with a follow-up time of at least 1 year

Author	Reference	Stenosis	Occlusion	Rebleeding
Rössle	1	33	15	18
LaBerge	2	19	9	18
Perarnau	3	47	0.7	6
Theilmann	4	56	7	7

patients with duplex-sonographic or endoscopic evidence of shunt failure.

Color coded duplex-sonography is a reliable means to non-invasively control shunt function (1, 9-10). A decrease in blood flow velocity in the stent-shunt and the portal vein by more than 50% of the immediate post-TIPS values is indicative of shunt insufficiency (1, 9). However, this does not indicate the need for radiological revision. In about 5% of the patients, varices do not reappear despite insufficient shunting. Thus, endoscopic assessment of the varices and determination of the potential risk of rebleeding is mandatory to decide whether radiological revision and redilatation is indicated or not. In another 10% of patiens treated by TIPS, hepatic encephalopathy was aggravated by the shunt and the spontaneous reduction of the shunt flow was appreciated.

REFRACTORY ASCITES

Portal hypertension is the major reason for the formation of ascites. Therefore, surgical shunts and TIPS may effectively reduce ascites formation. This is also true for refractory ascites. Previous studies in patients treated with surgical shunts showed good response to treatment; however, the high early mortality (5-20%) limits its applicability (11). Little is known about TIPS for refractory ascites. The results of the published studies (12, 13-14) are summarized in table 2. In general, TIPS seems to be an effective treatment for refractory ascites. Regarding survival, no conclusions can be drawn before data from randomized comparison with other current treatments are available.

HEPATIC ENCEPHALOPATHY (HE) AND LIVER FUNCTION

HE is inherent to the TIPS-treatment as it is for surgical shunts. Compared to surgical shunts TIPS has the advantage of a greater variability of shunt size with the feasibility of stepwise enlargement or reduction of the stent-shunt.

The effect of TIPS on the incidence of HE is given in table 3. Most patients with TIPS-induced HE respond to medical treatment with lactulose, branched chain amino acids and antibiotics.

HE correlates significantly with age and, in patients below 60, with Child-Pugh score (1, 15-16). In older patients HE does not correlate with Child-Pugh score (1, 15) indicating that other factors (e.g. cerebral circulation and function) may contribute to HE. In spite of this knowledge, TIPS-induced HE or aggravation of preexisting HE can not be prevented completely. Few patients with an apparently low risk of HE may develop severe mental disability after TIPS, and, in others, TIPS will be performed as a rescue treatment regardless of their high risk of HE. In these patients and in patients with progressive liver failure after TIPS the diameter of the shunt determines the severity and the progress of the syndrome. It is well known that smaller shunts have a lower risk of inducing HE and liver failure (17). In this regard, TIPS has the great advantage of variation of the shunt diameter at any time after its establish-

Table 2. Effect of TIPS on diurectic refractory ascites

Author	Reference	Number of patients	Response (%)	Complete resolution (%)
Ochs	12	49	92	74
Villarreal	13	7	100	
Ferral	14	14	50	50

Response is defined as complete resolution or improvement without need of further paracentesis.

Table 3. Effect of TIPS on hepatic encephalopathy (HE) in patients treated for variceal bleeding

Author	Reference	*De novo* HE (%)	Debilitating HE (%)
Rösle	1	15	5
LaBerge	2	25	3
Perarnau	3	9.5	1.4
Theilmann	4	27	3

ment. Implantation of small-size shunts eventually in combination with embolization of the varices, may prevent HE in patients at risk. Subsequent transjugular dilatation or reembolization is feasible if the patient rebleeds. On the other hand, in patients who develop TIPS-induced refractory HE, implantation of a reducing stent or occlusion using detachable balloon may cure the syndrome (18). In contrast, TIPS-induced liver failure, indicated by a progressive increase in bilirubin, is not reversible after implantation of a reducing stent (18).

CONCLUSIONS

1. Shunt stenosis and occlusion are frequent. Fortunately, variceal rebleeding is rare and reestablishment of the shunt is feasible in almost every patient.
2. Hepatic encephalopathy is the major clinical problem of TIPS. However, it seems to be manageable by preferential implantation of small diameter shunts in patients with a high risk of HE and by shunt reduction or occlusion in patients with refractory and debilitating HE or severe liver failure.

REFERENCES

1. Rössle M, Haag K, Ochs A, Sellinger M, Nöldge G, Perarnau, JM, Berger E, Blum U, Gabelmann A, Hauenstein KH, Langer M, Gerok W (1994): The Transjugular Intrahepatic Portosystemic Stent-Shunt Procedure for Variceal Bleeding. N Engl J Med 1994; 330:165-171.
2. LaBerge JM, Somberg KA, Lake JR, Gordon RL, Kerlan RK, Asher NL, Roberts JP, Ring EJ. Two-year outcome following transjugular intrahepatic portosystemic shunt for variceal bleeding: results in 90 patients. Hepatology (in press).
3. Perarnau JM. Transjugular intrahepatic portasystemic shunt. Technique and preliminary results. Gastroenterol Clin Biol 1993; 17:T22-27.
4. Theilmann L, Sauer P. Transjugular intrahepatic portosystemic stent shunt: Results and complications. Radiology 1994; 34:174-177.
5. Krause T, Siegerstetter V, Haag K, Hauenstein KH, Rössle M. Evaluation of thrombogenicity of metallic stents in patients with TIPS using Technetium 99m platelets. Eur J Nucl Med 1994; 21:741A.
6. Yamaguchi M, Diamond S, Watanabe H, Gallati H, Baur W, Sharefkin JB. Heparin and dibutyryl cAMP modulate gene expression in stimulated human saphenous vein smooth muscle cells. In Vitro Cell Biol 1993; 29A:867-872.
7. LaBerge JM, Ferrell LD, Ring EJ. Histopathologic study of stenotic and occluded transjugular intrahepatic portosystemic shunts. JVIR 1993; 4:779-786.
8. Uflacker R, Reichert P, D'Albuquerque LC, De Oliveira e Silva A. Liver anatomy applied to the placement of transjugular intrahepatic portosystemic shunt. Radiology 1994; 191:705-712.
9. Haag K, Nöldge G, Sellinger M, Ochs A, Gerok W, Rössle M. Transjugular intrahepatic portosystemic stent-shunt (TIPS): Monitoring of function by color duplex sonography. Gastroenterology 1992; 102:817A.
10. Lind CD, Malisch TW, Chong WK, Richards WO, Pinson CW, Meranze SG, Mazer M. Incidence of shunt occlusion or stenosis following transjugular intrahepatic portosystemic shunt placement. Gastroenterology 1994; 106:1277-1283.
11. Elcheroth J, Vons C, Franco D. Role of surgical therapy in the management of intractable ascites in cirrhosis. World J Surg 1994; 18:240-245.
12. Ochs A, Haag K, Sellinger M, Langer M, Gerok W, Rössle M. TIPS: Efficacy and survival in 49 patients with refractory and "untreatable" ascites. Hepatology 1993; 18(Pt. 2):292A.
13. Villarreal LG, Urmeneta JMZ, Vila JQ, Gómez-Acebo BS, Jaureguízar JIB, Areso JL, Valtuena JP. Portosystemic intrahepatic prothesis: PIP (TIPS) in the treatment of refractory ascites. A pilot study. Gastroenterol Hepatol 1993; 16:18-22.
14. Ferral H, Bjarnason H, Wegryn SA, Rengel GJ, Nazarian GK, Rank JM, Tadavarthy SM, Hunter DW, Castaneda-Zuniga WR. Refractory ascites: early experience in treatment with transjugular intrahepatic portosystemic shunt. Radiology 1993; 189:795-801.
15. Sellinger M, Ochs A, Haag K, Nöldge G, Gerok W, Rössle M. Incidence of hepatic encephalopathy and follow-up of liver function in patients with transjugular intrahepatic portosystemic stent-shunt (TIPS). Gastroenterology 1992; 102:883A.
16. Sanyal AJ, Freedman AM, Shiffman ML, Purdum PP, Luketic VA, Cheatham AK. Portosystemic encephalopathy after transjugular intrahepatic portosystemic shunt: results of a prospective controlled study. Hepatology 1994; 20:46-55.
17. Sarfeh IJ, Rypins EB, Conroy RM, Mason GR. Portocaval H-graft: relationship of shunt diameter, portal flow patterns and encephalopathy. Ann Surg 1983; 197:422-426.
18. Hauenstein KH, Haag K, Ochs A, Langer M, Rössle M. Reducing stent for TIPS-induced refractory hepatic encephalopathy and liver failure. Radiology 1995 (in press).

Therapeutic Paracentesis

R. Planas

INTRODUCTION

Ascites is the first sign of decompensation in most cirrhotic patients and is associated with a poor prognosis (1). The one-year survival probability rate of patients admitted to hospital for the treatment of an episode of ascites has been reported to be only 56% (2).

Since the introduction of modern diuretics in the 1960s, the treatment of ascites in patients with cirrhosis has been based on the combination of low-sodium diet and the administration of these drugs (3). This therapeutic schedule, however, is not entirely satisfactory since it is frequently associated with complications, particularly hepatic encephalopathy, renal impairment, and dilutional hyponatremia (4). In addition, between 5% to 10% of cirrhotics admitted to hospital for the treatment of an episode of tense ascites do not respond to diuretics. This condition, known as refractory ascites or diuretic-resistant ascites (5), is an important challenge and has stimulated investigations of alternative treatments for ascites in patients with cirrhosis. Until very recently, the prosthesis designed by LeVeen et al. in 1974 (6) was the only alternative treatment to diuretics for the management of cirrhotic patients with ascites. However, this procedure may induce serious complications, is associated with a high rate of obstruction of the prosthesis, and does not improve survival (7-9).

Since the reintroduction of therapeutic paracentesis by Ginés et al. (10) in 1985, numerous studies have demonstrated that this procedure is a rapid, effective, and safe therapy for tense ascites in patients with cirrhosis. It is, therefore, not surprising that contrary to previous clinical practice which was dictated by a fear of complications, at present therapeutic paracentesis is widely used in these patients.

COMPARISON OF PARACENTESIS PLUS INTRAVENOUS ALBUMIN WITH DIURETICS IN THE TREATMENT OF TENSE ASCITES

The first study reevaluating paracentesis as a treatment of ascites consisted of a randomized controlled trial comparing repeated large-volume paracentesis (4-6 l/day until the disappearence of ascites) plus intravenous albumin infusion (40 g after each tap) with standard diuretic therapy (furosemide plus spironolactone at increasing doses) in 117 cirrhotic patients with tense ascites and avid sodium retention who were admitted to several hospitals in the Barcelona area (10, 11). Patients who did not respond to the highest scheduled doses of diuretics (furosemide, 240 mg/day, and spironolactone, 400 mg/day) were treated with a LeVeen shunt. Patients with renal failure (serum creatinine over 1.5 mg/dl) were randomized separately to ensure a similar number of cases with renal failure in either treatment group. Patients with serious liver impairment (hepatic encephalopathy, serum bilirubin over 10 mg/dl, and prothrombin activity less than 40%) or severe renal failure (serum creatinine over 3 mg/dl) were not included in the study. Once ascites disappeared, patients were discharged from hospital with diu-

Table 1. Effects of paracentesis plus intravenous albumin treatment on plasma volume, renal function, endogenous vasoactive systems, and systemic and hepatic hemodynamics (mean ± SEM)*

Parameter	Before treatment	After treatment
Plasma volume (ml)	3,767 ± 160	3,442 ± 170
Glomerular filtration rate (ml/min)	65 ± 7	73 ± 8
Free water clearance (ml/min)	2.5 ± 0.6	2.9 ± 0.7
Plasma renin activity (ng/ml/h)	7.7 ± 3.3	8.7 ± 2.5
Norepinephrine (pg/ml)	630 ± 87	539 ± 70
Antidiuretic hormone (pg/ml)	4.6 ± 0.4	4.4 ± 0.5
Urinary PGE_2 (ng/day)	84 ± 19	105 ± 24
Urinary 6-keto-PGF_1 (ng/day)	257 ± 38	278 ± 46
Cardiac output (l/min)**	6.3 ± 0.6	6.1 ± 0.6
Peripheral resistance (dynes/sec/cm^{-5})**	1,110 ± 104	1,061 ± 108
Hepatic venous pressure gradient (mmHg)**	19.2 ± 1.9	20.3 ± 1.9

* No significant differences were found in any parameter before and after treatment.
** Measured in 7 patients; the remaining parameters were measured in 24 patients.

retics in order to prevent ascites reaccumulation. Cases developing tense ascites during follow-up were treated according to their initial schedule. The main results of this study were: *a*) Paracentesis was more effective than diuretics in eliminating ascites (96.5% versus 72.8%). *b*) Paracentesis plus intravenous albumin had no deleterous effect on systemic hemodynamics and renal function in the whole group of 58 patients treated with this procedure nor in the subgroups of patients with functional renal failure or without peripheral edema (table 1). Although mean arterial pressure decreased slightly after paracentesis treatment, no significant changes were observed in plasma volume, cardiac output, or peripheral vascular resistance. The observation that paracentesis treatment did not significantly modify the plasma levels of renin, norepinephrine and antidiuretic hormone, which are very sensitive to changes in effective intravascular volume, further indicates that therapeutic paracentesis associated with intravenous albumin does not impair systemic hemodynamics. As expected, ascites removal was associated with a marked reduction in free and wedged hepatic venous pressure. *c*) The incidence of hyponatremia, renal impairment, and hepatic encephalopathy was much lower in patients treated with paracentesis (5.1, 3.4 and 10.2%, respectively) than in those receiving diuretics (30, 27 and 29%). Other complications occurred with similar frequency in both groups of patients (table 2). The high incidence of hyponatremia, renal impairment, and encephalopathy in the diuretic group was comparable with that reported by Sherlock et al. (12) (41, 34 and 29%) in a large series of 112 patients with nonazotemic normonatremic cirrhosis with ascites treated with a variety of diuretic combinations. *d*) The duration of hospital stay, and therefore the cost of treatment, were lower in patients treated with paracentesis. *e*) There were no significant differences in the probability of readmission to the hospital during follow-up, causes of readmission, probability of survival, and causes of death between the two groups of patients. Most of these results were later confirmed in three further controlled trials, reported by Salerno et al. (13), Hagève et al. (14), and Solà et al. (15). In this latter sutdy dextran-40 was the plasma volume expander used.

Table 2. Complications during the first hospital stay in patients treated with paracentesis plus intravenous albumin (group 1) and patients treated with diuretics (group 2)

	Group 1 (n = 58)	Group 2 (n = 59)	p
Patients with complications	10	36	< 0.001
Hyponatremia (n patients)	3	18	< 0.001
Encephalopathy (n patients)	6	17	< 0.002
Renal impairment (n patients)	2	16	< 0.001
Hyperkalemia (n patients)	1	7	NS
Gastrointestinal bleeding (n patients)	2	6	NS
Peritonitis (n patients)	0	4	NS
Bacteremia (n patients)	2	0	NS
Others (n patients)	0	4	NS

In 38 cirrhotic patients with tense ascites (6 with renal failure and 16 without peripheral edema), Tító et al. (16) investigated whether ascites could be safely mobilized by total paracentesis (complete removal of ascites in a single tap) plus intravenous albumin infusion (6-8 g/l of ascites removed). The aim of this study was to assess whether cirrhotic patients with tense ascites could be treated in a 1-day hospitalization regime. With the aid of a suction pump, the volume of ascitic fluid removed and the duration of the procedure were 10.7 ± 0.5 l (mean ± SEM) and 60 ± 3 min, respectively. The incidence of hyponatremia, renal impairment, and hepatic encephalopathy in this series of patients (3, 0 and 10%, respectively) and the clinical course of the disease, as estimated by the probability of readmission to hospital, causes of readmission, probability of survival, and causes of death, were comparable with those reported by the same group of investigators in patients treated with repeated large-volume paracentesis (10).

In conclusion, these studies demonstrate that mobilization of ascitic fluid by repeated large-volume paracentesis or total paracentesis associated with intravenous albumin infusion does not impair systemic hemodynamics and renal function in patients with cirrhosis and tense ascites. Since therapeutic paracentesis is more effective than conventional diuretic therapy in mobilizing the ascitic fluid, besides being associated with lower incidence of complications and considerably reducing the duration of hospitalization, it should be considered as the treatment of choice for cirrhotic patients admitted to hospital with tense ascites. To avoid reaccumulation of ascites, patients treated with paracentesis require dietary sodium restriction and the administration of diuretics after the procedure.

PARACENTESIS PLUS INTRAVENOUS ALBUMIN INFUSION IN THE MANAGEMENT OF PATIENTS WITH REFRACTORY ASCITES. COMPARISON WITH PERITONEOVENOUS SHUNTING

Recently, a spanish multicenter randomized trial comparing therapeutic paracentesis with peritoneovenous shunting in cirrhotic patients with refractory ascites has been published (17). Forty-one patients were treated with repeated large-volume paracentesis plus intravenous albumin, and 48 with a LeVeen shunt. Diuretics were given after both treatments to avoid reaccumulation of ascites. Patients treated with paracentesis developing tense ascites during follow-up were treated by paracentesis, and those in the shunt group, by the insertion of a new prosthesis (in case of shunt obstruction) or with diuretics. During the first hospitalization, both treatments were equally effective in mobilizing the ascites, although the duration of hospital stay was significantly longer in the shunt group (19 ± 1 versus 11 ± 1 days). There were also no significant differences between both groups in the number of patients who developed complications (9 and 15) or died (3 and 6). During follow-up, 37 patients from each group were readmitted to hospital. The number of readmissions for any reason (174 versus 97) or for ascites (125 versus 38) was significantly higher, and the time to first readmission for any reason (1 ± 0.2 versus 2.3 ± 0.3 months) and for ascites (2.4 ± 0.3 versus 8 ± 2.6 months) significantly shorter in the paracentesis group than in the shunt group. However, the total time in hospital during follow-up was similar in the two groups (48 ± 8 and 44 ± 6 days; 19 ± 3 % and 22 ± 4 % of the follow-up period). Since the number of readmissions was higher among the patients treated with paracentesis, the mean duration of hospital stay during follow-up was significantly shorter in that group as compared to the peritoneovenous-shunt group (11 ± 8 versus 18 ± 14 days), particularly when ascites was the cause of readmission (10 ± 8 versus 23 ± 14 days). The peritoneovenous shunt was obstructed in 20 readmissions for ascites among 15 patients. The site of obstruction was the valve in 12 readmissions, the venous tube in 4, and thrombosis of the superior vena cava in 4; a superior vena cava syndrome developed in 2 patients. The probability of survival was similar in both groups (fig. 1). The probability of shunt obstruction at one and two years of follow-up was 40 and 52%, respectively (fig. 2).

A recent study in a large series of cirrhotics with ascites treated with a LeVeen shunt has suggested that the insertion of a 3 cm-long titanium tip into the venous end of the LeVeen

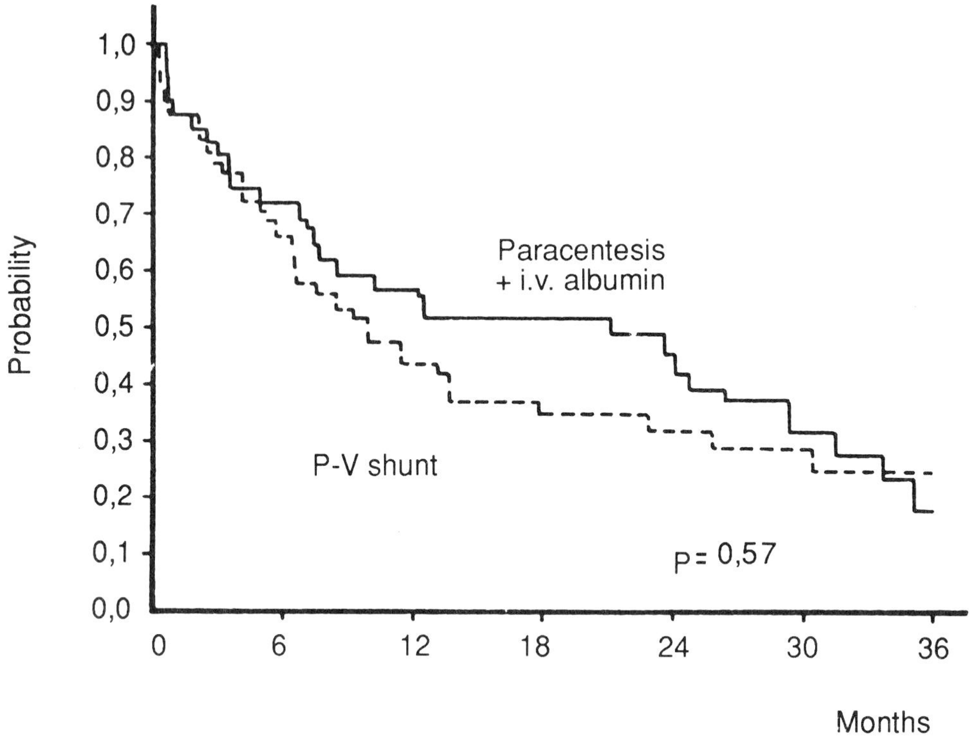

Fig. 1. Probability of survival after entry into the study in the two study groups. (Reprinted by permission from Ginès P et al. N Engl J Med 1991; 325:829-835.)

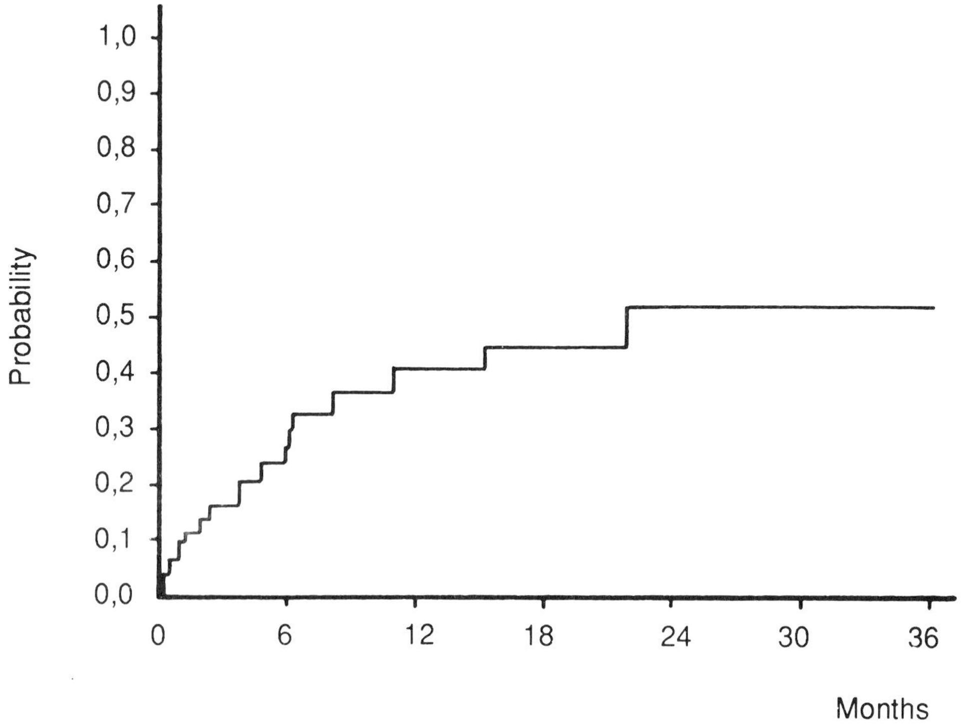

Fig. 2. Probability of peritoneovenous-shunt obstruction after entry into the study in patients with cirrhosis and ascites. (Reprinted by permission from Ginès P et al. N Engl J Med 1991; 325:829-835.)

shunt prevents thrombotic obstruction and development of superior vena cava thrombosis (18). This beneficial effect, however, has not been confirmed in an European multicentre randomized study comparing total paracentesis associated with intravenous albumin versus LeVeen shunt with titanium tip (19). In this study, 42 cirrhotic patients with refractory ascites were treated with total paracentesis plus intravenous albumin infusion and 39 with a LeVeen shunt with titanium tip. There were 22 cases of shunt obstruction in 14 patients, 40% occurring at the venous end. The one- and two-year probabilities of shunt obstruction were 47% and 60%, respectively. The results of this trial were very similar to those reported in the Spanish trial (17).

In conclusion, these trials show that although LeVeen shunt is more effective than paracentesis in the long-term control of refractory ascites, it does not reduce the total time in hospital or prolongs survival. Patients treated with peritoneovenous shunt require frequent reoperations due to obstruction of the prosthesis. This complication is not prevented by the insertion of a titanium tip at the venous end of the shunt. Therapeutic paracentesis, therefore, is an alternative treatment to LeVeen shunt in cirrhotic patients with refractory ascites.

IMPORTANCE OF INTRAVENOUS ALBUMIN INFUSION IN THE TREATMENT OF CIRRHOTICS WITH LARGE-VOLUME PARACENTESIS

Another randomized controlled trial, also from the Barcelona group, was aimed at investigating whether intravenous albumin administration is necessary in cirrhotic patients treated with therapeutic paracentesis (20). The inclusion criteria were identical to those of their first study (10). In this trial 52 cirrhotic patients with tense ascites (group 1) were treated by repeated large-volume paracentesis with intravenous albumin and 53 by paracentesis without albumin administration (group 2). There were no differences between the two groups in the number of patients with «complete» removal of ascites, loss of body weight and number of paracentesis performed per patient. Confirming previous studies, paracentesis plus intravenous albumin did not induce significant changes in standard renal function tests, plasma renin activity, and plasma aldosterone concentration. In contrast, paracentesis without albumin was associated with a significant increase in blood urea nitrogen, a constant and marked elevation in plasma renin activity (fig. 3) and plasma aldosterone concentration and a significant reduction in serum sodium concentration. Side effects occurred in 9 patients of group 1, and in 16 of group 2. This difference was due to a significantly higher incidence of hyponatremia and/or renal impairment in group 2 (20% versus 2%). The incidence of other complications was similar in the two groups (table 3). Serum sodium concentration returned to pretreatment values during follow-up in 6 of the 10 patients developing hyponatremia after treatment. However, renal function did not improve in any of the 6 patients developing renal impairment after paracentesis. Although the probability of survival was similar in the two groups, a multivariate analysis identified the development of hyponatremia or renal impairment, or both, after paracentesis and the occurrence of other complications during the first hospitalization (encephalopathy, gastrointestinal bleeding, and severe infections) as independent predictors of mortality.

The results of this study suggest that complete mobilization of ascites by paracentesis without plasma volume expansion is followed by an impairment in effective intravascular volume. This contention is supported by findings of several investigations assessing the effects of complete mobilization of ascites by large-volume of total paracentesis with and whitout albumin infusion on systemic hemodynamics, vasoactive hormones, and renal function (21-29). These studies also showed that the mobilization of ascites without plasma volume expansion was associated with an activation of the renin-aldosterone system and a suppression of the cardiac release of atrial natriuretic peptide. These abnormalities start within the first hours after complete mobilization of ascites and are constantly detected 48 hours after treatment. Despite the impairment in systemic hemodynamics in almost all patients treated with paracentesis without albumin infusion, only 20% of

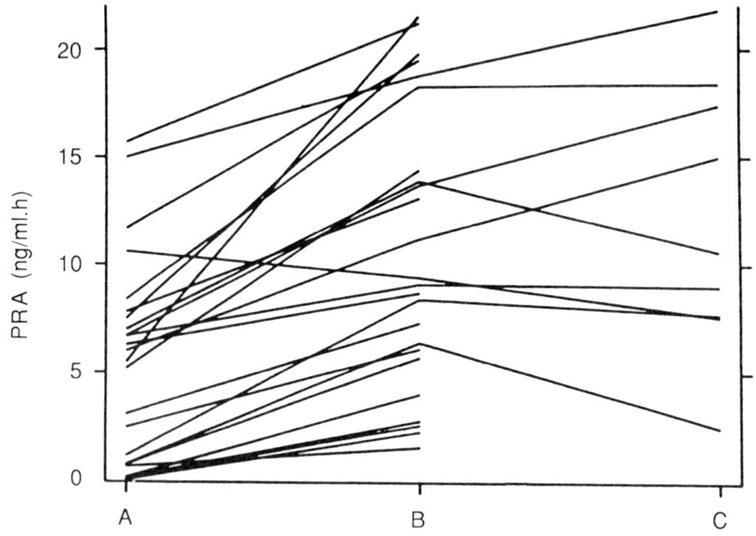

Fig. 3. Changes in plasma renin activity (PRA) in patients treated with paracentesis without i.v. albumin: A, before treatment (n = 24); B, 48 h after treatement (n = 24); C, five days after treatment (n = 9). (Reprinted by permission from Ginès P et al. Gastroenterology 1988; 94:1493-1502.)

patients develop renal or electrolyte complications, or both, probably because of intrarenal compensatory mechanisms (i.e., renal prostaglandins) that antagonize the effects of circulating hypovolemia on kidney function. Because renal impairment and dilutional hyponatremia following paracentesis are not reversible in many cases and are associated with a poor prognosis (20), the prevention of the impairment in effective blood volume by the intravenous infusion of albumin is an important measure in cirrhotic patients with tense ascites treated with repeated large-volume or total paracentesis.

Table 3. Complications during the first hospital stay in patients treated with paracentesis plus intravenous albumin (group 1) and patients treated with paracentesis without intravenous albumin (group 2)

	Group 1 (n = 52)	Group 2 (n = 53)	p
Patients with complications	9	16	NS
Hyponatremia and/or renal impairment	0	9	< 0.01
Hyponatremia and/or renal impairment plus other complications	1	2	NS
Other complications	8	5	NS
Number of complications	13	23	NS
Hyponatremia	1	9	< 0.01
Renal impairment	0	6	< 0.05
Hepatic encephalopathy	6	3	NS
Gastrointestinal hemorrhage	2	1	NS
Severe infection	4	4	NS

USE OF OTHER TYPES OF PLASMA EXPANDERS IN CIRRHOTIC PATIENTS TREATED WITH PARACENTESIS

The use of human serum albumin in cirrhotic patients treated with large-volume paracentesis is limited by its high price. It is, therefore, not surprising that several groups have investigated whether albumin could be substituted by less expensive plasma expanders in these patients.

Planas et al. (30) have compared in a randomized trial albumin versus dextran-70 (containing 6 g of dextran-70 per 100 ml of dextrose solution) as plasma expanders in 88 cirrhotic patients (16 with renal failure) with tense ascites treated by total paracentesis. Both substances were given at a dose of 8 g/l of ascitic fluid removed. After mobilization of ascites, patients were discharged from hospital with diuretics, and cases developing tense ascites during follow-up were treated according to their initial schedule. Neither paracentesis plus intravenous albumin nor paracentesis plus dextran-70 infusion were associated with significant changes in renal and hepatic function or serum electrolytes. The incidence of renal impairment (1 case in each therapeutic group), hyponatremia (3 and 4 cases, respectively) and other complications after paracentesis, and the clinical course of the disease, as estimated by the probability of readmission to hospital, causes of readmission, probability of survival and causes of death, were similar in the two groups of patients. The effect of paracentesis on effective intravascular volume was indirectly assessed by measuring plasma renin activity and aldosterone concentration before and 2 and 6 days after treatment with the patients being in hospital without diuretics. In patients treated with albumin, no significant changes in these parameters were observed during the entire period of observation. In contrast, both parameters increased significantly at the sixth day of treatment in patients receiving dextran-70 (fig. 4). A significant increase in renin and aldosterone (30% over baseline values) was observed in 51% of the 45 patients treated with dextran-70 and in only 15% of the 43 patients receiving albumin, which suggest that dextran-70 is less effective than albumin in the prevention of impairment in systemic hemodynamics induced by paracentesis.

Salerno et al. (31) performed a randomized controlled trial in 54 cirrhotic patients with refractory ascites treated by total paracentesis. Twenty-seven patients were given intravenous albumin (6 g/l of ascitic fluid removed) and 27 received an intravenous infusion of hemaccel (Emagel 3.5%, 150 ml/l of ascites evacuated). The mobilization of ascites in both groups was not associated with significant changes in renal and hepatic function, serum sodium concentration, plasma renin activity and plasma concentrations of aldosterone and atrial natriuretic peptide, which were determined 1, 3 and 6 days after treatment. Nine patients (4 in the albumin group and 5 in the hemaccel group) developed hyponatremia and 2 (one from each group) renal impairment after treatment. The probability of recurrence of massive ascites and survival during follow-up were similar in both groups.

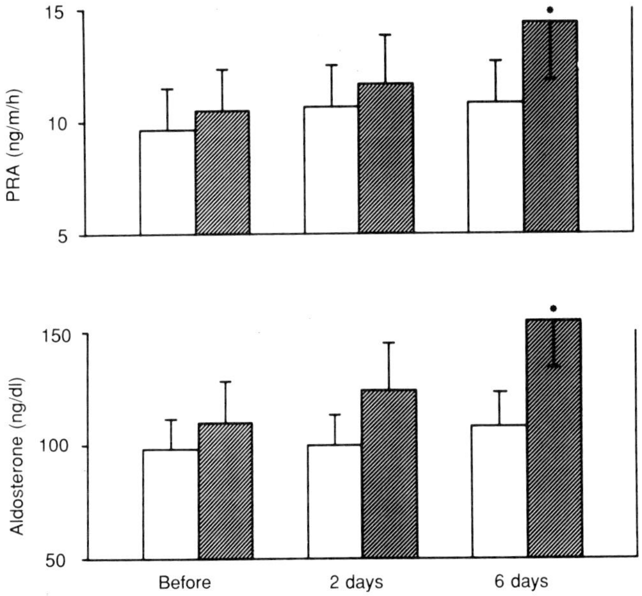

Fig. 4. Plasma renin activity (PRA) and plasma aldosterone concentration in patients treated with total paracentesis and i.v. albumin (open bars) and in those treated with total paracentesis and i.v. dextran-70 (shaded bars) before and 2 and 6 days after treatment (*$p < 0.02$ with respect to values obtained before treatment). Normal values in our laboratory: PRA 1.3 ± 0.2 ng/ml^{-1}; aldosterone, $10.5 \pm 1{,}1$ ng/dl. (Reprinted by permission from Planas R et al. Gastroenterology 1990; 99:1736-1744.)

Fassio et al. (32) performed a randomized controlled trial comparing dextran-70 (containing 6 g of dextran-70 per 100 ml isotonic saline solution) with human albumin in 41 cirrhotic patients treated daily with 5-liter paracentesis until resolution of the ascites. The criteria for inclusion in this study were similar to those in previous trials assessing the safety of paracentesis associated with albumin infusion. Dextran-70 was infused in the same amount as human albumin (6 g/l of ascites drained). Although the number of patients was relatively small, results indicate that dextran-70 was indeed a good substitute for albumin. This conclusion was based in the abscence of significant changes in renal and hepatic function, serum electrolytes and plasma renin activity 1 and 4 days after the last paracentesis in both groups. Four patients developed complications in each group, mainly hyponatremia, while one patient in each group developed renal impairment. The probability of survival and readmission to hospital because of tense ascites were similar in both groups of patients during the follow-up.

Solà et al. (15) treated 49 cirrhotic patients with tense ascites (7 with renal failure) with total paracentesis plus intravenous dextran-40 infusion (containing 10 g of dextran-40 per 100 ml of dextrose solution; the dose was 8 g per liter of ascitic fluid removed) and measured hepatic and renal function and plasma levels of renin and aldosterone prior to and 2 and 6 days after treatment. Plasma renin activity and plasma aldosterone concentration markedly increased after treatment in 70% of the patients. Of the 77 episodes of tense ascites treated with total paracentesis plus dextran-40 infusion during first hospitalization and follow-up, hyponatremia and/or renal impairment developed after treatment in 16 (21%) (hyponatremia on 14 occasions and renal impairment on 6). Cabrera et al. (33), in one study including 14 patients, have suggested that isotonic saline can also be a safe and cost-effective alternative plasma expander in cirrhotics with tense ascites treated with paracentesis.

These studies, therefore, suggest that dextran-70 and Hemaccel but not dextran-40 are as effective as albumin in preventing renal and electrolyte complications after therapeutic paracentesis in cirrhotic patients with tense ascites. They also suggest that plasma expanders in saline solution may be more effective than in dextrose solution in preventing the impairment of systemic hemodynamics induced by paracentesis. Nevertheless, further studies including larger number of patients are necessary to confirm these contentions. First, the results of Salerno et al. (31), Fassio et al. (32), and Cabrera et al. (33) need to be reproduced in trials including larger number of patients. Second, since in the study by Ginès et al. (20) renal impairment and/or dilutional hyponatremia developed in only 21% of the patients treated with paracentesis without intravenous albumin infusion, whereas plasma renin activity increased in 95%, it is possible that the number of patients treated with dextran-70 by Planas et al. (30) in whom a decrease in effective intravascular volume developed (51%) was not large enough to detect any possible adverse effect on renal function. In this regard, an international multicenter study which investigats the efficacy of albumin, dextran-70 and Hemaccel as plasma expanders in a large number of patients treated with therapeutic paracentesis is being performed.

CONCLUSIONS

Therapeutic paracentesis, either repeated large-volume paracentesis or total paracentesis, associated with the intravenous infusion of plasma expanders (albumin, dextran-70, Hemaccel) is a rapid, effective and safe treatment for ascites in patients with cirrhosis. Since therapeutic paracentesis is associated with lower incidence of complications than standard diuretic therapy and considerably shortens the duration of hospital stay, it should be considered the first-choice treatment for patients with marked sodium retention and tense ascites.

Although peritoneovenous shunt is more effective than therapeutic paracentesis in the long-term control of ascites in cirrhotic patients with refractory or recidivant ascites, a high proportion of patients treated with LeVeen shunt need reoperation due to obstruction of the prosthesis. The time in hospital as well as the probability of survival is identical with both therapeutic procedures. Therefore, therapeutic paracentesis is an alterantive treatment to peritoneovenous shunting in cirrhotic patients with refractory or recidivant ascites.

The mobilization of ascites by paracentesis without intravenous colloid administration is constantly associated with an impairment in the effective circulating blood volume, as estimated by the plasma levels or renin and aldosterone, and induces renal impairment and/or dilutional hyponatremia in approximately 20% of patients.

Therapeutic paracentesis does not improve systemic and renal hemodynamics or sodium retention. Therefore, cirrhotic patients treated with paracentesis require the administration of diuretics to avoid reaccumulation of ascites.

All studies on therapeutic paracentesis have excluded cirrhotics with severe impairment of liver and renal function. The safety of paracentesis in this subset of patients is, therefore, still unknown.

REFERENCES

1. Ginès P, Quintero E, Arroyo V, Terés J, Bruguera M, Rimola A, Caballería J, Rodés J, Rozman C. Compensated cirrhosis: natural history and prognostic factors. Hepatology 1987; 7:122-128.

2. Llach J, Ginès P, Arroyo V, Rimola A, Tító Ll, Badalamenti S, Jiménez W, Gaya J, Rivera F, Rodés J. Prognostic value of arterial pressure, endogenous vasoactive systems, and renal function in cirrhotic patients admitted to the hospital for the treatment of ascites. Gastroenterology 1988; 94:482-487.
3. Pérez-Ayuso RM, Arroyo V, Planas R, Gaya J, Bory F, Rimola A, Rivera F, Rodés J. Randomized comparative study of efficacy of furosemide versus spironolactone in nonazotemic cirrhotics with ascites. Gastroenterology 1983; 84:961-968.
4. Arroyo V, Ginès P, Planas R, Panés J, Rodés J. Management of patients with cirrhosis and ascites. Sem Liver Dis 1986; 6:353-369.
5. Arroyo V, Ginès P, Planas R. Treatment of ascites in cirrhosis. Gastroenterol Clin North Am 1992; 21:237-256.
6. LeVeen HH, Christoudias G, Moon JP. Peritoneovenous shunting for ascites. Ann Surg 1974; 180:580-591.
7. Smajda C, Franco D. The LeVeen shunt in the elective treatment of intractable ascites in cirrhosis: A prospective study on 140 patients. Ann Surg 1985; 201:488.
8. Stanley MM, Ochi S, Lee KK, Nemchausky BA, Greenlee HB, Allen JI, Allen MJ, Baum RA, Gadacz TR, Camara DS, Caruana JA, Schiff ER, Livingstone AS, Samanta AK, Najem AZ, Glick ME, Juler GL, Adham N, Baker JD, Cain GD, Jordan PH, Wolf DC, Fulenwider JT, James KE and the Veterans Administration Cooperative Study on Treatment of Alcoholic Cirrhosis with Ascites. Peritoneovenous shunting as compared with medical treatment in patients with alcoholic cirrhosis and masive ascites. N Engl J Med 1989; 321:1632-1638.
9. Bernhoft RA, Pellegrini CA, Way LW. Peritoneovenous shunt for refractory ascites: Operative complications and long-term results. Arch Surg 1982; 117:631-635.
10. Quintero E, Ginès P, Arroyo V, Rimola A, Bory F, Planas R, Viver J, Cabrera J. Paracentesis versus diuretics in the treatment of cirrhotics with tense ascites. Lancet 1985; i:611-612.
11. Ginès P, Arroyo V, Quintero E, Planas R, Bory F, Cabrera J, Rimola A, Viver J, Camps J, Jiménez W, Mastai R, Gaya J, Rodés J. Comparison of paracentesis and diuretics in the treatment of cirrhotics with tense ascites. Results of a randomized study. Gastroenterology 1987; 93:234-241.
12. Sherlock S, Senewiratne B, Scott A, Walker JG. Complications of diuretic therapy in hepatic cirrhosis. Lancet 1966; i:1049-1053.
13. Salerno F, Badalamenti S, Incerti P, Jempini S, Restelli B, Bruno S. Repeated paracentesis and IV albumin infusion to treat «tense» ascitis in cirrhotic patients: A safe alternative therapy. J Hepatol 1987; 5:102-108.
14. Hagève H, Ink O, Ducreux G, Pelletier G, Buffet C, Etienne JP. Traitement de l'ascite chez les malades atteints de cirrhose sans hyponatrémie ni insuffisance rénale. Gastroenterol Clin Biol 1992; 16:751-755.
15. Solà R, Vila C, Andreu M, Oliver MI, Coll S, Gana J, Ledesma S, Ginès P, Jiménez W, Arroyo V. Total paracentesis with dextran-40 vs diuretics in the treatment of ascites in cirrhosis. A randomized controlled trial. J Hepatol 1994; 20:282-288.
16. Tító Ll, Ginès P, Arroyo V, Planas R, Panés J, Rimola A, Llach J, Humbert P, Badalamenti S, Jiménez W, Rodés J. Total paracentesis associated with intravenous albumin in the management of patients with cirrhosis and ascites. Gastroenterology 1990; 98:146-151.
17. Ginès P, Arroyo V, Vargas V, Planas R, Casafont F, Panés J, Hoyos M, Viladomiu Ll, Rimola A, Morillas R, Salmerón JM, Ginès A, Esteban R, Rodés J. Paracentesis with intravenous infusion of albumin as compared with peritoneovenous shunting in cirrhosis with refractory ascites. N Engl J Med 1991; 325:829-835.
18. Hillaire S, Labianca M, Smajda C, Grange D, Franco D. Dérivation péritonéo-veineuse dans l'ascite irréductible de la cirrhose. Résultats d'une étude prospective sur les facteurs d'amélioration du pronostic. Gastroenterol Clin Biol 1988; 12:681-686.
19. Planas R, Ginés A, Angeli P, Guarner C, Salerno F, Vargas V, Bocchia S, Vinel J, Saló J, Ginès P, Domènech E, Gassull MA, Gatta A, Arroyo V, Rodés J. Controlled trial of total paracentesis (TP) plus iv albumin versus LeVeen shunt (LVS) with titanium tip in cirrhotic patients with refractory ascites. J Hepatol 1993; 18(Suppl):S60.
20. Ginès P, Tító Ll, Arroyo V, Planas R, Panés J, Viver J, Torres M, Humbert P, Rimola A, Llach J, Badalamenti S, Jiménez W, Gaya J, Rodés J. Randomized comparative study of therapeutic paracentesis with and without intravenous albumin in cirrhosis. Gastroenterology 1988; 94:1493-1502.
21. Simon DM, McCain JR, Bonkovsky HL, Wells JO, Hartle DK, Galambos JT. Effects of therapeutic paracentesis on systemic and hepatic hemodynamics and on the renal and hormonal function. Hepatology 1987; 7:423-429.
22. Panos MZ, Moore K, Vlavianos P, Chambers JB, Anderson JV, Gimson AES, Slater JDH, Rees LH, Westaby D, Williams R. Single, total paracentesis for tense ascites: sequential hemodynamic changes and right atrial size. Hepatology 1990; 11:662-667.
23. Terg R, Berreta J, Abecasis R, Romero G, Boerr L. Dextran administration avoids hemodynamic changes following paracentesis in cirrhotic patients. A safe and inexpensive option. Dig Dis Sci 1992; 37:79-83.
24. Luca A, Feu F, García-Pagán JC, Ginès A, Fernández M, Escorsell A, Jiménez W, Piera C, Arroyo V, Bosch J, Rodés J. Cambios hemodinámicos y humorales inmediatos y a las 24 horas de la paracentesis total con y sin albúmina. Gastroenterol Hepatol 1993; 16:230.
25. Pozzi M, Osculati G, Boari G, Serboli P, Colombo P, Lambrughi C, De Ceglia S, Roffi L, Piperno A, Negro Cusa E, D'Amico P, Grassi G, Mancia G, Fiorelli G. Time course of circulatory and humoral effects of rapid total paracentesis in cirrhotic patients with tense, refractory ascites. Gastroenterology 1994; 106:709-719.

26. Luca A, Fue F, García-Pagán JC, Jiménez W, Arroyo V, Bosch J, Rodés J. Favorable effects of total paracentesis on splanchnic hemodynamics in cirrhotic patients with tense ascites. Hepatology 1994; 20:30-33.
27. Kao HW, Rakov NE, Savage E, Reynolds TB. The effect of large volume paracentesis on plasma volume: A cause of hypovolemia? Hepatology 1985; 5:403-407.
28. Pinto PC, Amerian J, Reynolds TB. Large-volume paracentesis in nonedematous patients with tense ascites: its effects on intravascular volume. Hepatology 1988; 8:207-210.
29. Gentile S, Angelico M, Bologna E, Capocaccia L. Clinical, biochemical, and hormonal changes after a single, large-volume paracentesis in cirrhosis with ascites. Am J Gastroenterol 1989; 84:279-284.
30. Planas R, Ginès P, Arroyo V, Llach J, Panés J, Vargas V, Salmerón JM, Ginès A, Toledo C, Rimola A, Jiménez W, Asbert M, Gassull MA, Rodés J. Dextran-70 versus albumin as plasma expanders in cirrhotic patients with tense ascites treated with total paracentesis: Results of a randomized study. Gastroenterology 1990; 99:1736-1744.
31. Salerno F, Badalamenti S, Lorenzano E, Moser P, Incierti P. Randomized comparative study of Hemaccel vs albumin infusion after total paracentesis in cirrhotic patients with refractory ascites. Hepatology 1991; 13:707-713.
32. Fassio E, Terg R, Landeira G, Abecasis R, Salemne M, Podesta A, Rodríguez P, Levi D, Kravetz D. Paracentesis with Dextran-70 vs paracentesis with albumin in cirrhosis with tense ascites. Results of a randomized study. J Hepatol 1992; 14:310-316.
33. Cabrera J, Inglada L, Quintero E, Jiménez W, Losada A, Mayor J, Guerra C. Large-volume paracentesis and intravenous saline: effects on the renin-angiotensin system. Hepatology 1991; 14:1025-1028.

Advances in the Treatment of Renal Dysfunction in Cirrhosis

P. Ginès, J. Saló, A. Ginès

INTRODUCTION

The clinical course of patients with cirrhosis is frequently complicated by the development of abnormalities in renal function (1, 2). Although in some patients these abnormalities may be related to structural changes in the kidney, such as glomerular deposition of immunocomplexes in patients with chronic hepatitis B or C virus infection, in most cases the alterations in renal function occur in the absence of significant abnormalities in kidney histology.

The most common renal functional abnormalities in patients with cirrhosis are sodium and water retention and reduction in glomerular filtration rate (GFR) owing to an increased activity of sodium and water-retaining systems and a vasoconstriction of the renal circulation, respectively. The first two abnormalities are key factors in the development of ascites and dilutional hyponatremia, whereas the latter may lead to the development of hepatorenal syndrome.

At present, the only renal functional abnormality that can be managed satisfactorily in patients with cirrhosis is sodium retention. No effective therapy is yet available for the treatment of water retention and renal vasoconstriction in these patients. Nevertheless, the discovery of pharmacological agents with the ability to increase selectively renal water excretion, recent advances in the understanding of the pathogenesis of renal functional abnormalities in cirrhosis, and the introduction of new therapeutic modalities such as the transjugular intrahepatic portasystemic shunt (TIPS), open new perspectives in the management of these disturbances. This chapter describes these novel therapeutic options as well as the classical methods used in the management of renal dysfunction in cirrhosis. A brief discussion of the pathophysiology of renal functional abnormalities is also included.

PATHOPHYSIOLOGY OF RENAL FUNCTIONAL ABNORMALITIES

The most frequent alteration of renal function in patients with cirrhosis is sodium retention. In most cases, sodium retention is due to increased tubular sodium reabsorption since the amount of sodium filtered is normal due to normal GFR. The exact site of the nephron where this increased reabsorption occurs is not completely known, but it is likely that both proximal and distal tubules are involved. The increased tubular sodium reabsorption in cirrhosis is thought to be related, at least in part, to an activation of sodium-retaining systems, i.e., renin-angiotensin-aldosterone system and sympathetic nervous system (3, 4). Other factors, such as hemodynamic alterations in the peritubular capillaries may also participate since in some patients with ascites sodium retention occurs in the absence of activation of these antinatriuretic systems (5, 6). Cirrhotic patients with renal failure usually have more marked sodium retention than patients without renal failure due to both a reduction in filtered sodium load and increased tubular sodium reabsorption.

Water retention is another common abnormality of kidney function in cirrhotic patients with ascites. When mild, this abnormality can only be recognized by showing an impaired capacity to excrete an oral or intravenous water load. In severe cases, water retention leads to the development of dilutional hyponatremia due to an increased total body water relative to total body sodium. Several lines of evidences suggest that the most important pathogenic mechanism of water retention in cirrhosis is a hypersecretion of arginine vasopressin (AVP) which increases water reabsorption in the collecting tubules (7, 8).

Hepatorenal syndrome (HRS) or functional renal failure is the most severe abnormality of renal function that may occur in cirrhotic patients with ascites. This syndrome is characterized by marked reductions of renal blood flow (RBF) and GFR due to vasoconstriction of the renal circulation (9). The pathogenesis of HRS is uncompletely understood but it is probably related to an increased activity of renal vasoconstrictor systems (renin-angiotensin and sympathetic nervous systems). In addition, an inappropriately low production of vasodilator substances within the renal circulation, i.e., prostaglandins, relative to the increased activity of vasoconstrictor factors may also play a role (1, 2).

Several theories have been proposed to explain the pathophysiology of these functional renal abnormalities in cirrhosis. These theories have been discussed in detail in several recent reviews (10, 11). In the most recent theory, the arterial vasodilation hypothesis (12), the functional renal abnormalities are thought to be secondary to a primary disorder in the arterial circulation which results in an abnormal regulation of body fluid homeostasis. According to this theory, sinusoidal portal hypertension is the initial event with resultant arterial vasodilation, mainly located in the splanchnic circulation, causing underfilling of the arterial vascular compartment. This arterial underfilling is then sensed by high-pressure baroreceptors which results in the stimulation of renin-angiotensin and sympathetic nervous systems and non-osmotic AVP hypersecretion. The final consequence of this underfilling of the arterial circulation is renal sodium and water retention, which accumulates as ascites, and, in severe cases, renal vasoconstriction eventually leading to HRS (fig. 1).

THERAPEUTIC APPROACHES TO RENAL FUNCTIONAL ABNORMALITIES

Considering this proposed pathophysiological scheme, several potential therapeutic interventions are possible: blockade of neurohumoral mediators responsible for sodium and water retention, administration of renal vasodilator agents, administration of vasoconstrictor agents to increase systemic vascular resistance, reduction of portal pressure, and liver transplantation.

Natriuretic Agents

For many years, the pharmacological treatment of ascites in cirrhosis has been based on the administration of agents that increase urinary sodium excretion. Two types of natriuretic agents have been used, namely drugs that inhibit sodium transport in the ascending limb of the loop of Henle (loop diuretics, i.e., furosemide) and agents that block the sodium-retaining arm of the renin-angiotensin-aldosterone system (13). Loop diuretics act from the luminal compartment of the renal tubules and directly interfere with the Na^{+}-K^{+}-$2Cl^{-}$ cotransporter. The second type of agents, mainly represented by spironolactone, compete with aldosterone for the binding to the mineralocorticoid receptor in the cells of the collecting tubules. The combination of these two type of drugs is effective in increasing sodium excretion in approximately 90% of cirrhotic patients with ascites. In the remaining cases sodium retention cannot be overcome despite the administration of high doses of natriuretic agents. Currently, no effective pharmacological therapy exists for these patients.

No major advances in the field of natriuretic agents have occurred lately. Torasemide, a loop diuretic recently introduced in some european

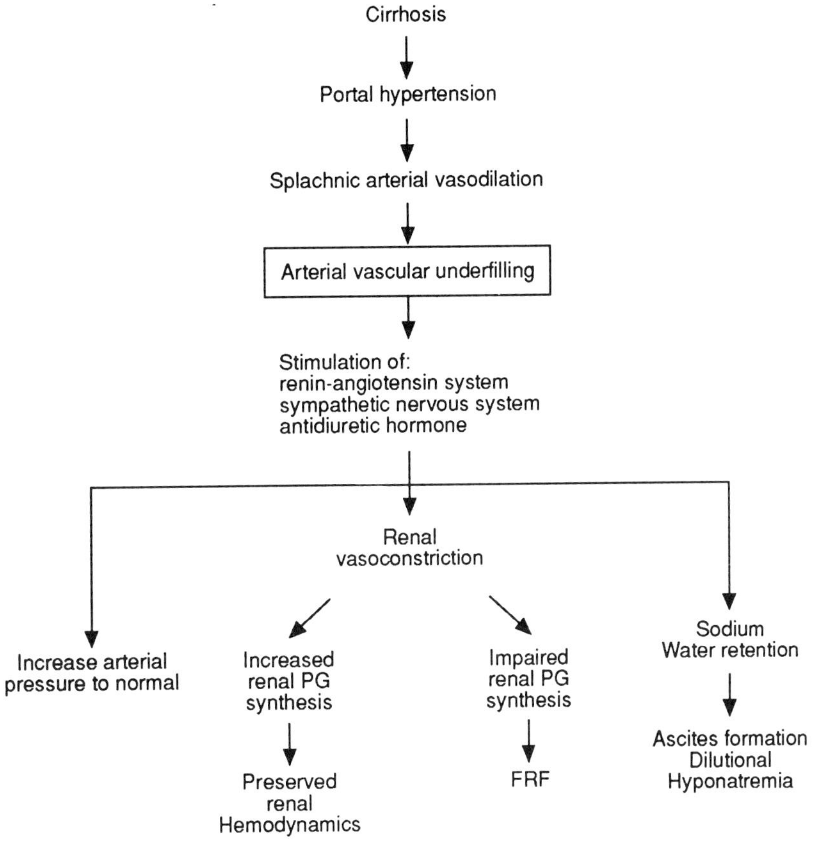

Fig. 1. Proposed pathogenesis of renal functional abnormalities in cirrhosis. FRF: functional renal failure.

countries, with a longer half-life and greater availability than furosemide, has been shown to induce a slightly higher natriuresis and diuresis than furosemide in patients with ascites and moderate sodium retention (14-16). However, it seems unlikely that torasemide could become an effective alternative to furosemide in patients resistant to the classical combination of furosemide and spironolactone. Atrial natriuretic peptide (ANP) has also been evaluated as natriuretic agent in patients with cirrhosis and ascites. The administration of pharmacological doses of ANP, that produce remarkably high plasma levels of this peptide, increases sodium excretion only in patients with mild-to-moderate sodium retention. No significant diuretic and natriuretic effect has been observed in patients with ascites and marked sodium retention treated with ANP (17-19). Therefore, ANP does not offer any therapeutic advantage over other natriuretic agents in the treatment of sodium retention in patients with cirrhosis.

Aquaretic Agents

As previously discussed, cirrhotic patients with ascites frequently develop water retention and dilutional hyponatremia. A non-osmotic hypersecretion of AVP is considered to play a major role in the pathogenesis of this abnormality (7, 8). At present, patients with dilutional hyponatremia are only managed with water restriction since no effective pharmacological therapy is available for this complication.

Recently, two types of drugs have been developed that selectively increase renal water excretion, antagonists of the V_2 receptor of AVP and selective kappa opioid agonists. In 1992, Yamamura et al (20) first described a nonpeptide compound, OPC-31260, that inhibits AVP binding to V_1 and V_2 receptors in a competitive manner but is about 100 times more selective for V_2 receptors. OPC-31260 has two major advantages over previously described peptide V_2 receptor antagonists: is effective after oral administration and has no antidiuretic agonist activity. This compound induces a dose-dependent increase in urine flow and free water clearance and decrease in urine osmolality in normal animals as well as in healthy subjects (20, 21). Its mode of action is different from classical natriuretic agents since the increase in urine volume is associated with only a mild increase in sodium excretion. Also, recent studies have demonstrated that k-opioid agonists increase urine volume and reduce urine osmolality in normal animals and healthy subjects (22-24). As with OPC-31260, this diuretic effect is associated with mild or no natriuresis. The increased water excretion following the administration of k-opioid agonists is accounted for both an inhibition of AVP release from the neurohypophysis and a direct intrarenal effect. Two recent investigations using single doses of OPC-31260 or the selective k-opioid agonist niravoline (RU 51599) have shown that both agents selectively increase water excretion in rats with experimental cirrhosis ascites and water retention (25, 26). Therefore, these compounds offer a novel therapeutic approach for the treatment of water retention and dilutional hyponatremia in cirrhotic patients with ascites.

Renal Vasodilators

Since renal vasoconstriction leading to reduced RBF and GFR is the pathogenic mechanism responsible for HRS, several therapeutic attempts have been made to reduce intrarenal vascular resistance by the administration of substances with renal vasodilator effect, specially prostaglandins. The rationale for the administration of prostaglandins to patients with cirrhosis was based on the observation that patients with HRS have low urinary excretion of vasodilator prostaglandins relative to the increased activity of renal vasoconstrictor systems (1, 2). Moreover, the inhibition of renal prostaglandins synthesis by the administration of non-steroidal antiinflammatory drugs to non-azotemic cirrhotic patients with ascites induces renal failure due to an acute renal vasoconstriction that mimics the renal abnormalities observed in patients with HRS. Unfortunately, however, the administration of prostaglandins, either orally or intravenously, to cirrhotic patients with ascites and HRS is not associated with any significant improvement of renal function (27-30).

Vasoconstrictor Agents

Since renal functional abnormalities in cirrhosis are related to a disturbance in the arterial circulation characterized by arterial vasodilation which leads to reduced systemic vascular resistance, it is not surprising that drugs with vasoconstrictor activity have been used in an attempt to improve renal function. The administration of vasoconstrictor agents (norepinephrine, metaraminol, angiotensin II, ornipressin) to cirrhotic patients with ascites induces arterial vasoconstriction which results in an increase in arterial pressure and systemic vascular resistance and reduction in cardiac output (31-38). A decrease in the degree of activation of endogenous vasoconstrictor systems (renin-angiotenin system, sympathetic nervous system) is also observed, although they remain still activated over normal values (36-38). Unfortunately, however, the administration of vasoconstrictors to cirrhotic patients with severe renal failure is only associated with mild or no increase in RBF and GFR (37-39). This lack of significant improvement of renal function despite the favorable effects observed in the systemic circulation may be related either to the vasoconstrictor effect of the drug on the renal circulation or persistent activation of endogenous vasoconstrictor systems.

A more rational therapeutic approach to the management of renal functional abnormalities in cirrhosis would be to induce vasoconstriction by antagonizing the substance(s) responsible for arterial vasodilation rather than to give vasoconstrictors. This quite simple approach has so far not been possible since the mediator(s) of arterial vasodilation is not known. However, investigations carried out over the last three years have improved our understanding of the mechanisms involved in the pathogenesis of arterial vasodilation. A number of studies have been focused on nitric oxide (NO) as possible mediator of arterial vasodilation in cirrhosis. NO is a very potent vasodilator agent synthetized in the vascular endothelium by the enzyme NO synthase from the aminoacid L-arginine

(39). NO is tonically produced under normal conditions in the vessels and is believed to play a major role in the maintenance of an active state of vasodilation in the arterial circulation. Several studies have been reported suggesting an increased synthesis of NO in animals with experimental cirrhosis and ascites. The activity of NO synthase, as estimated by the "in vitro" production of NO or by the concentration of cyclic guanosine monophosphate, the second messenger of NO, in vascular tissue is increased in rats with cirrhosis and ascites as compared to normal rats (40, 41). Consistent with these findings is the observation that the acute administration of an inhibitor of NO synthesis causes higher increase in arterial pressure in cirrhotic rats with ascites than in normal rats. This increase in arterial pressure induces natriuresis in cirrhotic rats but not in controls (42). Furthermore, the chronic administration of orally-active NO synthesis inhibitors to cirrhotic rats with ascites at a dose that normalizes the activity of NO synthase in the arterial wall, as estimated by aortic cyclic guanosine monophosphate concentration, is associated with normalization of the hyperdynamic circulation (43). Taken together, all these findings suggest that vascular NO synthesis is increased in experimental cirrhosis and plays an important role in the pathogenesis of arterial vasodilation. If an increased production of NO also exists in human cirrhosis, as suggested by a recent study (44), the administration of inhibitors of NO synthesis open new perspectives in the management of renal dysfunction in this condition.

Portasystemic Shunts

It has been known for many years that the relief of portal hypertension by side-to-side or end-to-side portacaval shunts is associated with increased sodium excretion and elimination of ascites in patients with cirrhosis (45). There are also isolated descriptions of reversal of HRS after these procedures (46, 47). Nevertheless, despite these favorable effects, portacaval anastomoses have not become a standard therapy in the management of ascites and/or renal dysfunction in cirrhosis due to the high morbidity and mortality associated with these surgical procedures.

Recently, a nonsurgical method of portal decompression, the transjugular intrahepatic portasystemic shunt (TIPS) has stepped in clinical hepatology (48). This therapeutic procedure consists in the placement of a self-expandable metal stent between an hepatic vein and the intrahepatic portion of the portal vein using a transjugular approach. The main advantage of TIPS over surgical portacaval shunts is the reduction of the operative mortality. The most frequent complications in patients treated with TIPS are hepatic encephalopathy and obstruction of the stent (49, 50). Despite these complications and the absence of controlled studies TIPS has become a popular therapy for patients bleeding from esophageal varices.

There is very limited information, most of which published in abstract form, on the use of TIPS for the treatment of ascites. As with surgical portasystemic shunts, TIPS is associated with favorable effects on renal function, such as increase in sodium excretion and/or improvement in GFR, which result in the elimination of ascites or decrease for diuretic requirements (51-54). The efficacy of TIPS in patients with ascites seems to depend on the status of liver function. Child B patients have good diuretic and natriuretic response whereas in Child C patients the response is usually very poor. In the only controlled study, performed in a small series of patients with refractory ascites, patients treated with TIPS had significantly shorter survival than those treated with paracentesis and intravenous albumin (55). Obviously, more controlled investigations including large groups of patients are needed to define the role of TIPS in the management of ascites in cirrhosis.

Peritoneovenous Shunt

Peritoneovenous shunt was widely used during the past in the treatment of refractory ascites and HRS in patients with cirrhosis (56). The insertion of the shunt causes the passage of ascitic fluid to the systemic circulation which leads to an increased cardiac output and expansion of the intravascular volume. These hemodynamic effects are associated with marked suppression of the activity of endogenous antinatriuretic systems and improvement of renal function (i.e., increased sodium excretion, RBF and GFR) resulting in a reduction of ascites and diuretic requirements in a significant proportion of patients. Despite these favorable effects, the use of the shunt is associated with a number of complications, some of them severe (i.e., coagulopathy, bacterial infection), which limit its clinical applicability. One of the most common and important complications is shunt obstruction (40% probability of obstruction at 1 year) which leads to reappearance of ascites in most patients (57). The obstruction of the shunt can be located either within the valve or at the venous end. This latter complication is frequently associated with superior vena cava thrombosis. The suggestion that the insertion of a titanium tip at the venous end of the shunt prevents thrombosis (58) has not been confirmed in a recent prospective study (59). Therefore, at present, the use of peritoneovenous shunt has markedly declined in most centers.

Paracentesis

A word on paracentesis seems appropriate since it has become a standard therapy for cirrhotic patients with large ascites in most hospitals (60). When performed in association with intravenous infusion of albumin, paracentesis, either total or repeated taps of 4-6 l/day, is more effective and is associated with lower incidence of complications than conventional diuretic treatment (61). The removal of ascites by paracentesis without albumin infusion constantly induces a reduction in the effective intravascular volume, as indicated by an increase in plasma renin activity, which is associated with the development of renal failure and/or hyponatremia in a significant proportion of patients (62). By contrast, paracentesis with intravenous albumin (6-8 g/l of ascites removed) is neither associated with changes in the effective intravascular volume nor with alterations in renal function or activity of antinatriuretic systems. It should be emphasized, however, that paracentesis plus intravenous albumin does not modify the preexisting renal function abnormalities. Neither sodium or water excretion nor GFR improve in patients treated with paracentesis plus intravenous albumin. Therefore, diuretics should be given after paracentesis to avoid the reaccumulation of ascites.

Liver transplantation

In recent years, it has become increasingly evident that abnormalities in the arterial circulation and renal function in patients with cirrhosis and ascites have very important prognostic significance (63, 64). Factors associated with poor prognosis include: arterial hypotension, increased plasma renin activity and norepinephrine concentration, reduced GFR, marked sodium retention, water retention and dilutional hyponatremia. Patients with at least one of these prognostic signs have a 1-year probability of survival of 50% or less. Moreover, in patients with ascites, these parameters are better predictors of survival than standard liver function tests (63). Therefore, cirrhotic patients with ascites and marked abnormalities of renal function or systemic hemodynamics should be evaluated for liver transplantation.

REFERENCES

1. Arroyo V, Ginès P, Rimola A, Gaya J. Renal Function Abnormalities, Prostaglandins, and Effects of Nonsteroidal Anti-inflammatory Drugs in Cirrhosis with Ascites. Am J Med 1986; 81:104-122.
2. Arroyo V, Ginès P, Jiménez W, Rodés J. Ascites, Renal Failure, and Electrolyte Disorders in Cirrhosis. Pathogenesis, Diagnosis, and Treatment. In: McIntyre N, Benhamou JP, Bircher J, Rizzetto M, Rodés J, eds. Oxford Textbook of Clinical Hepatology. Oxford: Oxford University Press, 1991; 427-470.
3. Bernardi M, Trevisani F, Gasbarrini A, Gasbarrini G. Hepatorenal Disorders: Role of the Renin-Angiotensin-Aldosterone System. Sem Liv Dis 1994; 14:23-34.
4. Henriksen JH, Ring-Larsen H. Hepatorenal Disorders: Role of the Sympathetic Nervous System. Sem Liv Dis 1994; 14:35-43.
5. Saló J, Clària J, Ginès A, Jiménez W, Rivera F, Arroyo V, Rodés J. Evidence for an Antinatriuretic Mechanism(s) other than the Renin-Aldosterone and the Sympathetic Nervous Systems in Cirrhosis with Ascites. J Hepatol 1993; 18:S61(Abstr).
6. Atucha NM, Cegarra M, Ramírez A, Quesada T, García-Estany J. Pressure Diuresis and Natriuresis in Cirrhotic Rats. Am J Physiol 1993; 265:G1045-G1049.
7. Arroyo V, Clària J, Saló J, Jiménez W. Antidiuretic Hormone and the Pathogenesis of Water Retention in Cirrhosis with Ascites. Sem Liv Dis 1994; 14:44-58.
8. Ginès P, Abraham WT, Schrier RW. Vasopressin in Pathophysiological States. Sem Nephrol 1994; 14:384-397.
9. Epstein M, Berk DP, Hollenberg NK, Adams DF, Chalmers TC, Abrams HL, Merrill JP. Renal Failure in the Patient with Cirrhosis: The Role of Active Vasoconstriction. Am J Med 1970; 49:175-185.

10. Levy M. Pathogenesis of Sodium Retention in Early Cirrhosis of the Liver: Evidence for Vascular Overfilling. Sem Liv Dis 1994; 14:4-13.
11. Schrier RW, Niederberger M, Weigert A, Ginès P. Peripheral Arterial Vasodilation: Determinant of Functional Spectrum of Cirrhosis. Sem Liv Dis 1994; 14:14-22.
12. Schrier RW, Arroyo V, Bernardi M, Epstein M, Henriksen JH, Rodés J. Peripheral Arterial Vasodilation Hypothesis: A Proposal for the Initiation of Sodium and Water Retention in Cirrhosis. Hepatol 1988; 8:1151-1157.
13. Ginès P, Arroyo V, Rodés J. Pharmacotherapy of Ascites Associated with Cirrhosis. Drugs 1992; 43:316-332.
14. Laffi G, Marra F, Buzzelli G, Azzena G, Meacci E, De Feo ML, La Villa G, Gentilini P. Comparison of the Effects of Torasemide and Furosemide in Nonazotemic Patients with Ascites: A Randomized, Double-blind Study. Hepatology 1991; 13:1101-1105.
15. Gerbes AL, Bertheau-Reiha U, Falkner C, Jüngst D, Paumgartner G. Advantages of the New Loop Diuretic Torasemide over Furosemide in Patients with Cirrhosis and Ascites. J Hepatol 1993; 17:353-358.
16. Fiaccadori F, Pedretti G, Pasetti G, Pizzaferri P, Elia G. Torasemide versus Furosemide in Cirrhosis: A Long-term, Double-blind, Randomized Clinical Study. Clin Investig 1993; 71:579-584.
17. Salerno F, Badalamenti S, Incerti P, Capozza L, Mainardi L. Renal Response to Atrial Natriuretic Peptide in Patients with Advanced Liver Cirrhosis. Hepatology 1988; 8:21-26.
18. Laffi G, Pinzani M, Meacci E, La Villa G, Renzi D, Baldi E, Cominelli F, Marra F, Gentillini P. Renal Hemodynamic and Natriuretic Effects of Human Natriuretic Factor Infusion in Cirrhosis With Ascites. Gastroenterology 1989; 96:167
19. Ginès P, Titó Ll, Arroyo V, Llach J, Salmerón JM, Ginès A, Jiménez W, Badalamenti S, Rivera F, Rodés J. Renal Insensitivity to Atrial natriuretic Peptide in patients with Cirrhosis and Ascites. Effect of Increasing Systemic Arterial Pressure. Gastroenterology 1992; 102:280-286.
20. Yamamura Y, Ogawa H, Yamashita H, Chihara T, Miyamoto H, Nakamura S, Onogawa T, Yamashita T, Hosokawa T, Mori T, Tominaga M, Yabuchi Y. Characterization of a Novel Aquaretic Agent, OPC-31260, as an Orally Effective, Nonpeptide Vasopressin V_2 Receptor Antagonist. Br J Pharmacol 1992; 105:787-791.
21. Ohnishi A, Orita Y, Okahara R, Fujihara H, Inoue T, Yamamura Y, Yabuchi Y, Tanaka T. Potent Aquaretic Agent. A Novel Nonpeptide Selective Vasopressin 2 Antagonist (OPC-31260) in Men. J Clin Invest 1993; 92:2653-2659.
22. Hamon G, Fatin M, Le Matret O, Jonquey S, Vincent JC, Bichet DG. Pharmacological Profile of Niravoline, a New Aquaretic Compound. J Am Soc Nephrol 1994; 5:272A(Abstr).
23. Sinnassamy P, Sultan P, Bichet DG. Aquaretic Effect of Niravoline (RU 51599), a Kappa-opioid Agonist in Healthy Volunteers. J Am Soc Nephrol 1994; 5:373A(Abstr).
24. Hamon G, Jouquey S. Kappa Agonists and Vasopressin Secretion. Horm Res 1990; 34:129-132.
25. Tsuboi Y, Ishikawa SE, Fujisawa G, Okada K, Saito T. Therapeutic Efficacy of the Non-peptide AVP Antagonist OPC-31260 in Cirrhotic Rats. Kidney Int 1994; 46:237-244.
26. Bosch M, Jiménez W, Angeli P, Leivas A, Clària J, Graziotto A, Arroyo V, Rivera F, Rodés J. Aquaretic Efficacy of the Kappa-opioid Receptor Agonist RU 51599 in Cirrhotic Rats with Ascites. J Hepatol 1994; 21(Suppl 1):S7(Abstr).
27. Fichman MP, Littenburg G, Brooker G, Horton R. Effect of Prostaglandin A1 on Renal and Adrenal Function in Man. Circ Res 1972; 30(Suppl 2):19-35.
28. Arieff AI, Chidsey CA. Renal function in Cirrhosis and the Effects of Prostaglandin A1. Am J Med 1974; 56:695-703.
29. Zussman RM, Axelrod L, Tolkoff-Rubin N. The Treatment of the Hepatorenal Syndrome with Intrarenal Administration of prostaglandin E1. Prostaglandins 1977; 13:819-30.
30. Ginès A, Salmerón JM, Ginès P, Arroyo V, Jiménez W, Rivera F, Rodés J. Oral Misoprostol or Intravenous Prostaglandin E2 Do Not Improve Renal Function in Patients with Cirrhosis and Ascites with Hyponatremia or Renal Failure. J Hepatol 1993; 17:220-226.
31. Gornel DL, Lancestremete RG, Papper S, Lowenstein LM. Acute Changes in Renal Excretion of Water and Solute in Patients with Laennec's Cirrhosis Induced by the Administration of the Pressor Amine Metaraminol. J Clin Invest 1962; 41:594-603.
32. Lancestremere RG, Klinger EL, Frisch E, Papper S. Simultaneous Determination of Cardiac Output and Renal Function in Patients with Laennec's Cirrhosis during the Administration of the Pressor Amine Metaraminol. J Lab Clin Med 1963; 61:820-825.
33. Laragh JH, Cannon PJ, Bentzel CJ, Sicinski AM, Meltser JL. Angiotensin II, Norepinephrine and Renal Transport of Electrolytes and Water in Normal Man and in Cirrhosis with Ascites. J Clin Invest 1963; 42:1179-1192.
34. Fischer JE, Balderssarini RJ. False Neurotransmitters and Hepatic Failure. Lancet 1971; 2:75-79.
35. Shapiro MD, Nicholls KM, Groves BM, Kluge R, Chung HM, Bichet DG, Schrier RW. Interrelationship between Cardiac Output and Vascular Resistance as Determinants of Effective Arterial Blood Volume in Cirrhotic Patients. Kidney Int 1985; 28:206-211.
36. Lenz K, Hörnatgl H, Druml W, Grim G, Laggner A, Schneeweisz B, Kleinberger G. Beneficial Effect of 8-Ornithin Vasopressin on Renal Dysfunction in Decompensated Cirrhosis. Gut 1989; 30:90-96.
37. Lenz K, Hörnatgl H, Druml W, Reither H, Schmid R, Schneeweisz B, Laggner A, Grimm G, Schneeweisz B, Gerbes AL. Ornipressin in the Treatment of Functional Renal Failure in Decompensated Liver Cirrhosis. Gastroenterology 1991; 101:1060-1067.
38. Saló J, Ginès A, Inglada L, Quer JC, Planas R, Ginès

P, Clària J, Jiménez W, Arroyo V, Rodés J. Ornipressin and Ornipressin plus Dopamine in Cirrhotic Patients with Renal Failure. J Hepatol 1993; 18:S145(Abstr).
39. Moncada S, Palmer RMJ, Higgs EA. Nitric Oxide: Physiology, Pathophysiology and Pharmacology. Pharmacol Rev 1991; 43:109-142.
40. Ros J, Jiménez W, Lamas S, Clària J, Arroyo V, Rivera F, Rodés J. Nitric Oxide Production in Arterial Vessels of Cirrhotic Rats. Hepatology (in press).
41. Niederberger M, Ginès P, Tsai P, Morris K, Weigert A, MacMurtry I, Schrier RW. Increased Aortic Cyclic Guanosine Monophosphate Concentration in Experimental Cirrhosis in Rats: Evidence for a Role of Nitric Oxide in the Pathogenesis of Arterial Vasodilation in Cirrhosis. Hepatology (in press).
42. Clària J, Jiménez W, Ros J, Asbert M, Castro A, Arroyo V, Rivera F, Rodés J. Pathogenesis of Arterial Hypotension in Cirrhotic Rats with Ascites: Role of Endogenous Nitric Oxide. Hepatology 1992; 15:343-349.
43. Martin PY, Niederberger M, Morris K, Tsai P, Ginès P, Schrier RW. Normalization of Vascular Nitric Oxide Production Corrects Arterial Vasodilation and Hyperdynamic Circulation in Rats with Cirrhosis and Ascites. J Am Soc Nephrol 1994; 5:89P(Abstr).
44. Guarner C, Soriano G, Tomas A, Bulbena O, Novella MT, Balanzo J, Vilardell F, Mourelle M, Moncada S. Increased Serum Nitrite and Nitrate Levels in Patients with Cirrhosis: Relationship with Endotoxemia. Hepatology 1993; 18:1139-1143.
45. Orloff MJ. Pathogenesis and Surgical Treatment of Intractable Ascites Associated with Alcoholic Cirrhosis. Ann N Y Acad Sci 1970; 170:213-238.
46. Schroeder ET, Numann PO, Chamberlain BE. Functional Renal Failure in Cirrhosis. Recovery after Portacaval Shunt. Ann Intern Med 1970; 72:923-928.
47. Ariyan J, Sweeney T, Kernstein MD. The Hepatorenal Syndrome: Recovery after Portacaval Shunt. Ann Surg 1975; 181:847-849.
48. Rössle M, Haag K, Ochs A, Sellinger M, Nöldge G, Perarnau JM, Berger E, Blum U, Gabelmann A, Hauenstein K, Langer M, Gerok W. The Transjugular Intrahepatic Portosystemic Stent-shunt Procedure for Variceal Bleeding. N Engl J Med 1994; 330:165-171.
49. Sanyal AJ, Freedman AM, Shifman ML, Purdum III PP, Luketic VA, Cheatham AK. Portosystemic Encephalopathy after Transjugular Intrahepatic Portosystemic Shunt: Results of a Prospective Controlled Study. Hepatology 1994; 20:46-65.
50. Freedman AM, Sanyal AJ. Complications of Transjugular Portosystemic Shunts. Semin Intervent Radiol 1994; 11:161-177.
51. García-Villarreal L, Zozaya JM, Quiroga J, Sangro B, Bilbao JI, Longo J, Prieto J. Prótesis Intrahepática Portosistémica en el Tratamiento de la Ascitis Refractaria. Estudio Piloto. Gastroenterol Hepatol 1993; 16:8-12.
52. Ochs A, Rössle M, Haag K, Gerber A, Morgenroth A, Deibert P, Hauenstein KH, Langer M, Gerok W. TIPS for Hepatorenal Syndrome. Hepatology 1994; 20(Pt 2):114A(Abstr).
53. Ferral H, Bjarnason H, Wegryn SA, Rengel GJ, Nazarian GK, Rank JM, Tadavarthy SM, Hunter DW, Castaneda-Zuniga WR. Refractory Ascites: Early Experience in Treatment with Transjugular Intrahepatic Portosystemic Shunt. Radiology 1993; 189:795-801.
54. Benner KG, Sahagun G, Saxon R, Barton RE, Keller F, Rabkin J, Reed M, Rösch J. Selection of Patients Undergoing Transjugular Intrahepatic Portosystemic Shunt for Refractory Ascites. Hepatology 1994; 20 (Pt 2):114A(Abstr).
55. Lebrec D, Giuily N, Hadengue A, Vilgrain V, Lassen C, Poynard T. Transjugular Intrahepatic Portosystemic Shunt vs Paracentesis for Refractory Ascites. Results of a Randomized Trial. Hepatology 1994; 20 (Pt 2):201A(Abstr).
56. Forns X, Ginès A, Ginès P, Arroyo V. Management of Ascites and Renal Failure in Cirrhosis. Sem Liv Dis 1994; 14: 82-96.
57. Ginès P, Arroyo V, Vargas V, Planas R, Casafont F, Panés J, Hoyos M, Viladomiu L, Rimola A, Morillas R, Salmeron JM, Ginès A, Esteban R, Rodés J. Paracentesis with Intravenous Infusion of Albumin as Compared with Peritoneovenous Shunting in Cirrhosis with Refractory Ascites. N Engl J Med 1991; 325:829-835.
58. Hillaire S, Labianca M, Borgonovo G, Smajda C, Grange D, Franco D. Peritoneovenous Shunting of Intractable Ascites in Patients with Cirrhosis: Improving Results and Predictive Factors of Failure. Surgery 1993; 113:373-379.
59. Ginès A, Planas R, Angeli P, Guarner P, Salerno F, Ginès P, Saló J, Rodríguez N, Doménech E, Soriano G, Anibarro L, Gassull MA, Gatta A, Arroyo V, Rodés J. Treatment of Patients with Cirrhosis and Refractory Ascites by LeVeen Shunt with Titanium Tip. Comparison with therapeutic paracentesis. Hepatology (in press).
60. Arroyo V, Ginès A, Saló J. A European Survey on the Treatment of Ascites in Cirrhosis. J Hepatol 1994; 21:667-672.
61. Ginès P, Arroyo V, Quintero E, Planas R, Bory F, Cabrera J, Rimola A, Viver J, Camps J, Jiménez W, Mastai R, Gaya J, Rodés J. Comparison of Paracentesis and Diuretics in the Treatment of Cirrhotics with Tense Ascites. Results of a Randomized Study. Gastroenterology 1987; 93:234-241.
62. Ginès P, Titó Ll, Arroyo V, Planas R, Panés J, Viver J, Torres M, Humbert P, Rimola A, Llach J, Badalamenti S, Jiménez W, Gaya J, Rodés J. Randomized Comparative Study of Therapeutic Paracentesis with and without Intravenous Albumin in Cirrhosis. Gastroenterology 1988; 94:1493-1502.
63. Llach J, Ginès P, Arroyo V, Rimola A, Titó Ll, Badalamenti S, Jiménez W, Gaya J, Rivera F, Rodés J. Prognostic Value of Arterial Pressure, Endogenous Vasoactive Systems, and Renal Function in Cirrhotic Patients Admitted to the Hospital for the Treatment of Ascites. Gastroenterology 1988; 94:482-487.
64. Arroyo V, Ginès P, Navasa M, Rimola A. Renal Failure in Cirrhosis and Liver Transplantation. Transplant Proc 1993; 25:1734-1739.

Advances in the Treatment of Hepatic Encephalopathy

A. T. Blei

INTRODUCTION

The importance of hepatic encephalopathy is recognized in the Child-Pugh classification as one of the factors influencing prognosis in cirrhosis (1). In fulminant hepatic failure, the presence of encephalopathy defines the syndrome and, in its advanced stage, is a key prognostic factor that becomes an indication for emergency liver transplantation (2). However, most cases seen in hepatological practice represent acute changes in mental state brought on by a precipitating event in cirrhotic individuals. For such episodes, removal of the inciting event as well as administration of available therapy is for the most part sufficient to reverse the abnormality. Thus, new developments in recent years originate from studies of the pathogenesis of this complex neuropsychiatric syndrome. From this approach, newer therapeutic avenues are being developed.

A rigorous evaluation of the efficacy of therapy in hepatic encephalopathy is a difficult task. Clinical trials in cirrhotic subjects have been carried out in the different clinical forms of presentation: acute encephalopathy, chronic portal-systemic encephalopathy and subclinical encephalopathy. The simultaneous presence of precipitating factors makes studies in acute encpehalopathy of cirrhotics very difficult to perform. Chronic encephalopathy, a prominent clinical problem when non-selective portacaval shunts were frequently performed, is less common as surgery for portal hypertension has become more selective. In subclinical encephalopathy, patients can be evaluated in a more stable condition, and this group is probably the best to evaluate the role of therapy. However, some of the neurochemical mechanisms present in subclinical states may not be the same as those operating in acute encephalopathy. There is even a terminology problem, as for some groups chronic encephalopathy represents more frequent episodes of precipitant-induced events, for others it is equated with «spontaneous» episodes while a permanent change in mental state is the definition for a few.

Treatment of hepatic encephalopathy can be directed at four different levels. We will mainly focus this review on *advances* in each of these target areas.

THE GUT

Clinical experience has taught that the neurotoxin(s) responsible for hepatic encephalopathy arise from the gut. These substances are of nitrogenous origin, as dietary protein indiscretion can precipitate changes in mental state. They are related to intestinal bacterial metabolism, as diverse antibiotics have shown to be effective therapy. When present in portal venous blood, these substances must undergo a high

Supported by a Merit Review from the Veterans Administration Research Service.

hepatic extraction, as construction of a surgical portal-systemic shunt will precipitate a change in mental state. Ammonia continues to meet these theoretical requirements, including recent evidence of very high portal venous levels, almost 10 fold over peripheral ones, with a normal hepatic extraction of approximately 0.9 (3).

Dietary Manipulation

Patients with cirrhosis have an increase in their protein requirements (4). In chronic hepatic encephalopathy, protein restriction should be avoided. Administration of vegetable protein has been clearly shown superior to animal protein. In a crossover study, 8 subjects with cirrhosis and chronic encephalopathy treated with lactulose underwent testing on equicaloric, equinitrogenic diets (5). There was a consistently better score on neuropsychological tests when vegetable protein was provided. The benefits of such an approach may be related to both an improved nitrogen balance (due to a reduced urinary nitrogen excretion) as well as the ability of dietary fiber to act as a substrate for colonic acidification. In this regard, a preliminary report suggests that it is the presence of fiber, rather than the source of protein, which makes the favorable impact (6). In countries with a traditionally high fiber content in their diet, such as Mexico (6), this approach may be better tolerated than in areas with a low fiber content and where such a diet may result in abdominal cramping and flatulence.

Oral Antibiotics

A double-blind study has examined the effects of neomycin in the treatment of hepatic encephalopathy (7). Patients with stages I to III were studied, with diverse precipitating factors; subjects were excluded if they had chronic hepatic encephalopathy or had multiorgan failure. Twenty patients received neomycin, 6g/day, and compared to 19 subjects with placebo. The time to regression to stage 0 was similar in both groups, 39 ± 23 hours with neomycin vs. 50 ± 22 hours with placebo. The study highlights the difficulty in performing clinical trials in such patients, as the course of the precipitating event cannot be controlled during randomization. The drug is generally not given on a chronic basis, because of concern with long-term ototoxicity and renal injury.

The mechanism of action of neomycin has traditionally been attributed to a reduction in aerobic, urease containing gram-negative bacilli. However, non-bacterial mechanisms have been proposed (8). These are based on a site of action of the drug in the small intestinal mucosa, where glutamine is broken down to ammonia and glutamate. In the rat small intestine, paromomycin had no effects on the generation of ammonia (9).

Other antibiotics have also been used in the treatment of acute episodes of encephalopathy. Metronidazole was as effective as neomycin in a study where the majority of the patients had chronic encephalopathy (10). The elimination half-life of metronidazole was almost tripled in cirrhotic patients in coma grade 2-4 (11) and the reduced clearance calls for a reduction of the starting dose of this drug to 250 mg bid. In 12 patients with chronic encephalopathy resistant to lactulose, vancomycin (2 g/day), administered in a double-blind crossover trial, improved the clinical status and the EEG findings (12). Of interest, vancomycin is effective against anaerobic Gram negative rods but not against aerobic bacteria. An interesting recent observation points at the presence of a slow colonic transit during early stages of encephalopathy (13). This aggravates the encephalopathic process and emphasizes the beneficial effects of colonic evacuation. An oral antibiotic, rifaximin, has been tested in Italy with greater patient tolerance than lactulose (14).

Non-Absorbable Disaccharides

The mechanisms by which these compounds exert their beneficial effects continue to be uncovered. In germ-free rats, administration of lactulose (β-galactosidefructose) and lactitol (β-galactosidesorbitol) did not result in the expected increase of fecal nitrogen and reduction of urinary nitrogen, confirming the central role of the gut flora in the mediation of lactulose's effects (15). An in vitro system was used to show that gut flora break down lactulose to acetate but not other short-chain fatty acids (C_{3-6}), substances that may have neurotoxic effects if absorbed. Although the fecal concentration of nitrogen was reduced with lactulose, nitrogen fecal excretion was increased due to a rise in stool mass (16, 17). A role for extraluminal effects of lactulose is uncertain; in support of it, the production of tumor necrosis factor by human monocytes exposed to endotoxin in vitro was reduced by co-incubation with lactulose (18).

A crystalline, pure preparation of lactulose, devoid of galactose and lactose contaminants seen in the usual formulation, was well tolerated in cirrhotics (19). Whether long term therapy with this compound will prevent the problem of flatulence and abdominal cramping, is unknown. Exposure to a non-diarrhogenic dose of lactulose appears to mitigate the severity of diarrhea when a larger dose is then administered (20).

Considerable interest has risen on whether lactitol, another synthetic non-absorbable disaccharide, has benefits over lactulose. Clinical efficacy in subclinical hepatic encephalopathy (21) and in chronic hepatic encephalopathy (22) was not different between the two drugs. Two meta-analyses concluded that lactitol was associated with less flatulence and was more palatable (23, 24), side-effects that interfere with patient compliance for long term therapy. Both drugs can increase fecal fat excretion to a mild to moderate degree (25).

Interest in prolonged treatment for chronic hepatic encephalopathy with non-absorbable disaccharides has been rekindled with the increasing application of TIPS (transjugular intrahepatic portal-systemic shunt) for the treatment of portal hypertension (26). In a controlled trial, up to 30% of patients had episodes of precipitant-induced encephalopathy (27), episodes that could be related to the placement of the TIPS itself, such as potential for infection or hemodynamic effects with alteration in renal function. Changes consistent with chronic encephalopathy were especially prominent in the first month afeter stent placement. This abnormality improved with time, reflecting in part the effects os stent stenosis/occlusion. Chronic, disabling encephalopathy appears to occur in a small percentage of patients, and may also be related to the development of liver failure after placement of the TIPS. Evaluation of prophylactic therapy for post-TIPS encephalopathy may be also extended to other drugs.

Combination Therapy

No formal double-blind study has evaluated the combination of non-absorbable disaccharides with neomycin. The available information from previous studies that indicates a potential additive effect of disaccharides with neomycin on nitrogen metabolism has been recently reviewed (28). Different bacterial populations appear involved in the action of the drugs. While obligate and facultative anaerobic flora may be responsible for the breakdown of lactulose, the effects of neomycin appear directed at a more selected aerobic population.

THE LIVER

Effects on the Urea Cycle

Ammonia is removed in the liver by two mechanisms: A low-affinity, high-capacity system located in periportal hepatocytes (the urea cycle) and a high-affinity, low capacity system in perivenous hepatocytes (glutamine synthesis). Two decades ago it was shown that some cirrhotics with encephalopathy have a reduced capacity for urea synthesis (29). Normal values, reported by others (30), may reflect different degrees of liver dysfunction as well as test conditions, especially as it concerns protein intake. Increasing the efficiency of the urea cycle may improve the clinical status of cirrhotic patients.

Oral zinc has been administered with this goal. Zinc is a cofactor in several enzymes that participate in the complex reactions of the urea cycle. Administration of zinc was shown to improve the activity of a key enzyme in the urea cycle or cirrhotic rats (31). In one trial, zinc acetate, 600 mg/day, improved the results of neuropsychological testing (32), while in a second study zinc sulfate had no appreciable effects (33). More recently, a patient in whom zinc deficiency was induced by oral histidine developed encephalopathy that was corrected by the administration of zinc (34). Also, there may be direct effects of zinc in the brain. Reduced zinc levels have been reported in autopsied brain tissue of cirrhotics dying in hepatic coma (35). In brain tissue, zinc may modulate glutamatergic neurotransmission (36). As nutritional deficiencies can be present in cirrhotics, especially in those with persistent alcohol intake, supplementation with zinc is an inexpensive and low-risk approach to the treatment of encephalopathy.

L-Ornithine-L-aspartate has received attention in Europe as a new approach to the treatment of encephalopathy. Each compound can act as a substrate for the urea cycle as well as glutamine synthesis in cirrhotics (37). Preliminary testing suggests a beneficial effect in cirrhotics with chronic encephalopathy when administered at doses of 18-27 g/day. The drug is practically void of side-effects and is available in an intravenous formulation. Full publication of these preliminary reports is awaited.

Alternative Pathways for Nitrogen Excretion

Children with urea cycle enzyme deficiences are chronically exposed to the deleterious effects of chronic hyperammonemia. Rational therapy is based on developing alternative pathways for nitrogen excretion. This approach has been now extended to the cirrhotic individual.

Sodium benzoate, after hepatic conversion to benzoyl CoA (fig. 1), combines with glycine to form hippurate, which es then eliminated via the urine. Ammonia is a direct precusor for the synthesis of glycine while glutamate can also be a precursor for glycine synthesis. As a result, one molecule of ammonia is eliminated with one molecule of hippurate. This is the basis for its successful use in children with urea cycle enzyme deficiencies (38).

In one study from New Delhi (30), sodium benzoate (10 g/day) was as effective as lactulose in improving the mental state of patients with acute encephalopathy. Normalization of the PSE (portal-systemic encephalopathy) index, ammonia levels and correction of neurophysiological parameters occurred in a similar proportion of patients; the time to improvement was also similar. Preliminary reports from Mexico confirm these findings and suggest a role for benzoate in chronic hepatic encephalopathy (40). An experience in the US is clouded by the concomitant administration of lactulose or neomycin (41). The sodium load is not negligible, and the drug may be difficult to administer in patients with ascites. Newer salts, like arginine-benzoate, are being developed.

Sodium phenylbutyrate (PB) has the advantage over benzoate of eliminating two molecules of nitrogen per molecule of drug (fig. 1). Phenylbutyrate is β-oxidized to phenylacetate, a compound so malodorous that cannot be administered directly. Phenylacetate is conjugated to glutamine (containing two nitrogen molecules derived from ammonia) to phenylacetylglutamine, a reaction that occurs in humans and subhuman primates in the liver and kidney. Phenylacetylglutamine (PAG) is excreted in the urine and studies in children with urea cycle enzyme deficiencies indicate an 85-90% efficiency in conversion of PB to PAG (42).

We have performed a preliminary study in cirrhotic individuals, looking at the efficiency of conversion. Five stable cirrhotic subjects received 10-20 g of sodium phenylbutyrate over a 3 day period in controlled metabolic conditions. With this dose, plasma glutamine levels were significantly reduced (fig. 2) and the efficiency of conversion ranged from 60 to 90%

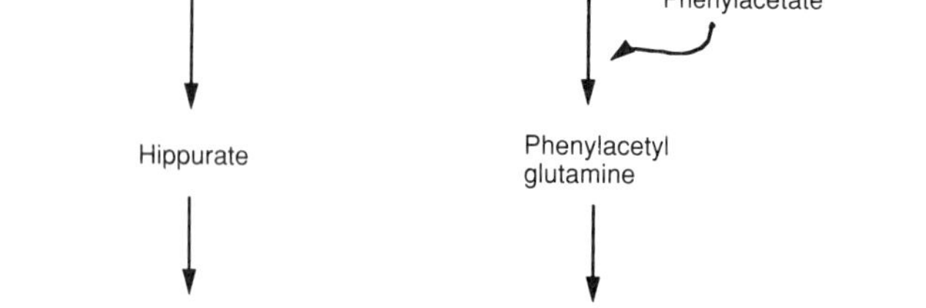

Fig. 1. Alternative pathways of nitrogen metabolism. When ammonia cannot be utilized in the urea cycle, sodium benzoate (after activation to benzoyl-CoA) can remove ammonia by conjugating with glycine; the hippurate formed is removed in the urine. Phenylbutyrate is beta-oxidized to phenylacetate, which is then conjugated in liver and kidney to phenylacetylglutamine, a product that is excreted in the urine.

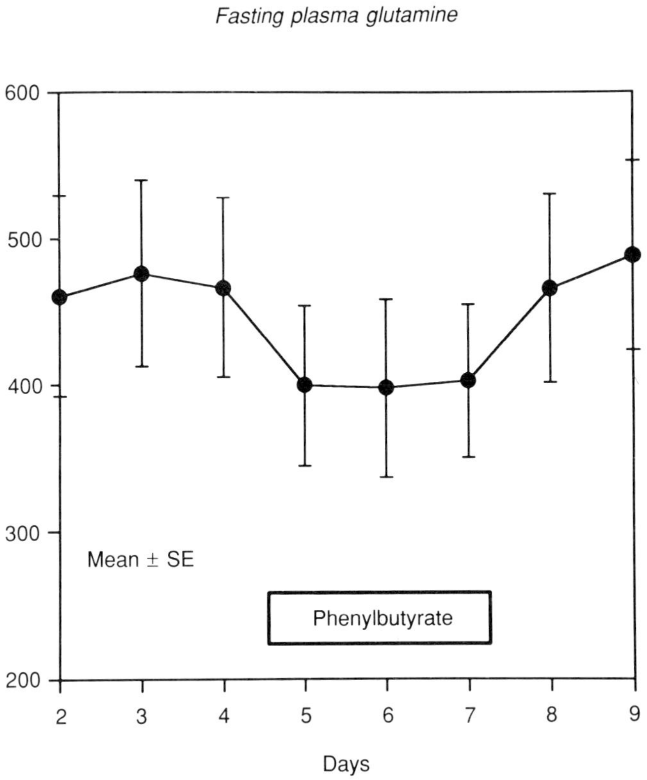

Fig. 2. Five cirrhotic patients were studied at our Clinical Research Center under constant metabolic conditions and a 40 g protein diet. Administration of oral sodium phenylbutyrate (20 g/day) during days 4 through 6 of the study resulted in a significant reduction in the next day's fasting plasma glutamine levels.

(43). Further studies are needed to delineate the role of phenylbutyrate in the treatment of encephalopathy in cirrhosis.

BLOOD-BRAIN BARRIER

The rationale for the use of *branched-chain amino acids* was based on a widely held view in the 70's, that has been recently re-examined by its proponent (44). It postulated that hepatic encephalopathy occurs as a result for an increased entry of aromatic amino acids into the brain, amino acids that are precursors of true and false neurotransmitters. This entry would be favored by two mechanisms: *a*) The imbalance of plasma amino acids seen in cirrhosis, where high levels of aromatic amino acids such as phenylalanine and tyrosine are present (due to a reduction in hepatic catabolism), in contrast to a reduction in branched chain amino acids like valine, leucine and isoleucine (due in part to a state of insulin resistance present in cirrhosis). *b*) Studies in rats after portacaval shunts suggest that the increased brain glutamine levels in hepatic encephalopathy (generated from ammonia) are exchanged with aromatic amino acids via a neutral amino acid carrier at the level of the blood-brain barrier (45), favoring the entry of the latter into brain.

Much controversy has surrounded the clinical use of branched chain amino acids. Their infusion improves the aromatic/branched chain amino acid plasma ratio. Recent human studies have even challenged the postulated increase of pehnyalanine entry into brain (46). A thorough review of the large clinical experience in all types of encepahlopathy has been reported (47). Even two meta-analyses of this experience have arrived at different conclusions. While one showed no clear benefit in mental state (48), the other concluded that the most seriously ill patients should receive the medication (49). A more recent double-blind evaluation in chronic encephalopathy compared the effects of branched chain amino acids to equicaloric casein (50). The former was more effective in providing an adequate nitrogen supply and in improving the mental state. In another recent double-blind study, cirrhotic patients were deemed more fit to drive (51), an assessment based on the results of psychometric tests. We have completed a study assessing the performance of cirrhotics «behind the wheel» and found no major deficit in a small group of selected patients with no prior history of encephalopathy and abnormal neuropsychological tests (52).

One can conclude that the benefits of the encephalopathic state are marginal and the cost-benefit relationship does not justify its widespread use. It is an effective nitrogen source for cirrhotic patients who are intolerant of dietary protein, and in this nutritional aspect, its use has a rationale.

BRAIN

Once the putative toxin(s) responsible for the alteration in mental state reach the brain, a cascade of neurochemical changes can be now detected. These will differ according to the clinical setting as well as exhibit inter individual variability. Even more strikingly, some subjects will not develop encephalopathy at all. It is not surprising, then, that drugs that alter a neurochemical mechanism will be effective only in a subset of patients.

Hepatic encephalopathy does not arise from a brain energy deficit, as would be the case of hypoglycemic-induced coma. An alteration of multiple neurotransmitter systems can be detected in animal models as well as in the brain of subjects dying in hepatic coma (53). Both excitatory and inhibitory neurotransmission is affected. A series of alterations described in excitatory pathways, such as those mediated via glutamatergic transmission, have not yet led to new therapeutic approaches. Most of the interest has focused on pharmacological manipulation of inhibitory systems, where alterations in GABAergic neurotransmission has received the greatest interest. Drugs that affect the dopaminergic and serotoninergic systems have also been examined.

Alterations in GABAergic Neurotransmission. Flumazenil

This antagonist of central benzodiazepine receptors would exert beneficial effects by displacing «endogenous benzodiazepines» from its binding site at the level of the $GABA_A$-receptor. The nature of these endogenous ligands is still controversial. Though diazepam and desmethyldiazepam have been found in the brain of subjects dying with fulminant hepatic failure who were reportedly never exposed to these drugs (54), it would appear that the nature of the largest group of compounds that react in a radioreceptor assay are not exactly benzodiazepines (55). The term «endozepines» has been coined to describe them. When present in the plasma of subjects with acute liver failure, they are highest in stage IV encephalopathy (56), raising doubts about a «classic» origin of a hepatic encephalopathy-related toxin from the intestinal tract. Their nature remains elusive and may even reflect compounds that are synthesized in the brain itself (57). A picture of idiopathic stupor responsive to flumazenil has been described in adults (58) and characterization of these endozepines may arise from these patients. It should be remembered that endogenous ligands with antagonistic properties, like diazepam-binding inhibitor, are also elevated in patients with hepatic encephalopathy (59).

An important double-blind study in cirrhotic patients with stage IV encephalopathy and in whom precipitating events had been excluded has shown that iv flumazenil resulted in a transient neurological improvement in 40% of subjects (60): There was no awakening in 14 episodes treated with placebo while improvement from stage IV to II-III in 6 of 13 episodes. The response ocurred in minutes to hours, a time frame that is uncommon with lactulose, where up to 48-60 hs pass before a beneficial effect is reportedly seen. There was no relationship between plasma benzodiazepine levels before therapy and the response to the drug. The crossover design confirmed the findings of the first group.

A second double-blind study has been reported as a preliminary communication (61) and confirms the findings of the earlier report. A preliminary report suggests a benefit for flumazenil in some patients with subclinical changes (62). A negative study in patients with overt encephalopathy was also reported in abstract form (63). A psychotic reaction was reported in one cirrhotic patient receiving flumazenil (64). It appears then that iv flumazenil has some beneficial effects in a subset of patients with deep encephalopathy. The benefit appears transient and the mechanisms by which the drug is effective remains to be elucidated. An oral formulation is not available in the US.

Alteration in Dopaminergic Neurotransmission

Considerable interest in the potential benefits to dopaminergic agonists in chronic hepatic encephalopathy led to trials with drugs like L-dopa and bromocriptine in the late 70's (reviewed in 65). Though L-dopa did not appear useful, bromocriptine, in one rigorous evaluation, benefited a few patients with chronic encephalopathy (66). This was not observed in another study (67). Bromocriptine can be administered to patients with chronic encephalopathy when other measures have failed.

Though a new clinical experience with a new dopaminergic drug is not available, neuroanatomical alterations in the globus pallidus, as seen with NMR spectroscopy (68) have rekindled interest in possible alterations of dopaminergic neurotransmission. Additional neurochemical alterations in these pathways have been reported (69). Extrapyramidal symptoms are prominent in chronic encephalopathy, again suggesting that the alteration in this neurotransmitter system may be more prominent in only a subset of individuals.

Alterations in Serotoninergic Neurotransmission

An increase in the uptake of tryptophan, the precursor of serotonin, has been well documented in animal models (45). Alterations in the concentration of serotonin metabolites, such as 5-HIAA, have been well described in the brain of cirrhotic patients dying in coma (69). The accelerated identification of serotonin receptor subtypes have been recently reviewed (70), each with different ligand specificity and with different second messenger systems. Ketanserin, an S2 receptor antagonist, was found to precipitate encephalopathy in some subjects when used for the treatment of portal hypertension (71). In a recent preliminary communication, a partial S1 receptor agonist was reported to improve the behavioral characteristics in an animal model (72). The development of agonists and antagonists to different receptor subtypes will allow a more selective testing of these pathways.

When All Else Fails

Intractable hepatic encephalopathy is an indication for liver transplantation in candidates for this procedure. In one case with hepatocerebral degeneration, with fixed neurological symptoms, a full recovery occurred after transplant (73). It may be premature to sanction this procedure on such patients without additional information.

Surgical treatment of intractable hepatic encephalopathy is seldom indicated, as concern exists about the ability of patients to tolerate a colectomy, the recommended procedure. A combined medical-surgical experience with colonic exclusion has been reported with acceptable surgical mortality and good clinical results (74).

With this last observation, we have come full circle in this review, that started and finished in the gut. Future advances in the treatment of encephalopathy, however, will arise from the «dissection» of neurochemical alterations in the brain of these patients. In the 90's, the «decade of the brain» (as per the WHO), hepatic encephalopathy is also a tool to unravel what lies «on the other side» of the blood-brain barrier.

REFERENCES

1. Pugh RN, Murray-Lyon IM, Dawson JL, Pietroni MC, Williams R. Transection of the esophagus for bleeding esophageal varices. Br J Surg 1973; 80:646-649.
2. Williams R, Wendon J. Indications for orthotopic liver transplantation in fulminant liver failure. Hepatology 1994; 20:55-58S.
3. Nomura F, Ohnishi K, Terabayashi H, Nakai T, Isobe K, Takekoshi K, Okuda K. Effect of intrahepatic portal-systemic shunting on hepatic ammonia extraction in patients with cirrhosis. Hepatology 1994; 20:1478-1481.
4. Swart GR, van den Berg JWO, Wattimena JLD, Rietveld JK, van Vuure JK, Frenkel M. Elevated protein requirements in cirrhosis of the liver investigated by whole body protein turnover studies. Clin Sci 1988; 75:101-107.
5. Bianchi GP, Marchesini G, Fabbri A, Rondelli A, Bugianesi E, Zoli M, Pisi E: Vegetable versus animal protein diet in cirrhotic patients with chronic encephalopathy. A randomized crossover comparison. J Int Med 1993; 233:385-392.
6. Uribe M, Conn HO, Dietary management of portal-systemic encephalopathy. In: Conn HO, Bircher J, eds. Hepatic Encephalopathy, Syndromes and Therapies. Bloomingtom: Medi-Ed Press, 1994; 331-350.
7. Strauss E, Tramote R, Silva EPS, Caly WR, Honain NZ, Maffei RA, de Sa MFG. Double-blind randomized clinical trial comparing neomycin and placebo in the treatment of exogenous hepatic encephalopathy. Hepato-Gastroenterol 1992; 39:342-345.
8. van Berlo CLH, van Leeuwen, PAM, Soeters, PB. Porcine intestinal ammonia liberation. Influence of food intake, lactulose, and neomycin treatment. J Hepatol 1988; 7:250-256.
9. Plauth M, Raible A, Graser TA, Noldeke IL, Furst P, Dolle W, Hartmann F. Lactulose or paramomycin do not affect ammonia generation in the isolated perfused rat small intestine. Zeitsch Gastroenterol 1994; 32:141-145.
10. Morgan MH, Read AE, Speller DCE. Treatment of hepatic encephalopathy with metronidazole. Gut 1982; 23:1-7.

11. Loft S, Sonne J, Dossing M, Buch Andreasen P. Metronidazole pharmacokinetics in patients with hepatic encephalopathy. Scand J Gastroenterol 1987; 22:117-123.
12. Tarao K, Ikeda T, Hayashi K, Sakurai A, Okada T, Ito T, Karube H et al. Successful use of vancomycin hydrochloride in the treatment of lactulose resistan chronic hepatic encephalopathy. Gut 1990; 31:702-706.
13. Van Thiel DH, Fagiuoli S, Wright HI, Chien MC, Gavaler JS. Gastrointestinal transit in cirrhotic patients: effect of hepatic encephalopathy and its treatment. Hepatology 1994; 19:57-71.
14. Bucci L, Palmieri GC. Double-blind, double-dummy comparison between treatment with rifaximin and lactulose in patients with medium to severe degree hepatic encephalopathy. Curr Med Res Opin 1993; 13:9-18.
15. Bird SP, Hewitt D, Ratcliff B, Gurr MI. Effects of lactulose and lacitol on protein digestion and metabolism in conventional and germ-free animal models: revelance of the results to their use in the treatment of portosystemic encephalopaty. Gut 1990; 31:1403-1406.
16. Mortensen PB. The effect of oral-administered lactulose on colonic nitrogen metabolism and excretion. Hepatology 1992; 16:1350-1356.
17. Mortensen PB, Holtug K, Bonnen H, Clausen MR. The degradation of amino acids, proteins, and blood to short-chain fatty acids in colon is prevented by lactulose. Gastroenterology 1990; 98:353-360.
18. Greve JW, Gouma DJ, Leeuwen PAM, Buurman WA. Lactulose inhibits endotoxin induced tumour necrosis factor production by monocytes. An in vitro study. Gut 1990; 31:198-203.
19. Vendemiale G, Palasciano G, Cirelli F, Altamura M, De Vincentiis A, Altomare E. Crystalline lactulose in the therapy or hepatic cirrhosis. Evaluation of clinical and immunological parameters. Preliminary results. Arzneimittel Forschung-Drug Res 1992; 42:969-972.
20. Flouric B, Briot F, Florent C, Pollier P, Maurel M, Rambaud JC. Can diarrhea induced by lactulose be reduced by prolonged ingestion of lactulose? Am J Clin Nutr 1993; 58:369-375.
21. Morgan MY, Alonso M, Stanger G. Lactitol and lactulose for the treatment of subclinical hepatic encephalopathy in cirrhotic patients. A randomised, cross-over study. J Hepatol 1989; 8:208-217.
22. Riggio O, Balducci G, Ariosto F, Merli M, TrAmiterra S, Ziparo V, Capocaccia L. Lactitol in the treatment of chronic hepatic encephalopathy —a randomized cross-over comparison with lactulose. Hepato-Gastroenterol 1990; 37:524-527.
23. Blanc P, Daures JP, Rouillon JM, Peray P, Pierruges R, Larrey D, Gremy F, Michel H. Lactitol or lactulose in the treatment of chronic hepatic encephalopathy: results of a meta-analysis. Hepatology 1992; 15:222-228.
24. Camma C, Fiorello F, Tine F, Marchesini G, Fabbri A, Plagliaro L. Lactitol in treatment of chronic hepatic encephalopathy. A meta-analysis. Dig Dis Sci 1993; 38:915-922.
25. Merli M, Caschera M, Piat C, Pinto G, Diofebi M, Riggio O. The effect of lactulose and lactitol administration on fecal fat excretion in patients with liver cirrhosis. J Clin Gastro 1992; 15:125-127.
26. Blei AT. Hepatic encephalopathy in the age of TIPS. Hepatology 1994; 20:249-252.
27. Sanyal AJ, Freedman AM, Shiffman ML, Purdum PP, Luketic VA, Cheatham AK. Portosystemic encephalopathy after transjugular intrahepatic portosystemic shunt: results or a prospective controlled study. Hepatology 1994; 20:45-55.
28. Weber F Jr. Combination therapy with lactulose or lactitol with antibiotics. In: Conn HO, Bircher J, eds. Hepatic Encephalopathy, Syndromes and Therapies. Bloomingtom. Medi-Ed Press, 1994; 285-294.
29. Rudman D, DiFulco D, Galambos JT et al. Maximal rates of excretion and synthesis of urea in normal and cirrhotic patients. J Clin Invest 1973; 52:2241-2249.
30. Weber FL Jr. The effect of lactulose on urea metabolism and nitrogen excretion in cirrhotic patients. Gastroenterology 1979; 77:518-523.
31. Riggio O, Merli M, Capocaccia L, Caschera M, Zullo A, Pinto G, Gaudio E et al. Zinc supplementation reduces blood ammonia and increases liver ornithine transcarbamylase activity in experimental cirrhosis. Hepatology 1992; 15:785-789.
32. Reding P, Duchateau J, Bataille C. Oral zinc supplementation improves hepatic encephalopathy. Results of a randomized controlled trial. Lancet 1984; 2:493-495.
33. Riggio O, Ariosto F, Merli M, Caschera M, Zullo A, Balducci G, Ziparo V. Short-term oral zinc supplementation does not improve chronic hepatic encephalopathy. Results of a double-blind crossover trial. Dig Dis Sci 1991; 35:1204-1208.
34. Van der Rijt CC, Schalm SW, Schat H, Foeken K, De Jong G. Overt hepatic encephalopathy precipitated by zinc deficiency. Gastroenterology 1991; 100: 1114-1118.
35. Pomier-Layargues G, Sparh L, Shapcott D, Michaud G, Lavoie J, Therrien G, Butterworth RF. Increased brain copper content in cirrhotic patients with hepatic coma. Hepatology 1994; 20:109A (Abstr).
36. Peters S, Koh J, Choi DW. Zinc selectively blocks the action of N-methyl-D-aspartate on cortical neurons. Science 1987; 236:589-593.
37. Kircheis G, Quack G, Erbler H. L-Ornithine-L-aspartate in the treatment of hepatic encephalopathy. In: Conn HO, Bircher J, eds. Hepatic Encephalopathy, Syndromes and Therapies. Bloomingtom: Medi-Ed Press, 1994; 373-386.
38. Brusilow SW, Valle DL, Batshaw ML. New pathways of nitrogen excretion in inborn errors of urea synthesis. Lancet 1979; 2:452-457.
39. Sushma S, Dasarathy S, Tandon RK, Jain S, Gupta S, Bhist SM. Sodium benzoate in the treatment of acute hepatic encephalopathy: A double-blind randomized trial. Hepatology 1992; 16:138-144.

40. Uribe M, Marin E, Cervera E, Huerta E, Bosque F, Santoyo R, Gil S. Sodium Benzoate Versus Disaccharides: A Controlled Multicenter Clinical Trial. Hepatology 1990; 12:445(Abstr).
41. Mendenhall CL, Rouster S, Marshall L, Weesner R. A new therapy for portal systemic encephalopathy. Am J Gastoenterol 1986; 81:540-543.
42. Brusilow SW: Phenylacctylglutamine may replace urea as a vehicle for waste nitrogen excretion. Ped Res 1991; 29:147-150.
43. Olafsson S, Brusilow SW, Blei AT. Phenylbutyrate decreases plasma glutamine in patients with cirrhosis. Hepatology 1994; 19:1111(Abstr).
44. Fischer JE. Branched-chain-enriched amino acid solutions in patients with liver failure: an early example of nutritional pharmacology. JPEN 1990; 14 (Suppl 1):249-256.
45. James JH, Jeppson B, Ziparo V, Fischer JE. Hyperammonaemia, plasma amino acid imbalance and blood brain amino acid transport: a unified theory of portal systemic encephalopathy. Lancet 1979; ii:772-775.
46. Knudsen GM, Schmidt J, Almdal T, Paulson OB, Vilstrup H. Passage of amino acids and glucose across the blood-brain berrier in patients with hepatic encephalopathy. Hepatology 1993; 17:987-992.
47. Morgan MY. Branched chain amino acids in the management of chronic liver disease. Facts and fantasies. J Hepatol 1990; 11:133-141.
48. Erikson LS, Conn HO. Branched-chain amino acids in the management of hepatic encephalopathy: an analysiss of variants. Gastroenterology 1989; 98:228-246.
49. Naylor CD, O'Rourke K, Detsky AS, Baker JP. Parenteral nutrition with branched-chain amino acids in hepatic encephalopathy: a meta-analysis. Gastroenterology 1989; 97:1033-1042.
50. Marchesini G, Dioguardi FS, Bianchi GP, Zoli M, Bellati G, Roffi L, Martines D, Abbiati R. Long term oral branched-chain amino acid treatment in chronic hepatic encephalopathy. A randomized double-blind casein-controlled trial. The Italian Multicenter Study Group. J Hepatol 1990; 11:92-101.
51. Plauth M, Egberts EH, Hamster W, Torok M, Muller PH, Brand O, Furst P, Dolle W. Long-term treatment of latent portosystemic encephalopathy with branched-chain amino acids. A double-blind placebo-controlled crossover study. J Hepatol 1993; 17:308-314.
52. Srivastava A, Mehta R, Rothke S, Rademaker F, Blei AT. Fitness to drive of patients with cirrhosis and portal-systemic shunting. A pilot study evaluating performance on the road. J Hepatol 1994; 21:1023-1028.
53. Butterworth RF. Pathogenesis and treatment of portal-systemic encephalopathy: an update. Dig Dis Sci 1992; 37:321-327.
54. Basile AS, Hughes RD, Harrison PM, Murata Y, Pannell L, Jones EA, Williams R, Skolnick P. Elevated brain concentrations of 1,4-benzodiazepines in fulminant hepatic failure. N Engl J Med 1991; 325:473-478.
55. Rothstein JD. Benzodiazepine-receptor ligands and hepatic encephalopathy: a causal relationship? Hepatology 1994; 19:248-250.
56. Basile AS, Harrison PM, Hughes RD, Gu ZQ, Pannell L, McKinney A, Jones EA, Williams R. Relationship between plasma bezondiazepine receptor ligand concentrations and severity of hepatic encephalopathy. Hepatology 1994; 19:112-121.
57. Yurdaydin C, Engler H, Walsh TJ, TeeHa J, Jones EA, Basile AS. Benzodiazepine receptor lingands (BRL) are synthesized de novo in the brain. Hepatology 1994; 20:109A(Abstr).
58. Rothstein JD, Guidotti A, Tinuper P, Cortelli P, Avoni P, Plazzi G, Lugaresi E et al. Endogenous benzodiazepine receptor ligands in idiopathic recurring stupor. Lancet 1992; 340:1002-1004.
59. Rothstein JD, Mekhann G, Guarneri P, Barbaccia ML, Guidotti A, Costa E. Cerebrospinal fluid content of diazepam binding inhibitor in chronic hepatic encephalopathy. Ann Nuerol 1989; 25:57-62.
60. Pomier-Layrargues G, Giguere JF, Lavoire J, Perney P, Gagnon S, D'Amour M, Wells J, Butterworth RF. Flumazenil in cirrhotic patients in hepatic coma: a randomized double-blind placebo-controlled crossover tiral. Hepatology 1994; 19:32-37.
61. Meier R, Gyr K, Haussler R and the PSE Study Group. Treatment of portosystemic encephalopathy with the benzodiazepine-receptor antagonist flumazenil. A randomized, double-blind placebo-controlled multicenter study. Gastroenterology 1994; 106:A942(Abstr).
62. Bruha R, Marecek Z, Brodanova M, Votruba M. Flumazenil as a diagnostic test for latent hepatic encephalopathy. J hepatology 1994; 19:844(Letter).
63. Van der Rijt CC, Schalm SW, Meulstee J, Stijnen TH. Flumazenil therapy for hepatic encephalopathy: A double-blind crossover study. Hepatology 1989; 10:590(Abstr).
64. Seebach J, Jost R. Flumazenil-induced psychotric disorder in hepatic encephalopathy [letter]. Lancet 1992; 339:488-489.
65. Morgan MY. The treatment of chronic hepatic encephalopathy. Hepatogastroenterol 1991; 38:377-387.
66. Morgan MY, Jakobovits AW, James IM, Sherlock S. Successful use of bromocriptine in the treatment of chronic hepatic encephalopathy. Gastroenterology 1980; 78:663-670.
67. Uribe M, Farca A, Márquez MA, García-Ramos G, Guevara L, Briones A, Gil S. Treatment of chronic portal-systemic encephalopathy with bromocriptine. A double-blind controlled trial. Gastroenterology 1979; 76:1347-1351.
68. Morgan MY. Cerebral magnetic resonance imaging and spectroscopy in the study of hepatic encephalopathy. In: Conn HO, Bircher J, eds. A Hepatic Encephalopathy, Syndromes and Therapies. Bloomingtom: Medi-Ed Press, 1994; 101-134.
69. Mousseau DD, Butterworth RF. Current theories on

the pathogenesis of hepatic encephalopathy. Proc Soc Exp Biol Med 1994; 205:329-344.

70. Hartig PR. Molecular pharmacology of serotonin receptors. EXS 1994; 71:93-102.

71. Vorobioff J, García-Tsao G, Groszmann RJ, Aceves G, Picabea E, Villavicencio R, Hernandez-Ortiz J. Long term hemodynamic effects of ketanserin, a 5-hydroxytryptamine blocker, in portal hypertensive patients. Hepatology 1989; 9:88-91.

72. Herneth AM, Steindl P, Ferenci P. Central acting serotonin (5-HT) ligands, which ameliorate hepatic encephalopathy, require partial 5-HT_{1A} agonistic properties. Hepatology 1994; 20:108A.

73. Powell EE, Pender MP, Chalk JB, Parkin PJ, Strong R, Lynch S, Kerlin P et al. Improvement in chronic hepatocerebral degeneration following liver transplantation. Gastroenterology 1990; 98:1079-1082.

74. Dagenais MH, Bernard D, Marleau D, Morgan S, Tasse D, Wassef R, Villeneuve, JP et al. Surgical treatment of severe postshunt hepatic encephalopathy. World J Surg 1991; 15:109-113.

Section 3

Treatment of Bacterial Infections in Liver Diseases

Diagnosis of Bacterial Infections in the Setting of Liver Disease

B. A Runyon

CIRRHOSIS AS A FORM OF ACQUIRED IMMUNODEFICIENCY

Patients with cirrhosis frequently have multiple defects in immune defense against bacterial infection (1-3). Although some relatively non-virulent bacteria, the so called «serum-sensitive» bacteria, can be killed by complement in the absence of phagocytes, most virulent organisms are first coated with host protein and are then killed by either motile phagocytes, such as neutrophils, or stationary phagocytes, such as Kuppfer cells (4). Pathogenic serum-resistant bacteria are usually not even recognized as foreign until they are «opsonized», i.e. coated, by host proteins (1). The most important opsonizing protein is complement, with globulin and fibronectin playing less important roles (5). Approximately two-thirds of patients with cirrhosis and ascites have subnormal serum total hemolytic complement activity (6). Because cirrhotic ascites is an ultrafiltrate of plasma with a dilution factor of 5-10, some ascitic fluid in this setting has undetectable complement activity (1, 6). Approximately two-thirds of patients with severe alcoholic liver disease have impaired neutrophil function (2, 7). Kuppfer cell function is also decreased in the setting of cirrhosis (3). To make matters even worse, the gut in the setting of cirrhosis appears to be more permeable to bacteria than is normal mucosa, resulting in frequent extra-intestinal dissemination of enteric bacteria (8). Cirrhosis is probably second only to diabetes mellitus as the most common form of acquired immunodeficiency—much more common than the acquired immunodeficiency syndrome caused by the human immunodeficiency virus (9).

In addition, acute liver failure, e.g. fulminant hepatic failure, has also been reported to be complicated by complement deficiency and defective opsonization (10).

PREVALENCE OF BACTERIAL INFECTION

These defects in immune defense would be predicted to predispose to frequent bacterial infections. It is not surprising that two recently published studies documented 46-47% cumulative frequency of bacterial infection during a single hospitalization of patients with cirrhosis (3, 11). Included among these infections was a cumulative frequency of spontaneous bacterial peritonitis (SBP) of 31%, urinary tract infection 25%, and pneumonia 21% (11).

Bacterial infections, especially bacteremia, also regularly complicate fulminant hepatic failure (12, 13).

SETTING IN WHICH INFECTION OCCURS

SBP essentially only complicates cirrhotic ascites; spontaneous infection of non-cirrhotic ascites is rare enough to be the subject of case reports (14). Patients usually develop infection when their liver disease is most severe. Eighty-one per cent of patients are jaundiced and 98% have an abnormal prothrombin time when SBP is documented (15). Patients usually develop infection of their ascitic fluid when the fluid is most voluminous and most dilute; an ascitic fluid protein concentration <1g/dl has been shown to be an important risk factor for development of SBP (16-18). This author has encountered only two episodes of ascitic fluid infection (out of ~500 total episodes) in which ascites was clinically undetectable; both were in children.

Two other important risk factors for bacteremia and ascitic fluid infection include variceal bleeding and urinary tract infection (19, 20). Variceal bleeding may lead to bacterial infection due to the increased permeability of the gut mucosa of cirrhotic animals (compared to normals) and the increased extra-intestinal dissemination of enteric bacteria that have been documented to occur in hemorrhagic shock (21). Infected urine may lead to urosepsis in these immunodeficient patients and result in ascitic fluid infection.

HIGH INDEX OF SUSPICION OF INFECTION

The high prevalence of immunodeficiency among patients with severe acute or chronic liver disease combined with the high prevalence of bacterial infection should lead to a high index of suspicion of bacterial infection on the part of the physicians caring for these patients. Although 87% of patients with SBP have signs or symptoms of infection (including 68% with fever, 49% with abdominal pain, and 54% with mental status change), 13% have no such findings and the change in mental status may be very subtle or misinterpreted as a manifestation of something other than infection (22). Bacterial infection may be manifested only by acidosis, azotemia, peripheral leukocytosis, or hypotension. A high index of suspicion of infection is required for early detection and early treatment of the infection—and maximum survival of the patient.

LOW «THRESHOLD» FOR OBTAINING CULTURES

In order to confirm the suspicion of bacterial infection, appropriate cultures must be obtained. Blood and urine should be cultured routinely. When evident, sputum should be obtained for Gram's stain and bacterial culture. When present, ascitic fluid should be sampled (see below).

ABDOMINAL PARACENTESIS

In the past many physicians were taught that abdominal paracentesis was a morbid procedure that was to be avoided if possible (23). However, more recent studies have demonstrated that this simple procedure is quite safe despite the 71% prevalence of coagulopathy in this patient population (24-26). Paracentesis-related transfusion-requiring bleeding occurs only after 0.2-0.9% of taps even when no prophylactic plasma infusions are given (24, 25). Paracentesis-related infection occurs approximately once per 1.000 taps —when the bowel is entered with the paracentesis needle (26, 27).

Because bowel may be adherent to the abdominal wall near surgical scars, it is best to avoid puncturing the abdominal wall near such scars. Sterile technique including an iodine cleansing of the skin should be used. This author uses sterile gloves but not sterile gown or cap.

ASCITIC FLUID CELL COUNT

Because *a*) the ascitic fluid bacterial culture takes at least 12 hours to demonstrate growth, *b*) the Gram's stain demonstrates bacteria in only 10% of SBP episodes, *c*) a decision to begin empiric antibiotics must be made as soon as possible to maximize survival, and *d*) the ascitic fluid polymorphonuclear leukocyte (PMN) count has been shown to be very sensitive in detecting bacterial infection, the ascitic fluid cell count is one of the most helpful ascitic fluid tests (26, 28). To avoid clotting of the specimen (especially infected specimens) the ascitic fluid should be injected into a tube containing anticoagulant, e.g., EDTA, immediately after the specimen is obtained (26). The tube should be rapidly transported to the laboratory; some laboratories refuse to process specimens received later than 30 minutes after the fluid is obtained. Neutrophils disintegrate rather rapidly at room temperature. Automated cell counters are not sensitive enough to count ascitic fluid; manual hemocytometers are used. The results are totally dependent on the skill of the technician performing the count. Occasionally, the fluid requires dilution because the cells are too numerous to be accurately counted. Similarly, the differential cell count is manual. The most important information obtained from the ascitic fluid cell count is the absolute PMN count (28). This is calculated by multiplying the total white cell count by the percentage of PMNs. If the absolute PMN count is ≥250 cells/cu mm, the patient is presumed to be infected. There is usually a predominance of PMNs among the white cells in the setting of SBP; frequently >90% of white cells are PMNs. A PMN count of 250 has been determined to be more sensitive than a count of 500 in detecting bacterial infection (28). The most common cause of an elevated PMN count is SBP (26). Peritoneal carcinomatosis, tuberculosis, pancreatitis, and hemorrhage into ascites can also lead to an elevated PMN count; in the former two conditions there is usually not a predominance of PMNs (26, 29-31).

ASCITIC FLUID BACTERIAL CULTURE

Before the insensitivity of the conventional method of ascitic fluid culture was recognized, there was much confusion about ascitic fluid analysis. Conventional bacterial cultures frequently grew no bacteria, despite elevated PMN counts. This led to a search for alternative tests for making a rapid diagnosis of ascitic fluid infection, e.g. pH, lactate, etc (see below). Improvements in ascitic fluid culture methods and reassessment of the sensitivity and specificity of the PMN count in detecting infection has documented the accuracy of this simple test and the inaccuracy of pH and lactate (28, 32).

The conventional method of ascitic fluid culture consists of submission of the fluid sample to the laboratory in a syringe or tube. A few drops of the fluid are then plated on three agar plates (at least one of which suppresses growth of gram-positive organisms) and a few more drops of fluid or centrifuged sediment are inoculated into broth. This method of culture assumes that infected ascitic fluid is usually a high-colony-count polymicrobial infection, as in the setting of gut perforation. However, >95% of episodes of ascitic fluid infection are SBP rather than secondary peritonitis. Spontaneously infected ascites is usually a low-colony-count monomicrobial infection, analogous to bacteremia; the median concentration of bacteria in SBP is only one organism per ml (33). We have known for >50 years that culturing blood on agar plates is too insensitive to be used to detect bacteremia. In fact, blood culture bottles were devised to detect low-colony-count monomicrobial infections; if one viable organism is present in the sample inoculated into the bottle, it should replicate and be detected. Therefore, culturing the fluid as if it were blood would be predicted to be sensitive in detecting bacterial growth. This, in fact, has been the case in all eight studies that have been published (33-40). The overall sensitivity of the blood culture bottles in detecting ascitic fluid infection was 82% in these studies, compared to only 51% for the conventional method (table 1). In addition bedside inoculation of blood culture bottles with ascitic fluid has been shown to be superior to delayed (four hours) inoculation of the bottles (41). Even a one-hour delay in inoculation leads to a statistically significant loss of culture-positivity (McHutchison J, Leal R, Runyon B, Akri-

Table 1. World literature of studies comparing blood culture bottle method of ascitic fluid culture to conventional method

Reference	Blood culture bottle (%) positive	Conventional (%) positive
33	93	43
34	91	58
35	91	42
36	81	52
37	74	44
38	77	57
39	76	53
40	84	35
Overall	227/277 (82%)	136/268 (51%)

viadis E, Antillon M, unpublished observations).

SUBTYPES OF ASCITIC FLUID INFECTION

Since the description and coining of the phrase «spontaneous bacterial peritonitis» 30 years ago, four other variants have been described (22, 27, 29, 42) (table 2). The natural history, prognosis, and treatment of patients with these forms of ascitic fluid infection may be different from patients with SBP. For example, patients with secondary bacterial peritonitis have a surgically-treatable source of infection in the abdomen. Yet these patients never (in this author's experience) develop a classic, rigid, «surgical abdomen» because the ascitic fluid itself prevents the visceral peritoneum from irritating the parietal peritoneum (42). It is not possible to distinguish spontaneous from secondary bacterial peritonitis by historical or physical examination data alone. This distinction is important because essentially 100% of patients with surgical peritonitis in the setting of ascites die without surgical intervention and 80% of SBP patients subjected to exploratory laparotomy die post-operatively (43). The ascitic fluid analysis provides clues that should lead to an emergency radiologic search for a surgical source of infection. Patients who meet two or more of the following criteria should receive plain and upright abdominal films, water-soluble contrast studies of the bowel, and computed tomographic scanning of the abdomen: ascitic fluid total protein >1g/dl, ascitic fluid glucose <50 mg/dl, and ascitic fluid LDH greater than the upper limit of normal for serum (42). Evidence for polymicrobial infection by Gram's stain or culture and/or an ascitic fluid bilirubin concentration greater than a simultaneous serum bilirubin can also provide evidence of gut perforation into ascitic fluid (42, 44). Although a markedly elevated, e.g., >100,000/cu mm, PMN count favors secondary peritonitis, it is not diagnostic.

Most examples of culture-negative neutrocytic ascites are explained by insensitive culture technique or recent antibiotic administration (even only one dose) (29, 33).

Monomicrobial nonneutrocytic bacterascites represents colonization of ascitic fluid with bacteria (22). This colonization is actually quite common in cirrhotic patients and cirrhotic rats and it may proceed to SBP or resolve spontaneously (22, 45).

Polymicrobial bacterascites occurs when an attempted paracentesis leads to needle perforation of the bowel and leakage of bacteria into ascitic fluid (27).

Table 2. Variants of ascitic fluid infection

Variant	Ascitic fluid culture	Ascitic fluid PMN count
Spontaneous bacterial peritonitis	Positive: monomicrobial	≥250/cu mm
Secondary bacterial peritonitis	Positive: polymicrobial	≥250/cu mm
Culture-negative neutrocytic ascites	Negative	≥250/cu mm
Monomicrobial non-neutrocytic bacterascites	Positive: monomicrobial	<250/cu mm
Polymicrobial bacterascites	Positive: polymicrobial	<250/cu mm

OTHER TESTING

In the future molecular biology techniques will be used to detect and identify bacterial genetic material in body fluids. This has already been accomplished in the setting of bacteremia; the «turn-around time» for such testing can be as short as 30 minutes (46).

As mentioned above, more sensitive culture techniques have validated the accuracy of the ascitic fluid PMN count and revealed the inaccuracy of ascitic fluid pH and lactate (28, 32). Other «humoral tests of infection» such as interleukin-6 and tumor necrosis factor have been proposed as helpful in detecting infection (47). However, until these high technology tests are shown to offer more information than a simple inexpensive PMN count, they should not and will not gain wide acceptance in the current climate of cost-effective health care.

REFERENCES

1. Runyon BA, Morrissey R, Hoefs JC, Wyle F. Opsonic activity of human ascitic fluid: a potentially important protective mechanism against spontaneous bacterial peritonitis. Hepatology 1985; 5:634-637.

2. Rajkovic IA, Williams R. Abnormalities of neutrophil phagocytosis, intracellular killing, and metabolic activity in alcoholic cirrhosis and hepatitis. Hepatology 1986; 6:252-262.
3. Rimola A, Soto R, Bory F, Arroyo V, Piera C, Rodés J. Reticuloendothelial system phagocytic activity in cirrhosis and its relation to bacterial infections and prognosis. Hepatology 1984; 4:53-58.
4. Reed WP, Albright EL. Opsonins in the hepatic clearance of pneumococci. Infect Immun 1986; 52:499-503.
5. Agnello V. Complement deficiency states. Medicine 1978; 57:1-23.
6. Runyon BA. Patients with deficient ascitic fluid opsonic activity are predisposed to spontaneous bacterial peritonitis. Hepatology 1988; 8:632-635.
7. Laffi G, Carloni V, Baldi E, Rossi ME, Azzari C, Gresele P, Marra F, Gentilini P. Impaired superoxide anion, platelet-activating factor, and leukotriene B4 synthesis by neutrophils in cirrhosis. Gastroenterology 1993; 105:170-177.
8. Runyon BA, Squier SU, Borzio M. Translocation of gut bacteria in cirrhotic rats to mesenteric lymph nodes partially explains the pathogenesis of spontaneous bacterial peritonitis. J Hepatol 1994; 21:792-796.
9. Runyon BA. Bacterial infections in patients with cirrhosis (Editorial). J Hepatol 1993; 18:271-272.
10. Wyke RJ, Rajkovic RA, Eddleston ALWF, Williams R. Defective opsonization and complement deficiency in serum from patients with fulminant hepatic failure. Gut 1980; 21:643-649.
11. Caly WR, Strauss E. A prospective study of bacterial infections in patients with cirrhosis. J Hepatol 1993; 18:353-358.
12. Wyke RJ, Canalese JC, Gimson AES, Williams R. Bacteraemia in patients with fulminant hepatic failure. Liver 1982; 2:45-52.
13. Gazzard BG, Portmann B, Murray-Lyon IM, Williams R. Causes of death in fulminant hepatic failure and relationship to qualitative histological assessment of parenchymal damage. Q J Med 1975; 176:615-626.
14. Wolfe GM, Runyon BA. Spontaneous *Salmonella* infection of high protein non-cirrhotic ascites. J Clin Gastroenterol 1990; 12:430-432.
15. Hoefs JC, Runyon BA. Spontaneous bacterial peritonitis. Disease-A-Month 1985; 31:1-48.
16. Runyon BA. Low-protein-concentration ascitic fluid is predisposed to spontaneous bacterial peritonitis. Gastroenterology 1986; 91:1343-1346.
17. Llach J, Rimola A, Navasa M, Ginès P, Salmerón JM, Ginès A, Arroyo V, Rodés J. Incidence and predictive factors of first episode of spontaneous bacterial peritonitis in cirrhosis with ascites: relevance of ascitic fluid protein concentration. Hepatology 1992; 16:724-727.
18. Andreu M, Solà R, Sitges-Serra A, Alia C, Gallén M, Vila MC, Coll S, Oliver MI. Risk factors for spontaneous bacterial peritonitis in cirrhotic patients with ascites. Gastroenterology 1993; 104:1133-1138.
19. Rimola A, Bory F, Teres J, Pérez-Ayuso RM, Arroyo V, Rodés J. Oral, nonabsorbable antibiotics prevent infection in cirrhotics with gastrointestinal hemorrhage. Hepatology 1985; 5; 463-467.
20. Ho H, Guerra LG, Zuckerman MJ, Pere JF, Polly SM. Urinary tract infection: a predisposing factor for spontaneous bacterial peritonitis. Gastroenterology 1990; 98:A593.
21. Hamdani R, Young S, Runyon BA. Increased bacterial translocation in cirrhotic rats undergoing hemorrhagic shock. Gastroenterology 1994; 106:A904.
22. Runyon BA. Monomicrobial nonneutrocytic bacterascites: a variant of spontaneous bacterial peritonitis. Hepatology 1990; 12:710-715.
23. Mallory A, Schaefer JW. Complications of diagnostic paracentesis in patients with liver disease. JAMA 1978; 239:628-630.
24. Runyon BA. Paracentesis of ascitic fluid: a safe procedure. Arch Intern Med 1986; 146:2259-2261.
25. McVay PA, Toy PTCY. Lack of increased bleeding after paracentesis and thoracentesis in patients with mild coagulation abnormalities. Transfusion 1991; 13:164-171.
26. Runyon BA. Paracentesis and ascitic fluid analysis. In: Yamada T, Alpers D, Owyang C, Powell D, Silverstein F, eds. Textbook of Gastroenterology. Philadelphia: JB Lippincott, 1991; 2455-2465.
27. Runyon BA, Canawati HN, Hoefs JC. Polymicrobial bacterascites: a unique entity in the spectrum of infected ascitic fluid. Arch Intern Med 1986; 146:2173-2175.
28. Runyon BA and Antillon MR. Ascitic fluid pH and lactate: insensitive and nonspecific tests in detecting ascitic fluid infection. Hepatology 1991; 13:929-935.
29. Runyon BA, Hoefs JC. Culture-negative neutrocytic ascites: a variant of spontaneous bacterial peritonitis. Hepatology 1984; 4:1209-1211.
30. Runyon BA, Hoefs JC, Morgan TR. Ascitic fluid analysis in malignancy-related ascites. Hepatology 1988; 8:1104-119.
31. Burack WR, Hollister RM. Tuberculous peritonitis: a study of 47 proved cases encountered by a general medical unit in 25 years. Am J Med 1960; 28:510-523.
32. Albillos A, Cuevas-Mons V, Millán I, Cantón T, Montes J, Barrios C, Garrido A, Escartín P. Ascitic fluid polymorphonuclear cell count and serum to ascites albumin gradient in the diagnosis of bacterial peritonitis. Gastroenterology 1990; 98:134-140.
33. Runyon BA, Canawati HN, Akriviadis EA. Optimization of ascitic fluid culture technique. Gastroenterology 1988; 95:1351-1355.
34. Kammerer J, Dupeyron C, Vuillemin N, Leluan G, Fouet P. Apport des examens cytologiques et bacteriologiques du liquide d'ascite cirrhotique au diagnostic de peritonite bactérienne. Med Chir Dig 1982; 11:243-251.
35. Runyon BA, Umland ET, Merlin T. Inoculation of blood culture bottle with ascitic fluid: Improved detection of spontaneous bacterial peritonitis. Arch Intern Med 1987; 147:73-75.
36. Bobadilla M, Sifuentes J, García-Tsao G. Improved

method for bacteriological diagnosis of spontaneous bacterial peritonitis. J Clin Microbiol 1989; 27:2145-2147.

37. Dalmau B, Nogueras A, Mas P, Segura F. Inoculation of blood culture bottles with ascitic fluid: improved detection of spontaneous bacterial peritonitis (correspondence). Arch Intern Med 1989; 147:1849-1850.
38. Castellote J, Xiol X, Verdaguer R, Ribes J, Guardiola J, Giménez A, Casais L. Comparison of two ascitic fluid culture methods in cirrhotic patients with spontaneous bacterial peritonitis. Am J Gastroenterol 1990; 85:1605-1608.
39. Sainz S, Soriano G, Coll P, Teixedo M, Alonso C, Such J, Guarner C. Peritonitis bacteriana espontánea: estudio comparativo de dos métodos de cultivo del líquido ascítico. Rev Esp Enf Digest 1990; 78:76-78.
40. Siersma PD, de Marie S, van Zeijl JH, Bac D-J, Wilson JHP. Blood culture bottles are superior to lysis-centrifugation tubes for bacteriological diagnosis of spontaneous bacterial peritonitis. J Clin Microbiol 1992; 30:667-669.
41. Runyon BA, Antillon MR, Akriviadis EA, McHutchison JG. Bedside inoculation of blood culture bottles with ascitic fluid is superior to delayed inoculation in the detection of spontaneous bacterial peritonitis. J Clin Microbiol 1990; 28:2811-2812.
42. Akriviadis EA, Runyon BA. The value of an algorithm in differentiating spontaneous from secondary bacterial peritonitis. Gastroenterology 1990; 98:127-133.
43. Garrison RN, Cryer HM, Howard DA. Clarification of risk factors for abdominal operations in patients with hepatic cirrhosis. Ann Surg 1984; 199:648-655.
44. Runyon BA. Ascitic fluid bilirubin concentration as a key to the diagnosis of choleperitoneum. J Clin Gastroenterol 1987; 9:543-545.
45. Runyon BA, Sugano S, Kanel G, Mellencamp M. A rodent model of cirrhosis and spontaneous bacterial peritonitis. Gastroenterology 1991; 100:1737-1742.
46. Davis TE, Fuller DD. Direct identification of bacterial isolates in blood cultures by using a DNA probe. J Clin Microbiol 1991; 29:2193-2196.
47. Byl B, Roucloux I, Crusiaux A, Dupont E, Devière J. Tumor necrosis factor alpha and interleukin 6 plasma levels in infected cirrhotic patients. Gastroenterology 1993; 104:1492-1497.

Prophylaxis and Treatment of Bacterial and Fungal Infection in Patients with Fulminant Hepatic Failure

N. Rolando, R. Williams

INTRODUCTION

Prophylaxis and treatment of infections in patients with fulminant hepatic failure (FHF) depend on the understanding of the immunological abnormalities present in this condition, the risk factors associated with the clinical management and the incidence, type and timing of these infections.

HOST DEFENSE MECHANISMS IN FULMINANT HEPATIC FAILURE

A variety of defects of host immune function arise as a direct consequence of FHF (1). The liver is the major site of complement synthesis and reduced levels of serum complement mainly C3 and C5 components have been reported by Wyke (2). Levels of complement correlated with low opsonisation index against bacteria and yeast (3) and opsonisation is significantly impaired in children (4) and adults (3) with this condition. A significant reduction in neutrophil adherence to nylon filters has been reported by Altin et al. (5). Abnormalities in neutrophil adherence in FHF may increase susceptibility to infection.

Chemotaxis of white cells is impaired in patients with FHF (2). Polymorphs from patients with FHF failed to migrate against normal serum, and Wyke (2) demonstrated that serum from FHF patients was a poor chemoatractact to normal polymorphs.

Although impaired phagocytosis and intracellular killing by polymorphs have been reported in patients with FHF (6, 7), Wyke (2) showed that these functions improved when a heat-labile fraction of normal serum was added. This suggested that the major defect is related to complement deficiency.

In addition, in patients with FHF, Kupffer cell function is significantly impaired (8). The low concentrations of plasma fibronectin found in FHF may explain impaired phagocytosis by Kupffer cells (8, 9).

INVASIVE PROCEDURES AND OTHER RISK FACTORS

Monitoring of patients with FHF requires the use of arterial, central venous pressure and Swanz-Ganz lines. Intra-vascular lines have been implicated as sources of bacteraemia in critically ill and in FHF patients (10).

In addition approximately 50% of these patients require haemodialysis. In other clinical conditions, the association between haemodialysis and bacteraemia has been reported (11). Endotracheal intubation and ventilation is necessary in 80% of FHF cases. The association between chest infection and endotracheal intubation has been reported in these patients (10). The presence of cerebral oedema in FHF precludes physiotherapy and the resulting accumulation of secretion may account for the high incidence of chest infections.

Insertion of an intracranial pressure monitor provides a further portal of entry for infection and the prophylactic administration of intravenous vancomycin to prevent gram positive infection in these patients has been suggested (12). Bladder catheters are another portal of entry for infection and should be removed in anuric patients.

The use of H_2 blockers to prevent gastrointestinal bleeding in patients with FHF (13) has been associated with the development of fungal infections. In addition, the modification of gastric pH may result in overgrowth of Gram negative bacilli in the stomach (14, 15). In ventilated patients colonization of the oropharynx with Gram negative bacilli commonly precedes the development of nosocomial pneumonia (16-18).

Another important factor is the suppression of the normal bacterial flora by antibiotics allowing proliferation of yeasts, that can translocate from the gut lumen to the bloodstream (19, 20). Finally corticosteroids use in these patients has been associated with disseminated aspergillosis (21).

INCIDENCE OF BACTERIAL INFECTIONS

The severe damage to the liver renders the patient with FHF at greatest risk of infection. An early retrospective post mortem study from our Institute documented major sepsis, endocarditis, meningitis, peritonitis and empyema, which were considered to have contributed to death in 11% of 105 cases (22).

Bacteraemia in FHF has been reported in up to 36% of adults (23-25) and 47% of children (26) with this condition.

A prospective study with extensive microbiological surveillance shows the real magnitude of the problem (10).

Bacteriologically-proven infections were recorded in 80% of patients and, in a further 10%, infection was suspected on clinical grounds (fig. 1). Fourteen percent of these patients had more than one episode of infection, and 8% had concomitant infections at different sites.

The most common infection was pneumonia, accounting for nearly 50% of episodes, followed by bacteraemia (26%) and urinary tract infection (22%) (fig. 2). Gram positive bacteria predominated causing 70% of infections. *S. aureus* was implicated in 52% of infections. Characteristically these infections occurred early during the disease (median of 5 days for pneumonia, 3 days for bacteraemia and 1.9 days for urinary tract infection).

Elevation in temperature and/or white cell counts were poor indicators of infection, and were absent in 30% of cases (fig. 3). Infection was present in all the majority of fatalities occurred in the first four days. Late death was di-

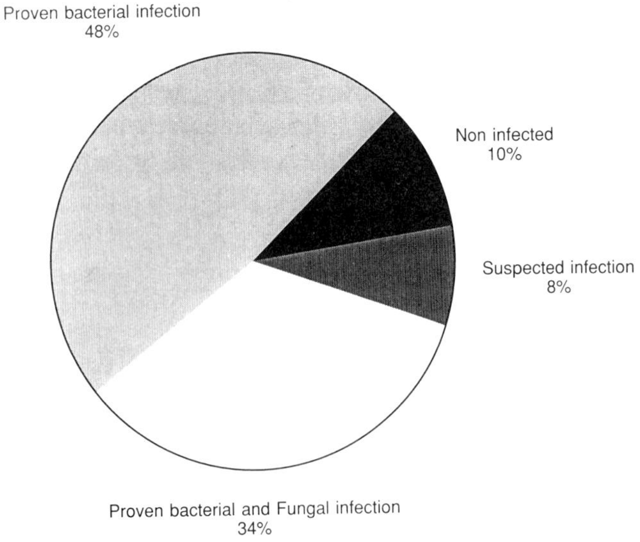

Fig. 1. Incidence of bacterial and fungal infection in fulminant hepatic failure.

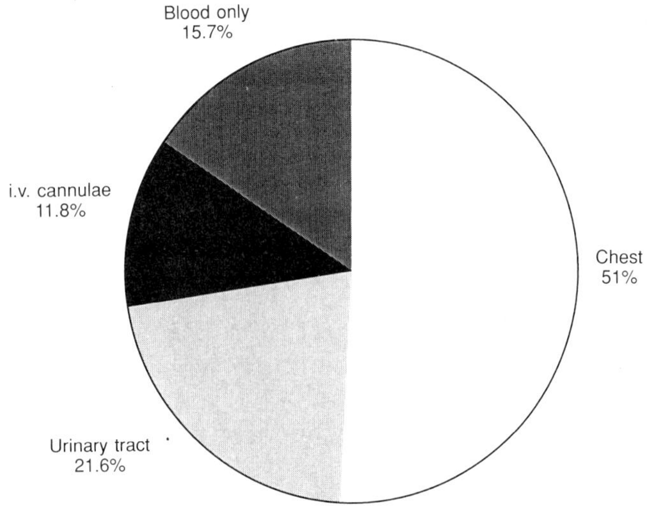

Fig. 2. Localization of bacterial infections in patients with fulminant hepatic failure.

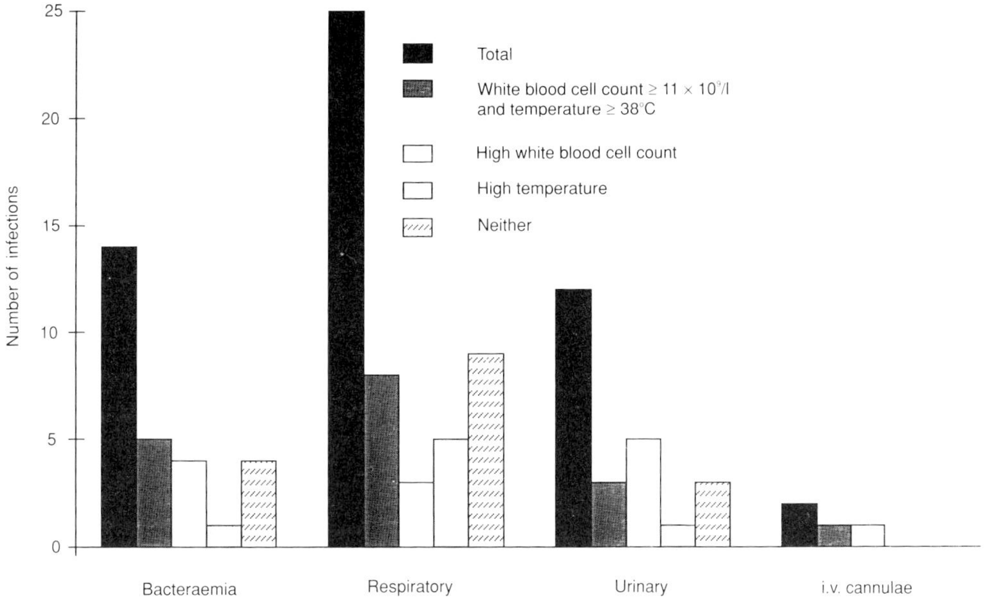

Fig. 3. Clinical signs of bacterial infection related to significant microbiological cultures in fulminant hepatic failure.

rectly attributable to overwhelming infection in a quarter of the cases.

INCIDENCE OF FUNGAL INFECTIONS

The assessment of the incidence of fungal infection in FHF by post mortem studies underestimated the true incidence. In a retrospective study in paediatric patients with FHF, fungal infections were implicated as the cause of death in 13% of patients (26). Disseminated aspergillosis complicating FHF was confined to a few case reports (27, 28). Aspergillosis has also been reported in patients with subacute hepatic necrosis who received corticosteroids as part of their management (27).

In a prospective study in our centre in patients in FHF, fungal infection was present in 32% of cases (29). All but one of the infections were caused by *Candida albicans*. In all cases concomitant bacterial infection was present.

Diagnosis of fungal infection during life in patients with FHF is difficult as obtaining tissue for microscopy and culture is often prohibited by clotting abnormalities. In this study diagnosis was based, on isolation of fungi from significant clinical sites. In addition a clinical syndrome characterized by deterioration in mental status, after an initial improvement; pyrexia (>38°C) unresponsive to broad-spectrum antibiotics; and a white cell count exceeding 20×10^9 at the time of diagnosis was present. Acute renal failure was present in all patients with fungal infection (table 1).

In some cases the diagnosis was made only at post mortem examination. In patients with FHF, fungal infection develops early, mainly in the second week after admission, and is not related to duration of antibiotic therapy. Mortality is high; when fungal infection is present 69% of patients with fungal infection died.

Table 1. Clinical and haematological features in patients with and without fungal infection

	Fungal infection	No fungal infection	p value
White cell counts at diagnosis	20.8×10^9	16.2×10^9	< 0.01
Coexistent bacterial infection	100%	80%	NS
Antibiotic resistant fever > 48 hr	75%	0	< 0.05
Acute renal failure	100%	0	< 0.05
Late deterioration in coma grade	75%	0	< 0.05

APPROACHES TO BACTERIAL AND FUNGAL INFECTION

General guidelines are those applicable to other patients in intensive care units. For the prevention of infection a close liaison between clinicians, nursing staff and the medical microbiologist is essential. Infection control policies relating to hand-washing, cleaning, disinfection and sterilization, should be regularly reviewed. Aseptic techniques are the first line of defense against infection and should be strictly enforced. An aseptic technique must be used when inserting or manipulating intra-vascular catheters or other invasive monitoring devices. Intravenous catheters should be changed every 72 hours and the catheter tips routinely send for culture.

Microbiological monitoring of FHF patients should be done on a daily basis. Daily cultures are justified since positive cultures can be obtained after one or two days after initiating antibiotic treatment (10). In addition, infection with multiresistant organisms and fungi may be detected (29). In units caring for patients with FHF where antimicrobial usage is high, surveillance for the emergence of bacteria resistant to clinically important antimicrobials is worthwhile.

Identification of patients colonized or infected with such organisms allows early implementation of policies to prevent cross-infection. Furthermore, in tertiary referral centres caring for this type of patients, screening on admission can identify those colonized by multiply-resistant bacteria.

Weekly surveillance includes swabs of nose, throat axillae and wounds for methicillin-resistant *S. aureus*. Surveillance for Enterobacteriaceae includes rectal swabs and urine sample. This kind of surveillance allowed us to document and control the emergence of both vancomycin-resistant *Enterococcus faecium* and *Enterococcus faecalis* on this unit (30). Other multiply-resistant bacteria in patients with FHF includes *Xanthomonas maltophilia*, *Pseudomonas cepacia* and *Enterobacter* sp.

Measures to control colonization and infection with resistant bacteria may require changes in antimicrobial policies to reduce selective pressures (31).

At King's College Hospital in London there has always been an enormous interest on infections in FHF patients. Since the 80's many approaches to infection in FHF patients have been undertaken, and I describe here the results of a series of studies, with different strategies. This constitutes a continuous evaluation of the problem where strategies were based on results from previous studies.

USE OF BROAD SPECTRUM ANTIBIOTICS WHEN INFECTION IS SUSPECTED OR ESTABLISHED

The severity of the underlying condition, the wide range of pathogens and the high mortality attributable to infection, are indications for the use of broad-spectrum antimicrobial agents. To evaluate the efficacy of two such regimens in patients with FHF, a prospective study was carried out in this Institute (32). Patients were allocated to receive aztreonam with vancomycin (A/V) or piperacillin with gentamicin (P/G). Antimicrobials were commenced when cultures yielded significant isolates or when bacterial infection was suspected. Fifty patients were enroled, 14 died within 48 h and were excluded from analysis. In the remaining 36 patients, there were 42 episodes of microbiologically-documented infection: 18 in the A/V group, and 24 in the P/G group. Changes were made to the antibacterial therapy in 10 patients in the A/V group and in 14 in the P/G group. The main indication for treatment modification was persisting pyrexia after 48 h, despite in vitro sensitivity of significant isolates to the trial drugs. The numbers of deaths attributable to infection were similar in both groups and there was no significant difference between the success rates of the regimens.

Despite the excellent anti-staphylococcal activities of gentamicin and vancomycin, there was a high incidence of *S. aureus* infections with a poor clinical response. The addition of flucloxacillin in an attempt to control these infections was the major cause of failure for both regimens.

Bacteriophage typing of *S. aureus* revealed that all but two isolates were distinguishable, which suggests that neither cross-infection nor an outbreak occurred.

The overall rate of bacterial infection during this study was 80% and the rate of fungal infection 17%.

The failure of broad-spectrum antibiotics when infection was suspected or established, encouraged to use prophylaxis. A regimen of gut sterilization and nasal Mupirocin for the eradication of *S. aureus* nasal carriage (31) was selected.

USE OF SELECTIVE PARENTERAL AND ENTERAL ANTISEPSIS REGIMEN (SPEAR)

The failure of broad-spectrum antibiotics once infection was suspected or established in patients with FHF (32) justified the use of an antimicrobial prophylaxis. In the intensive care setting, the use of SPEAR (selective parenteral and enteral antimicrobial regimen), was increasingly used at this time and showed a reduction of infection rates (33-36).

To evaluate this regimen we undertook a prospective SPEAR control randomized study. One hundred and one patients with FHF were enroled (37). Patients were allocated to two arms: *infected* at the time of admission or *non-infected*. Those allocated to the *infected* arm, were randomised to receive IV cefuroxime (group 1) or SPEAR (group 2). Patients in the *non-infected* arm were randomized to receive SPEAR (group 3) or no antimicrobials until clinical evidence of infection developed or significant positive cultures were obtained (group 4; control group).

A modification of SPEAR with intravenous cefuroxime was used. Also, Mupirocin 2% ointment was applied to the anterior nares and clotrimazole vaginal cream was used. The four groups were comparable in relation to age, sex, aetiology, maximum coma grade, intubation, renal failure and adverse prognostic factors.

Overall, bacteria was responsible for 80% of episodes of infection. Most of these were caused by Gram-positive bacteria and a third by *S. aureus*; gram-negative bacteria caused 30%, and fungi one fifth of infection episodes. In patients allocated to the non-infected arm there was a statistically significant reduction in episodes of infection between the patients that received SPEAR compared with those that received antimicrobials when clinically indicated. This difference was not observed in patients already infected on admission. Groups receiving SPEAR had a significant reduction in rates of infection compared with the control group ($p = < 0.005$). All groups receiving any early antimicrobial treatment had a lower incidence of infection compared with the control group (group 4) ($p = < 0.0005$).

Interestingly, there was no statistically significant difference in rates of infection between patients receiving antibiotics from admission (group 1) and those receiving SPEAR regimen (groups 2 and 3). The incidence of fungal infection was higher in the groups that did not receive SPEAR, but this was not statistically significant.

Thirty-seven clinical episodes of infection were documented; these were pneumonia and there were no statistically significant differences between the groups. Overall 55.5% of the patients survived and the proportion of survivors was higher, but not significantly so, in the groups receiving SPEAR (62.4% compared with the control group, 45.2%). Death related to sepsis was less frequent in the groups receiving SPEAR.

In this study, the chance of transplantation was higher in patients receiving SPEAR or early antimicrobials, suggesting that antimicrobial prophylaxis reduces the incidence of infection and improves the chances of transplantation. SPEAR did not alter the length of stay in the liver failure unit or result in a cost benefit.

The reduction of infection episodes in groups receiving SPEAR or antibiotics alone compared with the control group (group 4) seemed more closely related to the time of initiation of antimicrobials rather than gut decontamination per se.

In this study the overall rate of infection was 45% lower than in our previous study. The lower number of patients per group did not allow us to draw more conclusions. Therefore, we carried out a new study to confirm the advantages of SPEAR in these patients.

PROPHYLACTIC USE OF ANTIMICROBIALS WITH AND WITHOUT GUT DECONTAMINATION

The efficacy of prophylactic parenteral antibacterials, with or without selective decontamination (SSD) of the digestive tract (38), was assessed in 108 patients with FHF or severe paracetamol hepatotoxicity. These patients were randomized on admission to receive IV ceftazidime and flucloxacillin plus, either gut decontamination (group 1), or oral amphotericin B (group 2). They were 53 males and 55 females with a median age of 30 years (range 18-69). The main aetiology was paracetamol overdose in 86, viral infection in 15 and other causes in 7. The maximum INR reached was 15.3, mean 8.2. The maximum coma grades reached were I, II, III and IV in 7, 8, 3 and 60 patients, respectively. Thirty patients all with paracetamol overdose did not develop coma 10 in group 1 and 20 in group 2. Fifty-eight patients developed renal failure and 60 required mechanical ventilation.

Both groups were comparable in age, sex, aetiology, maximum INR, APACHE II score, renal failure, number of patients requiring ventilation, and early indicators of poor prognosis. There were no significant differences in maximum coma grade developed, between the two groups.

Patients were monitored for clinical and microbiological evidence of infection. There were 15 episodes of infection in 10 patients in group 1, and 17 episodes in 12 patients in group 2. All these infections except 3 were in patients who developed encephalopathy.

There were no differences in clinical episodes of chest infection 8/47 in group 1 and 16/61 in group 2.

Three episodes of infection were caused by multiply resistant bacteria: two were gentamicin-resistant *Klebsiella* spp. and one was a vancomycin-resistant *Enterococcus faecium*. There were 2 infections caused by *C. albicans* in group 1, and 1 in group 2.

The overall mortality in this study was 18/36 (33%). There was no significant difference in mortality between the two groups; 18 in each group. All deaths occurred in patients who developep grade III/IV encephalopathy. Infection was present or contributed to death in 21% of patients in group 1 and in 27% in group 2. Cerebral oedema and brain stem herniation was the main cause of death in 8 patients, 7 in group 1 and one in group 2 (p = 0.041). This study showed that the administration of oral non-absorbable antibacterials did not confer any additional benefit on FHF patients receiving prophylactic systemic antibacterials on development of infection. There was no difference in mortality between the two groups. Fifty per cent of patients with poor prognosis indicators underwent never transplantation: 5/13 (38%) in group 1 and 10/21 (47%) in group 2 (p = NS).

In this study we encountered the problem of emergence of multiresistant bacteria in particular multiresistant *Klebsiella* and *Enterobacter*. The use of third generation cephalosporins in the regimen used may account for this problem.

Although in this study we failed to demonstrated any additional benefit with the use of SDD, the use of antimicrobial prophylaxis reduced dramatically the risk of infection complication when compared with previous studies. The lack of efficacy of regimens containing SDD may be explained by the length of time required for the regimen to become effective and the shorter disease, combined with poor gut motility in these patients.

CONCLUSIONS

It has been stressed in this review why patients with FHF are so prone to infection. The continuous evaluation of the problem during recent years reassure us that FHF patients benefit greatly from the use of prophylactic intravenous antibiotics. The use of the different approaches mentioned above allowed us to reduce the incidence of bacterial infection from 80% as initially reported to 20% as reported in this last study (fig. 4).

When choosing a prophylactic regimen, it is important to balance the benefit of the regimen in high risk FHF patients and the risk of selecting resistant organisms through over-use of certain antibiotics. Avoidance of cephalosporins is recommended, but the prophylactic regimen should be adjusted to the microbiological problems in each centre.

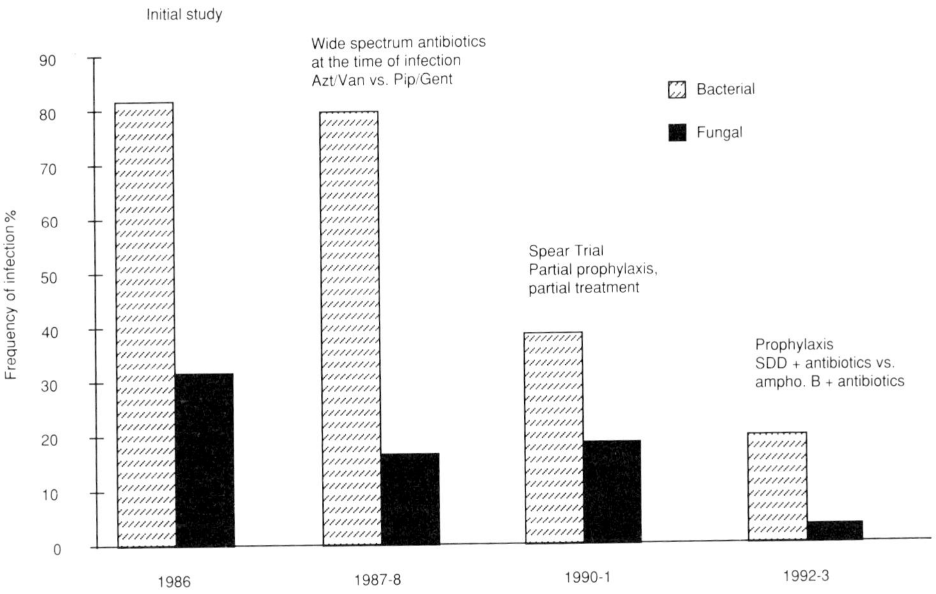

Fig. 4. Different approaches to bacterial and fungal infection in fulminant hepatic failure.

In our centre, after samples are taken for microbiology, prophylaxis with IV broad spectrum antibiotic with anti-staphylococcal activity is commenced. Routinely we use oral amphotericin B. Patients are constantly evaluated for infection, changes in antibiotics regimens and addition of antifungals (fig. 5). In FHF patients undergoing orthotopic liver transplantation, the addition of IV amphotericin B as prophylaxis is recommended. The combination of antimicrobial prophylaxis and measures to prevent infection improve the outcome in sepsis. However, in the severely inmunocompromised FHF patient, an approach aimed at improving the immunological defects found in these populations seems appropriate. In this context, the use of granulocyte colony stimulating factor (G-CSF) may reduce the incidence of infection by improving the microbicidal activity of mature neutrophils

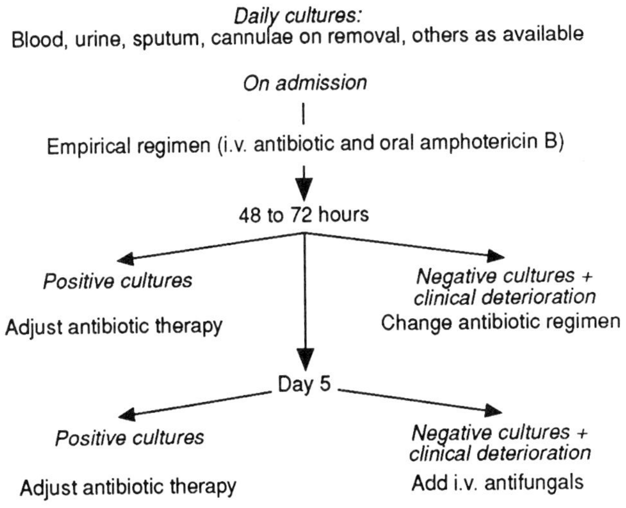

Fig. 5. Algorithm for prophylaxis and treatment of infection in fulminant hepatic failure patients.

It has been shown in other clinical condition that G-CSF enhances adhesion (39). Wang et al. demonstrated the chemotactic activity of G-CSF inducing migration of neutrophils (40). The *in vitro* administration of G-CSF rapidly increased expression of C3bi receptors on circulating granulocytes, improving opsonisation (41, 42). Roilides et al. reported the enhancement of phagocytic and bactericidal activity of normal and defective neutrophils (43, 44).

We are evaluating *in vitro* the effects of G-CSF on neutrophil function from FHF patients and our early data is encouraging. In the future a concomitant administration of G-CSF and antibiotic therapy will be indicated to reduce infection and mortality in FHF.

REFERENCES

1. Trey C, Davidson LS. The management of fulminant hepatic failure. In: Popper H, Schaffner F, eds. Progress in Liver Disease, vol III. New York: Grune & Stratton, 1970; 282-298.
2. Wyke RJ, Yousif-Kadaru AGM, Rajkovic IA, Eddles-

ton ALWF, Williams R. Serum stimulatory activity and polymorphonuclear leucocyte movement in patients with fulminant hepatic failure. Clin Exp Immunol 1982; 50:442-449.
3. Larcher VF, Wyke RJ, Mowat AP, Williams R. Mechanisms of serum defect in yeast opsonisation in children with fulminant hepatic failure. Clin Exp Immunol 1981; 46:406-411.
4. Wyke RJ, Rajkovic IA, Eddleston ALWF, Williams R. Defective opsonisation and complement deficiency in serum from patients with fulminant hepatic failure. Gut 1980; 21:643-649.
5. Altin M, Rajkovic I, Hughes R, Williams R. Neutrophil adherence in chronic liver disease and fulminant hepatic failure. Gut 1983; 24:746-750.
6. Bailey RJ, Woolf IL, Cullens H, Williams R. Metabolic inhibition of polymorphonuclear leucocytes in fulminant hepatic failure. Lancet 1976; i:1162-1163.
7. Alam AN, Poston LP, Wilkinson SP, Golindano CG, Williams R. A study in vitro of the sodium pump in fulminant hepatic failure. Clin Sci Mol Med 1978; 55:355-363.
8. Imawari M, Hughes R, Gove C, Williams R. Fibronectin and Kupffer cell function in fulminant hepatic failure. Dig Dis Sci 1985; 30:1028-1033.
9. Gonzales-Calvin J, Scully MF, Sanger Y, Fok J, Kakkar VV, Hughes RD, Gimson AES, Williams R. Fibronectin in fulminant hepatic failure. Br Med J 1982; 285:1231-1232.
10. Rolando N, Harvey F, Brahm J, Philpott-Howard J, Alexander G, Gimson AES, Casewell M. Williams R. Prospective study of bacterial infection in acute liver failure: an analysis of fifty patients. Hepatology 1990; 11:49-53.
11. Nsouli KA, Lazarus JM, Schoenbaum SC, Gottlieb MN, Lowrie EG, Shocair M. Bacteremic infection in haemodialysis. Arch Intern Med 1979; 139:1255-1258.
12. Muñoz SJ. Difficult management problems in fulminant hepatic failure. Semin Liver Dis 1993; 13:395-413.
13. Triger DR, Slater, DN, Goepel JR, Underwood JCE. Systemic candidiasis complicating acute hepatic failure in patients treated with cimetidine. Lancet 1981; ii:837-838.
14. Goularte TA, Lichtenberg DA, Craven DE. Gastric colonization in patients receiving antacids and mechanical ventilation: a mechanism for pharyngeal colonization. Am J Infect Contr 1986; 14:88.
15. Penn RG, Sanders WE, Sanders CC. Colonization of the oropharynx with gram negative bacilli: a major antecedent to nosocomial pneumonia. Am J Infect Control 1981; 9:25-34.
16. Craven DE, Kunches LM, Kilinsky V, Lichtenberg DA, Make BJ, McCabe WR. Risk factors for pneumonia and fatality in patients receiving continuous mechanical ventilation. Am Rev Res Dis 1986; 133:792-796.
17. Johanson WG, Pierce AK, Sanford JP, Thomas GD. Nosocomial respiratory infections with gram negative bacilli: The significance of colonization of the respiratory tract. Ann Inter Med 1972; 77:701-706.
18. Johanson WG, Pierce AK, Sanford JP. Changing pharyngeal bacterial flora of hospitalized patients. Emergence of gram negative bacilli. N Engl J Med 1969; 281:1137-1140.
19. Krause W, Matheis H, Wulf K. Fungemia and funguria after oral administration of Candida albicans. Lancet 1969; i:598-599.
20. Stone HH, Kolb LD, Currie CA, Geheber CE, Cuzzell JZ. Candida sepsis: Pathogenesis and principles of treatment. Ann Surg 1974; 179:697-710.
21. Walsh TJ, Hamilton SR. Disseminated aspergillosis complicating hepatic failure. Arch Intern Med 1983; 143:1189-1191.
22. Gazzard B, Portmann B, Murray-lyon IM, Williams R. Causes of death in fulminant hepatic failure and relationship to quantitative histological assessment of parenchymal damage. Q J Med 1975; 176:615-626
23. Nusinovici V, Crucibille C, Opolon P, Touboul JP, Darnis F, Caroli J. Hepatittes fulminantes avec coma. Revue de 137 cas. I Complications. Gastroenterol Clin Biol (Paris) 1977; 1:861-873.
24. Mummery RV, Bradley JM, Jeffries DJ. Microbiological monitoring of patients in hepatic failure with particular reference to extra corporeal porcine liver perfusion. Lancet 1971; ii:60-61.
25. Wyke RJ, Canalese JC, Gimson AES, Williams R. Bacteraemia in patients with fulminant hepatic failure. Liver 1982; 2:45-52.
26. Larcher VF, Wyke RJ, Mowat AP, Williams R. Bacterial and fungal infection in children with fulminant hepatic failure: possible role of opsonisation and complement deficiency. Gut 1982; 23:1037-1043.
27. Sesma P, Alvarez J, Linares P, Suarez MD. Disseminated aspergillosis complicating hepatic failure. Arch Inter Med 1984; 858:141-144.
28. Park GR, Drummond GB, Lamb D, Durie TB, Milne LJ, Lambie AT, Cameron EWJ. Disseminated aspergillosis occurring in patients with respiratory, renal, and hepatic failure. Lancet 1982; ii:179-83.
29. Rolando N, Harvey F, Brahm J, Philpott-Howard J, Alexander G, Casewell M, Williams R. Fungal infection: a common, unrecognised complication of acute liver failure. J Hepatol 1991; 12:1-9.
30. Wade J, Baillie L, Rolando N, Casewell M. Pristinamycin for *Enterococcus faecium* resistant to vancomycin and gentamicin. Lancet 1992; i:312-313.
31. Casewell MW, Hill RLR. Elimination of nasal carriage of *Staphylococcus aureus* with mupirocin («Pseudomonic acid») —a controlled trial. J Antimicrob Chemother 1986; 17:365-372.
32. Rolando N, Wade JJ, Fagan E, Philpott-Howard J, Casewell MW, Williams R. An open, comparative trial of aztreonam with vancomycin and gentamicin with piperacillin in patients with fulminant hepatic failure. J Antimicrob Chemother 1992; 30:215-220.
33. Stoutenbeek CP, van Saene HKF, Miranda DR, Zandstra DF. The effect of selective decontamination of the digestive tract on colonisation and infection rate in multiple trauma patients. Intensive Care Med 1984; 10:185-192.
34. Stoutenbeek CP, van Saene HKF, Miranda DR,

Zandstra DF, Langrehr D. The effect of oropharyngeal decontamination using topical non absorbable antibiotics on the incidence of nosocomial respiratory tract infections in multiple trauma patients. Trauma 1987; 27:357-364.
35. Unertl K, Ruckdeschel G, Selbmann HK, Jensen U, Forst H, Lenhart FP, Peter K. Prevention of colonization and respiratory tract infections in long-term ventilated patients by administration of local antimicrobial prophylaxis. Intensive Care Med 1987; 13:106-113.
36. Kerver AJ, Rommes JH, Mevissen-Verhage EA, Hulstaert PF, Vos A, Verhoef J, Wittebol P. Prevention of colonization and infection in critically ill patients: a prospective, randomized study. Crit Care Med 1988; 16:1087-1093.
37. Rolando N, Gimson AES, Wade JJ, Philpott-Howard J, Casewell M, Williams R. Prospective controlled trial of selective parenteral and enteral antimicrobial regimen in fulminant liver failure. Hepatology 1993; 17:196-201.
38. Rolando N, Wade JJ, Stangou A, Wendon J, Gimson AES, Philpott-Howard J, Williams R. Prospective study comparing prophylactic parenteral antimicrobials, with or witout enteral decontamination in patients with acute liver failure. Hepatology (Suppl in press).
39. Young KL, Linch DC. Differential effects of granulocyte- and granulocyte- macrophage colony-stimulating factors (G- and GM-CSF) on neutrophil adhesion in vitro and in vivo. Eur J Haematol 1992; 49:251-259.
40. Wang JM, Chen ZG, Collela S, Bonilla MA, Welte K, Bordigon C, Montovani A. Chemotactic activity of recombinant human granulocyte colony-stimulating factor. Blood 1988; 72:1456-1460.
41. Yuo A, kitagawa S, Ohsaka A, Ohta M, Miyasono K, Okabe T, Urabe A, Saito M, Takaku F. Recombinant human granulocyte colony-stimulating factor as an activator of human granulocytes: Potentiation of responses triggered by receptor-mediated agonist and stimulation of 3Cbi receptor expression and adherence. Blood 1989; 74:2144-2149.
42. Kitagawa S, You A, Souza LM, Saito M, Miura Y, Takaku F. Recombinant human granulocyte colony-stimulating factor enhances superoxide release in human granulocytes stimulated by chemotactic peptide. Biochem Biophys Res Commun 1987; 144:1143-1146.
43. Roilides E, Mertins S, Eddy J, Walsh TJ, Pizzo PA, Rubin M. Impairment of neutrophil chemotactic and bactericidal function in HIV-infected children and partial reversal after in vitro exposure to granulocyte-macrophage colony-stimulating factor. J Pediatr 1990; 117:531-540
44. Roilides E, Walsh T, Pizzo PA, Rubin M. Granulocyte colony-stimulating factor enhances the phagocytic and bactericidal activity of normal and defective human neutrophils. J Infect Dis 1991; 163:579-583.

Treatment of Spontaneous Bacterial Peritonitis and Other Severe Bacterial Infections in the Setting of Cirrhosis

M. Navasa

INTRODUCTION

Urinary tract infections, spontaneous bacterial peritonitis, respiratory infections and bacteremia are the most frequent infective complications in cirrhosis. Table 1 shows the overall incidence and the different types of infection found in several studies published in the last decade including large series of cirrhotic patients (1-17).

SPONTANEOUS BACTERIAL PERITONITIS

Spontaneous bacterial peritonitis (SBP), that is the spontaneous infection of the ascitic fluid without any apparent intra-abdominal source of the infection, is the most characteristic infective complication in cirrhosis (17). The incidence of SBP in cirrhotic patients admitted to hospital with ascites has been estimated to range between 7 and 23%. Recent studies have shown that the one-year probability of development of the first SBP in cirrhotic patients with ascites is of approximately 10%. This probability is higher in cirrhotic patients with low ascitic fluid protein concentration (< 1 g/dl) and/or severe hepatic insuficiency (18-20). The recent introduction of new effective treatments for the management of ascites and variceal bleeding in cirrhosis (sclerotherapy, variceal ligation, transjugular intrahepatic portocaval shunt, pharmacological treatment of portal hypertension, therapeutic paracentesis) has not been followed by a substantial improvement in the prognosis of patients with these complications. In contrast, the outcome of cirrhotic patients with SBP has dramatically improved during the last 15 years. In studies published before 1980, the rate of SBP resolution ranged between 25 and 50% and the survival of patients ranged between 0 and 20% (21, 22). The corresponding values in the latest studies are 70-90% and 50-70%, respectively (23). An early diagnosis of SBP due to a better knowledge of the signs and symptoms associated with the infections, the routine use of diagnostic paracentesis in patients admitted to hospital with ascites and, specially, the use of a more adequate antibiotic therapy are the most likely reasons for this improvement in prognosis.

Table 1. Incidence of bacterial infections in cirrhosis (%)

Patients with infection	39
Patients with	
Urinary tract infection	21
Spontaneous bacterial peritonitis*	15
Respiratory infections	8
Bacteremia	5
Other infections	5

* Percentage in relation to patients with ascites.

Table 2. Cefotaxime in the treatment of spontaneous bacterial peritonitis (SBP)

	SBP resolution (%)	Superinfection	Hospital survival (%)
Felisart et al. (26) (2 g/4 h)	86	–	73
Ariza et al. (31) (1 g/6 h)	81	–	42
Runyon et al. (27)			
5 days treatment	93	–	67
10 days treatment	91	–	42
Spanish Collaborative Group (28)			
2 g/6 h	75	–	69
2 g/12 h	79	–	79
Toledo et al. (29)	77	–	62

TREATMENT OF SBP WITH CEFOTAXIME (table 2)

Since SBP is a serious infection that may precipitate numerous potentially lethal complications (septic shock, progressive circulatory and renal impairment, liver failure), antibiotic administration must be started as soon as the diagnosis of the infection is established and, therefore, prior the identification of the responsible organism. Before 1985 the combination of an aminoglycoside, gentamicin or tobramycin, plus a beta-lactam antibiotic, ampicillin or cefalotin, was the most frequently used empiric antibiotic regime in cirrhotic patients with SBP (23). However, and despite of most organisms isolated in patients with SBP being susceptible in vitro to this antibiotic combination, resolution of the infection was obtained in less than 60% of cases. Moreover, several studies showed that cirrhotic patients with ascites are highly predisposed to develop nephrotoxicity and severe renal failure when treated with aminoglycosides. Cabrera et al. (24) reported an incidence of aminoglycoside nephrotoxicity of 31%, significantly higher than that reported in the general population (3-15%). On the other hand, Moore et al. (25), demonstrated in a large series of patients with different diseases treated with aminoglycosides that the presence of liver disease was one of the strongest independent predictors of aminoglycoside nephrotoxicity. It was, therefore, realized that empirical antibiotic regime in patients with SBP should consist in an antibiotic or antibiotic combination with adequate coverage against aerobic gram-negative bacilli and gram possitive cocci but without potential nephrotoxicity.

In 1985 Felisart et al. (26) published the first investigation assessing the efficacy of cefotaxime in patients with SBP. It consisted in a randomized controlled trial comparing cefotaxime (2 g every 4 h in patients without renal failure) versus the combination of ampicillin plus tobramycin in a large series of cirrhotic patients with SBP or other severe bacterial infections. As expected, 92% of the isolated bacteria in the group treated with ampicillin plus tobramycin and 98% in the group treated with cefotaxime were susceptible in vitro to the antibiotic regime administered. Resolution of the infection was achieved in 56% of the patients treated by ampicillin plus tobramycin and in 85% of patients treated by cefotaxime. The corresponding values in the patients with SBP included in the study were 61 and 86%, respectively. Nephrotoxicity and severe renal failure occurred in approximately 10% of patients receiving aminoglycosides whereas no patient treated with cefotaxime developed this complication. Finally, 15% of patients treated with ampicillin-tobramycin and none treated with cefotaxime developed superinfections caused by resistant organisms. Following this study, cefotaxime is considered as one of the first-choice antibiotics in the empirical treatment of SBP in patients with cirrhosis.

Two randomized controlled trials assessing the optimal duration of therapy and dosage of cefotaxime in cirrhotic patients with SBP have recently been reported. Runyon et al. (27) randomized 90 patients with SBP to receive cefotaxime (2 g i.v. every 8 hours) during 10 days (43 patients) or during 5 days (47 patients). Resolution of the infection (93.1% vs. 91.2%), recurrence of SBP during hospitalization (11.6% vs. 12.8%) and hospital mortality (32.6% vs. 42.5%) was comparable in the two groups. Short-course treatment with cefotaxime is, therefore, as efficacious as long-course therapy in cirrhotic patients with SBP. Rimola et al. (28) have reported the results of a randomized multicenter controlled trial in 143 patients with SBP treated with cefotaxime comparing two different dosages: 2 g every 6 h (71 cases) vs. 2 g every 12 h (72 cases). Peak serum levels and trough serum and ascitic fluid levels of cefotaxime were determined in both groups. The rate of SBP resolution (77% vs. 79%) and patient survival (69% vs. 79%) were similar in both groups. Peak serum levels of cefotaxime were not significantly different among the groups. As expected, trough serum and/or ascitic fluid levels were significantly lower or more frequently undetectable in patients receiving 2 g every 12 h of cefotaxime. These meassurements, however, did not correlate with SBP resolution or patient survival in any of the groups. Therefore, doses of cefotaxime lower than those usualy recommended are very effective in SBP.

PREDICTORS OF SBP RESOLUTION AND SURVIVAL IN PATIENTS TREATED WITH CEFOTAXIME

Two-hundred thirteen consecutive episodes of SBP empirically treated with cefotaxime in 185 cirrhotic patients were retrospectively analysed by Toledo et al. (29) to identify predictors of infection resolution and patients survival at the time of dignosis. One hundred sixty-five episodes (77%) resolved with cefotaxime alone, and 2 more episodes (1%), initially unresponsive to cefotaxime, were cured after modification of antibiotic therapy. Eighty-two patients died during hospitalization (38% mortality rate in relation to the 213 episodes of SBP). In a multivariate analysis 4 out of 51 clinical and laboratory variables considered at the time of diagnosis of infection (band neutrophils in white blood cell count, community-acquired vs. hospital acquired SBP, blood urea nitrogen and serum aspartate aminotransferase levels) were identified as independent predictors of infection resolution, and six (blood urea nitrogen serum aspartate aminotransferase level, community acquired vs. hospital acquired SBP, age, Child-Pugh score and ileus) as independent predictors of survival. Interestingly enough, no microbiological data, including *in vitro* susceptibility of cefotaxime of the isolated organism, had predictive value for infection resolution and survival.

A constant observation of the investigations concerning the treatment of SBP is that between 20 to 30% of patients die during hospitalization despite infection resolution. A recent study by Follo et al. (30) in 252 consecutive episodes of SBP has shown that the development of renal impairment following diagnosis of SBP is the strongest independent predictor of patient mortality in those episodes responding to cefotaxime. Renal impairment occurred in 83 episodes (33%) and in every instance it fullfilled the criteria of functional renal failure. Renal impairment was progressive in 35 episodes, steady in 27 and transient in 21. Mortality rate was 100% in episodes associated with progressive renal impairment, 31% in episodes associated with steady renal impairment, 5% in episodes with transient renal impairment and 7% in episodes without renal impairment. Other independent predictors of mortality in this series were age, blood urea nitrogen at diagnosis, isolation of the responsible organism in the ascitic blood culture and peak serum bilirubin during the antibiotic treatment.

TREATMENT OF SBP WITH OTHER PARENTERAL ANTIBIOTICS (table 3)

Following the study of Felisart et al. (26) proposing cefotaxime as the drug of choice in the empirical treatment of SBP in cirrhotic patients, several investigations have been carried out to assess the eficacy of other antibiotic regimes in these patients. In 1986, Ariza et al. (31) evaluated the use of aztreonam in 16 episodes of SBP caused by enterobacteria. Although the authors reported an initial positive response in all cases, 7 patients (44%) died during antibiotic treatment. Whether the cause of death in these patients was related to SBP or not is difficult to ascertain from the data offered by the

Table 3. Other parenteral antibiotics in the treatment of spontaneous bacterial peritonitis (SBP)

	SBP resolution (%)	Superinfection (%)	Hospital survival (%)
Ceftriaxone (32, 33)	91	–	70
Cefonicid (33)	94	–	63
Aztreonam (31)	66	16	50
Amoxicillin + clavulanic acid (34)	85	4	63

study. Overall mortality during hospitalization was 62%. Superinfections due to resistant organisms were detected in 3 cases (19%). These results, together with the fact that aztreonam is only capable of covering approximately 75% of the potential organism causing SBP, suggest that this antibiotic is probably not adequate for the empirical treatment of cirrhotic patients with SBP. In 1989, Mercader et al. (32) reported that ceftriaxone 2 g/day, a third generation cephalosporin with antibacterial activity similar to cefotaxime, was effective in 83% of 18 episodes of SBP in cirrhotic patients. Three patients developed superinfections (candida in 2 and enterococcus in one). More recently ceftriaxone (2 g/24 h) and cefonicid 2 g/12 h) have been compared in an open randomized trial (33). Both antibiotics showed similar efficacy in the treatment of SBP, with a resolution rate of 100% for ceftriaxone and 94% for cefonicid. Despite this high efficacy, hospital mortality rate was 30 and 37%, respectively. Three patients treated with ceftriaxone and two patients treated with cefonicid developed colonizations with Enterococcus faecalis or Candida albicans. Finally, in an investigation published in 1990 by Grange et al. (34), the administration of 1 g/6 h of amoxicillin associated to clavulanic acid was found to be effective in 85% of 27 episodes of SBP. One patient developed superinfection.

TREATMENT OF SBP WITH ORAL ANTIBIOTICS

Although SBP is occasionally diagnosed in patients with septic shock, ileus, gastrointestinal hemorrhage or hepatic encephalopathy and, therefore, requires to be treated with parenteral antibiotics, in most instances patients with SBP are in relatively good clinical condition and could be treated orally. Two studies have been reported assessing the effectiveness of oral antibiotics in SBP. Both studies used wide spectrum quinolones which are almost completely absorbed after oral administration and rapidly difuse to the ascitic fluid. Silvain et al. (35) reported the efectiveness of oral pefloxacin alone (1 case) or in combination with other oral antibiotics (cotrimoxazole, 9 cases; amoxicillin, 3 cases; cefadroxil, 1 case, and co-trimoxazole plus metronidazole, 1 case) in 15 SBP episodes. The rate of infection resolution was 87%, two patients developed superinfections and the survival at the end of hospitalization was 60%. Navasa et al. (36) have recently reported the results of a randomized controlled trial in 132 patients with non-severely complicated SBP (no septic shock, ileus or serum creatinine >3 mg/dl) comparing oral ofloxacin (400 mg/12 h) vs. intravenous cefotaxime (2 g every 6 h). The rate of infection resolution (78% vs. 79%) and patient survival (80% vs. 81%) were similar in the two groups. In addition, the incidence of superinfections an the length of antibiotic treatment were also similar in both groups, suggesting that oral ofloxacin is as effective as intravenous cefotaxime in the treatment of non-severely complicated SBP in cirrhosis.

URINARY TRACT INFECTIONS

Urinary tract infections are the most frequent infective complications in cirrhosis (table 1). As in the non-cirrhotic population, cirrhotics with indwelling catheters are highly predisposed to develop urinary tract infections. The incidence is markedly higher in female than in male cirrhotics (37).

Many urinary tract infections in cirrhosis are oligo-or asymptomatic, and bacteriüria alone is found in a high proportion of episodes in cirrhotics (37). However, its potential role in causing bacteremia should not be underestimated (17).

The majority of urinary tract infections in cirrhotic patients are caused by Gram-negative bacilli (4, 8, 37). Therefore, although urine cultures for identification and in-vitro sensitivity testing of causative organisms are always recommended, cases requiring immediate therapy should be given a modern quinolone (norfloxacin, ofloxacin, cyprofloxacin), or the ancient but effective co-trimoxazole, since these agents are very active against Gram-negative bacteria and reach high concentrations in urine. Other antibiotic regimes might include, amoxicillin plus clavulanic acid or an oral cephalosporin (38, 39).

PNEUMONIA

Community-acquired pneumonia is a frequent complication in subjects with active alcoholism (40). *Streptococcus pneumoniae* is the causative organism in most lower respiratory tract infections in alcoholics. However, a significant number of cases of pneumonia are caused by other pathogens normally present in the oropharyngeal area, especially anaerobic bacteria or *Haemophilus influenzae*, or by Gram-negative bacilli, particularly *Klebsiella pneumoniae* (40, 41). All these organisms, together with the possibility of *Mycoplasma pneumoniae* or *Legionella* sp., should be considered when selecting empiric therapy for lower respiratory tract infections in alcoholic subjects (42). In these subjects, a suggested primary antibiotic regime could include erythromycin combined with one of the following antibiotics: cefotaxime, ceftriaxone, amoxicillin-clavulanic acid, or imipenem. Although characteristics of community acquired pneumonia in non-alcoholic cirrhotic patients seems that do not differ from those seen in general population, the combination erythromycin plus a third generation cephalosporin might be adequate (42).

Hospital acquired pneumonia is predominantly caused by Gram-negative bacilli and staphylococci (43, 44). Some procedures or clinical conditions, such us tracheal intubation, esophageal tamponade or hepatic encephalopathy (45), are clearly predisposing factors for pneumonia in cirrhotic patients. Although the identification of the responsible organism in hospital acquired pneumonia is important for selection of antibiotic treatment, the empiric administration of third-generation cephalosporins (ie cefotaxime) should be considered as the first choice of antibiotic. In the case of suspicion of aspiration, clindamycin should be added (43, 44).

OTHER INFECTIONS

Soft tissue infections, particularly lymphangitis of the lower extremities and abdominal wall, are relatively frequent in cirrhotic patients with ankle edema or ascites. Although *Stafilococcus aureus* and *Streptococcus pyogenes* are the most frequent causative organisms, enterobacteriaceae and anaerobes may also be responsible for these infections (46). Cloxacillin has been considered the first choice antibiotic but considering these causative organisms, amoxicillin-clavulanic acid may be a more adequate empiric antibiotic treatment. More recently, quinolones such as ofloxacin have been proposed for the treatment of soft tissue infections.

Endocarditis complicating the course of cirrhosis usually arises on a previously normal endocardium. Gram-positive cocci, mainly *Streptococcus* spp. *(S. viridans, Enterococcus bovis)* and *Stafilococcus aureus* are the most common causative organisms, but the possibility of endocarditis caused by enterobacteria should not be underestimated (47, 48). The empiric treatment usually recommended includes ampicillin plus gentamicin.

Cirrhotic patients with hydtrotorax can develop spontaneous bacterial empyema (49). The pathogenesis of spontaneous bacterial empyema is thought to be the same as that of SBP, since the isolated bacteria are also the same. Therefore patients with spontaneous bacterial empyema may be treated with the same antibiotic regimes.

REFERENCES

1. Andreu M, Barrufet P, Force L, Solá R, Verdaguer A, Panadés A, Arán R. Fiebre en el enfermo con cirrosis hepática: estudio prospectivo durante 6 meses. Med Clin (Barcelona) 1985; 84: 433-436.
2. Clemente Ricote G, Barajas JM, Serrano MI, Pérez de Ayala MV, Menchén P, Senent MC, Castellanos D, Loeches N, Velo JL y Alcalá-Santaella R. Infecciones bacterianas en la cirrosis hepática. Gastroenterol Hepatol 1986; 9:285-290.
3. Ratnoff OD, Patek A. The natural history of Laennec's cirrhosis of the liver. An analysis of 386 cases. Medicine (Baltimore) 1942; 21:207-268.
4. Rimola A, Bory F, Planas R, Xaubet A, Bruguera M, Rodés J. Infecciones bacterianas en la cirrosis hepática. Gastroenterol Hepatol 1981; 4:453- 458.
5. Suárez C, Pajares JM. Epidemiología de las infecciones de la cirrosis hepática. Rev Clin Esp 1981; 160:299-303.
6. Dixon RE. Effects of infections on hospital care. Ann Intern Med 1978; 89:749-753.
7. Caly WR, Strauss E. A prospective study of bacterial infections in patients with cirrhosis. J Hepatol 1993; 18:353-358.

8. Gómez J, Vilardell F, Casais L, and Prats G. Infecciones urinarias del cirrótico. Rev Esp Enf Apar Dig 1979; 56:321-326
9. Lévy VG, Theis C, Denis C, Denis J. Critères cytologiques de l'infection de l'ascite au cours des cirrhoses. Gastroenterol Clin Biol 1982; 6:736-739.
10. Kammerer J, Dupeyron C, Vuillemin N, Leluan G, Fouet P. Apport des examens cytologiques et bactériologiques du liquide d'ascite cirrhotique au diagnostique de péritonite bactérienne. A propos de 610 prélèvements chez 156 malades. Med Chir Dig 1982; 11:243-251.
11. Pinzello G, Simonetti RG, Craxi A, DiPiazza S, Spano C, Pagliaro L. Spontaneous bacterial peritonitis: a prospective investigation in perdominatly nonalcoholic cirrhotic patients. Hepatology 1983; 3:545-549.
12. Attali P, Turne K, Pelletier G, Ink O, Etienne JP. pH of ascitic fluid. Diagnostic and prognostic value in cirrhotic and noncirrhotic patients. Gastroenterology 1986; 90:1255-1260.
13. Almdal TP and Skinhoj P. Spontaneous bacterial peritonitis in cirrhosis. Incidence, diagnosis and prognosis. Scand J Gastroenterol 1987; 22:295-300.
14. Graudal N, Milman N, Kikegaard E, Korner B, Thomsem AC. Bacteremia in cirrhosis of the liver. Liver 1986; 6:297-301.
15. Almdal T, Skinhoj P, Friis H. Bacteremia in patients suffering from cirrhosis. Infection 1986; 14:68-70.
16. Runyon BA. Bacterial infections in patients with cirrhosis. J Hepatol 1993; 18:271-273.
17. Rimola A. Infections in liver disease. In: McIntyre N, Benhamou JP, Bircher J, Rizzetto M, Rodés J, eds. Oxford Textbook of Clinical Hepatology. Oxford: Oxford Medical Press, 1991; 1272-1284.
18. Runyon BA. Low-protein-concentration ascitic fluid is predisposed to spontaneous bacterial peritonitis. Gastroenterology 1986; 91:1343-1346.
19. Llach J, Rimola A, Navasa M, Ginès P, Salmerón JM, Ginès A, Arroyo V, Rodés J. Incidence and predictive factors of first episode of spontaneous bacterial peritonitis in cirrhosis with ascites: relevance of ascitic fluid protein concentration. Hepatology 1992; 16:724-727.
20. Andreu M, Solá R, Sitges-Serra A, Alia C, Gallen M, Vila M.C, Coll S, Oliver MI. Risk factors for spontaneous bacterial peritonitis. Gastroenterology 1993; 104:1133-1138.
21. Conn HO. Spontaneous bacterial peritonitis and bacteremia in Laennec's cirrhosis caused by enteric organisms. A relatively common but rarely recognized syndrome. Ann Intern Med 1964; 60:568-580.
22. Conn HO, Fessel JM. Spontaneous bacterial peritonitis in cirrhosis: variations on a theme. Medicine (Baltimore) 1971; 50:161-197.
23. Rimola A. Treatment and prophylaxis of spontaneous bacterial peritonitis. In: Rodés J, Arroyo V, eds. Therapy in liver diseases. Barcelona: Doyma, 1992; 397-406.
24. Cabrera J, Arroyo V, Ballesta AM, Rimola A, Gual J, Elena M, Rodés J. Aminoglycoside nephrotoxicity in cirrhosis: value of β2-microglobulin to discriminate functional renal failure from acute tubular damage. Gastroenterology 1982; 82:97-105.
25. Moore RD, Smith CR, Lipsky JJ, Mellits ED, Lietman PS. Risk factors for nephrotoxicity in patients treated with aminoglycosides. Ann Intern Med 1984; 100:352-357.
26. Felisart J, Rimola A, Arroyo V, Pérez-Ayuso RM, Quintero E, Ginès P, Rodés J. Cefotaxime is more effective than is ampicillin-tobramycin in cirrhotics with severe infections. Hepatology 1985; 5:457-462.
27. Runyon BA, McHutchison JG, Antillon MR, Akriviadis EA, Montano AA. Short-course versus long-course antibiotic treatment of spontaneous bacterial peritonitis. A randomized controlled study of 100 patients. Gastroenterology 1991; 100:1737-1742.
28. Spanish Collaborative Group for Study of Spontaneous Bacterial Peritonitis. Two different dosages of cefotaxime in the treatment of spontaneous bacterial peritonitis in cirrhosis. Preliminary results of a multicenter randomize, comparative study. Hepatology 1992; 16:594.
29. Toledo C, Salmerón JM, Rimola A, Navasa M, Arroyo V, Llach J, Ginès A, Ginès P, Rodés J. Spontaneous bacterial peritonitis in cirrhosis: predictive factors of infection resolution and survival in patients treated with cefotaxime. Hepatology 1993; 17:251-257.
30. Follo A, Llovet JM, Navasa M, Planas R, Forns X, Francitorra A, Rimola A, Gassull MA, Arroyo V, Rodés J. Renal impairment after spontaneous bacterial peritonitis in cirrhosis: incidence, clinical course, predictive factors and prognosis. Hepatology 1994; 20.
31. Ariza J, Xiol X, Esteve M, Fernández F, Liñares J, Alonso T, Gudiol F. Aztreonam vs. Cefotaxime in the treatment of gram-negative spontaneous peritonitis in cirrhotic patients. Hepatology 1991; 14:91-98.
32. Mercader J, Gómez J, Ruiz J, Garre MC, Valdés M. Use of ceftriaxone in the treatment of bacterial infections in cirrhotic patients. Chemotherapy 1989; 35(Suppl 2):23-26.
33. Gómez-Jimenez J, Ribera E, Gasser I, Artaza MA, Del Valle O, Pamissa A, Martínez-Vázquez JM. Randomized trial comparing ceftriaxone with cefonicid for treatment of spontaneous bacterial peritonitis in cirrhotic patients. Antimicrob Agents Chemother 1993; 37:1587-1592
34. Grange JD, Amiot X, Grange V, Gutmann L, Biour M, Bodin F, Poupon R. Amoxicillin-Clavulanic acid therapy of spontaneous bacterial peritonitis: a prospective estudy of twenty-seven cases in cirrhotic patients. Hepatology 1990; 11:360-364.
35. Silvain C, Breux JP, Grollier G, Rouffineau J, Breq-Giraudon B, Breauchant M. Les septicémies et les infections du liquide d'ascite du cirrhotique peuvent-elles être traitées exclusivement par voie orale? Gastroenterol Clin Biol 1989; 13:335-339.
36. Navasa M, Planas R, Clemente G, Vargas V, Guarner C, Follo A, Viver J, Obrador A, Rodrigo L, Rimola A, Arroyo V, Rodés J, and members of the Collaborative Group for the Study of SBP, Spain. Oral ofloxacin vs.

intravenous cefotaxime in the treatment of non-complicated spontaneous bacterial peritonitis (SBP) in cirrhosis. Results of a multicenter, prospective, randomized trial. J Hepatol 1994; Suppl 1:S-11.

37. Burroughs AK, Rosenstein IJ, Epstein O, Hamilton-Miller JMT, Brumfit W, Sherlock S. Bacteriuria and primary biliary cirrhosis. Gut 1984; 25:133-137.
38. Lipsky B.A. Urinary tract infections in men. Epidemiology, pathophysiology, diagnosis and treatment. Ann Intern Med 1989; 110:138-150.
39. Westphal J-F, Jehl F, Vetter D. Pharmacological, toxicological, and microbiological considerations in the choice of initial antibiotic therapy for serious infections in patients with cirrhosis of the liver. Clin Infect Dis 1994; 18:324-335.
40. Adams HG, Jordan C. Infections in the alcoholic. Med Clin North Am 1984; 68:179-200.
41. Bradsher RW. Overwhelming pneumonia. Med Clin North Am 1983; 67:1233-1250.
42. Levy M, Dromer F, Brion N, Leturdu F, Carbon C. Community-acquired pneumonia. Chest 1988; 92:43-48.
43. Craven DE, Daschner F, Guiot L. Current topic: Nosocomial pneumonia. Eur J Clin Infec Dis 1989; 8:1-75.
44. Torres A, Celis R. Neumonías intrahospitalarias. Med Clin (Barcelona) 1987; 88:34-37.
45. Panés J, Terés J, Bosch J, Rodés J. Efficacy of balloon tamponade in treatment of bleeding gastric and esophageal varices. Results in 151 consecutive patients. Dig Dis Sci 1988; 33:454-459.
46. Swartz MN. Cellulitis and Superficial Infections. In: Mandel GL, Douglas RG Jr, eds. Principles and Practice of Infectious Diseases. 3rd ed. New York: Churchill Livingstone, 1990; 796-807.
47. Snyder N, Atterbury CE, Correia JP, Conn HO. Increased ocurrence of cirrhosis and bacterial endocarditis. A clinical and postmortem study. Gastroenterology 1977; 73:1107-1113.
48. Denton JH, Rubio C, Velázquez J. de Arellano GR. Bacterial endocarditis in cirrhosis. Dig Dis Sci 1981; 26:935-937.
49. Flaum MA. Spontaneous bacterial empyema in cirrhosis. Gastroenterology 1976; 70:416-417.

Prevention of Bacterial Infections in the Setting of Cirrhosis

C. Guarner

INTRODUCTION

Bacterial infection is a frequent and severe complication in the course of cirrhosis, as 30-60% of patients with cirrhosis are admitted to the hospital because of a bacterial infection or develop a nosocomial infection (1-8). The incidence of bacterial infections in cirrhotic patients is higher than in the general population (8) and depends on several factors such as severity of illness that is profound enough to require hospitalization (9-12) and multifactorial immunodeficiency (8-11). Frequently, the development of a bacterial infection may lead to other complications such as gastrointestinal hemorrhage, hepatic encephalopathy and hepatorenal syndrome (8, 13). Although the mortality rate (14-18) has decreased during the last decade as a consequence of an earlier diagnosis and advances in antibiotic therapy it remains very high (19-27). Also, the mortality rate of infected hospitalized cirrhotic patients is much higher than of non-infected hospitalized cirrhotic patients (28-30). Between 7 and 25% of the deaths of cirrhotic patients are related to bacterial infections (8, 31).

The most common causative agents isolated in bacterial infections in cirrhotic patients are gram-negative bacteria, especially *Escherichia coli* and *Klebsiella pneumoniae* (1-8). Gram-positive cocci are isolated less frequently and anaerobic bacteria are very uncommon (32). As these organisms are predominantly gut flora, it has been suggested that the gut may be the source of the bacteria (8, 18). However, a direct passage of intestinal flora to portal blood or to ascitic fluid has not been documented in cirrhotic patients, if the gut mucosa has not lost its integrity (33, 34). Bacterial translocation, defined as the passage of viable bacteria from the gastrointestinal tract to extraintestinal sites such as mesenteric lymph nodes (35), has been documented in other conditions in which gram-negative infections are frequent, such as hemorrhagic shock (36, 37), intestinal obstruction (38), obstructive jaundice (39), endotoxemia (40) and acute pancreatitis (41). Recently, bacterial translocation from the gut to cecal and mesenteric lymph nodes has been demonstrated in an experimental model of cirrhotic rats with ascites (42) and in an experimental model of acute surgically-induced portal hypertension (43). Interestingly, mesenteric lymph node cultures were positive in 4% of the control rats, in 53% of the cirrhotic rats without spontaneous bacterial peritonitis (SBP) or bacterascites and in all the cirrhotic rats with SBP or bacterascites (42). Therefore, these data suggest that bacterial translocation from gastrointestinal tract to cecum and mesenteric lymph nodes and other extraintestinal sites is an important step in the pathogenesis of bacterial infections in cirrhotic patients. Theoretically, decreasing bacterial translocation should diminish the incidence of bacterial infections in cirrhotic patients.

IMPORTANCE OF PROPHYLAXIS OF BACTERIAL INFECTIONS

Several measures have been proposed to reduce the incidence of bacterial infections in cirrhotic patients, such as discontinuing alcohol intake (44), reducing the hospitalization length (8-11), avoiding unnecessary instrumentation (9), improving the nutritional status (45) and preventing ascites formation, gastrointestinal hemorrhage and hepatic encephalopathy (8).

Since diuretic treatment increases the concentration of ascitic fluid complement components and the opsonic activity of ascitic fluid in cirrhotic patients (46), it has been suggested that diuretics could prevent the development of SBP (46). However, there are no available data in the literature confirming this hypothesis. In fact, the incidence of SBP in cirrhotic patients treated with diuretics was similar to that of patients treated with diuretics and paracentesis plus albumin, despite the fact that repeated paracentesis decrease the concentration of complement components, proteins and opsonic activity of ascitic fluid (47, 48).

Since enteric aerobic gram-negative bacteria are the most frequent causative agents isolated in bacterial infections in cirrhosis and since bacterial translocation seems to be an important step in its pathogenesis, inhibition of intestinal gram-negative bacteria should be an effective method of preventing bacterial infections in these patients. This has been evaluated in several studies detailed below.

THE CONCEPT OF SELECTIVE INTESTINAL DECONTAMINATION

Selective intestinal decontamination (SID) consists of the inhibition of the gram-negative flora of the gut with preservation of gram-positive cocci and especially anaerobic bacteria and, therefore, prevention of intestinal colonization, overgrowth and subsequent translocation of new potentially pathogenic bacteria (49). The gram-negative flora of the gut are responsible for bacterial infections in neutropenic (50-53) and in cirrhotic patients (1-8). Several clinical trials have shown a reduction in the incidence of infections caused by gram-negative bacilli in neutropenic patients submitted to SID, without overgrowth of resistant bacteria or important side effects (50-53).

In addition, SID with oral nonabsorbable antibiotics or with the poorly-absorbed quinolone, norfloxacin, increases complement factors and protein levels in ascitic fluid in cirrhotic patients with low ascitic fluid protein (54, 55) and in patients with schistosomal hepatic fibrosis and low protein ascitic fluid (56). These data suggest that SID may be useful in the prophylaxis of SBP, not only because it inhibits the aerobic intestinal flora, but also because it improves the antimicrobial capacity of the ascitic fluid in these patients (57).

Theoretical beneficial effects that should be expected of SID in the prevention of bacterial infections in cirrhotic patients are a decrease in the incidence of bacterial infections and an improvement in survival of the cirrhotic patients without side effects and minimal cost. In addition, prophylactic treatment should be more effective than strategies of early diagnosis and treatment.

Combinations of oral nonabsorbable antibiotics have been used in the prevention of bacterial infections in neutropenic patients (50-53) and in cirrhotic patients with gastrointestinal hemorrhage (58). However, combinations of oral nonabsorbable antibiotics have some disadvantages, such as the possible overgrowth of potentially pathogenic resistant bacteria, especially in those patients who should be treated for a long time, as well as an increase in side effects and cost (59, 60).

Norfloxacin is a quinolone that may be an ideal agent for SID because it is incompletely absorbed by the intestine, it is active against most aerobic gram-negative bacteria with little or no activity against gram-positive and anaerobic organisms (61, 62), as has been shown in volunteers (63), in neutropenic (64) and in cirrhotic patients (65). Emergence of resistance is low (65). Oral norfloxacin suppresses rapidly and strongly gram-negative bacilli from the fecal flora in cirrhotic patients. Fecal flora is totally recovered done week after the end of the treatment (66). Therefore, prophylactic treatment with norfloxacin in cirrhotic patients should be continued as long as patients are at high risk of bacterial infection (49, 66).

Several studies have demonstrated that oral norfloxacin reduces the incidence of infections caused by gram-negative bacilli in neutropenic patients, without overgrowth of resistant bacteria or important side effects (64, 67). However, it has been recently shown that long-term norfloxacin treatment reduces SBP incidence in cirrhotic rats, but it causes overgrowth of gut gram-positive bacteria and increases gram-positive cocci translocation and gram-positive cocci SBP (68).

Prophylactic SID should be considered in cirrhotic patients who are at high risk of developing bacterial infections (69, 70). Possible prophylactic SID indications, schedules and results are different in hospitalized patients than in outpatients and, therefore, are discussed separately below.

SELECTIVE INTESTINAL DECONTAMINATION IN HOSPITALIZED CIRRHOTIC PATIENTS

Clinical risk factors for developing bacterial infections in hospitalized cirrhotic patients are gastrointestinal bleeding (58, 71) and ascites with low protein concentration (72-76). Table 1 shows the results of different studies that have been performed to evaluate the efficacy of SID in preventing bacterial infection in hospitalized cirrhotic patients at high risk of bacterial infection.

Several studies have shown that cirrhotic patients with gastrointestinal hemorrhage have a high incidence of bacterial infections, especially during the first three to four days after admission (58, 71). The incidence of bacterial infections in these patients is about 20% at admission to the hospital and 40% during the hospitalization period. This high incidence of infections has been related to a marked reduction in the macrophage and Kupffer cell function (77) and to a higher bacterial translocation during the hemorrhagic shock (37). Recently, Runyon et al. (78) have shown that an hemorrhagic shock induced a significantly higher incidence of bacterial translocation ($p < 0.05$) in cirrhotic rats than in normal rats (67% vs. 14%, respectively).

In the first reported study of prevention of bacterial infection in cirrhotics with gastrointestinal hemorrhage, Rimola et al. (58) demonstrated a reduction in the incidence of infections caused by enteric bacteria during hospitalization in patients treated with oral nonabsorbable antibiotics. This randomized study compared the incidence of bacterial infection in 68 bleeding cirrhotic patients treated prophylactically with non-absorbable antibiotics (gentamicin, vancomycin and nystatin or neomycin, colistin and nystatin) since admission to hospital until 48 hours after stopping the hemorrhage with 72 control non-treated patients. The incidence of bacterial infections was significantly lower ($p < 0.05$) in treated group than in control group (16% vs. 34.7%), but hospital mortality was similar in both groups.

As it has been disussed previously, SID with oral non-absorbable antibiotics could have some disadvantages, especially if long-term treatment is required (59, 60). In order to assess the efficacy of SID with norfloxacin in the prevention of bacterial infections in cirrhotic patients with gastrointestinal hemorrhage, Soriano et al. (79) designed a prospective, randomized study in which 119 bleeding cirrhotic patients were included. Treated patients received norfloxacin orally or through a nasogastric tube 400 mg bid for 7 days beginning immediately after emergency gastroscopy and control group patients did not. The incidence of bacterial infections (10% vs. 37.2%), bacteremia and/or spontaneous bacterial peritonitis (3.3% vs. 16.9%) and urinary infections (0% vs. 18.6%) during the hospitalization period was significantly lower ($p = 0.001$, $p < 0.05$ and $p = 0.001$, respectively) in patients receiving norfloxacin than in control group, as a consequence of the decrease in the incidence of infections caused by aerobic gram-negative bacilli. No differences were observed in respiratory infections. No side effects related to norfloxacin treatment and/or infections by opportunistic bacteria were observed in this study. The decrease in mortality observed in the treated group (6.6% vs. 11.8%) did not reach statistical significance. In addition, the cost for antibiotic treatment showed a 62% reduction in the treated group when compared to the control group.

Recently, Blaise et al. (80) have evaluated the effect of systemic antibiotic therapy in the prevention of bacterial infection in cirrhotic pa-

Table 1. Prophylaxis of bacterial infection in hospitalized cirrhotic patients with high risk of bacterial infection

Risk group	Patients (n)	Treatment	Bacterial infection (%)		Survival (%)
Gastrointestinal hemorrhage patients[a, b, c]					
	140	Oral non-absorbable antibiotics			
Treated[a]	68		16[f]		73.5
Control	72		34.7		68
	119	Oral norfloxacin			
Treated[b]	60		10[g]		93.4
Control	59		37.2		88.2
	91	i.v. ofloxacin plus amoxicillin/clavulanic acid			
Treated[c]	46		20[g]		76
Control	45		66		65
Sclerotherapy patients[d]					
	97	i.v. imipenem/cilastatin			
Treated[d]	47		21.6		79
Control	50		28.9		72
Low ascitic fluid protein patients[e]					
	63	Oral norfloxacin			
			SBP	EPI[h]	
Treated[e]	32		0[f]	3.1[i]	93.8
Control	31		22.5	22.5	83.9

[a, b, c, d, e] References 58, 79, 80, 85 and 89, respectively. [f] $p < 0.05$. [g] $p < 0.01$. [h] EPI: extraperitoneal infections. [i] $p = 0.05$.

tients admitted to an intensive care unit for gastrointestinal bleeding by ruptured esophageal varices. Ninety one non-infected evaluable patients were randomized, 46 patients received ofloxacin 400 mg per day over a period of ten days, first intravenously then orally and an intravenous bolus of amoxicillin plus clavulanic acid (1g) before each endoscopy performed during hemorrhage, and 45 patients did not. The incidence of bacterial infections was significantly lower ($p < 0.001$) in the treated group than in the control (20% vs. 66%, respectively) and also the incidence of pulmonary tract infections (4% vs. 40%, respectively; $p < 0.001$). The incidence of pulmonary infection in this study was very high, probably because more than 30% of the patients required tracheal intubation and more than 35% a Blakemore tube to control hemorrhage. Mortality was higher in control group than in treated group (24% vs. 35%, respectively), but this difference was not significant.

As bacteremia and bacterial infections have been reported after sclerotherapy of esophageal varices (81-83), especially after emergency sessions (84), Rolando et al. (85) evaluated the incidence of bacterial infection after endoscopic sclerotherapy of esophageal varices and the role of systemic antibiotic prophylaxis in a prospective randomized control study. Ninety-seven cirrhotic patients with bleeding esophageal varices submitted to esophageal sclerotherapy were evaluable, 47 patients were treated with imipenem/cilastatin (500 mg i.v.) before each sclerotherapy session and 50 control patients with intravenous dextrose-saline. Early post-sclerotherapy bacteremia was similar in both groups (1.1% vs. 5.6% of sclerotherapy sessions, respectively), as well as late bacterial infections (20.5 and 23.4% of sclerotherapy sessions, respectively). Therefore, these authors do not recommend prophylactic parenteral antibiotic prior to sclerotherapy and suggest that the high incidence of bacterial infections in bleeding cirrhotic patients submitted to emergence sclerotherapy may be more related to gastrointestinal hemorrhage than to sclerotherapy.

Results of all these studies suggest that prophylactic antibiotics, preferentially norfloxacin, should be used to prevent bacterial infections in non-infected cirrhotics admitted to hospital because of gastrointestinal hemorrhage (71). Probably, systemic antibiotic should be evaluated in those patients who require tracheal intubation and/or balloon tamponade.

Several studies have shown that patients with cirrhosis with low ascitic fluid protein concentration have a high incidence of bacterial infections, especially SBP, during hospitalization (72-76). Between 10 and 25% of the hospitalized patients with ascites develop SBP (72-76). This high incidence of SBP in low ascitic fluid protein patients with cirrhosis has been attributed to a low antimicrobial activity of ascitic fluid (86-88), as bactericidal activity and total protein of ascitic fluid are directly related (57). Soriano et al. (89) performed a prospective randomized study in order to evaluate prophylactic SID in hospitalized patients with cirrhosis and low ascitic fluid protein. Thirty-two cirrhotic patients were treated with oral norfloxacin 400 mg day during all the hospitalization and 31 patients served as controls. Clinical and analytical characteristics were similar in both groups and most patients had been admitted for the treatment of ascites. The incidence of bacterial infections (3.1% vs. 41.9%) and SBP (0% vs. 22.5%) was significantly lower ($p < 0.005$ and $p < 0.05$, respectively) in patients receiving prophylactic norfloxacin. Also, the incidence of extraperitoneal infections was lower ($p = 0.052$) in the treated group than in the non-treated group (3.1% vs. 22.5%, respectively). The decrease in mortality observed in the group undergoing prophylactic SID did not reach statistical significance (6.2% vs. 16.1%, respectively). No cost-benefit evaluation was made in this study. Minimal side effects related to norfloxacin and no opportunistic bacterial infections were observed in the treated group. The authors concluded that prophylactic SID with norfloxacin should be used in hospitalized patients with cirrhosis and low ascitic fluid protein to prevent SBP and extraperitoneal infections.

Henrion et al. (90) evaluated the efficacy of SID in the prevention of bacterial infection in patients with cirrhosis admitted on an intensive care unit for different causes, such as gastrointestinal hemorrhage, ascites, encephalopathy and others. Ninety four non-infected patients at admission were randomized, forty five patients were treated with oral non-absorbable antibiotics (neomycin 1 g, colistin 1.500.000 U and nystatin 1.000.000 U every 6 hours) or norfloxacin 400 mg bid at least during five days and 49 served as control. The incidence of septicemia was significantly lower ($p < 0.05$) in treated group than in control (8.8% vs. 24.5%, respectively) and mortality was similar in both groups. These authors recommend SID for patients with cirrhosis admitted to an intensive care unit, particularly when hepatic function is poor.

Although mortality rate was not significantly decreased in any study, SID with norfloxacin should be considered in hospitalized cirrhotic patients with gastrointestinal hemorrhage or with low ascitic fluid protein. The incidence of bacterial infections is drastically reduced, no opportunistic bacterial infections and no significant side effects have been observed during short-term treatment and it is less expensive than the treatment of bacterial infections (91).

SELECTIVE INTESTINAL DECONTAMINATION IN CIRRHOTIC OUTPATIENTS

Table 2 shows the results of the studies of primary and secondary SBP prophylaxis in cirrhotic outpatients. Patients with cirrhosis who recover from SBP are predisposed to develop a new infection (92-95). The one year probability rate of SBP recurrence has been estimated between 32 and 69%. Therefore, long-term SID could be useful in preventing SBP recurrence in these patients. Gines et al. (96) carried out a double-blind, placebo controlled study to evaluate if long-term oral administration of norfloxacin prevents SBP recurrence in patients with cirrhosis. Forty cirrhotics were treated with oral norfloxacin (400 mg/day) and 40 did not. The incidence of SBP recurrence was significantly lower ($p < 0.05$) in the prophylactic group than in control group during follow-up

Table 2. Prophylaxis of spontaneous bacterial peritonitis in cirrhotic outpatients

Risk group	Patients (n)	Treatment	Bacterial infection (%)		Survival (%)
			SBP	EPI[e]	
Primary prophylaxis[a, b]					
	122	Oral norfloxacin			
Treated[a]	63		1.6[g]	30.1	70
Control[c]	59		15.2	25.4	68
	107	Oral norfloxacin			
Treated[b]	54		0[f]	13	85.2
Control	53		13	17	81.2
Secondary prophylaxis[d]					
	80	Oral norfloxacin			
Treated[d]	40		12[f]	7.5	82.5
Control	40		35	12	75

[a, b, d] References 102,106 and 96, respectively.
[c] Treated with norfloxacin only during hospitalary admissions.
[e] EPI extraperitoneal infections.
[f] $p < 0.05$.
[g] $p < 0.01$.

(12% vs. 35%, respectively), as a consequence of a lower incidence of gram-negative SBP ($p < 0.01$). The incidence of extraperitoneal infection was similar (7.5% vs. 12%, respectively). No differences were observed in number of hospital readmissions (36 and 42, respectively) or in survival during follow-up. Only an oral and esophageal candidiasis was observed in a patient after 7 months of norfloxacin treatment. These results show that long-term SID with norfloxacin is a highly effective and safe measure to prevent SBP recurrence. In spite of the bad prognosis of patients who survived to a SBP (92-95), some authors (97, 98) do not consider long-term norfloxacin therapy to be appropiate. Prophylactic treatment did not decrease hospital admissions or morbidity, did not improve survival and cost-effectiveness was not analyzed. However, patients with cirrhosis recovering from an SBP episode must be considered for liver transplantation (99) and treated prophylactically with norfloxacin while awaiting liver transplantation (100).

Low ascitic fluid protein patients with cirrhosis are predisposed to develop an SBP episode not only during hospitalization but also during follow-up (45, 101). Andreu et al. (101) followed up prospectively one-hundred and ten patients with cirrhosis with sterile ascites and without previous SBP to identify risk factors for first episode of SBP. Patients with low ascitic fluid protein concentration and/or high serum bilirubin had a high risk of developing the first SBP episode during follow-up. The probability of developing SBP was more than 50% after one year of follow-up in this group. Forty per cent of SBP episodes were acquired during hospitalization. Therefore, the authors suggest that these patients could benefit from prophylactic SID.

Recently, Novella et al. (102) have carried out a randomized study to evaluate primary prophylaxis of SBP with norfloxacin in cirrhotic patients with low ascitic fluid protein concentration or high serum bilirubin. In this study one-hundred and twenty-two patients were included, 63 patients were treated with oral norfloxacin 400 mg per day since the inclusion into the study and 59 patients were treated with norfloxacin only during hospitalization periods. This schedule was tried because these patients could benefit from short-term inpatient prophylaxis avoiding possible long-term SID side-effects or consequences. The chance of developing the first SBP episode was significantly higher ($p < 0.01$) in patients treated only during hospitalization than in continuosly treated patients (15.2% vs. 1.6%, respectively) and also the probability of first SBP episode at 18 months of follow-up was higher (31% vs. 9%, respectively, $p < 0.01$). However, the incidence of extraperitoneal bacterial infection was similar in both groups (25.4% vs. 30.1%, respectively) and no differences were observed in number of hospital readmissions, other complications of cirrhosis and survival (67.8% vs. 69.8%, respectively). Interestingly, in this study only 2 episodes of inpatient SBP were observed in more than 200 hospitalization, confirming that short-term SID is effective in preventing inpatient SBP (103), in spite of the increase of norfloxacin resistant flora (103-105).

Similar results have been observed by Grange et al. (106) in a multicentric, double-blind, placebo-controlled trial of primary prophylaxis of SBP in patients with cirrhosis with low ascitic fluid protein. In this study 107 patients were included, 54 patients treated with oral norfloxacin (400 mg/day) and 53 patients with placebo for 6 months. The incidence of first episode of SBP during these months was significantly lower ($p < 0.05$) in treated than in placebo group (0% vs. 7.5%, respectively), but mortality was similar (14,8% vs. 18,8%, respectively). Neither selection of resistant mutant bacteria to norfloxacin nor quantitative changes with respect to *Enterococcus* spp. in stool repeated samples were observed in the follow-up.

According to the results of both studies, SID with norfloxacin should be used in patients with cirrhosis with low ascitic fluid protein during hospitalization and probably in some patients during other extrahospitalary periods with high risk of SBP that have not been well-defined yet.

Recently, long-term antibiotic prophylaxis with a weekly dose of 750 mg ciprofloxacin is being evaluated in preventing primary or recurrence SBP (107).

The effectiveness of SID with norfloxacin might decrease with time because of the development or selection of resistance bacterial strains that subsequently colonize the gut and became a source of infection, especially in those patients submitted to a long-term prophylactic treatment (104, 105). In fact, SBP and pleural empyema by *Escherichia coli* resistant to norfloxacin has been reported (108). It is possible that in the future norfloxacin may be replaced by another drug, as bacterial resistance to norfloxacin is growing (104, 105).

REFERENCES

1. Rimola A, Bory F, Planas R, Xaubet A, Bruguera M, Rodés J. Infecciones bacterianas agudas en la cirrosis hepática. Gastroenterol Hepatol 1981; 4:453-458.
2. Suárez C, Pajares JM. Epidemiología de las infecciones en la cirrosis hepática. Rev Clin Esp 1981; 160:299-303.
3. Palazón JM, García A, Gómez A. Infecciones hospitalarias en pacientes con cirrosis hepática. Gastroenterol Hepatol 1984; 7:120-122.
4. Andreu M, Barrufet P, Force L, Solá R, Verdaguer A, Panadés A, Arán R. Fiebre en el enfermo con cirrosis hepatica: estudio prospectivo durante 6 meses. Med Clin (Barcelona) 1985; 84:433-436.
5. Clemente G, Barajas JM, Serrano MI, Pérez de Ayala MV, Menchón P, Senent MC, Castellanos D, Loaches N, Velo JL, Alcalá R. Infecciones bacterianas en la cirrosis hepática. Gastroenterol Hepatol 1986; 9:291-293.
6. Sánchez Tapias JM, Teres J, Arroyo V, Bosch J, Bruguera M, Rodés J. Infección peritoneal en la cirrosis hepática con ascitis. Cinco años de experiencia. Gastroenterol Hepatol 1978; 1:15-21.
7. Almdal TP, Skinhoj P. Spontaneous bacterial peritonitis in cirrhosis. Incidence, diagnosis and prognosis. Scand J Gastroenterol 1987; 22: 295-300.
8. Rimola A. Infecciones bacterianas en la cirrosis hepática. MTA-Medicina Interna 1987; 5:161-224.
9. Carey WD, Boayke A, Leatherman J. Spontaneous bacterial peritonitis: clinical and laboratory features with reference to hospital acquired-cases. Am J Gastroenterol 1986; 81:1156-1161.
10. Wyke RJ. Problems of bacterial infection in patients with liver disease. Gut 1987; 28:623-641.
11. Kremer A, Rios B, Moreno N, Allevato J, Calanni L, Chiocconi E, Formaro A, Schmidt G, Kremer C. Infections during the hospitalization of patients with liver cirrhosis. Acta Gastroenterol Latinoam 1993; 23:35-42.
12. Propst T, Propst A, Schauer G, Judmaier G, Braunsteiner H, Vogel W. Is spontaneous bacterial peritonitis a complication of hospitalization? J Hepatol 1993; 19:184-185.
13. Saez-Royuela F, Gómez-Rubio M, Fernández-Guerrero ML, Díaz-Curiel M, Hernández-Guio C. A microbiological and clinical study of 57 cases of spontaneous bacterial peritonitis in liver cirrhosis patients. Rev Clin Esp 1990; 187:321-324.
14. Rimola A, Soto R, Bory F, Arroyo V, Piera C, Rodés J. Reticuloendothelial system phagocytic activity in cirrhosis and its relation to bacterial infections and prognosis. Hepatology 1984; 4:53-58.
15. Pinzello G, Simonetti RG, Craxi A, Di Piazza S, Spano C, Pagliaro L. Spontaneous bacterial peritonitis: a prospective investigation in predominantly nonalcoholic patients. Hepatology 1983; 3:545-549.
16. Hoefs JC, Canawatti HN, Sapico FL, Hopkins R, Weiner J, Montgomerie JZ. Spontaneous bacterial peritonitis. Hepatology 1982; 2:399-407.

17. Tor J, Accarino A, Guarner ML, Arnal J, Crespo E, Sierra E. Infección espontánea del líquido ascítico en pacientes cirróticos; incidencia, características clínicas, bacteriológicas y mortalidad en un hospital general. Med Clin (Barcelona) 1983; 81:53-56.
18. Hoefs JC, Runyon BA. Spontaneous bacterial peritonitis. Disease-a-Month 1985; 31:1-48.
19. Runyon BA. Spontaneous bacterial peritonitis: an explosion of information. Hepatology 1988; 8:171-175.
20. Wyke RJ. Bacterial infections complicating liver disease. Baillieres Clin Gastroenterol 1989; 3:187-210.
21. Llovet JM, Planas R, Morillas R, Quer JC, Cabré E, Boix J, Humbert P, Guilera M, Domenech E, Bertrán X, Gassull MA. Short-term prognosis of cirrhotic patients with spontaneous bacterial peritonitis: multivariate study. Am J Gastroenterol 1993; 88:388-392.
22. Toledo C, Salmerón JM, Rimola A, Navasa M, Arroyo V, Llach J, Ginès A, Ginès P, Rodés J. Spontaneous bacterial peritonitis in cirrhosis: predictive factors of infection resolution and survival in patients treated with cefotaxime. Hepatology 1993; 17:251-257.
23. Felisart J, Rimola A, Arroyo V, Pérez-Ayuso RM, Quintero E, Ginès P, Rodés J. Cefotaxime is more effective than is ampicillin-tobramycin in cirrhotics with severe infections. Hepatology 1985; 5:457-462.
24. Ariza J, Xiol X, Esteve M, Fernández F, Linares J, Alonso T, Gudiol F. Aztreonam vs. cefotaxime in the treatment of gram-negative spontaneous peritonitis in cirrhotic patients. Hepatology 1991; 14:91-98.
25. Fong T, Akriviadis EA, Runyon BA, Reynolds TB. Polymorphonuclear cell count response and duration of antibiotic therapy in spontaneous bacterial peritonitis. Hepatology 1989; 9:423-426.
26. Grange JD, Amiot X, Grange V, Gutmann L, Biour M, Bodin F, Poupon R. Amoxicillin-clavulanic acid therapy of spontaneous bacterial peritonitis: A prospective study of twenty-seven cases in cirrhotic patients. Hepatology 1990; 11:360-364.
27. Runyon BA, Hutchinson JC, Antillon MR, Akriviadis EA, Montano A. Short-course versus long-course antibiotic treatment of spontaneous bacterial peritonitis. A randomized controlled study of 100 patients. Gastroenterology 1991; 100:1737-1742.
28. Kuo CH, Changchien CS, Yang CY, Sheen IS, Liaw YF. Bacteremia in patients with cirrhosis of the liver. Liver 1991; 11:334-339.
29. Mihas AA, Toussaint J, Hsu HS, Dotherow P, Achord JL. Spontaneous bacterial peritonitis in cirrhosis: clinical and laboratory features, survival and prognostic factors. Hepatogastroenterology 1992; 39:520-522.
30. Caly WR, Strauss E. A prospective study of bacterial infections in patients with cirrhosis. J Hepatol 1993; 18:271-272.
31. Schlichting P, Christensen E, Fauerholdt L, Poulsen H, Juhl E, Tygstrup N. Main causes of death in cirrhosis. Scand J Gastoenterol 1983; 18:891-898.
32. Targan SR, Chow AW, Guze LB. Role of anaerobic bacteria in spontaneous peritonitis in cirrhosis. Report of two cases and review of literature. Am J Med 1977; 62:397-403.
33. Schweinberg FB, Seligman AM, Fine J. Transmural migration of intestinal bacteria: a study based on the use of radioactive *Escherichia coli*. N Engl J Med 1950; 242:47-51.
34. Runyon BA. Fatal bacterial peritonitis secondary to nonobstructive colonic dilatation (Ogilvie's syndrome) in cirrhotic ascites. J Clin Gastroenterol 1986; 8:687-689.
35. Berg RD. Bacterial translocation from the gastrointestinal tract. J Med 1992; 23:217-244.
36. Rush BF, Sori AJ, Murphy TF, Smith S, Flanagan JJ, Machiedo GW. Endotoxemia and bacteremia during hemorrhagic shock. Ann Surg 1988; 207:549-554.
37. Deitch EA, Morrison J, Berg R, Specian RD. Effect of hemorrhagic shock on bacterial translocation, intestinal morphology, and intestinal permeability in conventional and antibiotic-decontaminated rats. Crit Care Med 1990; 18:529-536.
38. Maddaus MA, Wells C, Billiar T, Simmons RL. Simple mechanical intestinal obstruction induces translocation of gram-negative intestinal bacteria to the mesenteric lymph nodes. Surg Forum 1989; 40:186-188.
39. Deitch EA, Sittig K, Li M, Berg R, Specian RD. Obstructive jaundice promotes bacterial translocation from the gut. Am J Surg 1988; 159:79-84.
40. Deitch EA, Berg R, Specian R. Endotoxin promotes the translocation of bacteria from the gut. Arch Surg 1987; 122:185-190.
41. Runkel NSF, Moody FG, Smith GS, Rodríguez LF, La Rocco MT, Miller TA. The role of the gut in the development of sepsis in acute pancreatitis. J Surg Res 1991; 51:18-23.
42. Runyon BA, Squier S, Borzio M. Translocation of gut bacteria in rats with cirrhosis to mesenteric lymph nodes partially explains the pathogenesis of spontaneous bacterial peritonitis. J Hepatology 1994; 21:792-796.
43. García-Tsao G, Albillos A, Barden GE, West AB. Bacterial translocation in acute and chronic portal hypertension. Hepatology 1993; 17:1081-1085.
44. Adams HG, Jordan C. Infections in the alcoholic. Med Clin North Am 1984; 68:179-200.
45. Llach J, Rimola A, Navasa M, Ginès P, Salmerón JM, Ginès A, Arroyo V, Rodés J. Incidence and predictive factors of first episode of spontaneous bacterial peritonitis in cirrhosis with ascites: relevance of ascitic fluid protein concentration. Hepatology 1992; 16:724-727.
46. Runyon BA, Van Epps DE. Diuresis of ascites increases its opsonic activity and may prevent spontaneous bacterial peritonitis. Hepatology 1986; 6:369-399.
47. Runyon BA, Antillon MR, Montano AA. Effect of diuresis versus therapeutic paracentesis on ascitic fluid opsonic activity and serum complement. Gastroenterology 1989; 97:158-162.

48. Ljubicic N, Bilic A, Kopjar B. Diuretics vs. paracentesis followed by diuretics in cirrhosis: effect on ascites opsonic activity and immunoglobulin and complement concentrations. Hepatology 1994; 19:346-353.
49. van der Waaij D, Manson WL, Arends JP, de Vries Hospers HG. Clinical use of selective decontamination: the concept. Intensive Care Med 1990; 16(Suppl 3): S212-216.
50. Storring RA, McElwain TJ, Jameson B, Wiltshaw E, Spiers ASD, Gaya H. Oral non-absorbed antibiotics prevent infection in acute non lymphoblastic leukaemia. Lancet 1977; ii:837-840.
51. Hahn DM, Schimpff SC, Fortner CL, Smyth AC, Young VM, Wiernik PH. Infection in acute leukemia patients receiving oral nonabsorbable antibiotics. Antimicrob Agents Chemoter 1978; 13:958-964.
52. Wade JC, Schimpff SC, Wiernik Ph. Antibiotic combination- associated nephrotoxicity in granulocytopenic patients with cancer. Arch Intern Med 1981; 141:1789-1793.
53. Bosi A, Fanci R, Pecile P, Guidi S, Saccardi R, Vannucchi AM, Longo G, Donnini E, Orsi A, Rossi Ferrini P. Aztreonam versus colistin neomycin for selective decontamination of the digestive tract in patients undergoing bone marrow transplantation: a randomized study. J Chemother 1992; 4:30-34.
54. Soriano G, Teixidó M, Guarner C, Such J, Espinós JC, Sainz S, Enríquez J, Rodríguez JL, Vilardell F. Variación del C3 en líquido ascítico de pacientes cirróticos sometidos a esterilización intestinal o a descontaminación intestinal selectiva. Rev Esp Enf Apar Digest 1989; 75:123-126.
55. Such J, Guarner C, Soriano G, Teixidó M, Barrios J, Tena F, Méndez C, Enríquez J, Rodríguez JL, Vilardell F. Selective intestinal decontamination increases serum and ascitic fluid C3 levels in cirrhosis. Hepatology 1990; 12:1175-1178.
56. El Aggan HA, Abou Seif Helmy M, Guirguis TG. Selective intestinal decontamination in patients with schistosomal hepatic fibrosis and low-protein ascites. J Egypt Soc Parasitol 1993; 23:649-57.
57. Fromkes JJ, Thomas FB, Mekhjian HS, Evans M. Antimicrobial activity of human ascitic fluid. Gastroenterology 1977; 73:668-672.
58. Rimola A, Bory F, Terés J, Pérez-Ayuso RM, Arroyo V, Rodés J. Oral, nonabsorbable antibiotics prevent infection in cirrhotics with gastrointestinal hemorrhage. Hepatology 1985; 5:463-467.
59. Wiesner RH, Hermans PE, Rakela J, Washington II JA, Perkins JD, DiCecco S, Krom R. Selective bowel decontamination to decrease gramnegative aerobic bacterial and Candida colonization and prevent infection after orthotopic liver transplantation. Transplantation 1988; 45:570-574.
60. Vossen JM, Heidt PJ, van den Berg H, Gerritsen EJ, Hermans J, Dooren LJ. Prevention of infection and graft-versus-host disease by suppression of intestinal microflora in children treated with allogeneic bone marrow transplantation. Eur J Clin Microbiol Infect Dis 1990; 9:14-23.
61. Holmes B, Brogden RN, Richards DM. Norfloxacin. A review of its antimicrobial activity, pharmacokinetic properties and therapeutic use. Drugs 1985; 30:482-513.
62. Lee C, Ronald AR. Norfloxacin: its potential in clinical practice. Am J Med 1987; 82(Suppl 6B):27-34.
63. Nord CE. Effect of new quinolones on the human gastrointestinal microflora. Rev Infect Dis 1988; 10(Suppl 1):S193-196.
64. Karp JE, Wiliam GM, Hendricksen C, Laughon B, Redden Z, Bamberger BJ, Bartlett JG, Saral R, Burke PJ. Oral norfloxacin for prevention of Gram-negative bacterial infections in patients with acute leukemia and granulocytopenia. Ann Intern Med 1987; 106:1-7.
65. Ginès P, Rimola A, Marco F, Almela A, Marqués JM, Salmerón JM, Ginès A, Llach J, Jiménez de Anta MT, Arroyo V, Rodés J. Efecto de la administración de norfloxacino sobre la flora fecal en pacientes cirróticos. Gastroenterol Hepatol 1990; 13:325-328.
66. Soriano G, Guarner C, Tomás A, Anguera A, Mirelis B, Fernández C, Herrero M, Alonso C, Vilardell F. Duración del efecto de la norfloxacina sobre la flora fecal en pacientes cirróticos. Rev Esp Enferm Dig 1992; 81:322-326.
67. Winston DJ, Karp J, Talbot G, Levitt L, Corrado M, Ho WG, Champlin RE, Bartlett J, Finley RS, Joshi JH, Deresinski S. Norfloxacin for prevention of bacterial infections in granulocytopenic patients. Am J Med 1987; 82(Suppl 6B): 40-46.
68. Runyon BA, Borzio M, Young S, Squier SU. Norfloxacin leads to overgrowth of gram-positive gut flora and increases gram-positive bacterial translocation and SBP in an animal model. Hepatology 1993; 18:292A(Abstr).
69. Guarner C, Soriano G. Descontaminación intestinal y profilaxis de las infecciones en los enfermos hepáticos. Gastroenterol Hepatol 1990; 13:359-361.
70. Grange JD, Amiot X. La prophylaxie des complications infectieuses par decontamination bacterienne digestive selective chez les malades atteints de cirrhose. Gastroenterol Clin Biol 1992; 16:692-700.
71. Bleichner G, Boulanger R, Squara P, Sollet JP, Parent A. Frequency of infections in cirrhotic patients presenting with acute gastrointestinal haemorrhage. Br J Surg 1986; 73:724-726.
72. Runyon BA. Low-protein-concentration ascitic fluid is predisposed to spontaneous bacterial peritonitis. Gastroenterology 1986; 91: 1343-1346.
73. Bercoff E, Durrbach A, Manchon ND, Duranton Y, Senant J, Lacomte N, Bourreille J. Can the protein concentration of the ascitic fluid in ascites predict the ocurrence of an infection? Gastroenterol Clin Biol 1987; 11:636-638.
74. Such J, Guarner C, Enríquez J, Rodríguez JL, Seres I, Vilardell F. Low C3 in ascitic fluid predisposes to spontaneous bacterial peritonitis. J Hepatol 1988; 6:80-84.
75. Runyon BA. Patients with deficient ascitic fluid op-

sonic activity are predisposed to spontaneous bacterial peritonitis. Hepatology 1988; 8:632-635.
76. Rabinovitz M, Gavaler JS, Kumar S, Kajani M, Van Thiel DH. Role of serum complement, immunoglobulins, and cell-mediated immune system in the pathogenesis of spontaneous bacterial peritonitis (SBP). Dig Dis Sci 1989; 34:1547-1552.
77. Carr F, Loegering D. Reticuloendothelial system function and humoral deficiency following acute haemorrhage. Can J Physiol 1978; 56:299-303.
78. Hamdani R, Young S, Runyon BA. Increased bacterial translocation in cirrhotic rats undergoinghemorrhagic shock. Gastroenterology 1994; 106:A904 (Abstr).
79. Soriano G, Guarner C, Tomás A, Villanueva C, Torras X, González D, Sainz S, Anguera A, Cusso X,Balanzo J, Vilardell F. Norfloxacin prevents bacterial infection in cirrhotics with gastrointestinal hemorrhage. Gastroenterology 1992; 103:1267-1272.
80. Blaise M, Pateron D, Trinchet JC, Levacher S, Beaugrand M, Pourriat JL. Systemic antibiotic therapy prevents bacterial infection in cirrhotic patients with gastrointestinal hemorrhage. Hepatology 1994; 20:34-38.
81. Cohen LB, Korsten MA, Scherl EJ, Velez ME, Fiss RD, Elliot JA. Bacteremia after endoscopic injection sclerosis. Gastrointest Endosc 1983; 29:198-200.
82. Ayrs SJ, Goff JS, Warren GH. Endoscopy sclerotherapy for bleeding oesophageal varices: effects and complications. Ann Intern Med 1983; 98:900-903.
83. Schembre D, Bjorkman DJ. Post-sclerotherapy bacterial peritonitis. Am J Gastroenterol 1991; 86:481-486.
84. Bac DJ, de Marie S, Siersema PD, Snobl J, van Buuren HR. Post-sclerotherapy bacterial peritonitis: a complication of sclerotherapy or of variceal bleeding? Am J Gastroenterol 1994; 89:859-862.
85. Rolando N, Gimson A, Philpott-Howard J, Sahathevan M, Casewell M, Fagan E, Westaby D, Williams R. Infectious sequelae after endoscopic sclerotherapy of oesophageal varices: role of antibiotic prophylaxis. J Hepatol 1993; 18:290-294.
86. Akalin HE, Laleli Y, Telatar H. Bactericidal and opsonic activity of ascitic fluid from cirrhotic and non-cirrhotic patients. J Infect Dis 1983; 147:1011-1017.
87. Runyon BA, Morrissey RL, Hoefs JC, Wyle FA. Opsonic activity of human ascitic fluid: a potentially important mechanism against spontaneous bacterial peritonitis. Hepatology 1985; 5:634-637.
88. Mal F, Pham Huu T, Bendahou M, Trinchet JC, Garnier M, Hakim J, Beaugrand M. Chemoattractant and opsonic activity in ascitic fluid. A study in 47 patients with cirrhosis or malignant peritonitis. J Hepatol 1991; 12:45-49.
89. Soriano G, Guarner C, Teixidó M, Such J, Barrios J, Enríquez J, Vilardell F. Selective intestinal decontamination prevents spontaneous bacterial peritonitis. Gastroenterology 1991; 100:477-481.
90. Henrion J, Schapira M, Derue G, Heller FR. Prevention of bacterial infection using selective intestinal decontamination in patients with cirrhosis admitted to intensive care. Controlled study in 120 patients. Acta Gastroenterol Belg 1992; 55:333-340.
91. Press AG, Meyer zum Buschenfelde KH, Ramadori G. Z Gastroenterol 1992; 30:543-552.
92. Tító L, Rimola A, Ginès P, Llach J, Arroyo V, Rodés J. Recurrence of spontaneous bacterial peritonitis in cirrhosis: frequency and predictive factors. Hepatology 1988; 8:27-31.
93. Silvain Ch, Mannant PR, Ingrand P, Port E, Besson I, Beauchant M. Recidive de l'infection spontanée du liquide d'ascite au curs de la cirrhose. Gastroenterol Clin Biol 1991; 15:106-109.
94. Terg R, Levi D, López P, Rafaelli C, Rojter S, Abecasis R, Villamil F, Aziz H, Podesta A. Analysis of clinical course and prognosis of culture-positive spontaneous bacterial peritonitis and neutrocytic ascites. Evidence of the same disease. Dig Dis Sci 1992; 37:1499-1504.
95. Silvain C, Besson I, Ingrand P, Mannant PR, Fort E, Beauchant M. Prognosis and long-term recurrence of spontaneous bacterial peritonitis in cirrhosis. J Hepatol 1993; 19:188-189.
96. Ginès P, Rimola A, Planas R, Vargas V, Marcó F, Almela M, Forna M, Miranda ML, Llach J, Salmerón JM, Rodés J. Norfloxacin prevents spontaneous bacterial peritonitis recurrence in cirrhosis: Results of a double-blind, placebo-controlled trial. Hepatology 1990; 12:716-724.
97. Hoefs JC. Spontaneous bacterial peritonitis: prevention and therapy. Hepatology 1990; 12:776-781.
98. Schubert ML, Sanyal AJ, Wong ES. Antibiotic prophylaxis for prevention of spontaneous bacterial peritonitis? Gastroenterology 1991; 101:550-552.
99. Ink O, Pelletier G, Salmon D, Attali P, Pessione F, Hannoun S, Buffet C, Etienne JP. Pronostic de l'infection spontanée d'ascite chez le cirrhotique. Gastroenterol Clin Biol 1989; 13:556-561.
100. Holland DJ, Sorrell TC. Antimicrobial therapy and prevention of spontaneous bacterial peritonitis. J Gastroenerol Hepatol 1993; 8:370-374.
101. Andreu M, Solá R, Sitges A, Alia C, Gallen M, Vila MC, Coll S, Oliver MI. Risk factors for spontaneous bacterial peritonitis in cirrhotic patients with ascites. Gastroenterology 1993; 104:1133-1138.
102. Novella M, Gana J, Soriano G, Andreu M, Ortiz J, Guarner C, Coll S, Vila MC, Solá R, Vilardell F. Continuous vs. intermittent (nosocomial) prophylaxis of the first episode of spontaneous bacterial peritonitis in cirrhotic patients. Final results. J Hepatol 1994; 21(Suppl 1):S46(Abstr).
103. Tomás A, Soriano G, Guarner C, Portorreal R, Novella MT, Vilardell F. Hospital-acquired bacterial infections in patients with cirrhosis undergoing selective intestinal decontamination. J Hepatol 1993; 18: 262-263.
104. Daschner F. Emergence of resistance during selective decontamination of the digestive tract. Eur J Clin Microbiol Dis 1992; 11:1-3.

105. Dupeyron C, Mangeney N, Sedrati L, Campillo B, Fouet P, Leluan G. Rapid emergence of quinolone resistance in cirrhotic patients treated with norfloxacin to prevent spontaneous bacterial peritonitis. Antimicrob Agents Chemother 1994; 38:340-344.
106. Grange JD, Roulot D, Pelletier G, Pariente A, Denis J, Ink O, Blanc P, Richardet JP, Vinel JP, Amiot X, Delisle F, Fischer D, Bodin F. Primary prophylaxis of bacterial infections with norfloxacin in cirrhotic patients with ascites: Results of a double-blind, placebo-controlled trial. Gastroenterology 1994; 106:A901(Abstr).
107. Rolachon A, Cordier L, Bacq Y, Nousbaum JB, Franza A, Paris JC, Fratte S, Bohn B, Kitmacher P, Fournet J, Stahl JP, Zarski JP. Long term prevention of spontaneous bacterial peritonitis by weekly ciprofloxacin dose: A multicentric prospective study. Gastroenterology 1994; 106:A970(Abstr).
108. Castellote J, Xiol J, Rota R, Fernández G. Spontaneous bacterial peritonitis and empyema by *Escherichia coli* resistant to norfloxacine in a patient on selective intestinal decontamination with norfloxacine. J Hepatol 1994; 20:436.

Section 4

Treatment of Chronic Viral Hepatitis

Pharmacology of Interferon

D. L. Cutler

INTRODUCTION

The phenomenon of viral interference (1) had been described for several decades prior to the discovery of interferon. In 1957, Isaacs and Lindenmann (2) observed that cells from chick chorio-allantoic membranes incubated with heat-inactivated influenza virus released a factor which induced resistance by fresh membranes to infection by live influenza virus. This substance which they called interferon could not be sedimented by centrifugation at 100,000 g for 15 minutes, was non-dialyzable and was stable over the pH range of 1-10 (3, 4). Interferon activity was lost when the preparation was heated to 60°C for one hour (3) or subjected to digestion by trypsin (4) suggesting that interferon was a protein.

Purification and isolation of interferons from natural sources proved difficult because interferons are produced in minute quantities. Following the initial report by Gresser describing the production of interferon by human leukocytes (5), methodology was developed for the production and partial purification of leukocyte-derived interferon from pooled donor blood (6, 7, 8). The purity of this natural leukocyte interferon was less than 1% with an anti-viral specific activity of approximately 1×10^6 U/mg protein. It was not until one subtype of IFN, IFN-α_2 was cloned in an *E. coli* expression system (9) and purification methods were developed (10) that large amounts of IFN could be produced and large scale clinical trials could be initiated.

CLASSIFICATION

Initially interferons were classified based upon their resistance or sensitivity to inactivation by exposure to pH 2. Interferon preparations which retained anti-viral activity after exposure to pH 2 were designated class I. Interferon preparations which were labile at pH 2 were designated class II. Subsequently, class I interferons were further subdivided based upon their cellular origin into leukocyte and fibroblast interferon. The current classification of interferon is based upon the antigenic specificity of the proteins and divides interferons into three major classes; alpha interferon, beta interferon and gamma (immune) interferon (table 1).

There are at least 14 different non-allelic genes for alpha interferons located on the short arm of chromosome 9 (11). Interferon-β and γ

Table 1. Inteferon nomenclature

Cell of origin	Pre-1980 nomenclature	Acid stability	Current nomenclature
Leukocytes (macrophages, null-cells)	Type I leukocyte	pH 2 acid-stable	Alpha
Fibroblasts (connective tissue cells, epithelial cells)	Type I fibroblast	pH 2 acid-stable	Beta
T-lymphocytes (antigen-induced, mitogen-induced)	Type II immune	pH 2 acid-labile	Gamma

each have one gene located on chromosome 9 and 12, respectively. IFN-α and β have approximately 29% sequence homology; both, however, are structurally unrelated to IFN-γ (12). The degree of sequence homology between IFN-α and IFN-β genes suggest that they originated from a common ancestral gene and that they underwent evolutionary divergence 62 to 300 million years ago (9).

Analysis of the cDNA of numerous alpha interferon genes indicates an amino acid sequence homology of 75% or greater for the majority of IFN-α subtypes. IFN-α proteins have either 165 or 166 amino acids. IFN alfa-2b (Intron A; Schering-Plough) is comprised of 165 amino acids with a calculated molecular weight of 19,271 and an isoelectric point of 6.0. The molecule has four cysteines which occur at positions 1, 29, 98 and 138, a feature common to all IFN-α subtypes. Mass spectrometric analysis of proteolytic fragments has demonstrated two disulfide bonds between residues 1-98 and 29-138. The 29-138 disulfide bond is required for full expression of biologic activity whereas disruption of the 1-98 disulfide bond does not result in significant loss of potency (13). The majority of alpha interferons do not have N-linked glycosylation sites.

In contrast to the multiple species of IFN-α produced *in vivo*, commercial interferon produced by recombinant DNA techniques contains only single species of interferon. Currently, two recombinant human IFN-α preparations are approved by the FDA for sale in the United States, Roferon A (IFN alfa-2a; Roche) and Intron A (IFN alfa-2b; Schering-Plough). These two interferons differ by a single amino acid at position 23; IFN alfa-2a has a lysine at this position whereas IFN alfa-2b contains an arginine.

MECHANISM OF ACTION

Interferons exert their cellular activities after binding to specific receptors located on the cell surface. Interferon-α and β bind to the same receptor and can compete for the receptor site. Interferon γ binds to a receptor distinct from the IFN α/β receptor (14). The number of high-affinity receptors for IFN-α on human cells has been estimated, depending on the type of cell, to be between 650 and 13,000 per cell. The ligand and receptor form a high-affinity complex with a dissociation constant of 10^{-10} to 10^{-11} mol/L.

Once IFN-α binds to its receptor, the interferon-receptor complex is internalized by receptor mediated endocytosis and is degraded in lysosomes (15-17). Internalization of the interferon receptor complex results in temporary loss of cell surface receptors; recovery of cell surface receptor number takes several hours and is accompanied by protein synthesis. This process can be inhibited by cycloheximide suggesting that new receptors must be actively synthesized (18, 19). It has been hypothesized that this temporary decrease in cell surface receptors occurring after exposure to IFN represents a mechanism for down-regulation of cellular response to IFN. Although it was originally hypothesized that internalization of interferon was necessary for expression of interferon activity, it appears that internalization is not necessary.

In the past few years, several investigators have clarified the early steps involved in interferon signal transduction. The intervening events occurring between receptor binding and gene transcription have been summarized in three recent detailed review articles (20-22). Binding of IFN-α to its receptor leads to activation of receptor associated tyrosine kinases. These kinases (TYK-2 and JAK-1) separately or cooperatively phosphorylate three proteins designated p84, p91, p113. A fourth protein, p48, which possesses intrinsic DNA binding activity has been found in both the nucleus and cytoplasm. When phosphorylated, p84, p91 and p113 can associate with p48 to form a complex designated ISGF-3 (interferon-stimulated gene factor-3). ISGF-3 binds to interferon-stimulated response elements of DNA and results in transcription of mRNA for interferon induced proteins.

Binding of IFN-α to its receptor results in the induction of over 30 proteins many of which are responsible for the anti-viral activities of IFN. Some of the proteins induced by interferons (α, β, or γ) include (2'5')- oligoadenylate synthetase, β_2 microglobulin, indoleamine 2,3 dioxygenase (which results in tryptophan degradation), MHC class I antigen and an IFN-induced protein kinase. MHC class II antigen is induced by IFN-γ only. Two of these proteins, the (2'5')- oligoadenylate synthetase system and

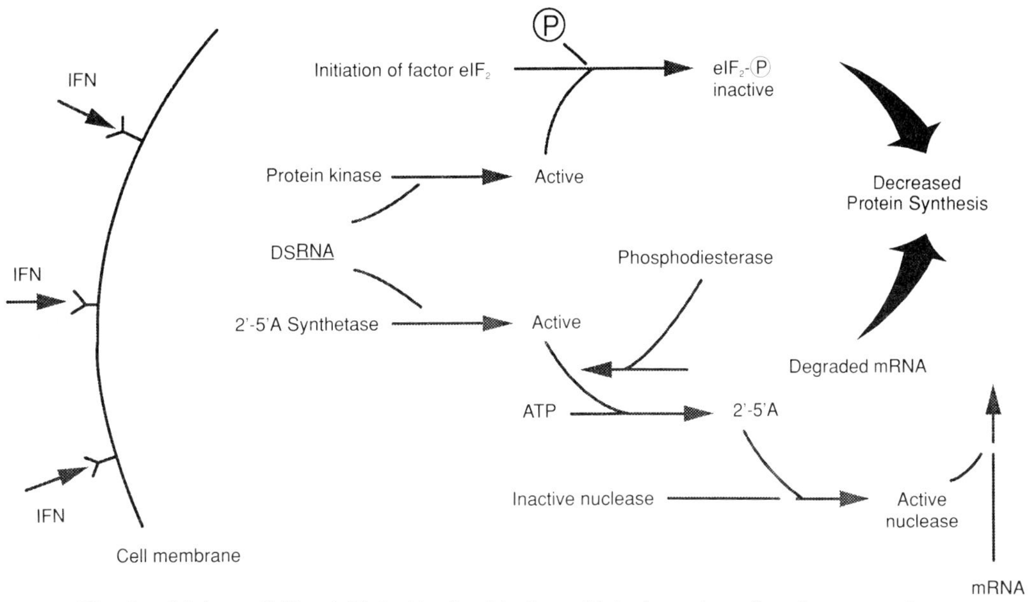

Fig. 1. Major activities initiated by the binding of interferon to cell surface receptors.

the eIF-2α protein kinase system will be briefly reviewed.

The (2'5') oligoadenylate synthetase system consists of a three enzyme pathway: (2'5')-oligoadenylate synthetase [(2'5') OAS] which catalyzes the production of 2'5' oligonucleotides (2'5'A) from ATP; an endoribonuclease (RNaseL) that is activated by 2'5'A, and a phosphodiesterase which results in hydrolysis of 2'5' oligonucleotides (fig. 1). Binding of IFN to its receptor results in a rapid increase in mRNA for (2'5') OAS and its subsequent translation. In the presence of dsRNA, (2'5') OAS is activated and catalyzes the conversion of ATP to 2'5' oligonucleotides (2'5'A). The increased concentration of 2'5'A activates a latent endoribonuclease (RNaseL) which cleaves both ribosomal and messenger RNA, thus inhibiting viral replication.

After administration of alpha interferon, there is a dose related increase in (2'5') OAS enzymatic activity measured in peripheral blood mononuclear cells from patients (23) and volunteers (24). Increased 2'5' OAS activity was observed for at least 72 hours post-dose, far longer than IFN was detected in serum (24). This may partially explain why anti-viral efficacy of IFN is observed even when interferon is dosed on a thrice weekly schedule.

eIF-2α protein kinase synthesis is another peptide induced by IFN (18). Like (2'5') oligoadenylate synthetase, it is synthesized in an inactive form and is activated in the presence of dsRNA (fig. 1). When activated, the induced protein kinase phosphorylates the enzyme eIF-2α resulting in inhibition of protein synthesis.

PHARMACOKINETICS OF INTERFERON ALFA-2B

Concentrations of IFN in serum have been quantified using sensitive and specific immunoassays (IRMA or ELISA). The bioactivity of the immunoactive peptide can be confirmed by its ability to inhibit cytopathic changes in a bioassay. Cells are incubated with the biological fluid containing IFN and subsequently washed and exposed to a cytopathic virus. The titre which results in 50 percent inhibition of the cytopathic effect is then recorded.

Because of the low IFN protein concentrations in serum obtained after SC administration, most pharmacokinetic studies of IFN alfa-2b have been performed at doses of 10 x 10^6 IU. After administration of 3 x 10^6 IU, the dose approved for treatment of hepatitis C, it is likely that serum IFN concentrations would be too low for rigorous pharmacokinetic analysis.

The pharmacokinetic profile of IFN alfa-2b in serum after single-dose administration has been characterized for the subcutaneous (s.c.), intramuscular (i.m.) and intravenous (i.v.) rou-

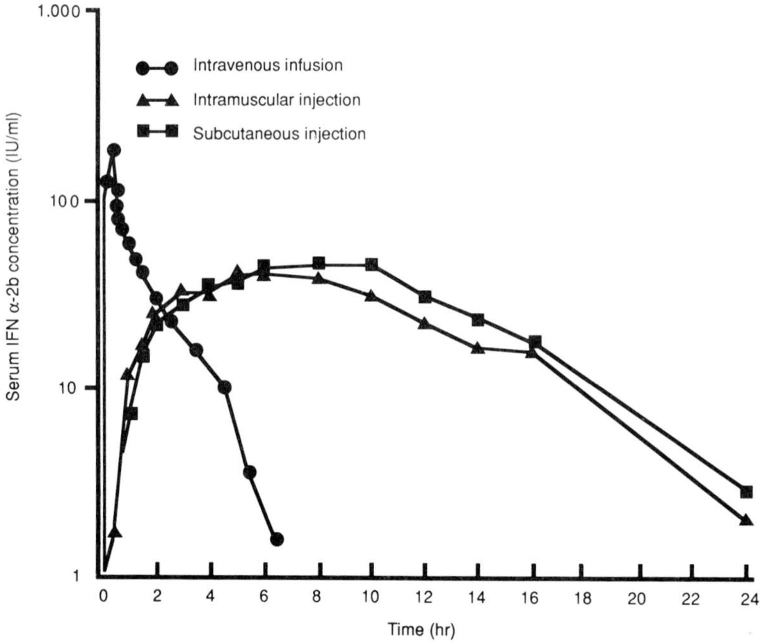

Fig. 2. Serum interferon alfa-2b concentrations after intravenous, intramuscular or subcutaneous administration of a single dose of interferon alfa-2b.

tes of administration (25). In a three-way cross-over design study, twelve healthy male volunteers received 5 x 10^6 IU/m^2 of IFN alfa-2b administered as a 30 minute intravenous infusion or by s.c. or i.m. injection. After subcutaneous or intramuscular injection the plasma concentration time curves were similar (fig. 2). Mean peak concentrations of IFN alfa-2b of approximately 50 IU/ml occurred between 7 and 8 hours after injection. The elimination half-lives following both i.m. and s.c. injections were calculated to be two to three hours. Serum concentrations of IFN alfa-2b were undetectable (< 10 IU/ml) by 16 hours post-injection.

After a 30 minute infusion of IFN alfa-2b mean peak serum concentrations of 188 IU/ml were observed (fig. 2). When the infusion was discontinued, serum concentrations of IFN declined rapidly in a biexponential manner with a distribution half-life of 0.1 hour and an elimination half-life of approximately 1.7 hours. Serum concentrations of IFN were undetectable by 4 hours post-infusion. The area under the plasma concentration-time curve (AUC) of interferon was greater after SC or IM injection than after intravenous administration. No IFN alfa-2b has been detected in urine samples from volunteers in human pharmacokinetic studies.

Pre-clinical data suggest that the kidney is the primary site of clearance of systemically administered interferons. Isolated perfused rabbit kidneys were used to investigate the clearance of IFN alfa-2 as well as natural human α and β interferons (26, 27). A large arteriovenous gradient was observed across the perfused kidneys compatible with extensive renal extraction of interferon. This is not unexpected as the glomerular membrane is permeable to low molecular weight (< 50,000 daltons) proteins. Recovery of interferon from the renal filtrate was less than 5% of the total administered dose indicating that greater than 90% of the interferon was reabsorbed at the tubular level. Available data suggest that IFN in the glomerular filtrate undergoes endocytosis and catabolism in lysozomes by cells of the proximal renal tubules (28, 29).

DRUG INTERACTIONS

Few formal studies of drug interactions have been performed with IFN alfa-2b. Preclinical data in rodents suggest that interferons reduce the concentration of cytochrome P450 in the liver and can decrease the clearance of theophylline (30). A study of the effect of alpha interferon performed in a small number of healthy volunteers and patients with hepatitis B demonstrated that single-dose administration of IFN-α decreased theophylline clearance and resulted in a statistically significant prolongation of theophylline half-life from 6.3 hours to 10.7 hours (31). Interferon administration has been shown to decrease hepatic clearance of antipyrine, an index of hepatic mixed function oxidase activity (32). Because of the potential for altered hepatic metabolism of drugs, appropriate caution is advised when interferon is administered to patients being treated with highly metabolized compounds such as theophylline or warfarin.

The effect of increasing doses of subcutaneously administered IFN alfa-2b on the pharmacokinetics of fluorouracil administered by continuous infusion has been investigated (33). Interpatient analysis showed no change in steady-state concentrations, elimination half-life, total body clearance or volume of distribution of fluorouracil. Analysis of intrasubject pharmacokinetics showed that IFN alfa-2b resulted in a 30% increase in steady-state concentrations of fluorouracil and that clearance of fluorouracil was decreased by 20 to 35%. Interferon has antiproliferative properties, and when administered in combination with cytotoxic agents or AZT may result in enhanced myelosuppression. These pharmacokinetic and pharmacodynamic interactions may require reduction in doses of cytotoxic agents when administered in combination with interferon.

ADVERSE EVENT PROFILE

As would be expected with a substance which physiologically functions in an autocrine or paracrine manner, systemic administration of pharmacologic amounts of IFN is associated with the occurrence of adverse events. Most frequently reported adverse reactions are flu-like symptoms such as fever, headache, rigors, fatigue, gastrointestinal disorders such as nausea, anorexia or diarrhea and alopecia. Table 2 lists the frequency of the more common treatment-related adverse events reported during clinical trials of IFN alfa-2b at a dose of 3×10^6 IU thrice weekly for the treatment of hepatitis C. Patients receiving a second course of IFN alfa-2b therapy for hepatitis C report a spectrum of adverse events similar to that reported during the initial course of therapy although the frequency of the acute flu-like adverse events is lower. Table 3 lists frequently observed adverse events in clinical trials of IFN alfa-2b in the treatment of hepatitis B. The frequency and severity of ad-

Table 2. Adverse events (%) reported by subjects enrolled in registration trials of IFN alfa-2b for the treatment of hepatitis C. Adverse events reported by greater than 10 % of subjets are listed

Fever	50
Headache	49
Myalgia	45
Fatigue	37
Asthenia	17
Rigors	34
Arthralgia	24
Dizziness	14
Influenza like-symptoms	6
Malaise	6
Diarrhea	14
Anorexia	15
Nausea	25
Depression	11
Irritability	13
Alopecia	17

Table 3. Adverse events (%) reported by subjects enrolled in registration trials of IFN alfa-2b for the treatment of hepatitis B. Adverse events reported by greater than 10 % of subjects are listed by dose regimens

	5×10^6 IU QD	10×10^6 IU TIW
Fever	66	86
Headache	61	44
Myalgia	59	40
Fatigue	75	69
Asthenia	5	15
Rigors	38	42
Arthralgia	19	8
Dizziness	13	10
Influenza-like symptons	13	10
Diarrhea	19	8
Anorexia	43	53
Nausea	50	33
Taste alteration	10	–
Vomiting	7	10
Depression	17	6
Irritability	16	12
Somnolence	14	9
Insomnia	11	6
Alopecia	26	38

verse events generally increases with the administration of higher doses or more intensive dosing regimens. With continued administration of IFN alfa-2b tachyphylaxis to the acute flu-like symptoms usually develops. These may however, be superceded by the development chronic adverse events such as non-specific malaise, asthenia or depression. These adverse events may be severe enough as to necessitate suspension of IFN therapy.

In healthy volunteers administered 10×10^6 IU of IFN alfa-2b by subcutaneous injection, the acute flu-like symptoms follow a time course similar to the mean serum concentrations of IFN, reaching a peak at approximately 6-10 hours post-dose and resolving by 16 to 24 hours after administration. The flu-like symptoms and fever seen in healthy volunteers appear to be associated with an increase in IL-6 concentrations in serum (34). Although mean peak IL-6 concentrations were low (19 pg/ml) this represented over a twenty-fold increase from pre-dose IL-6 concentrations. Serum IL-1, IL-2, IL-4, IL-8, IFN-γ, G-CSF, GM-CSF and TNF were either undetectable or showed no change from pre-dose concentrations.

Less frequently reported (< 5% of patients) but of clinical significance are metabolic and endocrine changes that can be associated with chronic interferon administration. The development of anti-thyroid antibodies (anti-microsomal or anti-thyroglobulin antibodies), sub-clinical or clinically evident hypothyroidism may occur during therapy (35, 36). More unusual is the development of hyperthyroidism. In a recent clinical review of the use of interferon alpha in the treatment of patients with hepatitis, 2.5% (6/237) of the patients developed thyroid abnormalities (37). Half of these patients developed hypothyroidism and three developed hyperthyroidism. The hypothyroidism associated with IFN therapy is usually, but not always reversible with discontinuation of therapy and can be managed during therapy by thyroxine supplementation. It is important to distinguish the symptoms of hypothyroidism from non-specific fatigue or malaise which can be observed during IFN therapy. Thyroid stimulating hormone (TSH) should be monitored during treatment and if it is elevated appropriate therapy should be initiated.

Interferons may also alter reproductive hormone physiology. Small studies conducted with partially purified natural leukocyte IFN have demonstrated statistically significant decreases in estrogen and progesterone in female volunteers (38) and decreases in serum testosterone concentrations in male volunteers (39). These changes occurred without affecting FSH, LH or prolactin.

Diabetes may be exacerbated during the course of interferon therapy. In addition, previously unrecognized subclinical diabetes may present for the first time during IFN treatment. Studies of peripheral insulin sensitivity using euglycemic clamp studies in healthy volunteers have demonstrated decreased glucose uptake by peripheral tissues after interferon administration which is compatible with insulin resistance. The insulin resistant state seen in healthy volunteers after administration of IFN is associated with elevated levels of the counter-regulatory hormones cortisol, glucagon and growth hormone (40). Thus, the decrease in insulin sensitivity observed after IFN administration mimics that observed in individuals with viral illnesses (41, 42). In addition, *in vitro* studies have shown that lymphoblastoid interferon can inhibit pro-insulin secretion by human pancreatic islets (43). This may also contribute to the development of diabetes.

Interferon administration results in moderate decreases in platelet and neutrophil counts which if severe may necessitate modification of the dose regimen. Discontinuation of IFN usually results in a prompt rise in hematologic parameters to baseline. Other adverse events seen on rare occasions include pulmonary infiltration, pneumonitis, pneumonia and retinal changes. The explanation for these findings has yet to be established.

Local injection site reactions are reported by approximately 10-15% of subjects receiving IFN alfa-2b for the treatment of hepatitis C. The reactions are characterized by tenderness, erythema or induration at the site of injection. The inflammation is self-limited and generally resolves within 24 hours.

Exogenously administered interferon may cause the development of anti-IFN antibodies. Antibodies which are directed against interferon can be divided into two broad categories;

non-neutralizing antibodies (binding antibodies) or neutralizing antibodies. Non-neutralizing antibodies bind to interferon epitopes but do not result in decreased IFN bioactivity in in vitro assays. These antibodies, however, may change the in vivo pharmacokinetics of interferon by altering its clearance or volume of distribution. Neutralizing antibodies bind to IFN epitopes involved in their recognition by IFN-specific receptors, or bind to the molecule elsewhere and still interfere with the binding of IFN to its receptor. Presumably, these antibodies inhibit IFN activity in vivo. Several recent publications have reviewed the frequency with which antibodies develop in response to different IFN preparations (44, 45). rIFN alfa-2a was associated with a 20% incidence of neutralizing antibodies and a 45% incidence of non-neutralizing antibodies while rIFN alfa-2b was associated with a 7% incidence of neutralizing antibodies and a 15% incidence of non-neutralizing antibodies (44). The reason for the apparently greater immunogenicity of rIFN alfa-2a is unclear. Interestingly however, in a recent study of the protein components of natural interferon from leukocytes derived from over 10,000 healthy individuals, the majority of the IFN alfa-2 protein was IFN alfa-2b. No IFN alfa-2a protein was expressed in these subjects (46). The same researchers investigated the gene frequency of IFN alfa-2 variant genes using pooled DNA from over 28,000 individuals residing in North America. In the population studied, the gene for IFN alfa-2b was the predominant variant while the gene for IFN alfa-2a could not be found. Thus, it is possible that the apparently higher immunogenicity of rIFN alfa-2a is related to the low frequency of its expression in nature. Alternatively, the apparent difference in the immunogenicity of rIFN alfa-2a and rIFN alfa-2b may be due to differences in the method of manufacturing.

CONCLUSION

In the thirty-seven years since its initial characterization, great progress has been made in the therapeutic use of interferons. Interferon alfa-2b is approved in the US for the treatment of selected patients with hepatitis B, hepatitis non-A/non-B/C, condyloma acuminata, hairy-cell leukemia and AIDS-related Kaposi's sarcoma. Use in the treatment of basal cell carcinoma is approved in several countries outside the United States. Oncologic indications in which Intron A (interferon alfa-2b) has shown clinically important activity but are not currently approved by the US Food and Drug Administration include chronic myelogenous leukemia, multiple myeloma, metastatic malignant melanoma, metastatic renal cell carcinoma, bladder cancer, low-grade non-Hodgkin's lymphoma and head and neck cancers. Efficacy has not been established in the treatment of advanced breast carcinoma, cervical, prostate, ovarian or pancreatic carcinoma or against small cell or non-small cell lung cancer. Research programs are ongoing to expand the range of disorders which can be successfully treated with interferon alfa-2b. Novel dosing regimens are also being explored with a view to enhancing the rate of patient response to interferon alfa-2b.

REFERENCES

1. Hoskins M. A Protective Action of Neurotropic Against Viscerotropic Yellow Fever in *Macacus rhesus*. Am J Trop Med Hyg 1935; 15:675-680.
2. Isaacs A, Lindenmann J. Virus Interference. I. The Interferon. Proc R Soc Lond Ser B 1957; 147:258-267.
3. Isaacs A, Lindenmann J, Valentine RC. Virus Interference. II. Some Properties of Interferon. Proc R Soc Lond Ser B 1957; 147:268-273.
4. Lindenmann J, Burke DC, Isaacs A. Studies on the Production, Mode of Action and Properties of Interferon. Br J Exp Pathol 1957; 38:551-562.
5. Gresser I. Production of Interferon by Suspensions of Human Leucocytes. Proc Soc Exp Biol Med 1961; 108:799-803.
6. Strander H, Cantell K. Production of Interferon by Human Leukocytes In Vitro. Ann Med Exp Fenn 1966; 44:265.
7. Cantell K, Hirvonen S. Large-Scale Production of Human Leukocyte Interferon Containing 10^8 Units per ml. J Gen Virol 1978; 39:541-543.
8. Cantell K, Hirvonen S, Morginsen K. Human Leukocyte Interferon Production, Purification and Animal Experiments. In: Waymouth C, ed. In Vitro, Baltimore Tissue Culture Association, 1975; 35-38.
9. Streuli M, Nagata S, Weissmann C. At Least Three Human Type-α Interferons: Structure of α_2. Science 1980; 209:1343-1347.
10. Nagabhushan TL, Leibowitz PJ. Recombinant DNA Technology and Characterization of Recombinant Alpha-2 Interferon. In Kisner DL, Smyth JF, eds. In-

terferon Alpha-2: Preclinical and Clinical Evaluation. Boston: Martinus Nijhoff, 1985.
11. Diaz M, Bohlander S, Allen G. Nomenclature of the Human Interferon Genes. J Interferon Res 1993; 13:243-244.
12. Gray P, Leung D, Pennia D, Yelverton E, Najarian R, Simonsen C, Derynck R, Sherwood P, Wallace D, Berger S, Levinson A, Goeddel D. Expression of Human Immune Interferon cDNA in *E. coli* and Monkey Cells. Nature 1982; 295:503-508.
13. Nagabhushan TL, Trotta PP. Interferons In: Ullman's Encyclopedia of Industrial Chemistry. 5th ed, vol A14. VCH VerlagsGesellschaft mbH, 1989; 365-378.
14. Branca AA, Baglioni C. Evidence That Types I and II Interferons Have Different Receptors. Nature 1981; 294:768-770.
15. Branca AA, Faltynek CR, D'Alessandro SB, Baglioni C. Interaction of Interferon with Cellular Receptors: Internalization and Degradation of Cell-Bound Interferon. J Biol Chem 1982; 257:13291-13296.
16. Zoon KC, Arnheiter H, Zur Nedden D, Fitzgerald D, Willingham MC. Human Interferon Alpha Enters Cells by Receptor-Mediated Endocytosis. Virology 1983; 130:195-203.
17. Yonehara S, Ishii A, Yonehara-Takahashi M. Cell Surface Receptor-Mediated Internalization of Interferon: Its Relation to the Antiviral Activity of Interferon. J Gen Virol 1983; 64:2409-2418.
18. Pestka S, Langer JA, Zoon KC, Samuel CE. Interferons and Their Actions. Annu Rev Biochem 1987; 56:727-777.
19. Branca AA, Baglioni C. Down-Regulation of the Interferon Receptor. J Biol Chem 1982; 257:13197-13200.
20. Pellegrini S, Schindler C. Early Events in Signalling by Interferons. Trends Biochem Sci 1993; 18:338-342.
21. Johnson HM, Bazer FW, Szente BE, Jarpe MA. How Interferons Fight Disease. Scientific American, May 1994; 68-75.
22. Sen GC, Lengyel P. The Interferon System: A Bird's Eye View of its Biochemistry. J Bio Chem 1992; 267:5017-5020.
23. Merritt JA, Ball LA, Sielaff KM, Meltzer DM, Borden EC. Modulation of 2',5'-Oligoadenylate Synthetase in Patients Treated with Alpha-Interferon: Effect of Dose, Schedule and Route of Administration. J Interferon Res 1986; 6:189-198.
24. Witter F, Barouki F, Griffin D, Nadler P, Woods A, Wood D, Lietman P. Biologic Response (anti-viral) to Recombinant Human Interferon Alpha 2a as a Function of Dose and Route of Administration in Healthy Volunteers. Clin Pharmacol Ther 1987;42:567-575.
25. Radwanski E, Perenteses G, Jacobs S, Oden E, Affrime M, Symchowicz S, Zampaglione N. Pharmacokinetics of Interferon α-2b in Healthy Volunteers. J Clin Pharmacol 1987; 27:432-435.
26. Bocci V, Pacini A, Muscettola M, Paulesu L, Pessina GP, Santiano M, Viano I. Renal Filtration, Absorption and Catabolism of Human Alpha Interferon. J Interferon Res 1981; 1:347-351.
27. Bocci V, Pacini A, Muscettola M, Pessina GP, Paulesu L, Bandinelli L. The Kidney is the Main Site of Interferon Catabolism. J Interferon Res 1982; 2:309-313.
28. Bino T, Edery H, Gertler A, Rosenberg H. Involvement of the Kidney of Catabolism of Human Leukocyte Interferon. J Gen Virol 1982; 59:39-45.
29. Bino T, Madar Z, Gertler A, Rosenberg H. The Kidney is the Main Site of Interferon Degradation. J Interferon Res 1982; 2:301-308.
30. Craig PI, Williams SJ, Cantrill E, Farrell GC. Rat but Not Human Interferons Suppress Hepatic Oxidative Drug Metabolism in Rats. Gastroenterology 1989; 97:999-1004.
31. Williams SJ, Baird-Lambert JA, Farrell GC. Inhibition of Theophylline Metabolism by Interferon. Lancet 1987; ii:939-940.
32. Williams SJ, Farrell GC. Inhibition of Antipyrine Metabolism by Interferon. Br J Clin Pharmacol 1986; 22:610-612.
33. Danhauser LL, Freimann JH Jr., Gilchrist TL, Gutterman JU, Hunter CY, Yeomans AC, Markowitz AB. Phase I and Plasma Pharmacokinetic Study of Infusional Fluorouracil combined with Interferon alfa-2b in Patients with Advanced Cancer. J Clin Oncol 1993; 11:751-761.
34. Sullivan L, Zhang Y, Cutler D, Narula S. Unpublished data.
35. Burman P, Karlsson FA, Öberg K, Alm G. Autoimmune Thryoid Disease in Interferon-Treated Patients. Lancet 1985; ii:100-101.
36. Fentiman IS, Thomas BS, Balkwill FR, Rubens RD, Hayward JL. Primary Hypothyroidism Associated with Interferon Therapy of Breast Cancer. Lancet 1985; i:1166.
37. Lisker-Melman M, DiBiscelgie AM, Usala SJ, Weintraub B, Murray LM, Hoofnagle JH. Development of Thyroid Disease During Therapy of Chronic Viral Hepatitis with Interferon Alfa. Gastroenterology 1992; 102:2155-2160.
38. Kauppila A, Cantell K, Jänne O, Kokko E, Vihko R. Serum Sex Steroid and Peptide Hormone Concentrations, and Endometrial Estrogen and Progestin Receptor Levels During Administration of Human leukocyte Interferon. Int J Cancer 1982; 29:291-294.
39. Orava M, Cantell K, Vihko R. Treatment with Preparations of Human Leukocyte Interferon Decreases Serum Testosterone Concentrations in Men. Int J Cancer 1986; 38:295-296.
40. Koivisto VA, Pelkonen R, Cantell K. Effect of Interferon on Glucose Tolerance and Insulin Sensitivity. Diabetes 1989; 38:641-647.
41. Rayfield EJ, Curnow RT, George DT, Beisel WR. Impaired Carbohydrate Metabolism During Mild Viral Illness. N Engl J Med 1973; 289:618-621.
42. Record CO, Alberti KG, Williamson DH, Wright R. Glucose Tolerance and Metabolic Changes in Human Viral Hepatitis. Clin Sci Mol Med 1973; 45:677-690.
43. Rhodes CJ, Taylor KW. Effect of Human Lymphoblastoid Interferon on Insulin Synthesis and Secretion in Isolated Human Pancreatic Islets. Diabetologia 1984; 27:601-603.
44. Antonelli G, Giannelli G, Pistello M, Maggi F, Vatte-

roni L, Currenti M, Del Vecchio S, Roffi L, Pastore G, Dianzani F. Clinical Significance of Recombinant Interferon-α_2 Neutralizing Antibodies in Hepatitis Patients. J Interferon Res 1994; 14:211-213.
45. Antonelli G, Currenti M, Turriziani O, Dianzani F. Neutralizing Antibodies to Interferon Alpha: Relative Frequency in Patients Treated with Different IFN Preparations. J Infect Dis 1991; 163:882-885.
46. Liao MJ, Lee N, Dipaola M, Hussain M, Brissette R, Ni D, Smith T, Desai M, Ferencz-Biro K, Testa D. Distribution of Interferon-α_2 Genes in Humans. J Interferon Res 1994; 14:183-185.

Interferon Therapy of Chronic Hepatitis B

R. P. Perrillo

INTRODUCTION

Chronic hepatitis B is a serious liver disorder that frequently results in cirrhosis, hepatocellular carcinoma, and death. It affects approximately 5% of the earth's population and is the ninth leading cause of death worldwide. The natural history of liver disease caused by persistent infection with hepatitis B virus (HBV) can be quite variable. Nonetheless, the frequent finding of chronic active hepatitis or cirrhosis and the strong link between HBV infection and hepatocellular carcinoma underscore the need for effective antiviral therapy. A number of studies have indicated that alpha interferon can be used successfully to treat chronic hepatitis B, and interferon is currently licensed to treat this condition in more than 40 countries worldwide. This chapter will review recent advances in interferon management of chronic hepatitis B.

SEROLOGICAL ENDPOINTS

The major goal of therapy for all forms of chronic viral hepatitis is to permanently suppress or eliminate the virus and thereby achieve a remission of the associated liver disease. A secondary, but nonetheless important goal is to diminish infectivity. The therapeutic endpoint of clinical trials in chronic hepatitis B has generally been the sustained elimination of circulating markers for viral replication such as HBeAg, HBV DNA and HBV DNA polymerase. The ability to test for HBV DNA has limited availability at the current time, however, and testing for HBV DNA polymerase remains a research tool. HBeAg seroconversion is generally accompanied by disappearance of HBV DNA polymerase and HBV DNA in serum (by dot blot or solution hybridization) (1), marked reduction in aminotransferase levels (2, 3) and improvement in liver histology (3, 4). Moreover, the loss of circulating HBeAg and HBV DNA is associated with a major decrease in the amount of HBV DNA in liver tissue and disappearance of replicative forms of the virus (5, 6). Clearance of hepatitis B surface antigen (HBsAg), implying termination of the HBV carrier state, has been more difficult to achieve and occurs in the minority of responders during the first year after completion of therapy. Recently, however, it has been shown that the number of patients who lose HBsAg tends to increase as the duration of follow up lengthens (7).

The conventional definition of a response has come to mean the sustained loss of both HBeAg and HBV DNA. In approximately 10% of treated patients in the US Multicenter Trial of interferon alfa, however, a sustained loss of HBV DNA occurred that was not associated with immediate HBeAg clearance (3). In that study, patients reaching this endpoint were termed «indeterminate responders». This term belies the importance of this result, however, because biochemical and histological improvement were documented in this situation. Moreover, several of the indeterminate responders exhibited delayed clearance of HBeAg during the second year of posttreatment observation (R. Perrillo, unpublished observations). Similar observations were recently made by Lok and colleagues in

Asian patients (8). In that study, the frequency of this phenomenon was substantially greater in patients who remained HBV DNA negative at the end of the first year of follow up (6 of 11 or 55% vs. 22 of 88 or 25%).

ROLE FOR LIVER BIOPSY

When considering antiviral therapy in a patient with chronic hepatitis B, it is important to obtain a baseline liver biopsy. This has three major advantages. First, it provides data on histologic severity and prognosis which leads to better education of the patient. Second, the biopsy provides useful information with regard to the relative urgency for treatment. For example, it is now recognized that HBV-associated chronic persistent hepatitis can occasionally evolve to more serious histological outcomes (9), but the rate at which this occurs is likely to be slow and more urgent therapy is need for a patient whose initial biopsy reveals incipient cirrhosis. Third, the extent of liver injury provides the clinician with information that may be indispensable in evaluating whether it is best to reduce or discontinue treatment should problems with tolerability be encountered.

The role for repeat liver biopsy is less clear. If the patient has not had a virologic response, the timing of a second biopsy should probably be dictated by the clinical course of the disease. If the patient has had a lasting biochemical, clinical, and virological response, there may be little, if any reason for a repeat biopsy. If a decision is made to repeat the biopsy in an individual with a sustained virological response and persistent mild aminotransferase elevations, it should probably be done several years after therapy so that the degree of histological change can be more accurately defined.

INTERFERON THERAPY

At the current time, interferon is the most extensively studied antiviral agent for chronic hepatitis B. The advent of recombinant DNA technology made commercial production feasible and laid the foundation for numerous clinical trials during the past 6 to 7 years. There are three major forms of interferon (alpha, beta, and gamma). Alpha interferon is produced by monocytes and transformed B cells in response to viruses and antigenic stimuli. Beta interferon is made by fibroblasts in response to double stranded RNA, polyribonucleotides and viruses. Gamma interferon, on the other hand, is produced by antigen or mitogen-stimulated T cells (10).

All forms (particularly alpha and beta) exert antiviral activity, but the majority of therapeutic trials have employed recombinant alpha interferon. Alpha interferon tends to have more striking antiviral effects and less pronounced immunological actions when compared to gamma interferon both *in vitro* and *in vivo* (11). More than 20 different subtypes of alpha interferon have been identified, the most biologically important being alpha-2 (10). On a conceptual basis, interferon should be an ideal agent for the treatment of this disorder because it is both immunomodulatory and antiviral. However, the early studies suggested that only 20 to 30% of patients responded to alpha or beta interferon (12, 13). The use of recombinant interferon alfa-2b has been more rigorously evaluated in a recent United States multicenter trial involving 169 patients (3). In this study, 37% of patients lost HBeAg and HBV DNA when treated with 5 million units of interferon given daily for 16 weeks. In contrast, the rate of HBeAg seroconversion in patients treated with 1 million units of interferon daily was not significantly different from that observed in untreated controls (17 and 7%, respectively). A nearly identical response to that achieved with 5 million units daily is obtained when patients are treated with 10 million units given three times weekly for 16 weeks (14, 15).

SHORT TERM AND LONG TERM RESPONSE TO INTERFERON THERAPY

Loss of HBeAg and HBV DNA is associated with biochemical, histological, and clinical improvement (tables 1 and 2). Normalization of elevated aminotransferase levels occurs in nearly 90% of patients who demonstrate a sustained loss of HBV DNA (3). In the remaining individuals, aminotransferase levels are generally

Table 1. Beneficial effects of alpha interferon treatment of chronic hepatitis B

Achieved to date	More data needed	Data not available
Sustained disappearance of viral replication	√	
Disappearance of HBsAg	√	
Eradication of virus in liver		√
Complete resolution of liver disase		√
Normalization of aminotransferase levels		√
Histologic improvement		
Short term	√	
Long term	√	
Decreased frequency of hepatoma		√
Improved survival		√

Adapted from Perrillo RP. Antiviral agents in the treatment of chronic viral hepatitis. In: Ockner R, Boyer T, eds. Progress in Liver Diseases. Vol. X. Philadelphia: W B Saunders, 1992; 286; with permission.

elevated less than twofold. Responders often report decreased symptoms, particularly lessening of fatigue, and liver biopsies done within 6 to 9 months of completion of therapy demonstrate improvement in piecemeal necrosis and lobular infiltrate (3, 4).

Reactivation of infection occurs in approximately 5 to 10% of individuals who undergo HBeAg seroconversion. This usually occurs within a year of completion of therapy. The great majority of responses appear to be sustained, however, even when patients are observed for intervals as long as 3 to 7 years (7), and patients in whom the disease reactivates have generally responded to a second course of therapy (16).

HBsAg clearance occurs in 10 to 15% of patients within the first year after treatment. This is generally observed during therapy or within the first 3 months after completion of treatment. Antibody to HBsAg is detectable in 75 to 90% of these patients, although this is often present in low titer (17). Some patients who become HBeAg negative as a result of therapy eventually lose HBsAg upon prolonged follow-up. In one study (7), the disappearance of HBsAg was documented in 13 of 20 responders (65%) during a mean follow up interval of 4 years. In approximately 80% of patients who become HBsAg-negative, HBV DNA is no longer detectable in serum by polymerase chain reaction (7, 18, 19). These data suggest that termination of the HBV carrier state may be possible in some patients. The application of polymerase chain reaction to the study of HBV DNA in liver tissue has provided further information about this situation. In studies conducted at Washington University (19) and the National Institutes of Health (18) investigators have been able to detect HBV DNA in liver tissue by polymerase chain reaction several years after spontaneous or treatment-induced HBsAg seroconversion. In one study, quantitation of the polymerase chain reaction product revealed low levels of HBV DNA that progressively decreased as the

Table 2. Immediate versus delayed effects in responders to interferon therapy

Effect monitored	Short term (≤12 months after response)	Long term (> 12 months after response)
ALT/AST	Improved or within normal limits	Improved or within normal limits
Symptoms	Absent or improved	Absent
Histology	Diminished periportal	Absent periportal
	Necrosis	Necrosis (17, 54)
	Diminished portal reaction	Slight or no portal reaction (17, 54)
	Similar degree of fibrosis	Diminished fibrosis
HBeAg	Remains negative	Remains negative
		Delayed clearance in HBV DNA negative patients
HBsAg	Clearance in minority	Clearance common
HBV nucleic acid by PCR		
Serum HBV DNA	Positive/negative	Usually negative
Liver Tissue		
HBV DNA	Positive	Usually positive
HBV RNA	Positive/negative	Usually negative
PBMC* HBV DNA	Positive/negative	Positive/negative

* Peripheral blood mononuclear cells.

Table 3. Clinical, serological, and histological features of long term HBeAg and HBV DNA negative patients

Age	Duration (in years)		Biopsy report	
	Negative HBeAg	Normal ALT	Initial	Follow up
63	0.75	0.60	CAH, possible C	Mildly active C
35	2.7	2.2	CPH, fibrosis	CPH, lobular inflammation
43	4.3	4.2	CAH, moderate severity	CPH
49	6.3	6.3	CAH	Within normal limits
43	0.25	0.25	CAH/C	CAH/C
	2.8	2.8		CPH
32	0.40	0.40	Mild CAH	CAH, severe fibrosis
	4.4	4.4		NSR, fatty change
51	0.90	1.0	CAH, R/O C	Mild CAH
	6.2	6.3		Mild portal and lobular inflammation
35	0.90	0.80	Mild CAH	CPH
	6.4	6.3		CPH

CAH: chronic active hepatitis; C: cirrhosis; CPH: chronic persistent hepatitis; NSR: non-specific reactive changes.

follow-up interval lengthened (19). The molecular form and transcriptional activity of this viral DNA has not been fully described, but the rare detection of HBV RNA in the liver tissue of some of these patients as well as the presence of low levels of HBV DNA in serum and peripheral mononuclear cells years after loss of HBsAg suggest that low level viral replication may continue indefinitely in some instances.

Long term histological observations (2 to 9 years) in HBsAg-negative patients with a past diagnosis of chronic hepatitis B have demonstrated the absence of disease progression and an even greater degree of histological improvement than that observed when patients are biopsied within a year after completion of therapy (18, 20). We have found the degree of histological improvement to be most marked 4 or more years after the disappearance of HBeAg and HBsAg; in some instances it was difficult to distinguish any histological abnormality (20). In a study conducted at the National Institutes of Health (18) patients were evaluated at intervals varying from 0.6 to 9 years after loss of HBsAg. A mild degree of inflammation along fibrous septae were observed in many of these patients. Nonetheless, this study also affirmed a marked overall improvement when compared to pretreatment biopsies. Recently, we have had the opportunity to histologically evaluate a group of patients who remained HBeAg negative but HBsAg positive years after a response was achieved (21). Multiple posttreatment biopsies were available in some instances. As can be seen in table 3, the histological appearance of biopsies obtained a few months after the disappearance of HBV DNA and HBeAg was not always interpreted as improved when compared to baseline assessments (patients 5 and 6). The same individuals, however, demonstrated marked resolution of inflammation in biopsies obtained approximately 2.8 and 4.4 years, respectively, after a response was achieved. These data, therefore, are reminiscent of the findings in patients who have lost the HBsAg marker.

DETERMINANTS OF RESPONSE

Several patient variables have been reported to negatively or positively influence the response to interferon. HBV carriers with high pretherapy aminotransferase values, active liver disease, and low levels of serum HBV DNA respond more frequently, presumably because these features reflect a greater immune response to HBV (2). The baseline HBV DNA level as determined by a solution hybridization assay was found to be the most reliable independent predictor of a response in the United States multicenter interferon trial (3). In that study, the rate of HBeAg seroconversion in treated patients with initial serum HBV DNA levels in excess of 200 pg per ml was comparable to that observed in untreated controls. These data suggest that patients with extremely high levels of viral replication

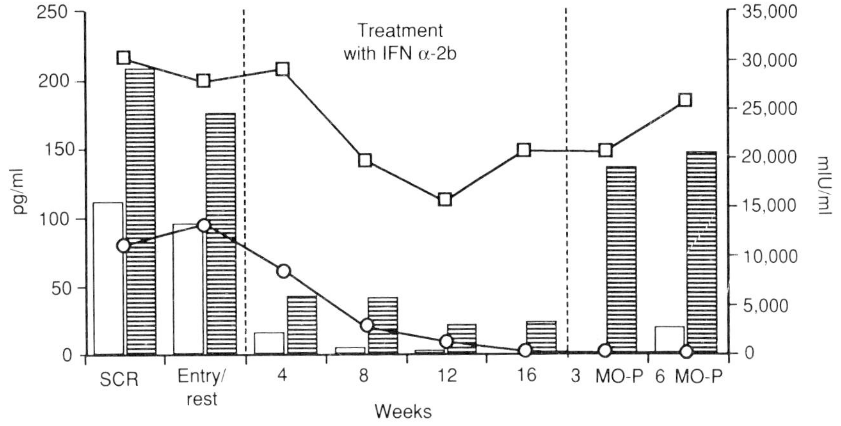

Fig. 1. Serial measurement of mean HBeAg concentrations (line graphs) and HBV DNA concentrations (bar graphs) by IMx methodology (Abbott®) in 16 responders (circles and open bars) and 13 nonresponders (squares and hatched bars). Patients were either treated with prednisone followed by interferon or interferon alone. Note the significantly lower HBeAg values at baseline in responders ($p = 0.005$ by Stepwise Cox Regression) and the similarity of the HBeAg and HBV DNA curves in both groups of patients.

do not appear to be good candidates for current regimens. Female patients appear to respond more frequently than do male patients, and individuals who acquire their infections during adulthood fare better than those exposed at birth (22, 23). In some series, heterosexuals have had substantially higher response rates than male homosexuals (2, 24), and homosexuals with antibody to human immunodeficiency virus appear to be particularly unlikely to respond (25).

Unfortunately, HBV DNA testing is not available to many physicians at the current time. This has recently prompted my associates and I to see if measurement of HBeAg concentration could be used in the same manner. HBeAg concentration was measured by a modification of a microparticle capture enzyme immunoassay which is currently in use in clinical laboratories and has the advantages of being fully automated with a rapid turnover time (1 hour). In this study, similar disappearance curves were observed for the two markers (fig. 1). Moreover, the baseline HBeAg concentration proved to be the best independent predictor of a response (26). Thus, measurement of HBeAg levels may provide a more convenient and readily available way of virologic monitoring in the future. New methods of quantitating HBV DNA in serum, including solid phase assays that utilize chemiluminiscent detection systems are currently under development. An important indicator that a response to interferon is likely is the presence of a transient increase in serum aminotransferase activity during treatment. Typically, this occurs during the second to third month of treatment and is associated with a progressive decline in serum HBV DNA levels. In a study conducted at the National Institutes of Health a transient increase in serum alanine aminotransferase (ALT) levels was observed in 7 of 10 patients who had a sustained loss of HBV DNA as a result of a 16-week course of recombinant alpha interferon (13). An even more striking example of the importance of this exacerbation of hepatitis activity was reported by investigators at King's College in London (27). In that study, AST levels increased to between 10 and 20 times the upper limit of normal in 6 of 23 patients treated with a 6 month course of lymphoblastoid interferon. Each of these patients lost HBeAg, and 5 of them became HBsAg negative as well. In the United States multicenter trial (3), twofold or greater elevations in ALT occurred in 37% of patients who were treated with interferon alfa-2b in a dose of 5 million units daily for 16 weeks (Perrillo, unpublished observations). As in the other trials cited above, the majority of responders (60%) were individuals in whom this phenomenon occurred. Taken together, these studies indicate that interferon is likely to be most effective when it acts in a dual fashion to augment the immune response of the host as well as inhibit viral replication.

INTERFERON SIDE EFFECTS

Adverse experiences occur frequently with all forms of interferon, usually in a dose-dependent fashion (28). These effects occur either early (within the first few hours to days) or late (appearing after the first two weeks). Early side effects include fatigue, fever, chills, myalgias, and arthralgias, often termed a «flu-like» syndrome. Nearly all patients experience these symptoms six to eight hours after the first dose of interferon alfa-2b when given in a dose of 5 MU daily or 10 MU three times weekly; however, fever, headache, and myalgia tend to abate after the first week. Patients are usually premedicated with acetaminophen to ameliorate these symptoms, and this can be continued at six hourly intervals if needed. Fatigue, the most prominent side effect of therapy, is generally reported throughout therapy but is often better tolerated as interferon is continued. The number of patients in whom fatigue led to dose modification or early discontinuation of therapy has been relatively small in the controlled, clinical studies. For example, in the US Multicenter Trial only 8 patients (9%) given the 5 MU dose of interferon alfa-2b required dose modification due to fatigue, and the drug was discontinued in a single patient due to this adverse experience. Interferon is mildly myelosuppressive, and this is more apt to be a clinical problem requiring dose reduction in patients with cirrhosis and hypersplenism. Other uncommon side effects include mild alopecia, impaired concentration, changes in mood, and frank depression (29, 30). Psychiatric side effects have been reported to occur in 17% of 58 patients who were treated with interferon alfa-2b in a dose of 10 MU every other day or 5 MU daily for 4 months (29). Most reports have not described major depressive symptoms attributable to interferon alfa-2b. This may be partially attributable to the difficulty in differentiating depression due to a chronic illness from that induced by therapy. Rarely, frank delirium and suicidal ideation have been reported (29).

The exacerbation of autoimmune hepatitis by interferon has been described (31) . This is not a clinical problem with hepatitis B, however, because the two disorders are usually easily distinguishable. There have also been reports of patients developing evidence of autoantibodies (e.g., anti nuclear antibody, smooth muscle antibody, or antibody to thyroid microsomal antigen) during interferon therapy (32, 33). Moreover, thyroid dysfunction (either hypothyroidism or less commonly, hyperthyroidism) and accompanying abnormalities in thyroid-stimulating hormone levels have been observed (34). Autoantibodies have been reported in more than 85% of cases (33), but clinically evident thyroid dysfunction appears to be relatively uncommon in patients treated for chronic hepatitis B. In a recent report involving 135 patients with malignant carcinoid tumors, however, 19% of patients either developed thyroid disease, systemic lupus erythematosus, pernicious anemia or vasculitis (35). Interferon has been reported to result in an autoimmune-like hepatitis, autoimmune thrombocytopenia, and symmetric polyarthropathy in a few cases (35-38). Moreover, there have been reports of worsening of psoriasis and rheumatoid arthritis. Until more is known, the data suggest the need for caution in treating patients with a preexisting, nonhepatic autoimmune disorder. In this situation, it seems reasonable to reserve interferon treatment for clinically and/or histologically severe liver disease.

Therapy with interferon appears to induce the formation of interferon antibody in a minority of patients. It is unclear whether these antibodies neutralize the antiviral effects of the drug, and their clinical significance remains controversial (3, 39-42). In the US Multicenter Study (3), neutralizing antibody to interferon alfa-2b as evaluated by ELISA appeared in 6 (7%) of patients who received 5 MU of interferon and none of the patients treated with 1 MU. The antibody titers were low (less than 1:20) in all patients and the presence of antibody did not preclude a response.

Relatively little is known of the interaction between various types of interferon and drugs *in vivo*. However, recent studies in humans have shown that recombinant alfa-2a interferon reduces the clearance of antipyrine and theophylline, which are primarily metabolized by the mixed-function oxidase system (cytochrome P450) in liver microsomes (43, 44). The extent, if any, to which recombinant interferon alfa-2b suppresses hepatic oxidative drug metabolism is currently unknown and no clinically significant drug interactions have been reported to date.

PATIENT GROUPS FOR FURTHER STUDY

Most of the existing clinical trials have focused attention on clinically stable adults with chronic active hepatitis and circulating markers for viral replication (HBeAg, HBV DNA, and/or elevated DNA polymerase). More information is needed, however, on the response to interferon in other patients with chronic hepatitis B. Molecular biological studies have led to the discovery of one or more mutations in the precore region of the HBV genome that inhibit the production of HBeAg (45). Patients who are infected with a precore mutant virus remain HBV DNA positive in serum and tend to have active liver disease. In Mediterranean countries such as Greece and Italy, approximately 40% of all treated patients with chronic hepatitis B fall into this category. Conflicting data have accumulated on the response to treatment in these cases. In one study from Italy, patients infected with a precore mutant virus demonstrated a high rate of relapse upon discontinuation of therapy (45), whereas in a second Italian study responses were generally sustained (46). Hadziyannis et al., on the other hand, have reported a high rate of relapse in the second year of follow up in similar patients in Greece (47). The response to interferon in children has also not been extensively evaluated. Asian children with normal aminotransferase levels do not respond (22). In Spain, in contrast, Ruiz-Moreno et al. have described response rates of approximately 50% in children with persistently elevated serum aminotransferase levels (48). Several small clinical trials have observed encouraging results in the treatment of chronic hepatitis B that is complicated by membranous nephropathy (49-51). In these studies, loss of HBeAg has been associated with decreased proteinuria as well as improvement in the liver disease.

PROBLEM PATIENTS

The above groups represent those in which there is a reasonable amount of data to suspect that interferon therapy may be effective. However, there is a large group of patients who are resistant to therapy and in whom therapy presents a special challenge. These could be classified as «problem patients». Nonresponders to interferon constitute the largest group of problem patients. Approximately 60% of treated patients do not respond to a 16 week course of interferon. A second course of therapy has been demonstrated to be nonsuccessful in most studies (52, 53). Recent data from Janssen et al suggest that prolongation of therapy may be helpful in inducing a response in patients who have failed to benefit from a standard course of interferon alfa (54). Accordingly, this has led to a large multicenter trial by the EUROHEP Study Group in which patients who remain HBeAg positive at the end of 16 weeks of therapy are randomly assigned to an additional 16 weeks of therapy or no treatment. Enrollment in this study has proceeded more slowly than anticipated, and the data are unlikely to become available before late next year. In the meantime, several alternate approaches currently seem feasible in patients who have failed to respond. One approach involves retreatment with interferon preceded by a short course of corticosteroids. This therapy has been shown to have greatest benefit for patients with low serum ALT at baseline (less than 100 IU/l) (3). Corticosteroid priming has been successfully applied in our medical center in patients who have failed interferon alone. Should a response not occur with a 6 week decremental course of prednisone, starting with a dose of 60 mg daily, I have had some success in retreating patients with a shorter cycle and initiating therapy with a higher dose . Another approach to improving outcome involves retreating patients when they appear to be better candidates for therapy, for example, when they have a higher ALT level and/or lower HBV DNA levels. This is possible in a number of instances, because the intensity of these markers often fluctuates in the natural history of the disease. Both of the latter approaches deserve further study in controlled clinical trials.

Patients who have persistently normal or mild aminotransferase elevations despite ongoing viral replication are the most difficult patients to treat successfully. This data has been most convincingly shown in Asian patients by Lok and colleagues. The response rate in healthy HBsAg carriers in Hong Kong approaches zero whereas in individuals with elevated ALT levels (averaging more than 1.5 times the upper limit of normal) responses occur significantly more frequently with rates that are comparable to those previously observed in Caucasians (55). Both the US Multicenter Trial of interferon alfa-2b and a smaller multicenter study in Europe (56) have demonstrated that response rates for patients with low ALT levels can be increased with the use of a short course of corticosteroids before administration of interferon. As the aminotransferase levels may be a poor reflection of the underlying histologic disease, however, one should be careful not to use this approach in patients who have not had a recent biopsy. Patients with evidence of active cirrhosis and borderline hepatic compensation are not good candidates because the ALT flare that follows the use of prednisone may increase the likelihood of clinical decompensation (57). In the future it may be possible to induce augmented cytotoxic T cell activity against HBV infected liver cells through the use of hepatitis B core peptide vaccines. Recently, it has been demonstrated by Chisari and associates that a number of core peptides can be identified that are capable of inducing cytotoxic T cell activity in transgenic mice with the HLA class 2.1 phenotype (58). Early studies in healthy human volunteers with synthetic peptides or retroviral core constructs are currently underway.

Evidence for hepatic decompensation is currently a contraindication to the treatment of patients with chronic hepatitis B because potentially lethal side effects, such as serious bacterial infections and flares of the hepatitis have been described (59, 60). In a recent study conducted at the National Institutes of Health, dramatic responses, including normalization of synthetic function, followed sustained clearance of HBV DNA in one third of cases (59). Despite these encouraging results, however, 50% of patients had one or more serious adverse effects that led to early discontinuation of treatment including spontaneous bacterial peritonitis, bacterial pneumonia, worsening of the hepatitis, and acute psychiatric syndromes. A multicenter study is currently nearing completion in the United States to access if a titratable, low dose regimen of interferon alfa is safer (table 4). The results of this study, only published in abstract form at the time of this writing have indicated that immunologic flares are much less common than with fixed, higher dose regimens but serious infections may, nonetheless, occur (60). Both clinical trials have demonstrated that a response is particularly unlikely to occur in patients with far advanced disease (Child's class C), a group in which severe side effects are more frequent. Low dose interferon therapy should only be administered in centers that are skilled in the management of patients with decompensated cirrhosis and where liver transplantation is available.

Table 4. Dose low titratable, interferon regimen for patients with decompensated cirrhosis

Week	Dose (MU)	Frequency
1	0.5×10^6	qod
2-3	1×10^6	qod
4-5	2×10^6	qod
3-7	3×10^6	qod
8-24	As tolerated	qod

Patients who are immunosuppressed also represent a very problematic group. The three largest groups are those with HIV infection, chronic renal failure, and those undergoing organ transplantation. Several features are encountered in these patients which make a response difficult to achieve. First, all such patients have high level viremia; second they have depressed cell mediated immunity; thirdly, there may be uncertain clinical advantages to treating such patients. For example, in patients with AIDS, death is more likely to occur due to the underlying disease rather than chronic hepatitis B. Studies are greatly needed in early, asymptomatic HIV positive patients, however, now that lengthening of the AIDS free interval is possible with early antiretroviral therapy (61). Several small series, including one conducted at our medical center a number of years ago, suggest that responses occur as frequently in patients with early HIV infection as in those with chronic hepatitis B alone. It should be borne in mind, however, that HIV positive patients are immunologically heterogeneous, and the absence of clinical signs and symptoms of disease may belie the true nature of the immunosuppressed state. In patients with advanced HIV disease it has been my impression that the stress of interferon therapy may actually hamper immunologic responses against hepatitis B virus.

Perhaps the most vexing group of immunosuppressed patients are those undergoing liver transplantation for chronic hepatitis B. Recurrent hepatitis B in the liver graft is the rule, particularly if patients are HBV DNA positive prior to transplantation. There are two ways of managing this situation, both of which have had only limited success. A recent study from Marcellin et al indicates that interferon treatment before transplantation may occasionally forestall the need for transplantation, but the routine application of this therapy does not generally improve outcome and may prove deleterious (62). Neither the rate of posttransplant infection, time to reinfection of the liver graft, or survival differed when compared to nontreated, historical controls. Interferon therapy given after transplantation has not been successful in dealing with the large viral burdens that these patients demonstrate once recurrent infection occurs, and until recently the role for high dose hepatitis B immunoglobulin or HBIg as a preventive measure was unclear. However, a recent study by Samuel and associates has convincingly shown that HBIg can successfully reduce the incidence of new infections when given in high doses (10,000 units given intravenously during the anhepatic phase; daily during the immediate postoperative period; and at least for 6 or more months to maintain high anti-HBs titers) (63). In this study, long term HBIg proved successful even if patients were HBeAg positive prior to transplantation. There are several problems encountered with this approach, however, including the lack of an intravenous preparation in the United States and the high cost involved (between $15,000 to $30,000 USD annually). Moreover, HBIg may have to be given indefinitely to prevent eventual infection of the graft due to the presence of extrahepatic reservoirs of infection (64). A number of new approaches to the treatment of chronic hepatitis B are currently under study, including the use of nucleoside analogues such as 3' thiacytidine (65). If this drug proves safe and effective in clinically stable patients, it may make a significant impact in treating chronic hepatitis B following liver transplantation, either given alone or in combination with reduced doses of HBIG.

COMBINATION ANTIVIRAL THERAPY

Various forms of combination therapy have been studied in the hope that additive or synergistic effects to interferon would be noted. One approach that has been tried involves the use of a combination of an immunomodulatory drug with interferon. Early reports had suggested that levamisole, an antihelminthic with T cell stimulating properties, might be useful in chronic hepatitis B (66), and it was hoped that a combination of this agent with interferon might prove to be more effective than interferon alone. However, in a recent study from Italy, the combination of levamisole given simultaneously with lymphoblastoid interferon for 6 months was actually associated with a lower response rate when compared to the same dose of interferon alone (67). Better results have been achieved when interferon is preceded by a short course of corticosteroids. The rationale for this approach is based on the observation that withdrawal of corticosteroid therapy frequently results in an acute hepatitis-like elevation of serum aminotransferase levels that is thought to represent an «immunologic rebound» against the virus. This enhancement of immunologic activity results in a transient decline in HBV DNA and DNA polymerase when corticosteroid withdrawal is used alone (68, 69). Early studies used a combination of a short course of corticosteroids followed by Ara-A or Ara-AMP (70-72). While the results were encouraging, the profound neuromuscular toxicity of these purine nucleosides limited further study. Subsequent studies used a short course of corticosteroids in conjunction with interferon therapy (2, 3). The combined regimen was seen to be generally well tolerated and effective in clinically stable patients. In contrast, corticosteroid withdrawal was shown to be potentially deleterious in patients with borderline synthetic function or overt hepatic decompensation, in which case it frequently exacerbated the disease and was occasionally associated with fatalities (57). The immunologic events following withdrawal of corticosteroids have not been extensively studied, and the mechanisms involved are, therefore, poorly understood. However, corticosteroids enhance the expression of HBcAg (73), and a corticosteroid-induced shift from nuclear to cytoplasmic HBcAg is thought to occur during the immune rebound. Theoretically, this might permit HBcAg peptides to become more appropriately displayed on the surfaces of infected hepatocytes in conjunction with HLA class I molecules and serve as a target for cytotoxic T cell responses.

The comparative efficacy of interferon alone to corticosteroid withdrawal followed by interferon has recently been evaluated in a United States multicenter trial (3). All patients met predefined criteria for virological and biochemical stability. This study demonstrated nearly identical rates of HBeAg seroconversion in the two treatment groups (approximately 40%). However, a trend was observed for patients with low pretherapy alanine aminotransferase levels (less than 100 IU per liter) to respond more frequently to the combination regimen when compared to the group that received interferon alone (44% vs. 18%, respectively). Of note, a similar pattern of response (57% vs. 17%) was reported in a double-blind European study that used the identical entry criteria and treatment protocols (56). Based on these results, it has become my practice to precede interferon therapy with 6 week course of corticosteroids in individuals with low levels of ALT. Should this fail to elicit an immunostimulatory effect, I have on occasion had success with a second course of therapy using a higher initial dose of corticosteroids and a shorter treatment cycle.

SUMMARY

Perhaps the most compelling reason to treat chronic hepatitis B with interferon resides in the disappearance of circulating HBsAg in one third of responders and further increases in the frequency of this phenomenon as follow up continues. Another important advantage to treatment is the striking degree of histological improvement that is frequently observed years after a response has been achieved. While a substantial number of patients do not respond to interferon, several promising agents are under study that should allow for a greater degree of success, either when used alone or in combination with interferon (discussed elsewhere in this symposium). A short course of corticosteroids prior to interferon appears to improve response rates in patients who have low ALT levels at baseline, and this has been the preferred approach for these patients at my medical center. Progress is being made in the development of safer interferon regimens for patients with mild to moderate hepatic decompensation. Nonetheless, even patients with marginal synthetic function, as reflected by albumin levels within the low normal range, appear to be at greater risk for complications during therapy and should preferably be referred for inclusion in research programs.

REFERENCES

1. Kuhns MC, McNamara AL, Perrillo RP, Cabal CM, Campbell CR. Quantitation of hepatitis B viral DNA by solution hybridization: comparison with DNA polymerase and hepatitis B e antigen during antiviral therapy. J Med Virol 1989; 27:274-281.
2. Perrillo RP, Regenstein FG, Peters MG, DeSchryver-Kecskemeti, Bodicky CJ, Campbell CR, Kuhns MC. Prednisone withdrawal followed by recombinant alpha interferon in the treatment of chronic type B hepatitis. A randomized, controlled trial. Ann Intern Med 1988; 109:95-100.
3. Perrillo RP, Schiff ER, Davis GL, Bodenheimer HC, Lindsay K, Payne J, Dienstag JL, O'Brien C, Tamburro C, Jacobson IM, Sampliner R, Feit D, Lekfowitch J, Kuhns M, Meschievitz C, Sanghvi B, Albrecht J, Gibas A. A randomized, controlled trial of interferon alfa-2b alone and after prednisone withdrawal, in the treatment of chronic hepatitis B. N Engl J Med 1990; 323:295 -301.
4. Brook MG, Petrovic L, McDonald JA, Scheuer PJ, Thomas HC. Histological improvement after anti-viral treatment for chronic hepatitis B virus infection. J Hepatol 1989; 8:218-225.
5. Di Bisceglie AM, Waggoner JG, Hoofnagle JH. Hepatitis B virus deoxyribonucleic acid in liver of chronic carriers. Correlation with serum markers and changes associated with loss of hepatitis B e antigen after antiviral therapy. Gastroenterology 1987; 1236-1241.
6. Lok ASF, Ma OCK, Lau JYN. Interferon alfa therapy in patients with chronic hepatitis B virus infection.

Effects on hepatitis B virus DNA in the liver. Gastroenterology 1991; 100:756-761.
7. Korenman J, Baker B, Waggoner J, Everhart JE, Di Bisceglie AM, Hoofnagle JH. Long-term remission of chronic hepatitis B after alpha-interferon therapy. Ann Intern Med 1991; 114:629-634.
8. Lok ASF, Chung HT, Liu VWS, Ma OCK. Long-term follow up of chronic hepatitis B patients treated with alpha interferon. Gastroenterology 1993: 105:1833-1838.
9. Fattovich G, Brollo L, Alberti A, Giustina G, Pontisso P, Realdi G, Ruol A. Chronic persistent hepatitis type B can be a progressive disease when associated with sustained viral replication. J Hepatol 1990; 11:29-33.
10. Peters M. Mechanisms of action of interferons. Semin Liver Dis 1989; 9:235-239.
11. Kirchner H. Interferons, a group of multiple lymphokines. Springer Semin Immunopathol 1984; 7:347-374.
12. Davis GL, Hoofnagle JH. Interferon in viral hepatitis: role in pathogenesis and treatment. Hepatology 1986; 6:1038-1041.
13. Hoofnagle JH, Peters M, Mullen KD, Jones DB, Rustgi V, Di Bisceglie A, Hallahan C, Park Y, Meschievitz C, Jones EA. Randomized, controlled trial of recombinant human alpha interferon in patients with chronic type B hepatitis. Gastroenterology 1988; 95:1318-1325.
14. Di Bisceglie AM, Bergasa NV, Fong TL, Fried MW, Swain M, Baker B, Korenman J, Waggoner JG, Park Y, Hoofnagle JH. A randomized, controlled trial of recombinant alpha interferon therapy for chronic hepatitis B. Hepatology 1991; 13:70A (Abstr).
15. Pérez V, Tanno H, Villamil F, Fay O. Recombinant interferon alfa-2b following prednisone withdrawal in the treatment of chronic type B hepatitis. Hepatology 1990; 11:S113-S117.
16. Perrillo RP. Treatment of chronic hepatitis B. In: Hollinger FB, Lemon SM, Margolis HS, eds. Viral Hepatitis and Liver Disease. Baltimore: Williams and Wilkins, 1991; 616-623.
17. Karayiannis P, Kanatakis S, Thomas HC. Anti-HBs response in seroconverting chronic HBV carriers following alpha-interferon treatment. J Hepatol 1990; 10:350-352.
18. Fong TL, Di Bisceglie AM, Gerber MA, Waggoner JG, Hoofnagle JH. Persistence of HBV DNA in the liver after loss of hepatitis B surface antigen in chronic hepatitis B. Hepatology (in press).
19. Kuhns M, McNamara A, Mason A, Campbell C, Perrillo R. Serum and liver hepatitis B virus DNA in chronic hepatitis B after sustained loss of surface antigen. Gastroenterology 1992; 103:1649-1656.
20. Perrillo RP, Brunt EM. Hepatic histologic and immunohistochemical changes in chronic hepatitis B after prolonged clearance of hepatitis B e antigen and hepatitis B surface antigen. Ann Intern Med 1991; 115:113-115
21. Perrillo RP, Mason AL. Long-term follow-up of interferon responders in chronic hepatitis B. In: Miguet JP, Dhumeaux D, eds. Progress in Hepatology 93. Paris: John Libbey Eurotext, 1993; 47-53.
22. Lai CL, Lok ASF, Lin HJ, Wu PC, Yeoh EK, Yeung CY. Placebo-controlled trial of recombinant alpha-2 interferon in Chinese HBsAg carrier children. Lancet 1987; ii:877-880.
23. Lok ASF, Lai CL, Wu PC, Lau JYN, Leung EKY, Wong LSK, Fung YL. Alpha interferon treatment in Chinese patients with chronic hepatitis B. Journal of Hepatology 1990; 11:S121-S125.
24. Novick DM, Lok ASF, Thomas HC. Diminished responsiveness of homosexual men to antiviral therapy for HBsAg-positive chronic liver disease. J Hepatology 1984; 1:29-35.
25. McDonald JA, Caruso L, Karayiannis P, Scully LJ, Harris JRW, Forster GE, Thomas HC. Diminished responsiveness of male homosexual chronic hepatitis B virus carriers with HTLV-III antibodies to recombinant alpha interferon. Hepatology 1987; 7:719-23.
26. Perrillo RP, Mimms L, Schechtman K, Robbins D, Campbell C. Monitoring of antiviral therapy by the quantitative evaluation of hepatitis B e antigen: A comparison to HBV DNA testing. Hepatology (in press).
27. Alexander GJM, Brahm J, Fagan EA, Smith HM, Daniels HM, Eddleston ALWF, Williams R. Loss of HBsAg with interferon therapy in chronic hepatitis B virus infection. Lancet 1987; ii:66-68.
28. Renault PRF, Hoofnagle JH. Side effects of alpha interferon. Semin Liv Dis 1989; 9:273-277.
29. Renault PF, Hoofnagle JH, Park Y, Mullen KD, Peters M, Brian-Jones D, Rustgi K, Jones EA. Psychiatric complications of long-term interferon alfa-therapy. Arch Intern Med 1987; 147:1577-1580.
30. McDonald EM, Mann AH, Thomas HC. Interferons as mediators of psychiatric morbidity. An investigation in a trial of recombinant gamma interferon hepatitis B carriers. Lancet 1987; ii:1175-1177.
31. Vento S, Di Perri G, Garofano T. Hazards of interferon therapy for HBV-seronegative chronic hepatitis [Letter]. Lancet 1989; ii:296.
32. Macfarland IG, Smith HM, Johnson PJ, Bray GP, Vergani D, Williams R. Hepatitis C virus antibodies in chronic active hepatitis: pathogenetic factor or false-positive result? Lancet 1990; 335:754-757.
33. Mayet WJ, Hess G, Gerken G, Rossol S, Voth R, Manns M, Meyer Zum Buschenfelde KH. Treatment of chronic type B hepatitis with recombinant alpha interferon induces autoantibodies not specific for autoimmune chronic hepatitis. Hepatology 1989; 10:24-28.
34. Fentiman IS, Thomas BS, Balkwill FR. Primary hypothyroidism associated with interferon therapy of breast cancer. Lancet 1985; ii:1166.
35. Roonblom LE, Alm GV, Oberg KE. Autoimmunity after alpha-interferon therapy for malignant carcinoid tumors. Ann Intern Med 1991; 115:178-183.
36. Conlon KC, Urba WJ, Smith JW, Steis RG, Longo DL, Clark JW. Exacerbation of symptoms of autoimmune disease in patients receiving alpha-interferon therapy. Cancer 1990; 65:2237-2242.
37. Shindo M, Di Bisceglie AM, Hoofnagle JH. Acute

exacerbation of liver disease during interferon alfa therapy for chronic hepatitis C. Gastroenterology 1992; 102:1406-1408.
38. Silva MO, Reddy KR, Jeffers LJ, Hill M, Schiff ER. Interferon induced chronic active hepatitis? Gastroenterology 1991; 101:840-842.
39. Craxi A, Di Marco V, Volpes R, Palazzao U. Anti-alpha interferon antibodies after alpha interferon treatment in patients with chronic viral hepatitis. Hepatogastroenterology 1988; 35:304-305.
40. Davis GL, Balart LA, Schiff ER, Lindsay K, Bodenheimer H, Perrillo R, Carey W, Jacobson IM, Payne J, Dienstag J, Van Thiel DH, Tamburro C, Lefkowitch J, Albrecht J, Meschievitz C, Ortego TJ, Gibas A. Treatment of chronic hepatitis C with recombinant interferon alfa. A multicenter randomized, controlled trial. N Engl J Med 1989; 321: 1501-1506.
41. Lok ASF, Lai CL, Leung EKY. Interferon antibodies may negate the antiviral effects of recombinant alpha interferon treatment in patients with chronic hepatitis B virus infection. Hepatology 1990; 12:1266-1270.
42. Porres JC, Carreno V, Ruiz M, Marron JA, Bartolome J. Interferon antibodies in patients with chronic HBV infection treated with recombinant interferon. J Hepatology 1989; 8:351-357.
43. Williams SJ, Baird-Lambert JA, Farrell GC. Inhibition of theophylline metabolism by interferon. Lancet 1987; ii:939-941.
44. Williams SJ, Farrell GC. Inhibition of antipyrine metabolism by interferon. Br J Clin Pharmacol 1986; 22:610-612.
45. Brunetto MR, Oliveri F, Rocca G, Criscuolo D, Chiaberge E, Capalbo M, David E, Verme G, Bonino F. Natural course and response to interferon of chronic hepatitis B accompanied by antibody to hepatitis B e antigen. Hepatology 1989; 10:198-202.
46. Alberti A, Fattovich G, Farci P, Brollo L, Pontisso P, Mandras A, Lai A, Belussi F, Giustina G, Balestrieri A, Ruol A. Favorable response to lymphoblastoid interferon of anti-HBe and HBV DNA positive chronic hepatitis B. In: Hollinger FB, Lemon SM, Margolis HS, eds. Viral Hepatitis and Liver Disease. Baltimore: Williams and Wilkins, 1991; 645-647.
47. Hadziyannis S, Bramou T, Makris A, Moussooulis G, Zigneno L, Papaioannou C. Interferon alfa-2b treatment of HBeAg negative/serum HBV DNA positive chronic active hepatitis type B. J. Hepatol 1990; 11:S133-S136.
48. Ruiz-Moreno M, Rua MJ, Molina J, Moraleda G, Moreno A, Aguada JG, Carreno V. Prospective, randomized controlled trial of interferon alpha in children with chronic hepatitis B. Hepatology 1991; 13:1035-1039.
49. García G, Scullard G, Smith C, Weissberg J, Alexander S, Robinson WS, Gregory P, Merigan TC. Preliminary observation of hepatitis B-associated membranous glomerulonephritis treated with leukocyte interferon. Hepatology 1985; 5:317-320.
50. Lisker-Melman M, Webb D, Di Bisceglie AM, Kassianides C, Martin P, Rustgi V, Waggoner JG, Park Y, Hoofnagle JH. Glomerulonephritis caused by chronic hepatitis B virus infection: treatment with recombinant human alpha interferon. Ann Intern Med 1989; 111:479-483.
51. Mizushima N, Kanai K, Matsuda H, Matsumoto M, Tamakoshi K, Ishii H, Nakajima T, Yoshimi T, Kimura M, Nagase M. Improvement of proteinuria in a case of hepatitis B associated glomerulonephritis after treatment with interferon. Gastroenterology 1987; 92:524-526.
52. Janssen HLA, Schalm SW, Berk L, de Man RA, Heijtink RA. Repeated courses of alpha interferon for treatment of chronic type B hepatitis. J Hepatol 1993; 17(Suppl 3):S47-S51.
53. Giacchino R, Timitelli A, Cristina E, Giambartolomei G, Leonardi D, Caocci F, Cirillo C. Repeated course of interferon treatment in chronic hepatitis B in childhood. Arch Virol 1992; 4(Suppl):273-7-276.
54. Janssen HLA, Berk L, Schalm SW, Heijtink RA, Hess G, Rossol S, Meyer zum Buschenfelde KH, Chamuleau RAFM, Janssen PLM, Reesink HW, Meyer B, Beglinger C, den Ouden-Muller JW, de Jong M, Mulder CJJ. Antiviral effect of prolonged intermittent lymphoblastoid alpha interferon treatment in chronic hepatitis B. Gut 1992; 33:1094-1098.
55. Lok ASF, Wu PC, Lai CL, Lau JYN, Leung EKY, Wong LSK, Ma OCK, Lauder IJ, Ng CPL, Chung HT A controlled trial of interferon with or without prednisone priming for chronic hepatitis B. Gastroenterology 1992; 102:2091-2097.
56. Fevery J, Elewaut A, Michielsen P, Nevens F, Van Eyken P, Adler M, Desmet V. Efficacy of interferon alfa-2b with or without prednisone withdrawal in the treatment of chronic viral hepatitis B. A prospective double-blind Belgian-Dutch study. J Hepatology 1990; 11:S108-S112.
57. Perrillo RP, Regenstein FG. Corticosteroid therapy for chronic active hepatitis B: Is a little too much? (Editorial). Hepatology 1986; 6:1416-1418.
58. Bertoletti A, Chisar FV, Penna A. Definition of a minimal optimal cytotoxic T cell epitope within the hepatitis B virus nucleocapsid protein. J. Virol 1993: 67:2376-2381.
59. Hoofnagle JH, Di Bisceglie AM, Waggoner JG, Park Y. Alpha interferon treatment of patients with clinically apparent cirrhosis due to chronic hepatitis B. Gastroenterology 1993; 104:1116-1121.
60. Perrillo R, Tamburro C, Regenstein F, Balart L, Bodenheimer H, Schiff E, Silva M, Albrecht J, Bodicky CJ, Campbell C, Miller B, Taylor B, Brodeur C, Roach K. Treatment of decompensated chronic hepatitis B (CHB) with a titratable, low dose regimen of recombinant interferon alfa-2b. Hepatology 1992; 16:126A (Abstr).
61. Volberding P, Lagakos SW, Koch MA, Pettinelli C, Myers MW, Booth DK, Balfour HH, Reichman RC, Bartlett JA, Hirsch MA, Murphy RL, Hardy WD, Soeiro R, Fischl MA, Bartlett JG, Meriagan TC, Hyslop NE, Richman DD, Valentine FT, Corey L. Zidovudine in asymptomatic human immunodeficiency virus infection. A controlled trial in persons with fewer than

500 CD-4 positive cells per cubic millimeter. N Engl J Med 1990; 322:941-949.
62. Marcellin P, Samuel D, Areias J, Loriot MA, Arulnaden JL, Gigou M, David MF, Bismuth A, Reynes M, Brechot C, Benhamou JP, Bismuth H. Pretransplantation interferon treatment and recurrence of hepatitis B virus infection after liver transplantation for hepatitis B end-stage liver disease. Hepatology 1994: 19:6-12.
63. Samuel D, Muller R, Alexander G, et al. Liver transplantation in European patients with the hepatitis surface antigen. N Engl J Med 1993; 329:1842-1847.
64. Yoffee B, Burns DK, Bhatt HS, Combes B. Extrahepatic hepatitis B virus DNA sequences in patients with acute hepatitis B infection. Hepatology 1990; 12:187-192.
65. Tyrell DLJ, Mitchell MC, De Man RA, Schalm SW, Main J, Thomas HC, Fevery J, Nevens F, Beranek P, Vicary C. Phase II trial of lamivudine for chronic hepatitis B. Hepatology 1993; 18:112A (Abstr).
66. Fattovich G, Brollo L, Pontisso P, Pornaro E, Rugge M, Alberti A, Realdi G. Levamisole therapy in chronic type B hepatitis. Results of a double-blind randomized trial. Gastroenterology 1986; 91:692-696.
67. Fattovich G, Giustina G, Brollo L, Guido M, Pontisso P, Noventa F, Alberti A. Therapy for chronic hepatitis B with lymphoblastoid interferon alfa and levamisole. Hepatology 1992; 16:1115-1119.
68. Rakela J, Redeker AG, Weliky B. Effect of short-term prednisone therapy on aminotransferase levels and hepatitis B virus markers in chronic type B hepatitis. Gastroenterology 1983; 84:956-960.
69. Scullard GH, Smith CI, Merigan TC, Robinson WS, Gregory PB. Effects of immunosuppressive therapy on viral markers in chronic viral hepatitis B. Gastroenterology 1981; 81:987-991
70. Omata M, Imazeki F, Yokosuka O, Ito Y, Uchiumi K, Mori J, Okuda K. Recombinant leucocyte A interferon treatment in patients with chronic hepatitis B virus infection. Pharmacokinetics, tolerance and biologic effects. Gastroenterology 1985; 88:870-880.
71. Perrillo RP, Regenstein FG, Bodicky CJ, Campbell CR, Sanders GE, Sunwoo YC. Comparative efficacy of adenine arabinoside 5' monophosphate and prednisone withdrawal followed by adenine arabinoside 5' monophosphate in the treatment of chronic active hepatitis type B. Gastroenterology 1985; 88:780-786.
72. Yokosuka O, Omata M, Imazeki F, Hirota K, Mora J, Uchiumi K, Ito Y, Okuda K Combination of short-term prednisolone and adenine arabinoside in the treatment of chronic hepatitis B. Gastroenterology 1985; 89:246-251.
73. Sagnelli E, Maio G, Felaco GM, Izzo CM, Manzillo G, Pasquale G, Filippini P, Piccinino F. Serum levels of hepatitis B surface and core antigens during immunosuppressive treatment of HBsAg-positive chronic active hepatitis. Lancet 1980; ii:395-397.

Interferon Therapy or Chronic Hepatitis C: Update 1995

G. L. Davis

In 1995, the topic of therapy of chronic hepatitis C must be focused largerly on interferon since other therapeutic alternatives remain limited. It is indeed remarkable that any treatment options are available since the therapy of chronic hepatitis C has a relatively short history. It was not until the approximately ten years ago that any therapeutic efforts were made for what was then referred to non-A, non-B hepatitis. Early studies demonstrated that corticosteroids and acyclovir were both ineffective (1, 2).

Interferon was first considered as an option because of its availability through studies of patients with hepatitis B and D. The first report of interferon's activity came from a small pilot study conducted at the NIH Liver Unit by Dr. Hoofnagle and colleagues (3). Although this study included only 10 patients and was done before the virus which caused non-A, non-B hepatitis was even identified, it made several very important observations which have served as the foundation for subsequent studies in the treatment of this disease. First, it was noted therapy normalized serum ALT levels, the only non-histological marker of disease at that time. Considering what we know today about response to interferon, it was remarkable that eight of the ten patients normalized their ALT levels. Second, low doses of interferon were required as compared to that required for the treatment of hepatitis B. The ten patients in the study received doses of interferon alfa-2b ranging from 0.5 to 5 million units given either daily, every other day, or three times per week. Third, relapse commonly occurred with discontinuation of treatment and, fourth, patients responded to retreatment. Finally, despite the preliminary nature of the study, Dr. Hoofnagle suggested that the data seemed to show that longer treatment periods might improve the durability of response.

Over the next 4 years, 4 randomized, controlled studies which used essentially identical protocols tested the effects of a fixed dose of 3 million units of interferon alfa-2b administered 3 times per week for 6 months (4-7). These trials also included a low dose and an untreated control group. Despite the fact that these studies were conducted in different parts of the globe, the results were remarkably similar with a mean of 42% achieving normal serum ALT levels by the end of treatment; this being termed «complete response». Response was also associated with histologic improvement primarily through reduction of lobular and periportal inflammation. These studies all confirmed a high rate of relapse after therapy was stopped such that only about 40% of the responders, 18% of all of the treated patients, had a durable or «sustained response» (8). By 1991, Fabio Tine and colleagues were able to review 17 randomized trials of interferon for chronic hepatitis C (9). All reported studies showed a significant response to treatment. Again, despite differences in the treatment regime and geographic location of the studies, the results were quite similar.

Shindo and colleagues, again at the NIH Liver Unit, showed that hepatitis C virus RNA, a measure of viral replication, fell in most patients who had a complete response to treatment, but not in non-responders to interferon (10). Additionally, they showed that relapse was inevitably associated with re-elevation of HCV-RNA. And finally, they showed what has now been repeatedly described. Namely, that some apparent sustained responders become viremic after stopping interferon despite maintaining normal ALT levels (11). The meaning of this discrepancy remains to be elucidated.

Thus, early treatment studies made several discoveries. They confirmed the results of the pilot study in large well-controlled trials and thereby documented the efficacy of interferon at about 40% in this disease, despite relatively low doses of interferon. This response was usually associated with a parallel fall in serum ALT and HCV-RNA, confirming that interferon acted as an apparant antiviral agent and seemingly suggesting that hepatitis C virus was a cytopathic virus. Although these studies represented a huge clinical step considering the absence of any therapeutic options prior to this time, they also made several observations which are critical to our subsequent discussions today. First, relapse was common and interferon appeared to eradicate infection in a minority of patients, about 18% of those treated. Thus, it appeared to only control the biochemical and histologic activity during the treatment period in most responders. And last, but not least, most patients did not respond to this interferon treatment regime. The obvious hope would be that higher doses or longer treatment periods might improve the response.

A large United States multicenter study reported by Lindsay and colleagues examined the question of whether higher doses of interferon might increase response (12). In fact, there was no difference in either initial or sustained response for doses of 3, 5 or 10 million units for 6 months. Not only did the higher doses have marginal, if any, effect on response rates, but they also increased the severity of side effects and would certainly increase cost. Although higher doses could hardly be recommended by this data, the study did appear to show a higher sustained response in patients initially treated with a high dose, 10 million units three times per week, and continued at a lower dose for a total of 12 months. Did longer treatment increase response?

In fact, several studies have now suggested that a longer treatment period increases the durability of the response (fig. 1). The best controlled of these from Metreau and colleagues in France showed a doubling of the sustained response rate from 14 to 29% with extension of the 3 million unit three times a week regime from 6 to 12 months (13). This was not seen with the study of Lindsay mentioned above, but the design of that study might have prevented such a discovery (12). Two other studies implied increased durability of response, but they were not controlled to a group treated with standard therapy (14, 15).

Many other studies have claimed superiority of a particular dose regime over what we usually consider standard therapy. However, these studies are generally small, uncontrolled, or biased by other important factors which might explain the differences. There is now clear evidence that response is significantly impacted by the degree of inflammation and fibrosis on liver biopsy, the level of viral replication, viral genotype, and the diversity of the virus in the individual, so called quasispecies.

The degree of histologic inflammation determines response to interferon. Several reports have empasized a higher response in mild disease than in cirrhotic patients. The original United States multicenter study or interferon for hepatitis C showed that nearly 65% of patients with chronic persistent hepatitis or mild chronic active hepatitis had normalization of serum ALT levels during treatment and about a third of these sustained the response (16). By contrast, patients with fibrosis or cirrhosis normalized their ALT levels in only about 30% of cases and about 90% relapsed after interferon was stopped. This in no way implies that those patients with fibrosis or cirrhosis should not be treated. It simply points out that the expectations from treatment may vary based on the initial histology.

The amount of viral replication in serum affects the response to interferon. Several studies have now shown that patients who achieved a complete and sustained response to interferon

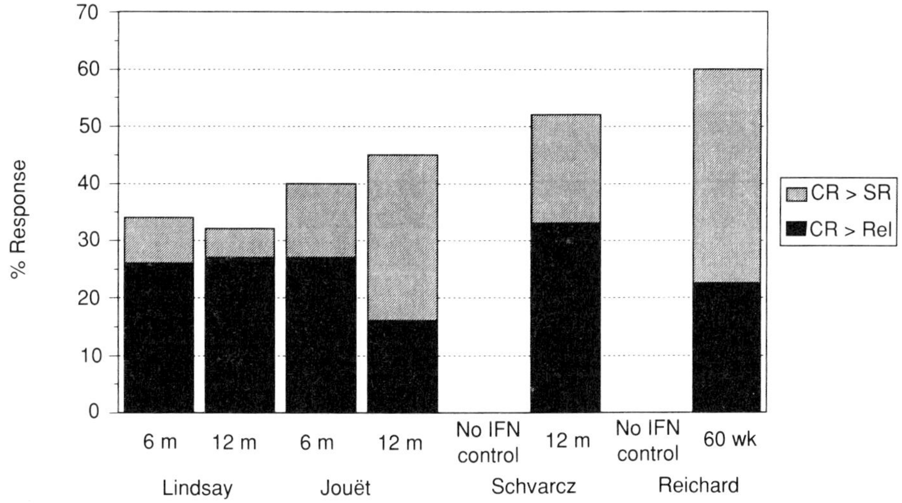

Fig. 1. Effect of longer interferon treatment period on initial and sustained response. The studies by Lindsay (12) and Jouët (13) both compared 6 to 12 months courses with a fixed dose of 3×10^6 units of interferon alfa. Neither Schvarcz (14) nor Reichard (15) compared their study groups to a control which was treated with a standard interferon regimen. Historical SR rate = 18% after 6 months of treatment.

had lower levels of HCV replication which were bellow the limit of detection of Chiron's branched DNA assay (17). Importantly, detectable HCV-RNA did not preclude response. Patients with detectable HCV-RNA simply tended not to sustain their response. Smilarly, Marcellin and colleagues found that patients with low level viremia, not detected by branched DNA, had a 57% complete and sustained response and those with less than about 3 million genomic equivalents had a 30% sustained response (18). In contrast, patients levels greater than 3 million had a very low sustained response rate. So, as with liver biopsy findings, viral levels should not be used to exclude patients from treatment, but may give a clue to which patients are less likely to relapse.

Certainly, one of the most critical determinant of response to interferon is the viral genotype (table 1) (18-24). There is little question that patients with genotypes 2 and 3 by the Simmonds classification method have a 2-to-4 fold higher response to interferon that do patients with genotype 1. Unfortunately, genotype 1 is the predominant genotype in the United States, representing about 85% of patients, and also in most parts of northern Europe.

Finally, it has been reported that viral diversity might influence natural history of HCV infection as well as response to treatment (25-27). The hepatitis C virus is a highly mutable virus. Each patient through mutation of his or her infecting virus develop minor genomic variations which are not different enough to classify as ge-

Table 1. Effect of HCV genotype on sustained response rates after interferon

	1a	1b	2a	2b	3a
Martinot (18)	2/11	2/54	5/19		15/38
Chemello (19)	0/6	11/64	16/39	4/7	15/19
Mita (20)		4/43	4/5	2/3	
Yamada (21)		7/29	7/11	1/3	
Ryff (22)	5/38	10/144	4/22	0/2	3/23
Zachoval (23)	1/11	1/30			8/14
Swanson (24)	5/25	0/12	0/2	0/2	11/31
Total	13/91 (14%)	35/376 (9%)	36/98 (37%)	7/16 (44%)	52/125 (42%)

notypic differences. These are called quasispecies. The greater this diversity, the greater the amount of hepatic inflammation, apparently due to greater immune response to different epitopes. ALT fluctuations may relate to immune mediated elimination of quasispecies. Response to interferon is more likely in patients with lesser degrees of HCV diversity. In addition, response to interferon is associated with a decrease in viral replication, a fall in the mutation rate, and a further corresponding decrease in viral diversity. Obviously, IFN resistent quasispecies persist during treatment and may be responsible for breakthrough elevations of the ALT. Relapse after treatment is stopped is usually associated with re-emergence of the original variants of the virus.

In summary, a number of investigators have shown that sustained response is high, greater than 30%, in patients with mild disease and either low level viremia or the responsive genotypes 2 or 3. Although the histologic severity might not otherwise compel us to treat these patients, we might consider a single 6 month course of interferon since the likelihood of a sustained response is high. On the other hand, the chance of a sustained response is low in patients with histologically more advanced disease, higher levels of viral replication, or genotype 1. These patients should be treated with standard therapy or perhaps longer initial therapy if this proves useful. Relapse after discontinuation should be anticipated and retreated. The search for the optimal retreatment regimen is currently underway in a international multicenter trial.

These proposals have obvious implications. Namely that geographical differences in viral genotype (28) necessarily imply that the optimal treatment regime will be different from country to country. This also means that we should not be quick to adopt the results of studies from areas where the genotypes differ from our own patients.

Table 2. **Potential adjuncts to interferon therapy for chronic hepatitis C**

Ribavirin (33, 34)
Thymosin
Quinolones (31)
Ursodeoxycholic acid (32)
N-acetyl cysteine (30)
NSAIDS
Iron reduction (29)
Prednisone

Several potential adjuncts to interferon treatment have been proposed (table 2) (29-32). None of these has yet been consistently confirmed to be of benefit, but further investigations are certainly necessary. However, two studies with ribavirin in combination with interferon deserve comment (33-34). This agent has shown antiviral activity against a number of viruses *in vitro* and pilot studies have suggested activity against HCV. Both appeared to increase the initial and sustained responses compared to interferon alone. The findings in these small studies must be confirmed in a large randomized controlled trial.

Future hopes lay in new agents and combinations of these with interferons. A promising direction is in inhibitors of the enzymes essential for viral replication. It has recently been suggested that there is a cellular immune response to HCV and augmentation of this mechanism may prove therapeutically useful.

In summary, currently recommended regimens of interferon are effective in about 40% of patients with chronic hepatitis C. Longer initial treatment may increase the durability of response, but this needs to be confirmed in well designed and controlled studies. Higher doses are of marginal, if any, benefit. There is little question that higher responses to treatment are seen in patients with mild disease, low viral levels, and genotypes 2 an 3. Future therapeutic regimens may be most appropriately tailored to the patient profile. Previously, many including myself would have suggested that those with mild disease had little chance of progressive liver disease and did not require treatment. Here a concept has been presented wherein a single 6 month course of interferon might be reasonable to consider in those with mild disease and viral factors predictive of a high likelihood of sustained response. On the other hand, longer treatment courses, retreatment of the anticipated relapse, adjuncts, and combination therapies must be considered for those with more advanced disease who we would otherwise anticipate to have little chance of long-term benefit from a single course. These patients are at increased risk of progression and liver failure. Discovery of effective treatment for them is a priority.

Finally, we must remember that what we do in our clinical practice must be based on well designed clinical trials that confirm these fascinating but preliminary data and ideas.

REFERENCES

1. Stokes P, López WC, Balart LA. Effects of short-term corticosteroid therapy in patients with chronic non-A, non-B hepatitis. Gastroenterology 1983; 92:1783 (Abstr).
2. Pappas SC, Hoofnagle JH, Young N, Strauss SE, Jones EA. Treatment of chronic non-A, non-B hepatitis with acyclovir: pilot study. J Med Virol 1985; 15:1-9.
3. Hoofnagle JH, Mullen KD, Jones DB et al. Treatment of chronic non-A, non-B hepatitis with recombinant human alpha interferon: A preliminary report. N Engl J Med 1986; 315:1575-1578.
4. Davis GL, Balart LA, Schiff ER et al. Treatment of chronic hepatitis C with recombinant interferon alfa: A multicenter randomized, controlled trial. N Engl J Med 1989; 321:1501-1506.
5. Marcellin P, Boyer N, Giostra E et al. Recombinant human alpha-interferon in patients with chronic non A non B hepatitis: a multicenter randomized controlled trial from France. Hepatology 1991; 13:393-397.
6. Causse X, Godinot H, Ouzan D et al. Comparison of 1 or 3 MU of interferon alfa-2b and placebo in patients with chronic non-A non-B hepatitis. Gastroenterology 1991; 101:497-502.
7. Saracco G, Rosina F, Torrani Cerenzia MR et al. A randomized controlled trial of interferon alfa-2b as therapy for chronic non-A, non-B hepatitis. J Hepatol 1990; 11(Suppl 2):43-49.
8. Davis GL. Interferon treatment of chronic hepatitis C. Am J Med 1994; 96(Suppl):41-46.
9. Tiné F, Magrin S, Craxi A, Pagliaro L. Interferon for non-A, non-B chronic hepatitis: a meta-analysis of randomized clinical trials. J Hepatol 1991; 13:192-199.
10. Shindo M, Di Bisceglie AM, Cheung L et al. Decrease in serum hepatitis C viral RNA during alpha-interferon therapy for chronic hepatitis C. Ann Intern Med 1991; 115:700-704.
11. Lau JYN, Davis GL, Ohno T, Diamond D, Kniffen J, Qian KP, Mizokami M. Discrepancy between virologic and biochemical response to interferon-α therapy in chronic hepatitis C virus infection. Lancet 1993; 342:1208-1209.
12. Lindsay KL, Davis GL, Schiff ER et al. Long-term response to higher doses of interferon alfa-2b treatment of patients with chronic hepatitis C: A randomized multicenter trial. Hepatology 1993; 18:106A.
13. Jouët P, Roudot-Thoraval F, Dhumeaux D, Metreau JM, and Le Groupe Français pour l'Etude du Traitement des Hepatites Chroniques NANB/C. Comparative efficacy of interferon alfa in cirrhotic and noncirrhotic patients with non-A, non-B, C hepatitis. Gastroenterology 1994; 106:686-690.
14. Schvarcz R, Glaumann H, Weiland O, Norkrans G, Wejstål R, Frydén A. Histological outcome in interferon alpha-2b treated patients with chronic posttransfusion non-A, non-B hepatitis. Liver 1991; 11:30-38.
15. Reichard O, Foberg U, Fryden A et al. High sustained response rate and clearance of viremia in chronic hepatitis C after treatment with interferon alfa-2b for 60 weeks. Hepatology 1994; 19:280-285.
16. Davis GL, Lindsay K, Albrecht J et al. Clinical predictors of response to recombinant alpha interferon treatment in patients with chronic non-A, non-B hepatitis (hepatitis C). J Viral Hepatitis 1994; 1:55-63.
17. Lau JYN, Davis GL, Kniffen J et al. Significance of serum hepatitis C virus RNA levels in chronic hepatitis. Lancet 1993; 341:1501-1504.
18. Martinot-Peignoux M, Marcellin P, Pouteau M et al. HCV genotype and pretreatment serum HCV RNA level are the main and independent prognostic factors of sustained response in alpha interferon in chronic hepatitis C. Hepatology (in press).
19. Chemello L, Bonetti P, Cavalletto L et al. Sustained response to interferon alfa in chronic hepatitis C is dependent on dose and duration of therapy and on the HCV genotype. Hepatology (in press).
20. Mita E, Hayashi N, Hagiwara H et al. Predicting interferon therapy efficacy from hepatitis C virus genotype and RNA titer. Dig Dis Sci 1994; 39:977-982.
21. Yamada G, Takahashi M, Miyamoto R, Tsuji T. Prediction of interferon effect in chronic hepatitis C by both quantification and genotyping of HCV RNA (letter). Dig Dis Sci 1994; 39:441-447.
22. Ryff JC, Smith P, Wolfe L. Interferon for chronic hepatitis C: when is a response a response. Hepatology 1994; 20:A1184.
23. Zachoval R, Hoffmann R, Nitschko H et al. Sustained response to interferon alpha in chronic hepatitis C may be predicted by HCV genotype and B cell response. Hepatology 1994; 20:A242.
24. Swanson NR, Lareu RR, Reed WD, Fox SA. An analysis of the influence of HCV genotype in short and long-term responses to alpha interferon therapy for chronic hepatitis C. Hepatology 1994; 20:A241.
25. Enomoto N, Kurosaki M, Tanaka Y, Marumo F, Sato C. Fluctuation of hepatitis C virus quasispecies in persistent infection and interferon treatment reveled by single-strand conformational polymorphism analysis. J Gen Virol 1994; 75:1361-1369.
26. Kanazawa Y, Hayashi N, Moribe T et al. Detection of genetic heterogeneity of hepatitis C virus quasispecies through single strand conformation polymorphism. Hepatology 1994; 20:A589.
27. Shindo M, Yoshimoto M, Arai K et al. Quasispecies of HCV genome detected by non-isotopic single strand conformation polymorphism (SSCP) in chronic hepatitis C responded differently to interferon therapy. Hepatology 1994; 20:A278.
28. Dusheiko G, Schmilovitz-Weiss H, Brown D et al. Hepatitis C genotypes: An investigation of type-spe-

cific differences in geographic origin and disease. Hepatology 1994; 19:13-18.
29. Olynyk J, Reddy R, di Bisceglie AM et al. Hepatic iron concentration as a predictor of response to alpha interferon therapy in chronic hepatitis C. Gastroenterology 1994; 107:90A.
30. Beloqui O, Prieto J, Suárez M, Gil B, Qian CH, Garcia N, Civeira MP. N-acetyl cysteine enhances the response to interferon alfa in chronic hepatitis C: a pilot study. J Interferon Res 1993; 13:279-282.
31. Takda A, Tsutsumi M. Efficacy of a combination therapy with interferon and ofloxacin in chronic type C hepatitis. Hepatology 1994; 20:A293.
32. Boucher E, Andre P, Jouanolle et al. Treatment of chronic viral C hepatitis by interferon plus ursodeoxycholic acid: results from a controlled randomized trial in 80 patients. Hepatology 1994; 20:A291.
33. Kakumu S, Yoshioka K, Wakita T, Ishikawa T, Takayanagi M, Higashi Y. A pilot study of ribavirin and interferon beta for the treatment of chronic hepatitis C. Gastroenterology 1993; 105:507-512.
34. Brillanti S, Garson J, Foli M et al. A pilot study of combination therapy with ribavirin plus interferon alfa for interferon alfa-resistant chronic hepatitis C. Gastroenterology 1994; 107:812-817.

Treatment of Chronic Hepatitis C by Interferon for Longer Duration than 6 Months

T. Poynard, V. Leroy, P. Mathurin, M. Cohard, P. Opolon, J. P. Zarski

INTRODUCTION

The most common dose and duration of alpha interferon in the treatment of chronic hepatitis C is 3 MIU TIW for 6 months. This dose and duration is specifically approved by some health autorities, ie the US FDA, and only recommended by others like in France. We have conducted a randomized clinical trial (RCT) of 18 months treatment with interferon alpha 2B in patients with chronic hepatitis C (1). We have also performed recently a meta-analysis of RCTs in the treatment of hepatitis C, with special reference to the efficacy of higher dose than 3 MIU-TIW and longer duration than 6 months. The original data of these two studies are submitted for publication and only summary of previously presented data will be discussed here, the other details will be given during the oral presentation at the international meeting on therapy in liver diseases in Barcelona, Spain.

OVERVIEW OF RCTS OF INTERFERON FOR LONGER DURATION THAN 6 MONTHS

A total of 67 RCTs of interferon in the treatment of chronic hepatitis C have been identified. In order to assess if longer duration of treatment is more effective than the classical 6 months («duration effect»), we have performed a meta-analysis of RCTs comparing directly different durations of treatment, but we have also indirectly compared the duration effect by comparing the respective efficacy of longer duration versus control to the efficacy of 6 months duration versus control.

Direct Comparisons

Among the 67 RCTs identified, 6 compared directly longer duration than 6 months to 6 months therapy (2-7). Details of this direct meta-analysis are given elsewhere. In summary there was a significant difference in favor of long duration (5 RCTs at 12 and one at 18 months) RCTs with interferon 3 MIU TIW in comparison to 6 months using the same dose, for sustained response for one year sustained ALT normalization with an increase of 10% (30% vs. 20%) and a trend for histological improvement (63% vs. 49%).

Indirect Comparisons

Details of this indirect meta-analysis are given elsewhere. Eight RCTs compared 3 MIU TIW for more than 6 months to a control group. Ten RCTs compared 3 MIU TIW for 6 months to a control group. In summary, there was a trend to a better improvement in the percentage of patients with sustained ALT response, relative to controls, among longer duration RCTs at 3 MIU TIW (30%) versus 6 months RCTs at 3 MIU TIW (20%). There was also a trend for histological improvement at the end of treatment in longer treatment, relative to controls, among longer duration RCTs at 3 MIU TIW (63%) versus 6 months RCTs at MIU TIW (20%). At the end of the treatment period, there was no difference, relative to controls, in longer duration RCTs (40%) versus 6 months (47%).

A preliminary analysis of two italian RCTs of 6 and 12 months period, but with 6 MIU TIW initially suggested also that 12 months administration was «superior to a 6-months schedule in reducing the probability or reactivation of liver disease after therapy withdrawal» (8).

A RANDOMIZED CLINICAL TRIAL OF 18 MONTHS THERAPY WITH INTERFERON α2B IN PATIENTS WITH CHRONIC HEPATITIS C

Because the details of this RCT are submitted for publication only the data presented in the abstract of a previous AASLD meeting (1): are given here. Other details will be presented during the meeting.

No trials have previously attempted to estimated the efficacy of 18-months treatment by interferon in patients with chronic non A non B hepatitis.

A total of 303 patients with histologically-proven chronic non-A non-B hepatitis were randomized into three groups after an initial 6-months treatment with 3 million units of interferon α2b three times a week: 103 patients (group I) received the same treatment for an additional 12 months; 101 patients (group II) received 1 million units three times a week for an additional 12 months; and 99 patients received no further treatment (group III), except if serum ALT was elevated at three consecutive monthly assays; in that case, patients received 3 millions units three times a week for up to 18 months. For 176 patients, a second biopsy was available at 18 months, 56 from group I, 63 from group II and 57 from group III. There were no significant differences at inclusion or at randomization among the groups or between patients with or without available final biopsy. Histological lesions were semiquantified using a grid including a previously validated score of disease activity. Biopsies were readed by two independent observers who were unaware of coded biopsy order, treatment received or biological and clinical data.

In group I, the percentage of patients who improved their histological activity score by at least one grade (39/56, 70%) was significantly higher (p = 0.003) than in group II (30/63, 48%) and group III (22/57, 39%). Among the 132 patients without cirrhosis at first biopsy, the incidence of cirrhosis during the follow-up period was 7% (3/44) in group I, 14% (6/44) in group II and 16% (7/44) in group III (p = 0.10). In group I, the percentage or patients with normal ALT values between 6 and 18 months (25/103, 24%) was significantly greater (p = 0.005) than in group II (15/101, 15%) and group III (12/99, 12%). The biological response estimated by serum ALT activity, athough significantly associated, did not enable prediction of the histological response. The percentage of patients with histological improvement in group I was 78% in patients whose ALT was higher than 2 times the normal value after 3 months of treatment, and 64% in patients with ALT higher than normal after 6 months of treatment.

In conclusion, 18 months treatment with interferon α2b at 3 million units three times a week improved histological lesions in comparison to a lower dose or a shorter duration, even in patients who did not normalize their ALT after 6 months of therapy.

Discussion

The efficacy of the standard schedule of interferon, 3 MIU TIW during 6 months in highly significant in comparison to controls, for normalizing serum ALT activity at the end of treatment (48% vs. 1%), for the improvement of histological lesions (68% vs. 21%) and also for the sustained ALT normalization (20% vs. 0%). To improve this efficacy of interferon, several strategies have been tested by RCTs: an increase of dose, an increase of duration and an increase of the total dose given either by increasing the dose or the duration.

Our overview of RCTs and our RCT of 18 months treatment duration were in favor of a long term treatment with 3 MIU TIW. At 12 months the advantage observed vs. 6 months was both for the histological improvement (63% vs. 49%) and for the one year sustained

ALT normalization with an increase of 10% (30% vs. 20%). Very few data are available for longer follow-up. With the 18 months treatment we have observed, two years after the end of the treatment and expressed in intention to treat 25% of complete ALT remission vs. 7% in the group treated during 6 months.

The two main concerns for long term treatment are the incidence of adverse effects and the increase of cost. For the adverse effects, we have observed 20% of patients who stopped interferon during the 18 months treatment because of adverse effects. In terms of compliance, we were surprised to observe a better compliance in the group treated continuously in comparison to the group treated by 6 months and retreated in case of ALT relapse. It is possible that some patients prefer a continuous treatment than a discontinuous treatment.

Overview of RCTs testing the dose effect does not demonstrate an advantage for histological improvement or for sustained ALT normalization. No study has clearly estimate the total dose received, whatever the duration or dose by injection. However, because of tolerance, its seems difficult to treat patients with this type of interferon TIW with greater dose than 3 MIU.

In the literature there no clear demonstration of predictive factors permitting to select patients who could benefit of 6 months, 12 months or 18 months IFN. At this time, there no evidence that genotype or virus quantity are independant predictive factors of sustained response in patients receiving long term interferon.

REFERENCES

1. Poynard T, Bedossa P, Chevallier M, Mathurin P, Lemonnier C and a Multicenter Study Group. Improvement of histological lesions by 18 months therapy with alpha-2b interferon(IFN 2b) in patients with chronic hepatitis C. A randomized clinical trial. Hepatology 1993; 18:90A(Abstr).
2. Craxi A, Di Marco O, Lo Iacono O, Almasio P, Bruno R, Camma C et al. Lymphoblastoid alpha-interferon for post transfusion chronic hepatitis C: a randomized trial of 6 vs. 12 months treatment. J Hepatol 1992; 16(Suppl 1):S8 (Abstr).
3. Lin R, Farrell GC for the Australian Hepatitis C Virus Study Group. Treatment of chronic active hepatitis C with interferon alpha 2b: interim report of a multicenter Australian trial (Abstr). In: Posters abstract book of viral hepatitis management: standards for the future. Cannes: Shering Plough International, 1992; 29.
4. Makris M, Preston FE, Triger DR. Randomized controlled trials of recombinant IFN alpha in chronic hepatitis C in hemophiliacs. Blood 1991; 78:1672-1677.
5. Metreau JM and the French Group for the Study of NANB/C Chronic Hepatitis Treatment. Results of long term interferon treatment in non-A non-B/C chronic active hepatitis. Gut 1993; 34(Suppl):S112-113.
6. Milella M, Santantonio T, Monno L, Pastore G. Comparison of short vs. long term treatment with recombinant alpha interferon in chronic hepatitis C (abstract). In: Abstract Book of the 1992 International Symposium on Viral Hepatitis and Liver Disease (the 8th Triennal Congress). Tokyo, 1993; 245.
7. Saracco G, Rosina F, Abate ML et al. Long term follow-up of patients with chronic hepatitis C treated with different doses of IFN alpha 2b. Hepatology 1993; 18:1300-1305.
8. Alberti A, Chemello L, Bonetti P, Casarin C, Diodati G, Cavaletto L et al. Treatment with interferon(s) of community-acquired chronic hepatitis and cirrhosis type C. J Hepatol 1993; 17(Suppl 3):S123-S126.

Treatment of Chronic Type B and C Hepatitis with Alpha Interferon. An Economic Appraisal

G. M. Dusheiko, J. A. Roberts

INTRODUCTION

Hepatitis B virus (HBV) and hepatitis C virus (HCV) have a propensity to cause chronic hepatitis, and morbidity due to chronic liver disease (1-3). Evidence suggests that both diseases may have a long natural history, which can be benign in some yet progress inexorably in others.

A proportion of patients with chronic type B or C hepatitis respond to therapy with alpha interferon (4, 5). It is possible that the reduction in disease activity and curtailment of viral replication in responsive patients could improve the long-term prognosis of the patients (6). There is growing concern over the burgeoning costs of medical therapy for treatment of chronic hepatitis, creating the need for an economic evaluation of alpha interferon. Ideally such a study should involve a prospective trial comparing cohorts throughout the natural history of disease. These data are not available, so it was necessary to construct a model to ascertain the likely benefits of therapy.

METHODS

In this model we have estimated the direct medical costs of the illness associated with ambulatory visits and in-patient admissions to hospital over the course of the disease. A Markov chain transitional model was constructed to estimate disease progression over a 30 year period in a hypothetical cohort of 1,000 patients with either chronic hepatitis B or C, treated with alpha interferon and to compare the outcome in these patients with a similar untreated cohort. These projections were based on the most reliable information available from published reports, and the advice of an international panel of hepatologists who attended a consensus conference in London in April 1993.

The economic evaluation undertaken includes a cost-effectiveness analysis assessing the costs in terms of lives saved, years of life saved, and quality-adjusted years of life saved as well as a cost-benefit analysis which includes some social costs and values of life.

The effect of intervention with alpha interferon upon the natural history of chronic hepatitis can be studied if it is assumed that a response to treatment, characterised by cessation of active viral replication, will prevent the development of cirrhosis and therefore progression to chronic liver disease.

The disease path in these patients includes five elements: *a*) chronic hepatitis, leading to, *b*) cirrhosis, *c*) clinically relevant sequelae of cirrhosis («decompensated cirrhosis») including hepatocellular carcinoma, *d*) death as a result of these sequelae, and *e*) transplantation is considered an option for selected patients with decompensated liver disease. Patient cohorts for hepatitis B and C have been defined and the rates of disease progression calculated by examining data from several sources.

The assumptions and estimates used in the model are briefly summarised:

1. Patients were defined according to age, sex, race and the symptoms of HBV and HCV infection and were all assumed to have chronic hepatitis.
2. Doses of alpha interferon were 10 mμ tiw for 16 weeks for hepatitis B and 3 mu tiw for 26 weeks for hepatitis C.
3. Final response rates to alpha interferon therapy were 35 and 25% for patients with hepatitis B and hepatitis C respectively; response to therapy halted disease progression.
4. In non-responders, and untreated patients: progress from chronic hepatitis to cirrhosis was at a rate of either 1 or 2% per year.
5. Probability of developing decompensation was 5% per year.
6. Probability of death in patients with decompensated cirrhosis was either 5 or 13% per year.

The costs were estimated for the therapy and subsequent monitoring and treatment of the disease, including transplantation, based on costing data from the Royal Free Hospital, London. The cost effectiveness of the therapy was expressed in terms of cost per life saved, cost per year of life saved and cost per quality adjusted year of life saved (QALYS). To explore the sensitivity of the model, the analysis included two rates of progression, two mortality rates, and estimates of either discounted or undiscounted costs.

RESULTS

The 30-year disease progression and numbers of surviving patients in each disease stage were calculated for two rates of cirrhosis and two rates of death, and after orthotropic liver transplantation following decompensation. There were fewer deaths among the treated cohorts, depending upon the rate of cirrhosis and the death rate. Fewer patients reached the cirrhotic or decompensated stage of the disease, and fewer transplants were required in the treated groups.

Direct Medical Costs

Direct medical costs for the treated cohorts are higher than for the untreated cohort in the first year, reflecting the costs of working up the patients prior to treatment. In subsequent years, the costs associated with the treated group are less than that of the untreated group, since fewer enter the later stages of the disease, requiring more intensive treatment and monitoring.

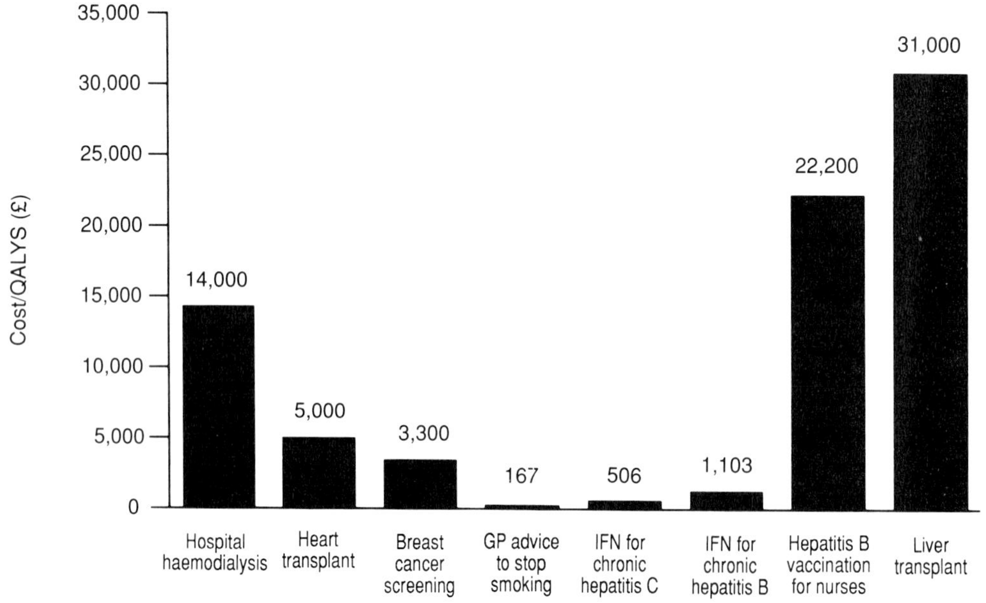

Fig. 1. Comparisons of cost effectiveness of alpha interferon therapy for hepatitis with other medical interventions. (Includes data from Maynard et al: Am Heart J 1990; 119:761-765; with permission.)

Cost effectiveness. Quality adjusted years of life saved have been estimated and costed in pounds sterling. The discounted costs per QALYS were between £500 and £1,000 for hepatitis B and C respectively; this can be compared to other interventions (fig. 1). Discounted costs per year of life saved ranged from £2,142 to £17,128. A cost benefit analysis indicated excess benefits over costs when values for life were included in the intervention.

CONCLUSIONS

In the hypothetical patient cohorts, alpha interferon therapy decreased the rate of disease progression and reduced the number of deaths compared to treatment. Costs for the treated groups are higher than the untreated group in the first year, reflecting costs of therapy, but in all subsequent years, the costs associated with treated groups are less than those of the untreated group.

These comparisons with other interventions provide interesting bench marks but must be interpreted with care because of the difficulties in ensuring the generalisation of the findings. The modelling structure is such that alternatives could be introduced, new approaches incorporated and assumptions changed as new and more reliable information accumulates. The study is offered as an exploratory model which in the absence of prospective long-term evaluation will enable decision makers to obtain some idea about the impact of intervention. These findings, together with the benefits that are likely to accrue from the reduction of the numbers of infectious individuals suggest that alpha interferon therapy has a role to play in public health policy to contain and limit hepatitis.

While alpha interferon is presently the mainstay of treatment for chronic viral hepatitis, approximately 50% of patients do not respond to therapy with this agent, and the search for additional therapies for this important human disease continues.

REFERENCES

1. Dusheiko GM. Pounder RE, eds. Recent Advances in Gastroenterology. 9th ed. Edinburgh: Churchill Livingstone, 1992; 195-216.
2. Hoofnagle JH, Alter HJ, Vyas GN, Dienstag JL, eds. Viral Hepatitis and Liver Disease. New York: Grune & Stratton, 1984; 97-113.
3. Alter MJ, Margolis HS, Krawczynski K, Judson FN, Mares A, Alexander WJ, Hu PY, Miller JK, Gerber MA, Sampliner RE et al. The natural history of community-acquired hepatitis C in the United States. N Engl J Med 1992; 327: 1899-1905.
4. Dusheiko G, Dibisceglie A, Bowyer S, Sachs E, Ritchie M, Schoub B, Kew M. Recombinant leukocyte interferon treatment of chronic hepatitis B. Hepatology 1985; 5:556-560.
5. Hoofnagle JH, Di Bisceglie AM, Shindo M. Antiviral therapy of hepatitis C—present and future. J Hepatol 1993; 17(Suppl 3):S130-136.
6. Korenman J, Baker B, Waggoner J, Everhart JE, Di-Bisceglie AM, Hoofnagle JH. Long-term remission of chronic hepatitis B after alpha-interferon therapy. Ann Intern Med 1991; 114:629-634.

Non Response to Interferon in Chronic Hepatitis B and C: Features and Mechanisms

A. Craxi, C. Linea, S. Magrin

INTRODUCTION

The introduction in clinical practice of interferon (IFN) therapy for chronic viral hepatitis has changed the attitude of physicians towards diagnosis and treatment of liver disease. Chronic hepatitis was previously felt to be an irreversible illness, with scarce likelihood to be cured even after an accurate etiologic and histologic assessment. Only a minority of patients with clearcut features of autoimmunity had, before the IFN era, a good chance of being cured by an etiologic therapy, namely immunosuppression with steroids and/or azathioprine.

Since the early pilot studies of α-interferon therapy for chronic hepatitis B and chronic non-A, non-B hepatitis, an enormous amount of experience on the use of interferons in chronic liver disease has accumulated through uncontrolled and controlled studies. Initial enthusiasm on antiviral treatment with IFN has however been progressively mitigated by the fact that not all patients with chronic hepatitis B or C respond to the drug, and that only a proportion of responders will maintain a long-lasting benefit, hence being truly cured of the disease.

Pooled results of controlled studies of IFN in chronic hepatitis B (1-3) show that the rate of response, measured as stable loss of HBeAg from blood, varies from less than 25% to over 60%. This wide range is mostly due to a variable rate of spontaneous seroconversion in the control group, since those studies reporting the best effect of IFN on viral replication also have the highest likelihood of HBeAg loss among control patients. Actually, the same clinical and laboratory features originally reported (4) as predictive of effectiveness of interferon were recently found, in a metaanalysis of individual data from ten published trials (3), to indicate also a good chance of spontaneous seroconversion. The latter study indicates that the overall benefit of IFN in chronic hepatitis B may be quantified as a relative risk of seroconversion 1.8 times higher than untreated cases, regardless of the initial chances of HBeAg loss. In other words, IFN will make things better for those who are already likely to stop HBV replication, but will only be of limited help in the other subjects.

Review by metaanalysis of therapeutic trials performed up to 1991 (5) shows that 50 to 60% of all patients with chronic hepatitis C receiving IFN at a dosage ≥ 3 MU tiw for at least six months reach normal alanine aminotransferase levels while on therapy. However half or more of these responders to IFN relapse to high ALT levels within a few months after stopping the drug, thus reducing the long-term response rate to 20-25%. Retreatment of relapsers may obtain a new response, usually followed again by relapse, in a substantial proportion of cases, while non-responders are refractory to retreatment.

Unsatisfactory results of IFN, and therefore the need for a better selection of patients to be treated and of alternative approaches for non-responders, might be mitigated by a better understanding of the mechanisms underlying the unresponsiveness to IFN.

MODES OF ACTION OF INTERFERON

Interferons are a part of a complex network interacting with other regulatory factors, such as cytokines and cellular growth factors, which serve as a defense mechanism against viral infections. The activity of α-IFN against hepatitis viruses is due to a direct antiviral effect, namely the induction of an antiviral state in the infected cell by enhancement of 2-5 oligoadenylate synthetase, protein kinase P1, ribonuclease L activities. Immune recognition and clearance of virus-infected cells is facilitated by IFN-induced enhancement of MHC class I antigens expression on the hepatocytes, in association with viral proteins. IFN can modify the cellular membrane, thus making difficult the release of virions. Moreover, the immunomodulatory activity of IFN, causing activation of NK cells and macrophages and also increased cytotoxic T cell function, is probably important in reducing the number of cells harboring replicating virus. These activities of IFN can be affected by many variables, related to the infecte host, to the virus and to the drug itself (fig. 1), mutually influencing themselves in a complex interplay. We shall review the knowledge available for HBV and HCV, aiming to point out approaches to enhance the response rate.

Host-Related Factors (table 1)

Stage of liver disease. The stage of liver disease is probably the most important factor in determining the response to IFN. Two different points need to be considered, i.e., the degree of inflammatory activity and the amount of fibrosis.

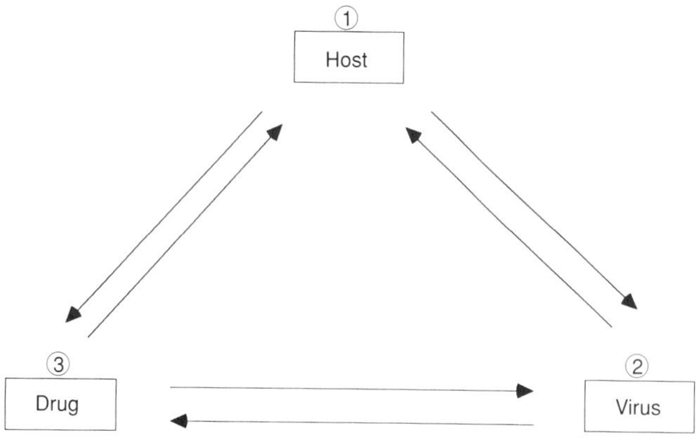

Fig. 1. Factors influencing the effectiveness of interferon in chronic viral hepatitis.

Table 1. **Causes of non-response. Host-related factors**

	HBV	HCV
Stage of liver disease		
Inactive necroinflamation	Yes	No
Presence of cirrhosis	No (?)	Yes
Timing of infection/(therapy)		
As age at the time of therapy	Yes (LR in young)	No (?)
As time elapsed since primary infection	?	Yes
Race		
Caucasian	Yes	No
Oriental	Yes	No
Sex		
M/F	Yes (?)	No
Male homosexuality	Yes	No
Associated disease		
Immunosuppression (HIV; iatrogenic)	Yes	No (?)
Iron overload	?	Yes (?)
Autoimmune phenomena		
Coexisting with infection	Yes	Yes
Secondary to viral infection	No	No
Cholestasis	No	Yes

In chronic hepatitis B, necroinflammation is due to the immune response to HBV (6). Hence, an «inactive» histology (portitis; absence of lobular inflammation) is predictive of a low likelihood of spontaneous or treatment-induced loss of viral replication (7). This reflects the lack of effectiveness of locally-acting cytotoxic mechanisms, allowing persistence of HBV replication (so-called «immune tolerance» phase) (8, 9). Chronic HCV infection causes liver cell damage by both direct cytopathic and immune-mediated mechanisms (10). Hence the relation between histological activity of liver disease and likelihood of response is less clearcut. Most studies in fact suggest that the effectiveness of IFN is similar in patients with chronic persistent and in those with chronic active hepatitis.

Fibrosis is a hallmark in the natural history of chronic hepatitis, signalling the evolution toward cirrhosis. Once severe fibrosis and cirrho-

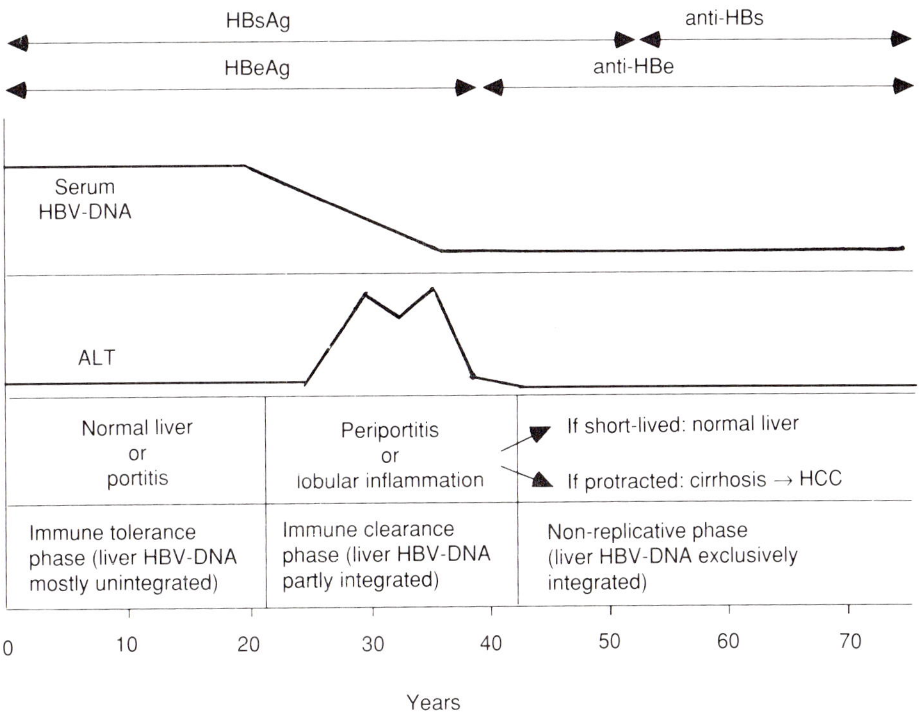

Fig. 2. Natural history of chronic hepatitis B (wild type virus).

tic nodules appear in the liver, the likelihood of response to IFN is diminished. This is much more evident in chronic hepatitis C than in chronic hepatitis B. Almost all large studies of prognostic factors in chronic hepatitis C (11-16) are concordant in establishing cirrhosis as the more important variable in predicting non-response to IFN. The long-term response rate in patients with cirrhosis can be as low as 5% (11). Unresponsiveness could be due to the long time elapsed since first contact with the virus, but also to infection with a more pathogenic and IFN-resistent strain of HCV. Selection of IFN-resistent viral mutants under the pressure of endogenous IFN is also conceivably involved (8, 9). Vascular factors intrinsic to cirrhosis might also conceivably alter the biovailability and pharmacokinetics of IFN. A recent study (17) and preliminary data (Ascione, Hepatology, 20, 294A, 1994) indicate that high serum levels of hyaluronate or laminin, both indicators of active collagen metabolism, are predictive of unresponsiveness to IFN in chronic hepatitis C, independently from cirrhosis. This suggests that increased collagen deposition on the sinusoidal pole of hepatocyte might affect IFN turnover in the liver. The importance of cirrhosis in reducing the response rate to IFN in chronic HBV infection is less clearcut. Most clinical trials have enrolled patients without cirrhosis, and even in the larger trials the proportion of cirrhotic patients is low. Although some studies report a lesser effect of α-IFN on seroconversion rates in cirrhotics, others do not find such an effect. A metaanalysis of 837 patients with chronic HBV infection (2), of whom 12.7% had cirrhosis, does not report a reduced response in cirrhotics. When spontaneous or treatment-induced HBeAg loss is obtained in a cirrhotic patient, this is usually irreversible and improves significantly the long-term outcome of the disease (7).

Timing of infection. Chronic hepatitis B and C infection display a complex kinetics of events, unfolding over many years with alternate phases of viral replication or quiescence and of immune tolerance or clearance to an heterogeneous viral population (18-20). In general, IFN is likely to be more effective when at the same time the immune mechanisms involved in viral clearance are already activated and the replicative drive of the virus is failing.

Chronic HBV infection in young patients has usually been acquired during the first years of life (fig. 2). These subjects have an «immune tolerance» pattern of infection (highly replicating virus; absence of liver necroinflammation). The response rate to IFN of HBV-infected children is, in an age-dependent fashion, less than that of adult subjects (21). A beneficial effect can be observed (22). During normal growth, the child enters the «immunoelimination phase» (HBV still replicating, but at lower level; liver necroinflammation). During this time a higher trend toward spontaneous (23) or IFN-induced seroconversion is observed. Children who did not respond to IFN when treated during the «immune tolerance» period may have a higher chance to lose HBV replication when retreated during the «immunoelimination phase». Actually, in these children immune potentiation with levamisole during IFN treatment seems to enhance the response rate (24, 25).

HCV infection of children is far less frequent than HBV infection, due to the ineffectiveness of mother-to-child transmission (26). Experience with treatment of pediatric HCV infection is hence limited. Published studies (27) report an incidence of non-response similar to adults.

The length of time elapsed since primary infection at the moment of starting IFN treatment is an important variable in determining response. The longer the virus has been in the host, the higher is the likelihood of selection of IFN-resistent viral strains. The probability of development of cirrhosis, which is in itself a major determinant of non-response, is clearly time-dependent. Long-term presence of virus-encoded proteins in the host might maintain and enhance mechanisms of inmunotolerance (28, 29). The effect of duration of infection on non-response is quite clear for HCV. A recent study from our group (11) identifies, besides the absence of cirrhosis, a short (lower than 24 months) disease duration as strongly predictive of primary and long-term response to IFN. In this study known hepatitis C infection since over 60 months was associated to a low chance of normalizing aminotransferases, independently from cirrhosis at multivariate analysis. This suggests that resistence to IFN, when HCV infection has been present for a long time, is due both to virus-related factors (selection of strains less sensitive to IFN) and to cirrhosis itself.

No direct data are available for HBV. It is known however that non-response to IFN is more common when the infection has been acquired early in life. Besides the problems of immune competence already discussed, this might suggest that a long time of replicative HBV infection leads to a reduced chance of spontaneous or IFN-induced clearance of viral replication. The progressive increase over the years in the number of liver cells with integrated viral DNA probably reduce the chances of a complete response (i. e., seroconversion from HBsAg to anti-HBs).

Race. Comparison of results obtained in chronic hepatitis B when treating Caucasians (2, 3) and Oriental patients (30) shows that the former are more sensitive to IFN treatment. Racial differences may be involved. It should be reminded that Oriental subjects who are chronic HBsAg carriers tend to remain in the «immune tolerance phase» more often than Caucasians. Non-response to IFN might only parallel the low trend to spontaneous seroconversion. The number of black subjects with chronic hepatitis B reported in IFN trials is small. Results suggest a strong trend to spontaneous and treatment-induced seroconversion (3). Interpretation of racial differences in response should take into account the different age at the time of infection. In the western world, with the exception of the Mediterranean basin (31), HBV infection occurs mostly in the young adult through high-risk practices (sex; i.v. drugs). The time elapsed since primary infection is hence usually quite short when IFN treatment is started. By contrast, Oriental patients (32) have almost always been infected early in their life, and have already a long duration of infection when treated.

Trials of IFN for chronic HCV infection in Oriental (mostly Japanese) patients show rates of response comparable to those of Caucasians. Some inconsistencies in the response rates can be attributed to the different pattern of infecting HCV types (33). Some Japanese trials have also used schedules of IFN administration which are not comparable for length and dosage to Western studies.

Sex. No clear effect of sex on the rate of response to IFN is seen in the metaanalyses performed in HBV- and HCV-infected patients (1-3, 5). The effect of sexual preference (i. e., a lower rate of response in HBeAg positive male homosexuals) formerly reported (4) is due to the high prevalence of infection with the human immunodeficiency virus (HIV) in this group. HBV-infected homosexuals who are not coinfected by HIV respond to IFN at the same rate as heterosexuals (3).

Associated diseases. *Immunosuppression.* A sizable proportion of subjects with chronic viral hepatitis of any etiology are coinfected by the human immunodeficiency virus (HIV). The drastical reduction in CD4 lymphocytes in the advanced phase of HIV infection causes profound hyporesponsiveness to HBV- and HCV-encoded proteins. The clinical expression, natural course and response to antiviral therapy of chronic hepatitis B and C are different in the HIV infected subject who already has clinical evidence of immunosuppression. Viral interference can be important, in these patients often harboring multiple infections, in determining loss of HBV, HDV or HCV replication (34, 35). Ultimately the prognosis and survival of the individual patient are strictly related to HIV infection and to the degree of immunosuppression.

Chronic HBV infection usually runs a mild course in these patients, most of them remaining indefinitely in the «immune tolerance» phase because of the lack of an effective immune response. In some cases however fibrosing cholestatic hepatitis, a severe and rapidly evolving lesion usually occurring in HBsAg positive liver transplantees under antirejection therapy, has been observed in AIDS patients (36). This suggests a direct cytopathic effect of HBV in the presence of high level of viral replication. Two metaanalyses (2, 3) showed that IFN treatment for chronic HBeAg positive hepatitis in HIV infected individuals gave no advantage over no treatment, as already previously reported by uncontrolled studies (4, 37). The failure of IFN in inducing viral clearance is related to the degree of immunosuppression, since a few responses can be observed in subjects with CD4 counts above 400/mm^3. Treatment of HIV infection with AZT (38), DDI or ACV (Martinot, ISVHLD, Tokio, A208, 1993) does not modify significantly the replication of HBV. New purine and pirimidine analogues (39-42) are being developed in the search for an effective anti-HIV agent. Testing in patients infected also by HBV is under way, with some promising results in terms of inhibition of HBV-DNA. Since the mechanism of action are different form IFN, they may circumvent non-response in such patients.

Table 2. Chronic hepatitis C in HIV-infected individuals: IFN trials[a]

Trial	Patients	CD4 Status	SR[b] ALT	SR[b] RNA	LR[c] ALT	LR[c] RNA
1	40	≥ 200	9	–	–	–
2	78	≥ 400	19	–	–	–
3	11	Any	1	–	–	–
4	6	Any	3	–	3	–
5	7	Any	5	–	–	–
6	14	≥ 400	5	3	4	4
7	12	Any	4	–	1	–
Overall	161		46 (29%)			

[a] Alfa-IFN ≥ 3 MU tiw for ≥ 6 months.
[b] Short-term response.
[c] Long-term response.

1. García-Samaniego. J Hepatol 1993; 18:S122.
2. Del Poggio. J Hepatol 1993; 18:S112.
3. Schwarz. Hepatology 1993; 18:254A.
4. Areias. Hepatology 1993; 18:222A.
5. Sangermano. Hepatology 1993; 18:253A.
6. Mariott. J Med Virol 1993; 40:107.
7. Boyer. J Inf Dis 1992; 165:723.

HCV-related chronic liver disease is less directly linked to immunopathogenetic mechanisms, and more dependent on direct viral cytotoxicity (10). Chronic hepatitis C in HIV infected subjects behaves similarly than in normally immunocompetent individuals. A more severe course of disease has been reported (43, 44), and might be due to the lack of mechanisms of suppression of HCV infection. It is difficult however to assess in these very sick patients the possible negative role of other cofactors. A summary of published results of IFN therapy in these patients is presented in table 2. The overall short-term response rate, measured on ALT normalization, is 29%. This compares unfavourably with the 50% response rate (5) reported in non-HIV infected patients, but still suggests some effect of IFN. In fact, the only study assessing long-term HCV-RNA loss reports disappearance of viraemia in 4/14 cases (29%), showing that HCV clearance can be obtained also in immunosuppressed hosts. These results are comparable to those obtained in subjects undergoing pharmacological immunosuppression after liver (45, 46) or kidney transplantation (47-49).

Iron overload. It has been recently reported that, in patients with chronic hepatitis B or C, the hepatic iron content was almost twice in non-responders to IFN therapy as compared to responders (50). The same study showed a weak correlation between serum ferritin and hepatic iron level. These findings are in line with previous studies (51) showing an altered iron metabolism in chronic HBV carriers. Since iron is a necessary cofactor for DNA and RNA synthesis, an excessive hepatocyte iron pool might facilitate the intracellular assembly of virions. Phlebotomy has been proposed as a mean to enhance response to IFN by causing depletion of liver iron. Clinical experience is still awaited. Results in subjects with massive iron overload, such as polytransfused β-thalassaemia patients with chronic hepatitis C, are conflicting. All published studies (52-54) have found a negative correlation between iron overload and likelihood of biochemical and histological response. However, in the absence of cirrhosis, the overall rate of long-term success is similar to that obtained in non-thalassaemic subjects. This shows that even in the presence of massive iron overload IFN can still affect HCV replication.

Autoimmune phenomena. Evidence of autoimmunity may coexist with chronic viral hepatitis, more often with HCV or HDV than with HBV (55-68). While earlier studies debated whether the presence of autoantibodies represented true autoimmunity or a secondary response to infection, it is now clear that up to 10% with otherwise typical chronic hepatitis C may have serum autoantibodies at significant titres in serum, coexisting with active HCV replication. These antibodies are mostly anti-liver/kidney microsomes (LKM), but sometimes anti-nuclear. IFN therapy in these subjects has usually been avoided, on the basis of possible reactivation of underlying autoimmune hepatitis. A small-scale study (F. Bianchi, unpublished) actually reports ineffectiveness of IFN treatment in 6 patients with LKM-positive chronic hepatitis C, with disease reactivation in 3. However in our experience no significant differences in the rate of response to IFN are observed when treating such patients. It is conceivable that, among a vast majority of cases with «true» hepatitis C and secondary immune phenomena, a few subjects with autoimmune hepatitis and associated HCV infection may hide.

Cholestasis. Mild features of biochemical cholestasis are not uncommon in chronic hepatitis C. These consist mostly in a raised gammaglutamyltransferase and alkalyne phosphatase, without hyperbilirubinemia or symptoms. Bile duct damage and epithelioid granulomas around biliary structures in the portal tract are often seen in liver biopsies from patient with HCV-related liver disease (69). Cholestatic features and the presence of bile duct damage are variably related to HCV replicative levels (70-72). Elevated levels of gammaglutamyltransferase are predictive of a poor response to IFN (15, 73, 74), albeit less strongly than cirrhosis or HCV-RNA level (11). Subjects with chronic hepatitis C and cholestasis might be infected by a more resistent HCV strain. No association with a specific HCV genotype has been demonstrated. In these patients a moderate efficacy of ursodexoycholic acid (UDCA) in normalizing liver tests and improving liver biopsy features has already been demonstrated (75, 76). No convincing effect on HCV viraemia was howe-

Table 3. Causes of non-response. Virus-related factors

	HBV	HCV
Viral type	?	Genotype 1
Mutants		
De novo mutation under therapy		Hypervariable E2/NS1
Selection of unfavourable strain from mixed infection (escape mutant; antigen drift; replication-competent virus)	HBeAg minus mutant	Hypervariable E2/NS1
Original infection with resistent mutant	HBeAg minus muntant	Hypervariable E2/NS1
Virus load		
In relation to the way of infection		PTH vs. sporadic
In relation to the time of infection		Early vs. late (?)
In relation to viral type	?	Genotype 1 (?)
In relation to coexisting disease/immunosuppression	Yes	Yes
Coexisting infection		
With hepatotropic viruses	HDV, HCV	HBV + HDV
With limphotropic viruses	HIV	HIV
Viral persistence		
In the liver	Yes	Yes (?)
In lymphoid cells	Yes	Yes
In extrahepatic, non-lymphoid tissues	Yes (?)	Yes (?)
Virus-induced immune alterations		
In cytokine expression		
In adhesion molecules		
In IFN and IFN receptors synthesis		
In IFN-inducible gene products		

ver found. Randomized trials exploring combined therapy with UDCA and IFN are under way.

Virus-related Factors (table 3)

Viral type. HCV is a highly heterogeneous viral agent, encompassing a range of different viral types and subtypes (33, 77, 78). Many classifications of HCV types based on sequence variations of different HCV region have been proposed. Thus, studies dealing with the relationship between HCV type and response to IFN are not strictly comparable, since different region of the HCV genome have been used for genotyping. Earlier studies mostly used Okamoto's classification (79), while the most recent attempts of HCV classification have been performed on the 5' UTR region (80). The following comments relate to HCV classification based on 5' UTR. Differences in the pathogenicity of the various types of HCV have been reported. Some studies show a higher prevalence of cirrhosis among subjects infected with type 1b (81-83), but other workers (84) do not confirm this issue. Geographical heterogeneity of distribution of HCV infection (33, 85-87) might be partly responsible for discordance, since the prevalence of genotypes supposed to be less pathogenic (types 1a, 2 and 3) is low in some countries (33, 85). The relationship between HCV type and response to IFN is also controversial. In fact, there is clear evidence that subjects infected with genotype 1b responde less well to IFN treatment than those infected by genotype 1a, 2a or 3 (88-94). This difference in response might be at least in part related to the level of pre-treatment viraemia and to the stage of liver disease (level of histological fibrosis and/or presence of cirrhosis). Studies assessing clinical and virological variables of responsiveness to IFN have shown that pretreatment viraemia and cirrhosis are independent predictive factors of response to IFN. However, there are conflicting results for the inclusion of HCV type as an independent predictive factor. In fact, the link between HCV type and response to IFN is more evident in some geographical areas where the infection is frequently due to HCV of non-1b genotype. In areas of high HCV type 1 endemicity such as Southern Europe, the majority of responders to IFN are actually infected by HCV type 1 (85, 95), confirming that unresponsiveness of this viral type is a relative, rather than absolute, phenomenon. In these patients, typing of the virus in regions other than the currently used 5' non coding terminus might disclose other viral (sub)types. The biological mechanisms linking a specific viral type to IFN responsiveness is currently unknown.

HBV genotypes, which have a peculiar geographical distribution (96-112), have never

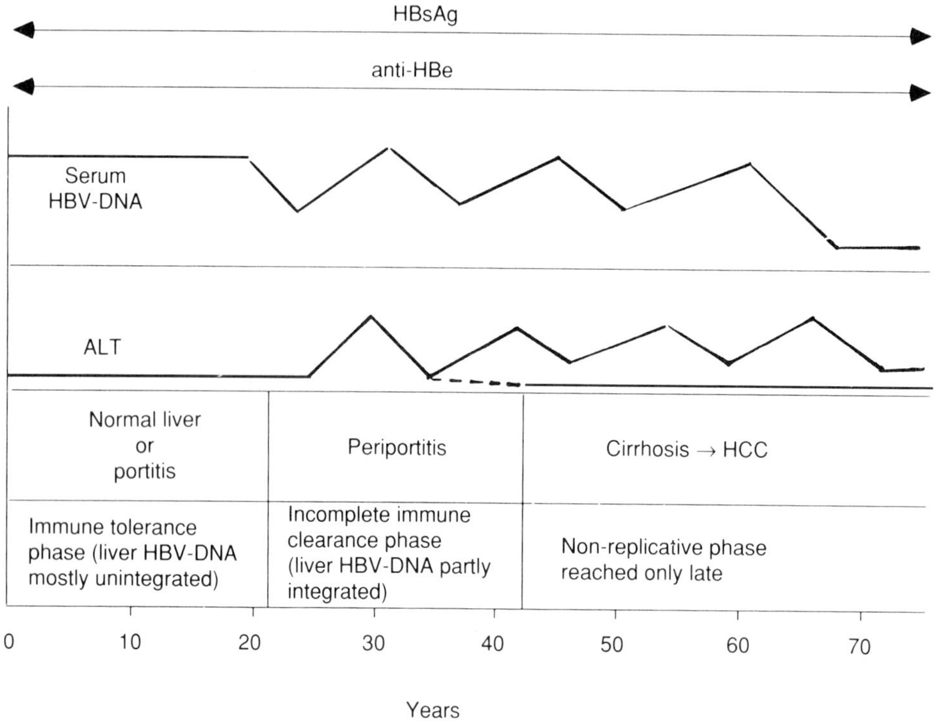

Fig. 3. Natural history of chronic hepatitis B (pre-core mutant).

been clearly related to a variable pattern of disease expression or to a difference in sensitivity to IFN therapy.

Viral mutants. Occurrence of viral mutation during chronic infection is a well-known phenomenon, affecting both HBV (113-128) and HCV (129-135). Mutations may exert a profound influence on viral replicative ability, pathogenicity and sensitivity to endogenous and exogenous antiviral actions.

The infection may be due to a viral strain whose likelihood of responding to IFN is already low at the time of starting therapy. This is particularly evident for the HBV pre-core mutant, the so-called HBeAg-minus variant (136). Prevalence of the pre-core mutant in an individual chronically infected with HBV can be associated to a worse disease outcome than infection with wild-type HBV (136-171) (fig. 3). The absence of an efficient target for immune response, due to the defective expression of HBV nucleocapsid epitopes on the liver cell membrane, leads to an altered immune clearance phase, lasting for years with active necroinflammation but inefficient viral elimination. This in turn leads to earlier development of cirrhosis. IFN treatment has been reported to be less effective in subjects infected with the HBeAg minus variant (136, 161, 172-176), although few reports (177, 178) might indicate an efficacy similar to that on wild-type virus. Overall analysis of reported studies indicates a likelihood of loss of HBV viraemia during IFN administration ranging from 20 to 60%. Long-term results are however disappointing, since less than 10% of HBeAg negative, HBV-DNA positive subjects who have been treated with IFN remain with normal ALT and non-viraemic (by dot-blot techniques) when evaluated few months after stopping therapy. Results of antiviral therapy are even worse if more sensitive techniques for detection of HBV genomes, such as PCR, are used. The causes of this poor efficacy of IFN may be the same underlying the protracted HBV replicative phase in untreated patients, namely the lack of an efficient target for the immune clearance of the virus. Appearance of the HBeAg-minus variant under IFN treatment has also been reported, in association with failure to respond to IFN (141). This is likely to be due to a selection effect (i. e., expansion of a pre-existing mutant viral population after suppression of wild-type HBV) rather than to *de novo* apparence of the mutation in the individual receiving treatment.

Variations of the HCV quasispecies under IFN therapy are known to occurr. This is especially frequent in the hypervariable E2/NS1 region (179, 180), and seems to correlate both to reactivation of liver disease and to IFN resistance.

Coexisting infections. Concurrent hepatitis B and hepatitis C are sometimes found in subjects with parenteral risk factors (181). Replication of one of the two viruses (usually HBV) is almost always suppressed, unless the patient is also coinfected by HIV. Effectiveness of IFN in dual infections has not been formally assessed. Anecdotal evidence suggests that ALT normalization is difficult to obtain. HBV reactivation after successful treatment of HCV has been reported (182).

Drug-related Factors (table 4)

Dosage and schedule of IFN. Interferon is currently the only agent of proven efficacy in the treatment of chronic hepatitis B and C.

In chronic hepatitis B, α-interferon obtains cessation of viral replication and of the ensuing necroinflammation at a higher rate than in untreated controls (1-3). In a recent meta-analysis (3), ten randomized controlled trials showed concordantly that therapy with α-IFN increased the *a priori* likelihood of HBeAg loss by a factor of 1.76. This study also clearly indicated a dose-response effect. When a cut-off was set at 200 MU/sqm for the total dose received (equivalent, for a subject with a body surface of 1.75 sqm, to 7.3 MU thrice weekly for 16 week or 4.5 Mu thrice weekly for 26 weeks) meta-analysis showed that treatment schedules administering total doses below this cut-off were inferior to those above the cut-off (increase of likelihood of HBeAg loss 1.35 vs. 2.05). Currently recommended regimens of IFN in chronic hepatitis B are 6 to 10 MU tiw for 16-24 weeks.

Patients with chronic hepatitis C usually receive α-IFN at dose of 3 MU tiw for 6 months, according to the experience accumulated in the earlier trials. Since only one every four treated subjects obtain a sustained remission (5) and at least another one relapse after therapy, patients who respond and relapse may require retreatment. Efficacy of retreatment in obtaining long-term remission is actually unknown. Some investigators suggest that prolonged treatment (up to 12 months or more) might reduce the relapse rate in subjects obtaining complete ALT normalization (183). Our experience in patients predominantly infected by genotype 1b suggests that treatment with high doses of α-IFN over a brief period (total dose of 420 MU in 6 months) is equivalent, in terms both of response rate and of prevention of relapses, to a longer treatment period (total dose of 600 MU in 12 months) (184, 185). Prolonged interferon administration to patients with chronic hepatitis C is poorly accepted and might favour drug resis-

Table 4. Causes of non-response. Drug related factors

	HBV	HCV
Dosage of interferon		
Schedule of interferon (daily, alternate days, weekly continuous infusion)		
Way of administration (i.m., s.l., e.v., continuous infusion)		
Type of IFN		
α_2-Recombinants		
α_2-Lymphoblastoid	Equivalent	Equivalent
α_2-Leukocytes		
β-IFN	Only Effective i.v.	Only Effective i.v.
IFN antibodies		
Total Abs	No	No
Neutralizing Abs	?	?
Primary resistance to IFN		
Scarce activation of intracellular pathways		
Down regulation of IFN receptors (after therapy)		
Side effects/disease reactivation (IFN hepatitis [?])		

* Assessed only for interferon.

tante. A pulse-treatment schedule would be preferred for compliance and costs. Preliminary evidence (186) suggests a comparable sustained response rate. The intermittent administration can be proposed not only to elicit a sustained biochemical and virological remission but also to circumvent the development of drug resistance due, e.g., to selection of drug resistant strains or to drug adaptation and even toxicity. Alternative approaches such as escalating dosages or weekly administration do not alter the likelihood of response (187-190). Escalation of the dose may achieve response in some non-responders.

One of the early RCTs (191) showed that a low dose of α-IFN (1 MU tiw) is inferior to a higher dose (3 MU tiw) in promoting a decrease of hepatic necroinflammation. This was later confirmed by studies using dose-adjustment regimens, where reduction of the dose at 1 MU often caused «breakthrough» ALT elevations (192).

We recently compared the results of trials performed at our Institution with different doses of α-IFN, and found a clearcut dose-effect relationship with a peak effectiveness at a schedule of 6 MU tiw (193).

Type of IFN. Recombinant (α_{2a} or α_{2b}) and lymphoblastoid (αn_1) interferons have been used in most studies. Natural human leukocyte (αn_3) interferon is also effective in normalizing ALT in chronic hepatitis C (194). The results obtained with this kind of IFN are similar to that observed using different IFN preparations (191, 195, 196). A trial comparing recombinant α_{2a} and lymphoblastoid αn_1 IFN did not show any difference in the rate of response or relapse (197).

β-Interferon has been used, chiefly by Japanese investigators, in chronic hepatitis B and C (198-200). It should be administered only by intravenous injection, since intramuscular or subcutaneous injections do not give detectable serum levels (201). When this condition is fulfilled, the effectiveness seems to be comparable to that of α-IFN in chronic HBV or HCV infection. Intramuscular injection of β-IFN was, in a comparative study with α_{2b} or αn_3-IFN, rather ineffective in obtaining response in chronic hepatitis C (202).

Anti-interferon antibodies (anti-IFN). The appearance of anti-IFN antibodies has been documented in treated patients with chronic hepatitis B and C (204-206). The prevalence of such antibodies, classified as neutralizing or non-neutralizing according to their ability to block the biological effects of IFNs, is highly variable in published studies, ranging from 1 to 20% in relation to schedule of IFN and also to the assay used for their detection (207, 208). When enzyme immunoassays (EIA) and the antiviral neutralization bioassay (ANB) are compared, anti-IFN antibodies occur earlier by EIA than by ANB. The higher sensitivity of the former test (208) is however counterbalanced by the lack of clinical significance of non-neutralizing antibodies. The latter are detected by EIA, but not by ANB, which discloses only blocking factors (i.e., neutralizing antibodies).

The influence of IFN antibodies on the therapeutic effectiveness of IFN is still controversial (209), and at least partly related to the discordance between assay systems. High titers of anti-IFN antibodies seem to modulate the biological properties of IFN, reducing its antiviral effect and immunomodulatory actions. Actual interference on the clinical course of infection may depend from the timing of onset of the antibody response. In chronic hepatitis C appearance of anti-IFN antibodies after ALT normalization is not associated to a significant loss of IFN effect (209). Anti-IFN antibodies have also been included among the causes of ALT elevation during IFN treatment (so-called *breakthrough*) when high titers are produced (210). Breakthrough hepatitic reactivations are found in less than 5% of subjects with chronic hepatitis C treated with doses of α-IFN ≥ 3 MU tiw. Failure of IFN therapy can be attributed to anti-IFN antibodies only if the biochemical reactivation is concomitant with the appearance of antibodies (211). In chronic hepatitis B a breakthrough phenomenon is exceedingly rare.

Anti-IFN antibodies may have a role in the failure of response to IFN both in patients who show an initial response and in those who never respond to therapy. However only a small minority of subjects who do not respond have anti-IFN antibodies, confirming that blocking of IFN actions occurs only in selected cases. Antibodies to IFN are on the other hand found also in patients with a complete and long-lasting response. Hence the appearance of anti-IFN should not be considered as an indication to stop treatment, when otherwise effective.

Primary resistance to IFN. This phenomenon must be distinguished from the secondary resistance to IFN caused by the appearance of anti-IFN antibodies. IFNs interact with cell surface receptors to elicit a response in the target cells. The transmembrane signalling mechanisms of the receptor are still unknown. It is however established that, upon treatment with IFN, most genes are quickly and transiently induced and others are inhibited by down-regulation (212-214). There are conflicting views as to the nature of the signalling pathways, but probably the scarce activation of this intracellular pathways may be responsible for the primary resistence to IFN. Probably a down-regulation mechanism is also implicated in resistance to IFN. High levels of circulating α-IFN may cause receptor down-regulation, with a lower expression of these glycoproteins on the hepatocyte membranes (215, 216).

REFERENCES

1. Tine F, Liberati A, Craxi A, Almasio P, Pagliaro L. Interferon treatment in patients with chronic hepatitis B: A meta-analysis of the published literature. J Hepatol 1993; 18:154-162.
2. Wong DKH, Cheung AM, O'Rourke K, Naylor CD, Detsky AS, Heathcote J. Effect of alpha-interferon treatment in patients with hepatitis B e antigen-positive chronic hepatitis B: A meta-analysis. Ann Intern Med 1993; 119:312-323.
3. Krogsgaard K, Bindslev N, Christensen E, Craxi A, Schlichting P, Schalm S, Carreño V, Trepo C, Gerken G, Thomas HC, Andersen PK, Ring-Larsen H and EUROHEP. The treatment effect of alpha interferon in chronic hepatitis B is independen of pretreatment variables. Result based on individual patient data from 10 clinical controlled trials. J Hepatol 1994; 21:646-655.
4. Thomas HC, Karayiannis P, Brook G. Treatment of hepatitis B virus infection with interferon. Factors predicting response to interferon. J Hepatol 1991; 13(Suppl 1):S4-S7.
5. Tine F, Magrin S, Craxi A, Pagliaro L. Interferon for non-A, non-B chronic hepatitis. A meta-analysis of randomised clinical trials. J Hepatol 1991; 13:192-199.
6. Naumov NV, Eddleston ALWF. Host immune response and variations in the virus genome: Pathogenesis of liver damage caused by hepatitis B virus. Gut 1994; 35:1013-1017.
7. Realdi G, Fattovich G, Hadziyannis S, Schalm SW, Almasio P, Sánchez-Tapias J, Christensen E, Giustina G, Noventa F and EUROHEP. Survival and prognostic factors in 366 patients with compensated cirrhosis type B: a multicenter study. J Hepatol 1994; 21:656-666.
8. Foster GR, Thomas HC. Effects of hepatitis B and hepatitis C virus replication on the actions of interferon. Antiviral Res 1994; 24:131-136.
9. Foster GR, Thomas HC. Recent advances in the molecular biology of hepatitis B virus: Mutant virus and the host response. Gut 1993; 34:1-3.
10. González-Peralta RP, Davis GL, Lau JYN. Pathogenetic mechanisms of hepatocellular damage in chronic hepatitis C virus infection. J Hepatol 1994; 21:255-259.
11. Pagliaro L, Craxi A, Camma C et al. α-Interferon for chronic hepatitis C: An analysis of pretreatment clinical predictors of response. Hepatology 1994; 19:820-828.
12. Camps J, Crisóstomo S, García-Granero M, Riezu-Boj JI, Civeira MP, Prieto J. Prediction of the response of chronic hepatitis C to interferon alfa: A statistical analysis of pretreatment variables. Gut 1993; 34:1714-1717.
13. Camps J, García-Granero M, Riezu-Boj JI et al. Prediction of sustained remission of chronic hepatitis C after a 12-month course of alfa interferon. J Hepatol 1994; 21:4-11.
14. Davis GL. Prediction of response to interferon treatment of chronic hepatitis C. J Hepatol 1994; 21:1-3.
15. Serfaty L, Giral P, Loria A, Andréani T, Legendre C, Poupon R. Factors predictive of the response to interferon in patients with chronic hepatitis C. J Hepatol 1994; 21:12-17.
16. Tsubota A, Chayama K, Ikeda K et al. Factors predictive of response to α-interferon therapy in hepatitis C virus infection. Hepatology 1994; 19:1088-1094.
17. Matsunaga T, Kojima J, Inoue A, Matsumiya K. Serum hyaluronate levels predict responsiveness to alpha interferon therapy in patients with chronic hepatitis C. Clin Chim Acta 1994; 229:191-195.
18. Bonino F, Brunetto MR. Hepatitis B virus heterogeneity, one of many factors influencing the severity of hepatitis B. J Hepatol 1993; 18:5-8.
19. Brunetto MR, Cerenzia MT, Oliveri F et al. Monitoring the natural course and response to therapy of chronic hepatitis B with an automated semi-quantitative assay for IgM anti-HBc. J Hepatol 1993; 19:431-436.
20. Brunetto MR, Calvo PL, Oliveri F et al. Hepatitis C virus infection and liver disease: Peculiar epidemiological and clinicopathological features. FEMS Microbiol Rev 1994; 14:259-266.
21. Bruguera M, Amat L, García O et al. Treatment of chronic hepatitis B in children with recombinant alfa interferon: Different response according to age at infection. J Clin Gastroenterol 1993; 17:296-299.

22. Barbera C, Bortolotti F, Crivellaro C et al. Recombinant α_{2a}-interferon hastens the rate of HBeAg clearance in children with chronic hepatitis B. Hepatology 1994; 20:287-290.
23. Bortolotti F, Cadrobbi P, Crivellaro C et al. Long-term outcome of chronic type B hepatitis in patients with acquired hepatitis B virus in infection in childhood. Gastroenterology 1990; 99:805-810.
24. Ruiz-Moreno M, García R, Rua MJ et al. Levamisole and interferon in children with chronic hepatitis B. Hepatology 1993; 18:264-269.
25. Fattovich G, Giustina G, Brollo L et al. Therapy for chronic hepatitis B with lymphoblastoid α-interferon and levamisole. Hepatology 1992; 16:1115-1119.
26. Roudot-Thoraval F, Pawlotsky J-M, Thiers V et al. Lack of mother-to-infant transmission of hepatitis C virus in human immunodeficiency virus-seronegative women: A prospective study with hepatitis C virus RNA testing. Hepatology 1993; 17:772-777.
27. Ruiz-Moreno M, Rua MJ, Castillo I et al. Treatment of children with chronic hepatitis C with recombinant α-interferon: A pilot study. Hepatology 1992; 16:882-885.
28. Botarelli P, Brunetto MR, Minutello MA et al. T-lymphocyte response to hepatitis C virus in different clinical courses of infection. Gastroenterology 1993; 104:580-587.
29. Mondelli MU, Cerino A, Boender P et al. Significance of the immune response to a major, conformational B-cell epitope on the hepatitis C virus NS3 region defined by a human monoclonal antibody. J Virol 1994; 68:4829-4836.
30. Lok ASF. Antiviral therapy of the Asian patient with chronic hepatitis B. Semin Liver Dis 1993; 13:360-366.
31. Craxi A, Tine F, Vinci M et al. Transmission of hepatitis B and hepatitis delta viruses in the households of chronic hepatitis B surface antigen carriers: A regression analysis of indicators of risk. Am J Epidemiol 1991; 134:641-650.
32. Lok ASF. Natural history and control of perinatally acquired hepatitis B virus infection. Dig Dis 1992; 10:46-52.
33. Bukh J, Purcell RH, Miller RH. At least 12 genotypes of hepatitis C virus predicted by sequence analysis of the putative E 1 gene of isolates collected worldwide. Proc Natl Acad Sci USA 1993; 90:8234-8238.
34. Govindarajan S, Cassidy WM, Valinluck B, Redeker AG. Interactions of HDV, HBV and HIV in chronic B and D infections and in reactivation of chronic D infection. Prog Clin Biol Res 1991; 364:207-210.
35. Monno L, Angarano G, Santantonio T et al. Lack of HBV and HDV replicative activity in HBsAg-positive intravenous drug addicts with immune deficiency due to HIV. J Med Virol 1991; 34:199-205.
36. Fang JWS, Wright TL, Lau JYN. Fibrosing cholestatic hepatitis in patient with HIV and hepatitis B. Lancet 1993; 342:1175.
37. McDonald JA, Caruso L, Karayannis P, Scylly LJ, Harris JR, Forster GE, Thomas HC. Diminished responsiveness of male homosexuals chronic hepatitis B virus carriers with HTLV-III antibodies to recombinant α-interferon. Hepatology 1987; 7:719-723.
38. Gilson RJC, Hawkins AE, Kelly GK, Gill SK, Weller IVD. No effect of zidovudine on hepatitis B virus replication in homosexual men with symptomatic HIV-1 infection. AIDS 1991; 5:217-220.
39. Hung L-F, Brumbaugh AE, Bhatia G et al. Effects of purine nucleoside analogues with a cyclobutane ring and erythromycin A oxime derivatives on duck hepatitis B virus replication in vivo and in cell culture and HIV-1 in cell culture. J Med Virol 1991; 35:180-186.
40. Beach JW, Jeong LS, Alves AJ et al. Synthesis of enantiomerically pure (2'*R*, 5'*S*)-(–)-1-[2-(hydroxymethyl)-oxathiolan-5-yl]cytosine as a potent antiviral agent against hepatitis B virus (HBV) and human immunodeficiency virus (HIV). J Org Chem 1992; 57:2217-2219.
41. Lin T-S, Luo M-Z, Liu M-C, Balakrishna Pai S, Dutschman GE, Cheng Y-C. Synthesis and biological evaluation of 2', 3'-dideoxy-L-pyrimidine nucleosides as potential antiviral agents against human immunodeficiency virus (HIV) and hepatitis B virus (HBV). J Med Chem 1994; 37:798-803.
42. Lin T-S, Luo M-Z, Liu M-C. A stereospecific synthesis of 2', 3'-dideoxy-β-L-cytidine (β-L-ddC), a potent inhibitor against human hepatitis B virus (HBV) and human immunodeficiency virus (HIV). Tetrahedron Lett 1994; 35:3477-3480.
43. Martin P, Di Bisceglie AM, Kassianides C, Lisker-Melman M, Hoofnagle JH. Rapidly progressive non-A, non-B hepatitis in patients with human immunodeficiency virus infection. Gastroenterology 1989; 97:1559-1561.
44. Telfer P, Sabin C, Devereux H, Scott F, Dusheiko G, Lee C. The progression of HCV-associated liver disease in a cohort of haemophilic patients. Br J Haematol 1994; 87:555-561.
45. Lavine JE, Lake JR, Ascher NL, Ferrell LD, Ganem D, Wright TL. Persistent hepatitis B virus following interferon alfa therapy and liver transplantation. Gastroenterology 1991; 100:263-267.
46. Van Thiel DH, Wright HI, Gavaler JS, Fung J, Starzl TE. Interferon therapy of hepatitis following liver transplantation under FK 506 or cyclosporine. Transplant Proc 1991; 23:3052-3053.
47. Thervet E, Pol S, Legendre C, Gagnadoux M-F, Cavalcanti R, Kreis H. Low-dose recombinant leukocyte interferon-α treatment of hepatitis C viral infection in renal transplant recipients: A pilot study. Transplantation 1994; 58:625-628.
48. Chan T-M, Lok ASF, Cheng IKP, Ng IOL. Chronic hepatitis C after renal transplantation: Treatment with α-interferon. Transplantation 1993; 56:1095-1098.
49. Harihara Y, Kurooka Y, Yanagisawa T, Kuzuhara K, Otsubo O, Kumada H. Interferon therapy in renal allograft recipients with chronic hepatitis C. Transplant Proc 1994; 26:2075.

50. Van Thiel DH, Friedlander L, Fagiuoli S, Wright HI, Irish W, Gavaler JS. Response to α-interferon therapy is influenced by the iron content of the liver. J Hepatol 1994; 20:410-415.
51. Lustbader ED, Hann H-WL, Blumberg BS et al. Serum ferritin as a predictor of the host response to hepatitis B virus infection. Science 1983; 220:423-425.
52. Clemente MG, Congia M, Lai ME et al. Effect of iron overload on the response to recombinant interferon-alfa treatment in transfusion-dependent patients with thalassemia major and chronic hepatitis C. J Pediatr 1994; 125:123-128.
53. Di Marco V, Lo Iacono O, Capra M et al. α-Interferon treatment of chronic hepatitis C in young patients with homozygous β-thalassemia. Haematologica 1992; 77:502-506.
54. Donohue SM, Wonke B, Hoffbrand AV et al. Alpha interferon in the treatment of chronic hepatitis C infection in thalassaemia major. Br J Haematol 1993; 83:491-497.
55. Garson JA, Lenzi M, Ring C et al. Hepatitis C viraemia in adults with type 2 autoinmune hepatitis. J Med Virol 1991; 34:223-226.
56. Magrin S, Craxi A, Fabiano C et al. Hepatitis C virus replication in «autoimmune» chronic hepatitis. J Hepatol 1991; 13:364-367.
57. Miyakawa H, Kako M, Nagai K et al. HCV-RNA in type 2 autoimmune hepatitis. Am J Gastroenterol 1991; 86:1688-1689.
58. Magrin S, Craxi A, Fabiano C et al. Serum hepatitis C virus (HCV)-RNA and response to alpha-interferon in anti-HCV positive chronic hepatitis. J Med Virol 1992; 38:200-206.
59. Mehta SU, Mishiro S, Sekiguchi K et al. Immune response to GOR, a marker for non-A, non-B hepatitis and its correlation with hepatitis C virus infection. J Clin Immunol 1992; 12:178-184.
60. Michel G, Ritter A, Gerken G, Meyer zum Büschenfelde K-H, Decker R, Manns MP. Anti-GOR and hepatitis C virus in autoinmune liver diseases. Lancet 1992; 339:267-269.
61. Abuaf N, Lunel F, Giral P et al. Non-organ specific autoantibodies associated with chronic C virus hepatitis. J Hepatol 1993; 18:359-364.
62. Fried MW, Draguesku JO, Shindo M et al. Clinical and serological differentiation of autoimmune and hepatitis C virus-related chronic hepatitis. Dig Dis Sci 1993; 38:631-636.
63. Seelig R, Renz M, Bünger G, Schröter H, Seelig HP. Anti-LKM-1 antibodies determined by use of recombinant P450 2D6 in ELISA and Western blot and their association with anti-HCV and HCV-RNA. Clin Exp Immunol 1993; 92:373-380.
64. Vergani D, Mieli-Vergani G. Type II autoimmune hepatitis. What is the role of the hepatitis G virus. Gastroenterology 1993; 104:1870-1873.
65. Mackie FD, Peakman M, Yun M et al. Primary and secondary liver/kidney microsomal autoantibody response following infection with hepatitis C virus. Gastroenterology 1994; 106:1672-1675.
66. Michitaka K, Durazzo M, Tillmann HL, Walker D, Philipp T, Manns MP. Analysis of hepatitis C virus genome in patients with autoimmune hepatitis type 2. Gastroenterology 1994; 106:1603-1610.
67. Zhang ZX, Chen M, Wallhagen K et al. Molecular basis for antibody cross-reactivity between the hepatitis C virus core protein and the host-derived GOR protein. Clin Exp Immunol 1994; 96:403-409.
68. Magrin S, Provenzano G, Almasio P, Vaccaro A, Fabiano C, Pinzello GB, Craxi A. Treatment of chronic hepatitis C with features of autoimmunity. Ital J Gastroenterol 1993; 25:458-459.
69. Emile JF, Sebagh M, Féray C, David F, Reynès M. The presence of epithelioid granulomas in hepatitis C virus-related cirrhosis. Hum Pathol 1993; 2:1095-1097.
70. Yamada G, Takahashi M, Endo H et al. Quantitative hepatitis C virus RNA and liver histology in chronic hepatitis C patients treated with interferon alfa. Gut 1993; 34Suppl:S133-S134.
71. Gordon SC, Kodali VP, Silverman AL et al. Levels of hepatitis C virus RNA and liver histology in chronic type C hepatitis. Am J Gastroenterol 1994; 89:1458-1461.
72. Navas S, Castillo I, Bartolomé J, Marriott E, Herrero M, Carreño V. Positive and negative hepatitis C virus RNA strands in serum, liver and peripheral blood mononuclear cells in anti-HCV patients: Relation with the liver lesion. J Hepatol 1994; 21:182-186.
73. Mazzella G, Salzetta A, Casanova S et al. Treatment of chronic sporadic-type non-A, non-B hepatitis with lymphoblastoid interferon: Gamma GT levels predictive for response. Dig Dis Sci 1994; 39:866-870.
74. Battezzati PM, Podda M, Bruno S et al. Factors predicting early response to treatment with recombinant α_{2a}-interferon in chronic non-A, non-B hepatitis. Preliminary report of a long-term trial. Ital J Gastroenterol 1992; 24:481-484.
75. Puoti C, Pannullo A, Annovazzi G, Filippi T, Magrini A. Ursodeoxycholic acid and chronic hepatitis C infection. Lancet 1993; 341:1413-1414.
76. Takano S, Ito Y, Yokosuka O et al. A multicenter randomized controlled dose study of ursodeoxycholic acid for chronic hepatitis C. Hepatology 1994; 20:558-564.
77. Simmonds P, Holmes EC, Cha T-A et al. Classification of hepatitis C virus into six major genotypes and a series of subtypes by phylogenetic analysis of the NS-5 region. J Gen Virol 1993; 74:2391-2399.
78. Simmonds P, Alberti A, Alter HJ et al. A proposed system for the nomenclature of hepatitis C viral genotypes. Hepatology 1994; 19:1321-1324.
79. Okamoto H, Sugiyama Y, Okada S et al. Typing hepatitis C virus by polymerase chain reaction with type-specific primers: Application to clinical surveys and tracing infectious sources. J Gen Virol 1992; 73:673-679.
80. Stuyver L, Rossau R, Wyseur A et al. Typing of hepatitis C virus isolates and characterization of new

subtypes using a line probe assay. J Gen Virol 1993; 74:1093-1102.
81. Ichimura H, Tamura I, Kurimura O et al. Hepatitis C virus genotypes, reactivity to recombinant immunoblot assay 2 antigens and liver disease. J Med Virol 1994; 43:212-215.
82. Pozzato G, Kaneko S, Moretti M et al. Different genotypes of hepatitis C virus are associated with different severity of chronic liver disease. J Med Virol 1994; 43:291-296.
83. Qu D, Li J-S, Vitvitski L et al. Hepatitis C virus genotypes in France: Comparison of clinical features of patients infected with HCV type I and type II. J Hepatol 1994; 21:70-75.
84. Yamada M, Kakumu S, Yoshioka K et al. Hepatitis C virus genotypes are not responsible for development of serious liver disease. Dig Dis Sci 1994; 39:234-239.
85. Dusheiko G, Schmilovitz-Weiss H, Brown D et al. Hepatitis C virus genotypes: An investigation of type-specific differences in geographic origin and disease. Hepatology 1994; 19:13-18.
86. Takada N, Takase S, Takada A, Date T. Differences in the hepatitis C virus genotypes in different countries. J Hepatol 1993; 17:277-283.
87. McOmish F, Yap PL, Dow BC et al. Geographical distribution of hepatitis C virus genotypes in blood donors: An international colllaborative survey. J Clin Microbiol 1994; 32:884-892.
88. Gerolami V, Halfon P, Bourliere M et al. Hepatitis C virus genotypes in chronic hepatitis and response to α-interferon therapy. J Infect Dis 1993; 168:1328-1329.
89. Hino K, Sainokami S, Shimoda K et al. Genotypes and titers of hepatitis C virus for predicting response to interferon in patients with chronic hepatitis C. J Med Virol 1994; 42:299-305.
90. Matsumoto A, Tanaka E, Suzuki T, Ogata H, Kiyosawa K. Viral and host factors that contribute to efficacy of α_{2a}-interferon therapy in patients with chronic hepatitis C. Dig Dis Sci 1994; 39:1273-1280.
91. Mita E, Hayashi N, Hagiwara H et al. Predicting interferon therapy efficacy from hepatitis C virus genotype and RNA titer. Dig Dis Sci 1994; 39:977-982.
92. Orito E, Mizokami M, Mizoguchi N et al. Hepatitis C virus serotype II responds more favorably to α-interferon therapy. J Hepatol 1994; 21:130-132.
93. Qu D, Li J-S, Vitvitski L et al. Hepatitis C virus genotypes in France: Comparison of clinical features of patients infected with HCV type I and type II. J Hepatol 1994; 21:70-75.
94. Yamada M, Kakumu S, Yoshioka K et al. Hepatitis C virus genotypes are not responsible for development of serious liver disease. Dig Dis Sci 1994; 39:234-239.
95. Magrin S, Craxi A, Fabiano C et al. HCV viraemia, viral genotypes and response to IFN in patients with chronic hepatitis C from Sicily. J Hepatol 1994; 21:S24.
96. Chirara MM, Chetsanga CJ. Variant or hepatitis B virus isolated in Zimbabwe. J Med Virol 1994; 42:73-78.
97. Crowe JS, Gewert DR, Barber KA et al. α_2-Interferon (IFN) genotype analysis of Chinese chronic hepatitis B patients undergoing recombinant α_{2a}-IFN therapy. J Infect Dis 1994; 169:875-878.
98. Norder H, Couroucé A-M, Magnius LO. Complete genomes, phylogenetic relatedness, and structural proteins of six strains of the hepatitis B virus, four of which represent two new genotypes. Virology 1994; 198:489-503.
99. Shrestha SM, Tsuda F, Okamoto H et al. Hepatitis B virus subtypes and hepatitis C virus genotypes in patients with chronic liver disease in Nepal. Hepatology 1994; 19:805-809.
100. Lauder LJ, Lin H-J, Lau JYN, Siu T-S, Lai C-L. The variability of the hepatitis B virus genome: Statistical analysis and biological implications. Mol Biol Evol 1993; 10:457-470.
101. Uy A, Wunderlich G, Olsen DB, Heermann K-H, Gerlich WH, Thomssen R. Genomic variability in the pre-S1 region and determination of routes of transmission of hepatitis B virus. J Gen Virol 1992; 73:3005-3009.
102. Fiordalisi G, Cariani E, Mantero G et al. High genomic variability in the pre-C region of hepatitis B virus in anti-HBe, HBV DNA-positive chronic hepatitis. J Med Virol 1990; 31:297-300.
103. Crawford DH. Hepatitis B virus «escape» mutants. Br Med J 1990; 301:1058-1059.
104. Blum HE, Galun E, Liang TJ, Von Weizsäcker F, Wands, JR. Naturally occurring missence mutation in the polymerase gene terminating hepatitis B virus replication. J Virol 1991; 65:1836-1842.
105. Cuthbert JA. Southwestern Internal Medicine Conference: Hepatitis B –Molecular variants with clinical significance. Am J Med Sci 1991; 302:396-403.
106. Faruqi AF, Roychodhury S, Greenberg R, Israel J, Shih C. Replication-defective missence mutations within the terminal protein and spacer/intron regions of the polymerase gene of human hepatitis B virus. Virology 1991; 183:764-768.
107. Foster GR, Carman WF, Thomas HC. Replication of hepatitis B and delta viruses: Appearance of viral mutants. Semin Liver Dis 1991; 11:121-127.
108. Lai ME, Melis A, Mazzoleni AP, Farci P, Balestrieri A. Sequence analysis of hepatitis B virus genome of a new mutant of ayw subtype isolated in Sardinia. Nucleic Acids Res 1991; 19:5078.
109. Lee H-S, Ulrich PP, Vyas GN. Mutations in the S-gene affecting the immunologic determinants of the envelope protein of hepatitis B virus. J Hepatol 1991; 13(Suppl4):S97-S101.
110. Moriyama K, Nakajima E, Hohjoh H, Asayama R, Okochi K. Immunoselected hepatitis B virus mutant. Lancet 1991; 337:125.
111. Omata M, Ehata T, Yokosuka O, Hosoda K, Ohto M. Mutations in the precore region of hepatitis B virus DNA in patients with fulminant and severe hepatitis. N Engl J Med 1991; 324:1699-1704.
112. Roychoudhury S, Faruqi AF, Shih C. Pregemonic RNA

encapsidation analysis of eleven missense and nonsense polymerase mutants of human hepatitis B virus. J Virol 1991; 65:3617-3624.
113. Wang Y-J, Lee S-D, Wu J-C, Lo K-J. Acute hepatitis B viral infection in a patient with anti-HBs. J Med Virol 1991; 35:133-135.
114. Chen Y, Robinson WS, Marion PL. Naturally occurring point mutation in the C terminus of the polymerase gene prevents duck hepatitis B virus RNA packaging. J Virol 1992; 66:1282-1287.
115. Condreay LD, Wu T-T, Aldrich CE et al. Replication of DHBV genomes with mutations at the sites of initiation of minus- and plus-strand DNA synthesis. Virology 1992; 188:208-216.
116. Ehata T, Omata M, Yokosuka O, Hosoda K, Ohto M. Variations in codons 84-101 in the core nucleotide sequence correlate with hepatocellular injury in chronic hepatitis B virus infection. J Clin Invest 1992; 89:332-338.
117. Waters JA, Kennedy M, Voet P et al. Loss of the common «A» determinant of hepatitis B surface antigen by a vaccine-induced escape mutant. J Clin Invest 1992; 90:2543-2547.
118. Blum HE. Hepatitis B virus: Significance of naturally occurring mutants. Intervirology 1993; 35:40-50.
119. Foster GR, Thomas HC. Recent advances in the molecular biology of hepatitis B virus: Mutant virus and the host response. Gut 1993; 34:1-3.
120. Antoni BA, Rodríguez-Crespo I, Gómez-Gutiérrez J, Nieto M, Peterson D, Gavilanes F. Site-directed mutagenesis of cysteine residues of hepatitis B surface antigen –Analysis of two single mutants and the double mutant. Eur J Biochem 1994; 222:121-127.
121. Lau JYN, Wright TL. Emerging viral mutants in hepatitis B, reply. Lancet 1994; 343:355-356.
122. Melegari M, Bruno S, Wands JR. Properties of hepatitis B virus pre-S1 deletion mutants. Virology 1994; 199:292-300.
123. Petit M-A, Zoulim F, Berthillon P et al. PreS1 antigen/antibody patterns following interferon therapy in acute and chronic hepatitis B. J Hepatol 1994; 20:47-56.
124. Schödel F. Emerging viral mutants in hepatitis B. Lancet 1994; 343:355.
125. Uchida T, Aye TT, Shikata T et al. Evolution of the hepatitis B virus gene during chronic infection in seven patients. J Med Virol 1994; 43:148-154.
126. Uchida T, Shimojima M, Gotoh K, Shikata T, Tanaka E, Kiyosawa K. «Silent» hepatitis B virus mutants are responsible for non-A, non-B, non-C, non-D, non-E hepatitis. Microbiol Immunol 1994; 38:281-285.
127. Yamamoto K, Horikita M, Tsuda F et al. Naturally occurring escape mutants of hepatitis B virus with various mutations in the S gene in carriers seropositive for antibody to hepatitis B surface antigen. J Virol 1994; 68:2671-2676.
128. Zuckerman AJ, Harrison TJ, Oon C-J. Mutations in S region of hepatitis B virus. Lancet 1994; 343:737-738.
129. Ogata N, Alter HJ, Miller RH, Purcell RH. Nucleotide sequence and mutation rate of the H strain of hepatitis C virus. Proc Natl Acad Sci USA 1991; 88:3392-3396.
130. Murakawa K, Esumi M, Kato T, Kambara H, Shikata T. Heterogenity within the nonstructural protein 5-encoding region of hepatitis C viruses from a single patient. Gene 1992; 117:229-232.
131. Müller HM, Pfaff E, Goeser T, Theilmann L. Genetic variability of German hepatitis C virus isolates. J Med Virol 1993; 40:291-306.
132. Tanaka T, Kato N, Hijikata M, Shimotohno K. Base transitions and base transversions seen in mutations among various types of the hepatitis C viral genome. FEBS Lett 1993; 315:201-203.
133. Finkelstein SD, Sayegh R, Uchman S, Christensen S, Swalski PA, Bodenheimer H. Disease activity of hepatitis C correlates with single-stage polymerase chain reaction detection of hepatitis C virus. Am J Clin Pathol 1994; 101:321-326.
134. Komoda Y, Hijikata M, Tanji Y et al. Processing of hepatitis C viral polyprotein in *Escherichia coli*. Gene 1994; 145:221-226.
135. Shimizu YK, Hijikata M, Iwamoto A, Alter HJ, Purcell RH, Yoshikura H. Neutralizing antibodies against hepatitis C virus and the emergence of neutralization escape mutant viruses. J Virol 1994; 68:1494-1500.
136. Bonino F, Brunetto MR, Rizzetto M, Will H. Hepatitis B virus unable to secrete e antigen. Gastroenterology 1991; 100:1138-1141.
137. Akahane Y, Yamanaka T, Suzuki H et al. Chronic active hepatitis with hepatitis B virus DNA and antibody against e antigen in the serum. Disturbed synthesis and secretion of e antigen from hepatocytes due to a point mutation in the precore region. Gastroenterology 1990; 99:1113-1119.
138. Raimondo G, Stemler M, Schneider R, Wildner G, Squadrito G, Will H. Latency and reactivation of a precore mutant hepatitis B virus in a chronically infected patients. J Hepatol 1990; 11:374-380.
139. Ulrich PP, Bhat RA, Kelly I, Brunetto MR, Bonino F, Vyas GN. A precore-defective mutant of hepatitis B virus associated with e antigen-negative chronic liver disease. J Med Virol 1990; 32:109-118.
140. Lyra L, Parana R, Cotrim H. Knowledge of the precore mutation variant of the hepatitis B virus. Am J Gastroenterol 1991; 86:1851-1852.
141. Santantonio T, Jung M-C, Schneider R, Pastore G, Pape GR, Will H. Selection for a pre-C stop codon mutation in a hepatitis B virus variant with a pre-C initiation codon mutation during interferon treatment. J Hepatol 1991; 13:368-371.
142. Santantonio T, Jung M-C, Miska S, Pastore G, Pape GR, Will H. Prevalence and type of pre-C HBV mutants in anti-HBe positive carriers with chronic liver disease in a highly endemic area. Virology 1991; 183:840-844.
143. Tong S, Diot C, Gripon P et al. *In vitro* replication competence of a cloned hepatitis B virus variant with a nonsense mutation in the distal pre-C region. Virology 1991; 181:733-737.

144. Tur-Kaspa R, Klein A, Aharonson S. Hepatitis B virus precore mutants are identical in carriers from various ethnic origins and are associated with a range of liver disease severity. Hepatology 1992; 16:1338-1342.
145. Benjelloun S, Tong S, Li J, Menfalout L, Trépo C, Benslimane A. Pre-core mutation associated with lack of hepatitis B e antigenaemia in Moroccan asymptomatic carriers of the virus. Res Virol 1993; 144:159-167.
146. Bortolotti F, Crivellaro C, Brunetto MR, Cadrobbi P, Bertolini A, Alberti A. Selection of a precore mutant of hepatitis B virus and reactivation of chronic hepatitis B acquired in childhood. J Pediatr 1993; 123: 583-585.
147. Chuang W-L, Omata M, Ehata T, Yokosuka O, Ohto M. Concentrating missence mutations in core gene of hepatitis B virus: Evidence for adaptive mutation in chronic hepatitis B virus infection. Dig Dis Sci 1993; 38:594-600.
148. Chuang W-L, Omata M, Ehata T et al. Precore mutations and core clustering mutations in chronic hepatitis B virus infection. Gastroenterology 1993; 104:263-271.
149. Ehata T, Omata M, Chuang W-L et al. Mutations in core nucleotide sequence of hepatitis B virus correlate with fulminant and severe hepatitis. J Clin Invest 1993; 91:1206-1213.
150. Féray C, Gigou M, Samuel D, Bernuau J, Bismuth H, Bréchot C. Low prevalence of precore mutations in hepatitis B virus DNA in fulminant hepatitis type B in France. J Hepatol 1993; 18:119-122.
151. Gramegna M, Lampertico P, Lobbiani A, Colucci G. Detection of the hepatitis B virus major pre-core mutation by the amplification refractory mutation system technique. Res Virol 1993; 144:307-309.
152. Li J-S, Tong S-P, Wen Y-M, Vitvitski L, Zhang Q, Trépo C. Hepatitis B virus genotype A rarely circulates as an HBe-minus mutant: Possible contribution of a single nucleotide in the precore region. J Virol 1993; 67:5402-5410.
153. Manzin A, Paolucci S, Lampertico P et al. Direct detection of HBV preC mutants in heterogeneous viral populations by a modified DNA sequencing method. Res Virol 1993; 144:303-306.
154. Ogata N, Miller RH, Ishak KG, Purcell RH. The complete nucleotide sequence of a pre-core mutant of hepatitis B virus implicated in fulminant hepatitis and its biological characterization in chimpanzees. Virology 1993; 194:263-276.
155. Seifer M, Standring DN. Stability governs the apparent expression of «particulate» hepatitis B e antigen by mutant hepatitis B virus core particles. Virology 1993; 196:70-78.
156. Tong S-P, Li J-S, Vitviski L, Kay A, Trépol C. Evidence for a base-paired region of hepatitis B virus pregenome encapsidation signal which influences the patterns of precore mutations abolishing HBe protein expression. J Virol 1993; 67:5651-5655.
157. Uchida T, Aye TT, Becker SO et al. Detection of precore/core-mutant hepatitis B virus genome in patients with acute or fulminant hepatitis without serological markers for recent HBV infection. J Hepatol 1993; 18:368-372.
158. Wen Y-M. Hepatitis B virus precore and core gene mutations in chronic hepatitis B and hepatocelular carcinoma patients. J Intern Med 1993; 234:441-445.
159. Akarca US, Greene S, Lok ASF. Detection of precore hepatitis B virus mutants in asymptomatic HBsAg-positive family members. Hepatology 1994; 19:1366-1370.
160. Aye TT, Uchida T, Becker SO et al. Variations of hepatitis B virus precore/core gene sequence in acute and fulminant hepatitis B. Dig Dis Sci 1994; 39:1281-1287.
161. Barbera C, Calvo P, Coscia A et al. Precore mutant hepatitis B virus and outcome of chronic infection and hepatitis in hepatitis B e antigen-positive children. Pediatr Res 1994; 36:347-350.
162. Goergen B, Meyer zum Büschenfelde K-H, Gerken G. Mutation specific PCR and direct solid phase sequencing assay for the detection of hepatitis B virus pre-C/C mutants in anti-HBe-positive, chronic hepatitis B. J Med Virol 1994; 43:97-102.
163. Hamasaki K, Nakata K, Nagayama Y et al. Changes in the prevalence of HBeAg-negative mutant hepatitis B virus during the course of chronic hepatitis B. Hepatology 1994; 20:8-14.
164. Hawkings AE, Gilson RJC, Bickerton EA, Tedder RS, Weller IVD. Conservation of precore and core sequences of hepatitis B virus in chronic viral carriers. J Med Virol 1994; 43:5-12.
165. Hawkins AE, Gilson RJC, Beath SV et al. Novel application of a point mutation assay: Evidence for transmision of hepatitis B viruses with precore mutations and their detection in infants with fulminant hepatitis B. J Med Virol 1994; 44:13-21.
166. Kim SK, Jang SK, Rho HM. Effect of frameshift mutation in the pre-C region of hepatitis B virus on the X and C genes. J Gen Virol 1944; 75:917-923.
167. Lai ME, Solinas A, Mazzoleni AP et al. The role of precore hepatitis B virus mutants on the long-term outcome of chronic hepatitis B virus hepatitis. A longitudinal study. J Hepatol 1994; 20:773-781.
168. Laskus T, Rakela J, Tong MJ, Nowicki MJ, Mosley JW, Persing DH. Naturally occurring hepatitis B virus mutants with deletions in the core promoter region. J Hepatol 1994; 20:837-841.
169. Lee J-H, Di Bisceglie AM, Baker BL, Zeldis JB. The development of a mutation in the precore region of the hepatitis B virus in a chronically infected individual. Gastroenterology 1994; 106:243-247.
170. Lok ASF, Akarca U, Greene S. Mutations in the precore region of hepatitis B virus serve to enhance the stability of the secondary structure of the pre-genome encapsidation signal. Proc Natl Acad Sci USA 1994; 91:4077-4081.
171. McIvor C, Morton J, Bryant A, Cooksley WG, Durrant S, Walker N. Fatal reactivation of precore mutant hepatitis B virus associated with fibrosing cholestatic after bone marrow transplantation. Ann Intern Med 1994; 121:274-275.

172. Xu J, Brown D, Harrison T, Lin Y, Dusheiko G. Abscence of hepatitis B virus precore mutants in patients with chronic hepatitis B responding to α-interferon. Hepatology 1992; 15:1002-1006.
173. Pastore G, Santantonio T, Milella M et al. Anti-HBe-positive chronic hepatitis B with HBV-DNA in the serum response to a 6-month course of lymphoblastoid interferon. J Hepatol 1992; 14:221-225.
174. Hadziyannis S, Bramou T, Makris A, Moussoulis G, Zignego L, Papaioannou C. Interferon alfa-2b treatment of HBeAg negative/serum HBV DNA positive chronic active hepatitis type B. J Hepatol 1990; 11(Suppl1):S133-S136.
175. Brunetto MR, Oliveri F, Demartini A et al. Treatment with interferon of chronic hepatitis B associated with antibody to hepatitis B e antigen. J Hepatol 1991; 13(Suppl1):S8-S11.
176. Brunetto MR, Giarin M, Saracco G et al. Hepatitis B virus unable to secrete e antigen and response to interferon in chronic hepatitis B. Gastroenterology 1993; 105:845-850.
177. Fattovich G, Farci P, Rugge M et al. A randomized controlled trial of lymphoblastoid α-interferon in patients with chronic hepatitis B lacking HBeAg. Hepatology 1992; 15:584-589.
178. Alberti A, Fattovich G. Interferon therapy for the anti-HBe positive form of chronic hepatitis B. Antiviral Res 1994; 24:145-153.
179. Kanazawa Y, Hayashi N, Mita E et al. Influence of viral quasispecies on effectiveness of interferon therapy hepatitis C patients. Hepatology 1994; 20:1121-1130.
180. Honda M, Kaneko S, Sakai A, Unoura M, Murakami S, Kobayashi K. Degree of diversity of hepatitis C virus quasispecies and progression of liver disease. Hepatology 1994; 20:1144-1151.
181. Martin P. Hepatitis C infection in patients with chronic hepatitis B: Curiosity or co-factor. Am J Gastroenterol 1994; 89:1139-1141.
182. Villa E, Grottola A, Trande P et al. Reactivation of hepatitis B virus infection induced by interferon (IFN) in HBsAg-positive, antiHCV-positive patients. Lancet 1993; 341:1413.
183. Reichard O, Foberg U, Fryden A et al. High sustained response rate and clearance of viremia in chronic hepatitis C after treatment with interferon alpha-2b for 60 weeks. Hepatology 1994; 19:280-285.
184. Craxi A, Di Marco V, Lo Iacono O et al. Lymphoblastoid α-interferon for post-transfusion chronic hepatitis C: a randomized trial of 6 vs. 12 months treatment. J Hepatol 1992; 16:S8.
185. Craxi A, Lo Iacono O, Di Marco V et al. Community-acquired chronic hepatitis C in an area of high serotype 1 endemicity: interferon for 6 or 12 months? Hepatology 1994; 20:162A.
186. Negro F, Baldi M, Mondardini A et al. Continuous versus intermitent therapy for chronic hepatitis C with recombinant interferon alfa-2a. Gastroenterology 1994; 107:479-485.
187. Bosch O, Tapia L, Quiroga JA, Carreño V. An escalating dose regimen of combinant interferon-alpha 2A in the treatment of chronic hepatitis C. J Hepatol 1993; 17:146-149.
188. Kagawa T, Morizane T, Saito H et al. A randomized, controlled trial of weekly administration of lymphoblastoid interferon in patients with chronic hepatitis C. J Hepatol 1993; 17:91-96.
189. Gómez-Rubio M, Porres JC, Castillo I et al. Prolonged treatment (18 months) of chronic hepatitis C with recombinant alpha-interpheron with a control group. J Hepatol 1990; 11:S63-S67.
190. Picciotto A, Varagona G, Valle F et al. Interferon therapy in chronic hepatitis C. Evaluation of low dose maintenance schedule in responder patients. J Hepatol 1993; 17:359-363.
191. Davis GL, Balart LA, Schiff ER et al. Treatment of chronic hepatitis C with recombinant interferon alpha. A multicenter randomized controlled trial. N Engl J Med 1989; 321:1501-1506.
192. Diodati G, Bonetti P, Noventa F et al. Treatment of chronic hepatitis C with recombinant human alpha-2a: result of a randomized controlled clinical trial. Hepatology 1994; 19:1-5.
193. Almasio P, Craxi A, Di Marco V et al. Dose-effect relationship for α-interferon in hepatitis C. Hepatology 1994; 20:155A.
194. Milella M, Santantonio T, Monno L et al. Human leukocyte alpha interferon in the treatment of chronic hepatitis C. Medit J Inf Parasit Dis 1993; 7:20.
195. Pastore G, Milella M, Monno L et al. Biochemical, virological and histological response to long-term treatment with rIFNa2a in chronic hepatitis C. Ital J Gastroenterol 1992; 24:296.
196. Marcellin P, Boyer N, Giostra E et al. Recombinant human alpha interferon in patients chronic non-A non-B hepatitis: a multicenter randomized controlled trial from France. Hepatology 1991; 13:393-397.
197. Rumi MG, Romeo R, Parravicini ML et al. Randomized comparative study of recombinant alpha and lymphoblastoid interferon in patients with chronic active hepatitis C. J Hepatol 1994; 18:S27.
198. Kagawa T, Morizane T, Saito H et al. A pilot study of long-term weekly interferon beta administration for chronic hepatitis B. Am J Gastroenterol 1993; 88:212-216.
199. Kobayashi Y, Watanabe S, Konishi M et al. Quantitation and typing of serum Hepatitis C virus RNA in patients with chronic hepatitis C treated with interferon beta. Hepatology 1993; 18:1319-1325.
200. Kakamu S, Yoshioka K, Wakita T et al. Pilot study of Ribavirin and Interferon beta for chronic hepatitis B. Hepatology 1993; 18:258-263.
201. Kobayashi H, Komita T, Hakozaki M et al. Circulating interferon in cancer patients after administration of human fibroblast interferon by different routes. Jpn J Cancer Chemoter 1980; 7:614-20.
203. Villa E, Trande P, Grottola A, Manenti F. Alpha, but not Beta interferon is useful in non-A, non-B chronic active hepatitis: final report of a comparative prospective randomized study. J Hepatol 1993; 18:S186.
204. Craxi A, Di Marco V, Volpes R, Palazzo U. Anti-α in-

terferon antibodies after α-interferon treatment in patients with chronic viral hepatitis. Hepato-gastroenterology 1988; 35:304-305.

205. Porres JC, Carreno V, Ruiz M et al. Interferon antibodies in patients with chronic HBV infection treated with recombinant interferon. J Hepatol 1989; 8; 341-357.

206. Lok A S-F, Lai C-L, Leung E K-Y. Interferon antibodies may negate the antiviral effects of recombinant α-interferon treatment in patients with chronic hepatitis B virus infection. Hepatology 1990; 12; 1266-1270.

207. Antonelli G, Currenti M, Turriziani O, Dianzani F. Neutralizing antibodies to interferon-a: relative frequency in patients with different interferon preparations. J Infect Dis 1991; 163:882-885.

208. Hennes U, Jucker W, Fisher EA et al. The detection of antibodies to recombinant alpha-2a interferon in human serum. J Biol Stantard 1987; 15:231-244.

209. Bonetti P, Diodati G, Drago et al. Interferon antibodies in patients with chronic hepatitis C virus infection treated with recombinant alpha-2a interferon. J Hepatol 1994; 20:416-420.

210. Bonetti P, Diodati G, Drago C et al. Anti-interferon antibodies during interferon therapy for chronic hepatitis C. J Hepatol 1994; 20:315-321.

211. Milella M, Antonelli G, Santantonio T et al. Neutralizing antibodies to recombinant alpha-interferon and response to therapy in chronic hepatitis C virus infection. Liver 1993; 13:146-150.

212. Aguet M. High affinity binding of 125-I labeled mouse IFN to a specific cell surface receptors. Nature 1980; 284:459.

213. Langer J, Pestka S. IFN receptors. Immunol Today 1990; 9:393.

214. Pfeffer LM. Mechanisms of IFN action. Boca Raton: CRC Press, 1987.

215. Nakajima S, Kuroki T, Shintani M et al. Changes in interferon receptors on peripheral blood mononuclear cells from patients with chronic hepatitis B being treated with interferon. Hepatology 1990; 12:1261-1265.

216. Lau JYN, Sheron N, Morris AG, Bomford AB, Alexander GJM, Williams R. α-Interferon receptor expression and regulation in chronic hepatitis B virus infection. Hepatology 1991; 13:332-338.

Interferon Therapy for Atypical or Unusual Patients with Chronic Viral Hepatitis

J. M. Geders, A. S. F. Lok

Clinical trials on interferon therapy in chronic hepatitis B virus (HBV) and hepatitis C virus (HCV) infection have focused on a subset of patients that fulfill strict inclusion and exclusion criteria. Data on the safety and efficacy of α-interferon therapy in patients who do not meet these criteria are limited. This article reviews our current knowledge on the role of α-interferon therapy in patients with atypical clinical or serological picture and in patients with significant concurrent medical illnesses.

CHRONIC HBV INFECTION

Oriental Patients

Constitute 80% of patients with chronic HBV infection on a world wide basis. Thus, the practical value of any form of treatment for chronic hepatitis B depends on its efficacy in Oriental patients. In an initial study, Oriental patients were reported to respond poorly to α-interferon therapy. In this randomized controlled trial, 72 Chinese adults were randomized to receive no treatment or α2a-interferon in doses of 2.5, 5, or 10 MU/m^2 given intra-muscularly thrice weekly for 12 to 24 weeks (1). Only 8 (15%) of 54 treated patients and none of the 18 controls had sustained clearance of hepatitis B e antigen (HBeAg). None of the patients lost hepatitis B surface antigen (HBsAg).

Several factors may contribute to the poor response in this trial. At least 50% of Chinese HBV carriers are believed to be infected perinatally. Delay in treatment until adulthood may have permitted integration of HBV DNA into the host genome, thus making eradication of HBV difficult. Against this hypothesis were findings from Southern blot hybridization analysis of the pre-treatment liver biospies, which failed to demonstrate integration of HBV DNA. Alternatively, the poor response may be related to the high proportion (44%) of patients who had normal pre-treatment serum aminotransferase (ALT) levels. The natural course of perinatally acquired HBV infection has an additional initial phase of immune tolerance in which liver disease is inactive despite active virus replication, patients in this phase may be more resistant to treatment. Another factor that may have contributed to the poor long-term response in this trial was the high frequency (47%) of reactivation, possibly secondary to a high incidence (39%) of interferon neutralizing antibodies (2).

The marked difference in response between patients in the immune tolerant and immune clearance phase was clearly demonstrated in a recently reported randomized controlled trial in which 115 Chinese adults with elevated ALT levels were separately randomized from those with normal ALT levels to receive: *a*) prednisone priming followed by α-interferon for 16 weeks, *b*) α-interferon alone, or *c*) no treatment (3). Fifteen (39%) of 39 treated patients who had elevated ALT levels cleared HBeAg, compared with 2 (5%) of 38 patients who had normal ALT levels, $p < 0.0005$. The spontaneous HBe seroconversion rate was also higher among the patients with elevated ALT levels: 3 (19%) of 16 compared with none of 20 with normal ALT levels, but the difference was not statistically significant, p = 0.16. Among the interferon treated patients, prednisone priming did not improve the overall response rate: 23% vs. 21%. This study confirmed previous findings that Oriental patients with normal pre-treatment serum ALT levels respond poorly to interferon therapy. However, the response was significantly better in patients with elevated ALT levels and comparable to that in Caucasian patients. These data suggest that the difference in response to interferon therapy between Oriental and Caucasian patients is not related to genetic differences. Prednisone priming has been used to induce rebound in immune function and to improve the response to subsequent treatment with α-interferon. The overall results in European and American studies showed that prednisone priming has no additional benefit over interferon alone (4, 5). The results of prednisone priming in Oriental adults is conflicting (3, 6). Thus, the role of prednisone priming remains to be confirmed.

A recent report showed that 65% of American patients who had sustained loss of HBeAg after interferon therapy lost HBsAg during a mean follow-up period of 4.3 years (7). However, none of 128 Chinese adults who responded to interferon therapy with loss of HBeAg lost HBsAg during a similar period of follow-up (8). The exact reason(s) for the difference is unclear but may be related to a longer duration of infection, re-infection, or inability of the immune system to completely eliminate the virus even after the virus load has been reduced in the Chinese patients.

Children

Ideally, treatment should be instituted as early as possible before there is significant irreversible liver damage. Studies in Caucasian adults showed that patients with a shorter duration of infection are more likely to respond to α-interferon therapy. A better antiviral response may be achieved in Oriental patients by initiating treatment at an earlier age. Results from randomized controlled trials of α-interferon therapy with or without prednisone priming in Chinese children were however, disappointing (table 1) (9, 10). In the initial study, 24 Chinese children, age 1.5 to 5 years, were randomized to receive α2a-interferon in doses of 10 MU/m^2 thrice weekly for 12 weeks or placebo (9). All the children were asymptomatic, only two had elevated ALT levels. All 24 children remained HBeAg positive at 12 months. Thus, the antiviral response to α-interferon alone was poor in Oriental patients even when treatment was initiated within 5 years of infection. This poor response could not be attributed to an inadequate dose or duration of treatment since similar dose regimen has been used in Caucasian adults and children with greater success.

To determine if rebound recovery in immune response following abrupt steroid withdrawal can overcome immune tolerance in Oriental children, 90 asymptomatic Chinese children, age 2 to 17 years, were randomized to receive: *a*) prednisone priming followed by a2b-interferon in doses of 5 MU/m^2 for 16 weeks, *b*) α2b-interferon alone, or *c*) no treatment (10). All except 8 children had normal ALT levels at entry. A higher proportion of children who received interferon after prednisone priming cleared HBeAg: 4 (13%) of 31 vs. 1 (3%) of 29 who received interferon only, but the response was still far from satisfactory (table 1). None of the control children lost HBeAg. In contrast, the response in European children all of whom had elevated ALT levels were similar to that in adults (table 1) (11-13). The higher response and the more active liver disease in European children are probably related to the difference in age at infection, with most European children being infected during childhood rather than perinatally.

Patients with Pre-Core Mutations

Most anti-HBe positive patients have inactive liver disease and no evidence of HBV replication, and will not benefit from interferon therapy. However, a small proportion, with mutations in the pre-core region of HBV that prevent the secretion of HBeAg, continue to have active liver disease and are positive for HBV DNA in serum. The predominant mutation in these patients is a G to A change at nucleotide 1896, cre-

Table 1. Antiviral response to α-interferon therapy in children with chronic HBV infection

Author	Dose (MU/m² tiw)	Duration (wk)	Age (yr)	ALT (IU/l)	N. of patients	N. lost (%)	
						HBeAg	HBsAg
Lai, 1987	10	12	3.5	12	12	0 (0)	0 (0)
(9)	–	–	3.5	13	12	0 (0)	0 (0)
Lai, 1991	Pred. + 5	16	6	14	31	4 (13)	0 (0)
(10)	5	16	6.5	12	29	1 (3)	0 (0)
	–	–	6	9	30	0 (0)	0 (0)
Ruiz–Moreno,	10	24	8.7	147	12	7 (58)	0 (0)
1991 (11)	5	24	7.3	138	12	5 (42)	0 (0)
	–	–	8.5	115	12	2 (17)	0 (0)
Sokal, 1993	9	16	8.3	113	29	11 (38)	2 (7)
(12)	–	–	8.7	58	25	2 (8)	0 (0)
Utili, 1994	Pred. + 3	52	12	100	22	9 (41)	2 (9)
(13)	–	–	12	102	21	2 (9.5)	0 (0)

ating a stop codon in codon 28 (14). Interferon therapy can suppress HBV replication and induce remission of liver disease in these patients, but the relapse rate is high (15-17). Pre-core stop codon mutations can also be detected in HBeAg positive patients, its presence being predictive of imminent HBeAg clearance.

In a retrospective analysis on pre-core HBV sequence in Italian patients who received α-interferon therapy (18), the authors concluded that response to α-interferon was impaired when pre-core stop codon mutant reaches significant levels. However, a larger scale study on 106 HBeAg positive Chinese patients found that patients with the stop codon mutation were significantly more likely to respond than those with wild type sequence: 55% vs. 17% ($p = 0.02$) (19). The patients with the stop codon mutation were also more likely to have elevated ALT levels: 86% vs. 46% of those with wild type sequence ($p = 0.01$). Thus, the association between pre-core stop codon mutation and response to interferon therapy may be indirect.

Cirrhotic Patients

HBV replication is usually quiescent by the time patients develop end stage cirrhosis, so interferon is of no benefit to these patients. Rarely, patients with established cirrhosis continue to have replicative infection. In a retrospective analysis of 18 patients who received α-interferon in doses of 2 MU tiw to 5 MU daily for a mean of 12 weeks, 6 (33%) patients responded and had marked clinical improvement, 4 subsequently lost HBsAg (20). Among the 12 non-responders, 6 died and 4 required liver transplantation. Thus, interferon therapy can inhibit HBV replication with improvement in liver disease even in patients with established cirrhosis. However, there is a high risk of precipitating liver failure and infectious complications. Nine (50%) patients in that study developed significant side effects that required premature termination of treatment. Similar findings have been reported in a US multi-center trial. α-interferon may have a role in the treatment of patients with established cirrhosis who continue to have replicative infection, but these patients should only be treated in specialized centers with very careful monitoring and the back up of liver transplantation, and the starting dose of interferon should be very low: 0.5-1 MU tiw.

CHRONIC HCV INFECTION

Serologic tests for HCV infection are limited. Tests for HCV antigen and IgM HCV antibody (IgM anti-HCV) are not yet available.Most tests for serum HCV RNA are poorly standardized and at best semi-quantitative. The branched chain DNA assay is currently the most reliable test for quantitation of serum HCV RNA level, but it is expensive and less sensitive than polymerase chain reaction (PCR) assays. Thus, it is difficult to define «atypical» serology in patients with chronic HCV infection.

Hepatitis C «Carriers» with Normal ALT Levels

These subjects may have: *a*) falsely positive hepatitis C antibody (anti-HCV) test result, *b*) recovery from HCV infection, *c*) chronic hepatitis C with fluctuating ALT levels, or *d*) «carrier» state with normal ALT levels, intermittent or persistent viremia, and liver histology ranging from non-specific hepatitis to chronic hepatitis and cirrhosis (21). The role of interferon therapy in the last category of patients is hotly debated. The arguments for treatment include: histologic finding of significant liver disease in some patients and possibility of progression to more severe liver disease in others, potential for higher response rate since «carriers» may be younger, have lower serum HCV RNA level, and are less likely to have cirrhosis. However, the risks and rate of progression of liver disease in these subjects is unknown, the potential for higher response is purely speculative, interferon treatment is expensive and not completely free of side effects, the long-term benefit of interferon treatment even in successful responders is uncertain, and the only way to monitor response in these subjects is to perform serial tests for serum HCV RNA level, which would further increase the expense of treatment. Clearly, randomized controlled trials to determine the short- and long- term efficacy of interferon therapy in «carriers» are needed. In addition, the natural history of HCV infection has to be better defined before recommendation on treatment of «carriers» can be made.

Patients with Concurrent Human Immunodeficiency Virus (HIV) Infection

A significant proportion of patients with HCV infection (intravenous drug users and hemophiliacs) have concurrent HIV infection. These patients tend to have higher serum HCV RNA levels, possibly related to HIV-induced immunosuppression (22). This is supported by a recent report in which significantly higher serum HCV RNA levels were found only in HIV positive patients with reduced CD4 counts (23). Some studies also found that concurrent HIV infection accelerates the progression of HCV-induced chronic liver disease (24).

Several small-scale studies have shown that patients with concurrent HCV and HIV infection have similar response rates to interferon therapy as HIV negative patients. In general, the initial response and relapse rates did not seem to correlate with the stage of HIV infection or baseline CD4 counts. However, the majority of the patients treated had no or early clinical manifestations of acquired immunodeficiency syndrome, and CD4 counts >300/mm^3. In addition, an HIV negative control group was seldom included. Interpretation of the results of many of these studies were further complicated by the concomitant use of zidovudine (AZT) although there is no data to suggest that AZT has any effect on HCV replication or HCV-induced liver disease. The details of two studies that have been published are shown in table 2 (25, 26).

The results of the early studies cannot be extrapolated to patients with more advanced HIV infection. The more profound immunosuppression in advanced HIV infection may reduce the efficacy of interferon treatment. Many patients with advanced HIV infection have leucopenia, further decrease in cell counts during interferon therapy may increase the risk of opportunistic infections as has been reported in two patients (27). In addition, a rapid decline in CD4 counts during interferon therapy was recently reported in three patients (28).

Hemophiliac Patients

The majority of hemophiliac patients who received untreated clotting factor concentrates have chronic HCV infection, and many of them have concurrent HIV infection. Two studies in hemophiliac patients (most of whom were HIV negative) showed that the response to interferon therapy was similar to other patients (29, 30). One study also demonstrated an improvement in liver histology (29). Recent studies sug-

Table 2. Response to α-interferon therapy in patients with concomitant HCV and HIV infection

Author	Interferon Rx		N. of patients	N. of patients with no symptoms of HIV infection	CD4 count mm^{-3}	N (%) with	
	Dose (MU)	Duration (months)				Complete response	Sustained response
Boyer, 1992	3 or 5 tiw	4	3	1	352 ± 257	1	0
	3 or 5 tiw	6	9	5	352 ± 257	3	1
Marriott, 1993	9qd	3	9	9	584 ± 283	5*	4
	9 tiw	3					
	6 tiw	3					
	3 tiw	3					

* 3 became serum HCV RNA negative.

gest that response to interferon therapy may be related to HCV genotype: patients infected with type 2a (Simmond's classification) respond better than those with type 1b, and those infected with a single genotype respond better than those with mixed genotypes. Hemophiliac patients are more likely to be infected with mixed genotypes because of their exposure to huge donor pools. Larger scale studies are needed to confirm if the efficacy of interferon therapy in hemophiliacs is similar to other patients and to determine if the response is related to HCV genotype.

Hemodialysis Patients

Twenty to fourty percent of hemodialysis patients are positive for anti HCV. Interferon is normally excreted by the kidneys, and is not removed by dialysis. There has been very few studies on the use of interferon in patients with renal failure because of the concern that serious adverse effects may develop due to accumulation of interferon. In one study, 10 patients received interferon for 1 year (3MU tiw tapered to 1.5 MU tiw), nine patients had complete biochemical response, but only one became serum HCV RNA negative (31). In another study, 13 patients (with chronic non-A, non-B hepatitis) 11 of whom were anti-HCV positive, received interferon (3MU tiw) for 6 months (32). Ten (77%) patients had normal ALT levels at the end of treatment, seven had sustained biochemical remission. Improvement in histological activity index was also observed, but tests for serum HCV RNA were not performed. No undue side effect was observed in both studies. These preliminary data suggest that interferon in doses of 3MU tiw may be safe in hemodialysis patients, and that the efficacy is similar to other patients. However, larger-scale studies that include pharmacokinetic monitoring are needed before interferon can be recommended for use in patients with end stage renal failure.

Renal Transplant Recipients

HCV-induced chronic liver disease has been reported to occur in approximately 50% of renal transplant recipients. Limited data exists on the safety and efficacy of interferon in these patients because of the concern that the effectiveness of interferon may be reduced by the immunosuppression associated with anti-rejection treatment, and the possibility of interferon induced rejection. Interferon enhances histocompatibility antigen (HLA) expression (especially class II antigens), and may potentially increase the risk of rejection. Early studies on the prophylactic use of interferon against cytomegalovirus infection in renal transplant recipients found a high incidence of steroid-resistant rejection and allograft loss (33) but recent studies on the use of interferon in recurrent HBV/HCV infection in liver transplant recipients failed to confirm an increased risk of rejection in these patients (34).

Interferon was reported to be safe and effective in inducing sustained biochemical, histological, and virological remission in one renal transplant recipient (35). However, two recent studies reported deterioration in renal function in 30-40% patients and high relapse rate (36, 37). Thus, until further data become available, interferon therapy cannot be recommended for renal transplant recipients with chronic hepatitis C.

CONCLUDING PERSPECTIVE

It is clear that studies on the safety and efficacy of interferon therapy in chronic viral hepatitis have to be extended to patients with atypical serology or concomitant medical problems since these patients constitute a large proportion of patients with chronic viral hepatitis and data on the «usual» patients that meet all inclusion and exclusion criteria may not be applicable to these «unusual» patients.

REFERENCES

1. Lok ASF, Lai CL, Wu PC, Leung EKY. Long-term follow-up in a randomized controlled trial of recombinant alpha interferon in Chinese patients with chronic hepatitis B infection. Lancet 1988; ii:298-302.
2. Lok ASF, Lai CL, Leung EKY. Interferon antibodies may negate the antiviral effects of recombinant alpha-interferon treatment in patients with chronic hepatitis B virus infection. Hepatology 1990; 12:1266-1270.
3. Lok ASF, Wu PC, Lai CL et al. A Controlled Trial of Interferon With or Without Prednisone Priming for Chronic Hepatitis B. Gastroenterology 1992; 102:2091-2097.
4. Fevery J, Elewant A, Michielsen P et al. Efficacy of interferon alfa-2b with or without prednisone withdrawal in the treatment of chronic viral hepatitis B. A prospective double-blind Belgian-Dutch study. J Hepatol 1990; 11(Suppl):S108-S112.
5. Perrillo RP, Schiff ER, Davis GL and the Hepatitis Interventional Therapy Group. A randomized, controlled trial of interferon alfa-2b alone and after prednisone withdrawal for the treatment of chronic hepatitis B. N Engl J Med 1990; 323:295-301.
6. Liaw YF, Lin SM, Chen TJ et al. Beneficial effect of prednisolone withdrawal followed by human lymphoblastoid interferon on the treatment of chronic type B hepatitis in Asians: a randomized controlled trial. J Hepatol 1994; 20:175-180.
7. Korenman J, Baker B, Waggoner J et al. Long-Term Remission of Chronic Hepatitis B after Alpha-Interferon Therapy. Ann Inter Med 1991; 114:629-634.
8. Lok ASF, Chung HT, Liu VWS, Ma OCK. Long-Term Follow-Up of Chronic Hepatitis B Patients Treated With Interferon Alfa. Gastroenterology 1993; 105:1833-1838.
9. Lai CL, Lok ASF, Lin HJ et al. Placebo-controlled trial of recombinant α2-interferon in Chinese HBsAg-carrier children. Lancet 1987; ii:877-880.
10. Lai CL, Lin HJ, Lau JYN et al. Effect of Recombinant Alpha2 Interferon With or Without Prednisone in Chinese HBsAg Carrier Children. Q J Med 1991; 78:155-163.
11. Ruiz-Moreno M, Rua MJ, Molina J et al. Prospective, Randomized Controlled Trial of Interferon-α in Children with Chronic Hepatitis B. Hepatology 1991; 13:1035-1039.
12. Sokal EM, Wirth S, Goyens et al. Interferon alfa-2b therapy in children with chronic hepatitis B. Gut 1993; Suppl:S87-S90.
13. Utili R, Sagnelli E, Gaeta GB et al. Treatment of chronic hepatitis B in children with prednisone followed by alfa-interferon: a controlled randomized study. J Hepatol 1994; 20:163-7.
14. Carman WF, Jacyna MR, Hadziyannis S et al. Mutation preventing formation of e antigen in patients with chronic HBV infection. Lancet 1989; ii:588-591.
15. Brunetto MR, Oliveri F, Rocca G et al. Natural Course and Response to Interferon of Chronic Hepatitis B Accompanied by Antibody to Hepatitis B e Antigen. Hepatology 1989; 10:198-202.
16. Pastore G, Santantonio T, Milella M et al. Anti-HBe-positive chronic hepatitis B with HBV-DNA in the serum response to a 6-month course of lymphoblastoid interferon. J Hepatol 1992; 14:221-225.
17. Fattovich G, Farci P, Rugge M et al. A Randomized Controlled Trial of Lymphoblastoid Interferon-α In Patients with Chronic Hepatitis B Lacking HBeAg. Hepatology 1992; 15:584-589.
18. Brunetto MR, Giarin M, Saracco G et al. Hepatitis B Virus Unable to Secrete e Antigen and Response to Interferon in Chronic Hepatitis B. Gastroenterology 1993; 205:845-850.
19. Lok ASF, Akarca US, Greene S. Predictive value of pre-core hepatitis B virus mutations in spontaneous and interferon induced hepatitis B e antigen clearance. Hepatology (in press).
20. Hoofnagle JH, Di Bisceglie AM, Waggoner JG, Park Y. Interferon Alfa for Patients with Clinically Apparent Cirrhosis Due to Chronic Hepatitis B. Gastroenterology 1993; 104:1116-1121.
21. Esteban JI, Lopez-Talavera JC, Genesca J et al. High rate of infectivity and liver disease in blood donors with antibodies to hepatitis C virus. Ann Intern Med 1991; 115:443-9.
22. Sherman KE, O'Brien J, Gutierrez AG et al. Quantitative evaluation of hepatitis C virus RNA in patients with concurrent human immunodeficiency virus infections. J Clin Microbiol 1993; 31:2679-82.
23. Ghany MG, Leissinger C, Laiger R, Sanchez-Pescador R, Lok ASF. Interaction between HCV and HIV infection in a hemophiliac population. Hepatology 1994; 20:255A.
24. Martin P, DiBisceglie AM, Kassianides C, Lisker-Melman M, Hoofnagle JH. Rapidly progressive non-A, non-B hepatitis in patients with human immunodeficiency virus infection. Gastroenterology 1989; 97:1559-1561.
25. Boyer N, Marcellin P, Degott C, Degos F, Saimot AG, Erlinger S, Benhamou JP. Recombinant interferon-α

for chronic hepatitis C in patients positive for antibody to human immunodeficiency virus. J Infect Dis 1992; 165:723-726.
26. Marriott E, Navas S, del Romero J, Garcia S, Castillo I, Quiroga JA, Carreño V. Treatment with recombinant a-interferon of chronic hepatitis C in anti-HIV-positive patients. J Med Virol 1993; 40:107-111.
27. Pesce A, Rosenthal E, Vinti H et al. Opportunistic infections and CD4 lymphocytopenia with interferon treatment in HIV-1 infected patients. Lancet 1993; 341:1597.
28. Vento S, DiPerri G, Cruciani M et al. Rapid decline of CD4+ cells after IFNa treatment in HIV-1 infection. Lancet 1993; 341:958-959.
29. Makris M, Preston FE, Triger DR et al. A randomized controlled trial of recombinant interferon-α in chronic hepatitis C in hemophiliacs. Blood 1991; 78:1672-1677.
30. Bresters D, Mauser-Bunschoten EF, Cuypers HTM et al. Disappearance of hepatitis C virus RNA in plasma during interferon alpha-2b treatment in hemophilia patients. Scand J Gastroenterol 1992; 27:166-168.
31. Taltavull TC, Baliellas C, Sese´ E et al. Interferon (IF) may be useful in hemodialysis (HD) patients with HCV chronic infection who are candidates to kidney transplant (KT). Hepatology 1994; 20:337A.
32. Ellis ME, Alfurayh O, Halim MA et al. Chronic non-A, non-B hepatitis complicated by end-stage renal failure treated with recombinant interferon alpha. J Hepatol 1993; 18:210-216.
33. Hirsch MS, Schooley RT, Cosimi AB et al. Effects of interferon-alpha on cytomegalovirus reactivation syndromes in renal-transplant receipents. N Engl J Med 1983; 308:1489-1493.
34. Wright HI, Gavaler JS, Van Thiel DH. Preliminary experience with α-2b-interferon therapy of viral hepatitis in liver allograft recipients. Transplantation 1992; 53:121-124.
35. Chan TM, Lok ASF, Cheng IKP, Ng IOL. Chronic hepatitis C after renal transplantation. Transplantation 1993; 56:1095-1098.
36. Pol S, Thervet E, Legendre C et al. Hepatitis C viral infection in renal transplant recipients: a pilot study of low-dose recombinant leukocyte interferon-alpha (α-2b IFN). Hepatology 1994; 20:160A.
37. Izopet J, Rostaing L, Dubois M et al. Failure of HCV RNA clearance in kidney transplant recipients treated with alpha-interferon. Hepatology 1994; 20:165A.

Liver Transplantation for Chronic Viral Hepatitis

D. Samuel, C. Feray, H. Bismuth

INTRODUCTION

Liver transplantation is the best available treatment for end-stage liver disease. Liver disease due to hepatitis B (HBV) or C virus (HCV) is the main cause of liver disease in patients candidates to liver transplantation. The risk of viral recurrence and reinfection of the graft is the main issue in these patients. Viral reinfection of the graft may be responsible for the occurrence of acute or chronic liver disease leading to graft failure, death or retransplantation (1, 2). We will discuss herein the mechanisms involved in viral recurrence, the graft lesions due to hepatitis viruses, the current methods of prevention of viral reinfection, and the treatment of viral reinfection after liver transplantation.

HBV AND LIVER TRANSPLANTATION. MECHANISMS INVOLVED IN HBV REINFECTION AFTER LIVER TRANSPLANTATION

The risk of HBV reinfection after transplantation is close to 80% when no preventive measures are taken (3, 4). Reappearance of HBsAg is associated with HBV reactivation, as estimated by reappearance of HBV DNA in serum and, in most of the cases, occurrence of acute hepatitis (5) leading to chronicity. In some cases, acute liver failure can develop leading either to death or to emergency retransplantation. Three mechanisms of recurrence have been postulated: *a*) immediate reinfection of the graft due to circulating HBV particles during or soon after transplantation; *b*) reinfection of the graft due to the presence of HBV in extrahepatic sites with replication and excretion of HBV; *c*) combination of both mechanisms. We think that the second mechanism is mainly involved in the reinfection of the graft of patients receiving anti-HBs immunoglobulins. In a previous work, we demonstrated the presence of replicative forms of HBV in the peripheral blood mononuclear cells (PBMC) whereas these forms were absent from serum suggesting that HBV replication arising from PBMC was involved in the mechanisms of graft reinfection (6). Supporting this hypothesis, we found that, in 11 HBsAg positive transplanted patients who became HBsAg negative while receiving anti-HBs imunoglobulins, HBV DNA could be detected, using PCR method, either in serum or PBMC while it was not demonstrated in the liver graft (7). This last observation suggests that HBV remains in the organism after liver transplantation and is the basis of the long term administration of anti-HBs immunoglobulins to protect the graft from HBV reinfection.

Role of the Initial Liver Disease and of the Pretransplant Viral B Replication Level on HBV Recurrence after Liver Transplantation

In our experience, the rate of HBV recurrence is higher in patients with HBV-associated than with HBV-Delta (HDV) associated cirrhosis or fulminant hepatitis B (5). This was largely confirmed in a European multicenter study wihch showed that, whatever the treatment administered, HBV recurrence was 67% in HBV cirrhosis, 40% in HDV fulminant hepatitis, 32% in HDV cirrhosis, and 17% in HBV fulminant hepatitis (8).

The role of HBV replicative status on post-transplant HBV recurrence was emphasized in a study from Pittsburgh including patients who did not receive long term passive immunoprophylaxis. Eight out of 45 patients cleared completely HBsAg and all of them were anti-HBe positive prior to transplantation (2). In a study from King's College, the rate of HBV recurrence was 7/9 in non replicative patients, vs. 10/10 in replicative patients (3). In our series and in the series from Hannover (9), the pretransplant HBV DNA status detected using non PCR technique was the best accurate predictor of recurrence. In an European multicenter study on 372 HBsAg-positive patients transplanted, HBV recurrence rate was dependent on the presence of HBV replication at time of transplantation: 83% in HBV DNA and HBeAg positive HBV-cirrhosis; 66% in HBV DNA negative and HBeAg positive HBV-cirrhosis; and 58% in HBV DNA and HBeAg negative HBV-cirrhosis ($p = 0.05$). The lower recurrence rate of HBV infection was observed in HDV cirrhotic patients (10, 11) and in fulminant hepatitis B patients (12). This low recurrence rate may be due to the fact that most of these patients were HBV DNA negative at time of liver translantation.

Graft Lesions Due to HBV

The outcome of HBV infection of the graft after liver transplantation is relatively specific: *a*) After reappearance of HBsAg in serum, most patients developed graft lesions (2, 13); *b*) the reappearance of HBsAg is frequently associated with the occurrence of acute hepatitis and evolution to chronic active hepatitis; *c*) development of acute liver failure can be observed few weeks after the occurrence of the hepatitis; *d*) occurrence of cirrhosis within 12 months after the reappearance of HBsAg has been reported. This severe evolution may be due to the immunosuppression which enhances HBV replication. When HBV reinfection recurred, the levels of HBV DNA and of HBsAg in serum are very high. High amounts of HBsAg and HBeAg are present in the cytoplasm and high amounts of HBcAg are present in the nuclei of hepatocytes (2, 13). HBV histologic lesions in the graft are remarkable by the paucity of the inflammatory infiltrate and the rapid development of fibrosis. The King's College group have described an unusual clinicopathological pattern in some patients with a particularity severe clinical evolution called fibrosing cholestatic hepatitis (FCH) (14). The histologic features are characterized by extensive periportal fibrosis, canalicular and cellular cholestasis, enlargement of hepatocytes associated with extensive cytoplasmic HBsAg expression, variable degree of HBcAg and HBeAg cytoplasmic expression, and HBcAg and HBeAg nuclear expression. In contrast, in patients with usual patterns of HBV-induced liver lesions of the graft (i.e., non FCH), there was a high expression of HBcAg in nuclei without diffuse extensive expression of HBsAg. It was suggested, that the extensive presence of HBsAg in these cases of fibrosing cholestatic hepatitis (FCH) are indicative of a non immunologically mediated mechanism of hepatocyte damage. Higher amounts of liver HBsAg, HBcAg and preS1/preS2 are present in FCH as compared to non FCH (15). Demetris et al. reported that in some patients hepatocyte degenerative changes are associated with marked viral expression in the absence of inflammation (1, 2). Thus, these authors suggested that, in this particular circumstance, HBV was directly cytopathic as it was described in models of transgenic mouse and HBV-transfected HepG2 cell lines (16, 17). On the contrary, patients who become and remain serum HBsAg negative after transplantation usually have normal liver histology (5). This underscores the importance of remaining HBsAg negative after liver transplantation.

METHODS OF PREVENTION OF HBV REINFECTION

Anti-HBs Passive Immunoprophylaxis

Polyclonal anti-HBs immunoglobulins. The use of anti-HBS immunoglobulins (Ig) in liver transplantation to prevent HBV reinfection was first described by the King's College/Cambridge group (18) in a patient receiving anti-HBs Ig during the anhepatic phase and at day 6 post-transplant. However, the administration of anti-HBs Ig during the anhepatic phase and the immediate post-transplantation period gave disapointing results since most of patients either remained HBsAg positive or became again HBsAg positive after a short period of time (3, 4), the rate of HBsAg reappearance being up to 80%. The failure of this type of therapy may be related to the low amount of anti-HBs Ig administrated, insufficient to neutralize the amount of HBsAg and to the fact that it did not take into account the persistence of HBV in extrahepatic sites. The Hannover group has suggested to administer very high doses of anti-HBs Ig during the first 6 post-transplant days to neutralize HBsAg, followed by new doses of anti-HBs Ig until the 6th month after transplantation. Interestingly, in some patients receiving anti-HBs Ig for 6 to 12 months, HBsAg reappeared in serum, either immediately or after several months following discontinuation of anti-HBs Ig (9, 19). In 1986, we decided to use a similar protocol but without discontinuation of anti-HBs Ig administration. Our patients received 10,000 IU during the anhepatic phase and 10,000 IU of anti-HBs Ig daily during the first 6 post-operative days. Afterwards, the level of anti-HBs was assessed weekly and 10,000 IU of anti-HBs Ig were readministered when anti-HBs levels were lower than 100 IU/l. Using this protocol, the actuarial rate of reappearance of HBsAg was 17 and 29% at 1 and 2 years of follow-up, respectively (8). The 2-year recurrence rate of HBV infection was significantly higher in patients with HBV cirrhosis (59%) than in those with fulminant hepatitis (0%) or with viral HBV and HDV cirrhosis (13%); the recurrence rate was significantly higher in patients with HBV cirrhosis who were serum HBV DNA positive before transplantation than in those who were HBV DNA negative (96% vs. 29%). In the European multicenter study (8), the rate of HBV recurrence was 75% in patient receiving no or short term anti-HBs Ig as compared to 33% in those receiving long term administration of anti-HBs Ig ($p < 0.001$). The beneficial effect of long term administration of anti-HBs Ig was found in patients transplanted for HBV cirrhosis, HDV cirrhosis and HBV fulminant hepatitis. Long-term administration of anti-HBs Ig did not reduce the rate of HBV recurrence in patients with HBV DNA positive HBV-cirrhosis. In a multivariate analysis, long-term administration of anti-HBs Ig was associated with a reduced rate of HBV recurrence and longer survival.

Monoclonal anti-HBs immunoprophylaxis. There is only on report on the use of monoclonal anti-HBs Ig: seven patients were treated with a human monoclonal anti-HBs Ig and HBsAg reappeared in 4 patients (20). In 3 of these cases of recurrent HBV infection, a HBV mutant was described (21). This mutation occurred in the pre-S region of the genome coding for the HBs envelope and may be due to a pressure of selection of the monoclonal anti-HBs.

Anti-HBs Vaccination. Active anti HBV immunisation was used after the liver transplantation either alone or in combination with passive anti-HBs immunoprophylaxis. Various protocols were proposed and discordant results were obtained. Anti-HBV vaccination was not proven to be sucessful in this setting.

Antiviral Treatment

Antiviral treatment prior to transplantation. The above results have shown the role of HBV replication at time of liver transplantation, as a predictive factor for HBV recurrence. Thus it seemed logical to try to stop HBV replication before liver transplantation. Antiviral treatment is used widely in patients with chronic active hepatitis or well compensated liver cirrhosis. In patients with severe decompensated liver disease with neutropenia and thrombocytopenia, such as candidates for transplantation, interferon has not been frequently used (22). A deterioration of liver function may be observed in this particular group of patients, when HBV replication is stopped.

Alpha recombinant interferon (IFN). In a pilot study, we have treated patients with HBV DNA negative or HBV DNA positive viral B cirrhosis waiting for transplantation in order to reduce the rate of HBV replication after transplantation (23). Patients have received IFN at a dosage of 3 MU tiw for at least 2 months until the transplantation. The patients received after the transplantation the same anti-HBs passive immunoprophylaxis protocol as described above. Patients with active sepsis, bilirubin level > 50 μmol/l, platelets < 20,000/mm^3, white blood cell count < 1,500/mm^3, or rapidly deteriorating condition were not included in this study. The tolerance to IFN was relatively good. However the dosage had to be reduced from 3 MU to 1.5 MU in 8 out of 22 patients due to neutropenia and/or thrombocytopenia. Also, IFN was discontinued definitively in 1 patient because of spontaneous bacterial peritonitis, and temporarily in 2 because of transient encephalopathy. Before starting IFN therapy, 8 patients were HBV DNA positive and 15 were HBV DNA negative. The antiviral effect before transplantation was satisfactory since 7 out of 8 HBV DNA positive patients became HBV DNA negative prior to transplantation. However, the rate of HBV recurrence was not different from that usually observed in patients receiving only post-transplant passive immunoprophylaxis without IFN prior to transplantation. This suggests that the duration of treatment was not sufficient; however, the use of IFN at higher doses or for longer periods may be very difficult in these patients.

In the future new direct antiviral agents should be evaluated in this setting.

Treatment of HBV Reinfection after Liver Transplantation

Ara-A or Ara-AMP. We have treated some patients reinfected with HBV after liver transplantation with Ara-AMP. Briefly, patients received a dose of 10 mg/kg/d for 5 days followed by 10 mg/kg for 21 days via intramuscular route and, more recently, Ara-AMP 10 mg/kg/day for 15 days. The treatment was relatively well tolerated, the main adverse effects being asthenia in all patients and myalgias in 45%. These adverse effects were always transient. An antiviral effect was observed during Ara-AMP treatment in all patients, but in most of these cases, this effect was transient (24). At the end of Ara-AMP treatment all patients remained HBsAg positive and 90% were still HBV DNA positive. Some of our patients have been subsequently treated with a second course of Ara-AMP. A loss of HBsAg and HBV DNA in 10 and 30% of patients, respectively, was observed several months after the end of the second course of Ara-AMP.

Recombinant alpha interferon. Interferon is an immunostimulating agent. Irreversible acute rejection of the kidney in renal transplant patients have been reported. For this reason, interferon was used cautiously after liver transplantation. The Pittsburgh group reported the results of the treatment with recombinant alpha interferon during 6 months at a dose of 3 MU three times a week in 13 patients with HBV reinfection after liver transplantation. Transaminase levels were not modified by the treatment, and all patients remained HBsAg positive. No information was given on the effect of interferon on serum HBV DNA level in these patients (25). New antiviral treatments such as ganciclovir, famciclovir and lamivudin are currently being evaluated.

LIVER TRANSPLANTATION IN PATIENTS WITH HDV LIVER CIRRHOSIS

As described above, patients chronically infected with HBV and HDV have lower risk of HBsAg reappearance than patients chronically infected with HBV alone. The rate of HBsAg reappearance in patients with HBV-HDV cirrhosis was around 50% in the series of O'Grady et al. and Ottobrelli et al. in which patients did not receive long term administration of anti-HBs Ig (10, 26). In our series of 76 patients, 72 of whom received chronic anti-HBs Ig treatment, the rate of HBsAg reappearance was only 13% (11). In the European multicenter study, HBV recurrence was less frequent in delta cirrhotic patients than in HBV cirrhotic patients. The recurrence rate was 60% in patients receiving no or short-term anti-HBs immunoprophylaxis, as compared to 17% in those receiving long-term anti-HBs immunoprophylaxis (8). The lower HBV recurrence rate in HBV-HDV cirrhotic patients compared to HBV patients is probably due to several reasons: *a*) almost all patients with HDV cirrhosis are HBV DNA negative at time of liver transplantation, and *b*) HDV has an inhibitory effect on HBV replication (27).

A very interesting aspect is HDV reinfection after liver transplantation. In our experience, HDV reinfection, as estimated by the presence of HDV RNA in serum or liver and HDAg in serum or liver was about 80% in the first post-transplant months. The course of HDV reinfection is different depending on HBsAg reappearance. HBsAg recurrence was associated with a simultaneous HBV and HDV replication with presence of HBV DNA and HDV RNA and/or HDAg. In most cases, an acute hepatitis develops with presence of HBV and HDV markers in the liver leading to chronic hepatitis (11, 26). In the European multicenter study, HBV recurrence was less severe in delta cirrhotic patients than in HBV cirrhotic patients (8). In most patients who became HBsAg negative, HDV RNA was found in serum and HDV Ag in liver. Liver transplantation is a unique model where HDV, known to be a defective virus needing HBV for replication, is detected in HBsAg negative patients. Several points should be noted: *a*) In these patients, in contrast to patients with reappearance of HBsAg, the liver graft was histologically normal; *b*) HDV markers were frequently detected in the first post-transplant months but were detected in only 5% of patients after 2 years (11). The hypotheses for presence of HDV replication in HBsAg negative patients are as follows: *a*) HBV markers could be present, but not detectable. It has been suggested that the administration of anti-HBs Ig prevents HBsAg detection from serum by formation of HBsAg-Anti-HBs Ab immune complexes. However, the Torino group has reported the same observation in patients transplanted not receiving anti-HBs Ig (10, 26); in addition, among 7 of our patients without HBsAg in serum, HBV DNA was found positive in the liver in only one case by PCR. *b*) HDV is present in the hepatocytes in the absence of HBsAg but cannot replicate. *c*) In our experience the level of HDV RNA in liver was lower in patients without HBsAg than with HBsAg; the level of delta virus in the absence of hepatitis B virus, may be too low to cause hepatic injury.

In conclusion, the risk of HBsAg reappearance after liver transplantation in HBV-HDV cirrhotic patients is low, particularly in those receiving long term anti-HBs immunoprophylaxis and the 3 year survival in our series is 88%. Patients in whom HBsAg reappeared have simultaneous HBV and HDV replication with occurrence of chronic hepatitis in most of the cases. Markers of HDV replication have been found in patients without detectable serum HBsAg and HBV markers in the liver and these patients have a normal liver graft.

LIVER TRANSPLANTATION FOR HCV CIRRHOSIS

Before HCV tests were available, the risk of viral recurrence after transplantation for socalled non-A, non-B cirrhosis was considered to be low and one year survival after liver transplantation was similar to other forms of liver disease. In fact, the development of anti-HCV testing and detection of HCV RNA in serum showed that the risk of HCV recurrence is high and was underestimated.

Liver Transplantation in HCV Cirrhosis

With the appearance or second generation tests for anti-HCV antibodies, it appeared that anti-HCV Ab persisted in 90% of cases after liver transplantation. Since anti-HCV was almost universally present after transplantation for HCV cirrhosis, this test could not be considered reliable for the diagnosis of HCV recurrence (28, 29). The detection of HCV RNA in serum by PCR appeared as the best method to diagnose HCV recurrence (30-32). We and others have shown that HCV RNA is detected after transplantation in some patients demonstrating the presence of HCV after transplantation. In a previous work, we demonstrated the recurrence of HCV infection by comparing in 2 patients the hypervariable domain of the E2/NS1 region before and after liver transplantation (32). In these 2 patients, we found a 95% nucleotide sequences homology in the hypervariable domain of the 5' part of the E2/NS1 region between the HCV pre- and post-transplant strain in each of these 2 patients demonstrating that the same strain of HCV was present in the serum of these 2 patients before and after transplantation. In our experience and in most studies, HCV RNA is found in 80-90% of patients with HCV cirrhosis at time of transplantation (31-34). After transplantation, HCV RNA was detected in the serum in 85-90% of the patients transplanted for HCV cirrhosis. HCV RNA was detected as soon as the first post-transplant week in some patients (33). In our experience, the actuarial rate of occurrence of acute lobular hepatitis was 57% at one year and 72% at 4 year post-transplant. The actuarial rate of occurrence of chronic active hepatitis was 25% at one year and 60% at 4 year after the occurrence of acute lobular hepatitis. After 4 years of follow-up, the development of liver cirrhosis was observed in only one case. Our results are in accordance with those of the San Francisco group who showed a 51% rate of occurrence of hepatitis; in their experience, the rate of occurrence of hepatitis was 22/43 (51%); 18 patients having either mild chronic hepatitis or persistent hepatitis and 4 patients having severe forms of chronic hepatitis with portal fibrosis or cirrhosis (31, 35).

Factors Influencing the Rate of HCV Recurrence and the Severity of Graft Disease

The pretransplant level of viremia was not predictive of HCV recurrence: in our experience the rate of acute hepatitis on the graft was similar in patients with and without detectable HCV viremia by PCR before transplantation (34). In contrast, Chazouilleres et al. have found an association between the pretransplant HCV viremia, detected by the branched DNA assay, and HCV recurrence (36). In our studies, the severity of HCV recurrence was related to the level of HCV viremia post-transplantation: when the graft was almost normal the level of viremia was much lower than when there was hepatitis on the graft (34). However, the level of viremia was not different between patients with acute and chronic hepatitis. We have found an association between genotype 1b and occurrence of severe graft hepatitis: the rate of acute and chronic hepatitis was higher in patients infected with genotype 1b than with other genotypes (37). This finding was recently reported by the King's College group (38). The pathogenicity of HCV genotype 1b was not dependent of the level of viremia in comparison with the level of viremia of other genotypes suggesting that the HCV genotype 1b was more pathogenic for hepatocytes than other genotypes.

Survival of HCV-Positive Transplant Recipients

In our experience, the 5 year survival of HCV positive recipients was 80%, a figure similar to that of patients transplanted for other liver diseases. The rate of retransplantation of patients with HCV cirrhosis with a mean follow-up of 30 months was not different than that for other liver diseases. In our experience, HCV chronic hepatitis was present in some cases of graft failure leading to retransplantation but was associated in all cases but one with either acute or chronic rejection or hepatic vessels thrombosis.

Histological Features of HCV Hepatitis on the Graft

The histological features of hepatitis C in liver transplant recipients are the presence of mononuclear parenchymal infiltrates, acidophilic necrosis, and hepatocyte swelling in most of cases in the acute hepatitis phase. In the chronic phase lymphocytes aggregates are seen. In both phases, fatty changes and duct damage are frequently observed. It should be noted that signs of rejection can be present together with signs of hepatitis. Some atypical histological signs were noted by Feray et al. including hepatocyte swelling with minimal inflammation, centrilobular ballooning mimicking ischemia, florid ductal proliferation with acute pericholangitis mimicking biliary obstruction, hepatitis coexistent with rejection, and duct or ductule damage without rejection. In these cases, the diagnosis of hepatitis due to HCV infection may be difficult especially when rejection is suspected. In our experience, the resolution of chronic hepatitis C infection on the graft was not observed (32).

Prevention of HCV Infection in Liver Transplant Recipients

In contrast to HBsAg positive recipients of liver transplants, no methods of prevention of recurrence of HCV infection have been reported.

Treatment of HCV Infection after Liver Transplantation

The most effective treatment against HCV infection is recombinant alpha interferon. However, interferon is an immunostimulating agent which enhances the expression of HLA class I molecules on hepatocytes and has been reported to facilitate the occurrence of rejection in renal transplant recipients. In a report from Pittsburgh on the use of recombinant alpha interferon in patients with HCV hepatitis on the graft, the rate of complete response (as assessed by the normalization of transaminases) was 9%, and the authors reported no cases of acute or chronic rejection. However, no data concerning HCV RNA in serum was given and few histological data were available. In our experience, 2 out of 14 patients treated with interferon had a normalization of liver tests and HCV RNA remained positive in all. In addition, 5 patients developed a severe ductopenia requiring retransplantation in 3 (39). Others have found an antiviral effect in patients treated with interferon without occurrence of severe rejection. However, we think that the use of interferon in liver transplant recipients should be at least cautious or contraindicated.

CONCLUSIONS

The prevalence of HBV recurrence after liver transplantation is higher in patients with HBV cirrhosis than in patients with HBV-HDV cirrhosis of fulminant hepatitis B and is related to the presence of HBV replication prior to transplantation. Long-term passive anti-HBs immunoprophylaxis is the best current way of preventing HBV reinfection and improves long-term survival.

The rate of recurrence of HCV infection is high reaching 85% and the rate of HCV hepatitis on the graft is around 75%. In most cases, this hepatitis leads to chronic hepatitis. The severity of hepatitis on the graft is related to the level of viremia at time of hepatitis and to genotype 1b. The methods of prevention of HCV infection after liver transplantation are to be found. The treatment of HCV hepatitis on the graft with interferon should be carefully evaluated. Other antiviral treatments without immunostimulating effect are needed.

Finally, patients transplanted for hepatitis B without HBV replication, receiving post-transplant long term anti-HBs immunoprophylaxis and patients transplanted for HCV cirrhosis have a similar 5 year survival than other groups of liver transplanted patients.

REFERENCES

1. Demetris AJ, Jaffe R, Sheahan DG et al. Recurrent hepatitis B in liver allograft recipients. Differenciation between viral hepatitis B and rejection. Am J Pathol 1986; 125:161-172.
2. Demetris AJ, Todo S, Van Thiel DH et al. Evolution of hepatitis B virus liver disease after hepatic replacement. Practical and theoretical considerations. Am J Pathol 1990; 137:667-676.
3. Todo S, Demetris AJ, Van Thiel D, Teperman L, Fung J, Starzl TE. Orthotopic liver transplantation for patients with hepatitis B virus related liver disease. Hepatology 1991; 13:619-626.
4. O'Grady JG, Smith HM, Davies SE et al. Hepatitis B reinfection after orthotopic liver transplantation. Serological and clinical implications. J Hepatol 1992; 14:104-111.
5. Samuel D, Bismuth A, Mathieu D et al. Passive immunoprophylaxis after liver transplantation in HBsAg-positive patients. Lancet 1991; 337: 813-815.
6. Zignego AL, Samuel D, Gugenheim J et al. Hepatitis B virus replication and mononuclear blood cells infection after liver transplantation. In: Zuckermann AJ, eds. Viral Hepatitis and Liver Disease. New York: Alan R Liss, 1988; 808.
7. Feray C, Zignego AL, Samuel D et al. Persistent hepatitis B virus infection of mononuclear cells without concomitant liver infection: the liver transplantation model. Transplantation 1990; 49:1155-1158.
8. Samuel D, Müller R, Alexander G, Fassati L, Ducot B, Benhamou JP, Bismuth H and the investigators of the European concerted action on viral hepatitis study. Liver transplantation in European patients with the hepatitis B surface antigen. N Engl J Med 1993; 329:1842-1847.
9. Müller R, Gubernatis G, Farle M et al. Liver transplantation in HBs antigen (HBsAg) carriers. Prevention of hepatitis B virus (HBV) recurrence by passive immunisation. J Hepatol 1991; 13:90-96.
10. Rizzetto M, Chiaberge E, Negro F et al. Liver transplantation in hepatitis delta virus disease. Lancet 1987; ii:469-471.
11. Samuel D, Zignego AL, Reynes M, Feray C, Arulnaden JL, David MF, Gigou M, Bismuth A, Mathieu D, Gentilini P, Benhamou JP, Brechot C, Bismuth H. Long-term clinical and virologic outcome after liver transplantation for cirrhosis due to chronic delta hepatitis. Hepatology; 1995(in press).
12. Brechot C, Bernuau J, Thiers V et al. Multiplication of hepatitis B virus in fulminant hepatitis B. Br Med J 1984; 288:270.
13. Philips MJ, Cameron R, Flowers MA et al. Post-transplant recurrent hepatitis B viral liver disease.

Viral-burden, steato-viral, and fibroviral hepatitis I. A J Pathol 1992; 140:1295-1308.
14. Davies SE, Portmann BC, O'Grady JG, Aldis PM, Chaggar K, Alexander GM, Williams R. Hepatic histologic findings after transplantation for chronic hepatitis B virus infection, including a unique pattern of fibrosing cholestatic hepatitis. Hepatology 1991; 13:150-157.
15. Lau JYN, Bain VG, Davies SE, O'Grady JG, Alberti A, Alexander GJM, Williams R. High-level expression of hepatitis B viral antigens in fibrosing cholestatic hepatitis. Gastroenterology 1992; 102:956-962.
16. Chisari FV, Filippi P, Buras J et al. Structural and pathological effects of synthesis of hepatitis B virus large envelope polypeptide in transgenic mice. Proc Nat Acad Sci USA 1987; 84:6909-6913.
17. Roingeard P, Romet-Lemonne JL, Leturcq D, Goudeau A, Essex M. Hepatitis B virus core antigen (HBc Ag) accumulation in an HBV nonproducer clone of HepG2-transfected cells is associated with cytopathic effect. Virology 1990; 179:113.
18. Johnson PJ, Wansbrough-Jones MH, Portmann B, Eddleston ALWF, Williams R, D'A Maycock W, Calne RY. Familial HBsAg-positive hepatoma: treatment with orthotopic liver transplantation and specific immunoglobulin. Br Med J 1978; 1:216.
19. Lauchart W, Müller R, Pichlmayr R. Long-term immunoprophylaxis of hepatitis B virus (HBV) reinfection in recipients of human liver allografts. Transplant Proc 1987; 19:4051-4053.
20. Fung J, Ostberg L, Shapiro R, Todo S, Demetris A, Starzl TE. Human monoclonal antibody against hepatitis B surface antigen in preventing recurrent hepatitis B following liver transplantation. In: Hollinger FB, Lemon SM, Margolis HS, eds. Viral hepatitis and liver disease. Baltimore: Williams and Wilkins, 1991; 651.
21. MacMahon G, Ehrlich PH, Moustafa ZA et al. Genetic alterations in the gene encoding the major HBsAg: DNA and immunological analysis of recurrent HBsAg derived from monoclonal antibody-treated liver transplant recipients. Hepatology 1992; 15:757-766.
22. Di Bisceglie AM. Interferon therapy of complicated hepatitis B virus infection. Semin Liver Dis 1989; 9:254-258.
23. Marcellin P, Samuel D, Areias J, Gigou M, Benhamou JP, Bismouth H. Pretransplant interferon treatment and recurrence of Hepatitis B virus infection after liver transplantation for hepatitis B-related end-stage liver disease. Hepatology 1994; 19:6-12.
24. Marcellin P, Samuel D, Loriot MA, Areias J, Bismuth H, Benhamou JP. Anti-viral effect of adenine arabinoside monophosphate (ARA-AMP) in patients with recurrence of hepatitis B virus (HBV) infection after liver transplantation. Hepatology 1990; 12:966(Abstr).
25. Wright HI, Gavaler JS, Van Thiel DH. Preliminary experience with alpha 2b interferon therapy of viral hepatitis in liver allograft recipients. Transplantation 1992; 53:121-124.
26. Ottobrelli A, Marzano A, Smedile A et al. Patterns of hepatitis delta virus reinfection and disease in liver transplantation. Gastroenterology 1991; 101:1649-1655.
27. Krogsgaard K, Kryger P, Aldershvile J et al. Delta infection and suppression of hepatitis B virus replication in chronic HBsAg carriers. Hepatology 1987; 7:42-45.
28. Martin P, Muñoz SJ, Di Bisceglie AM, Rubin R, Wagooner JG, Armenti VT, Moritz MJ, Jarell BE, Maddrey WC. Recurrence of hepatitis C virus infection after orthotopic liver transplantation. Hepatology 1991; 13:719-721.
29. Read AE, Donegan E, Lake J, Ferrell L, Galbraith C, Kuramoto IK, Zeldis JB, Ascher NL, Roberts J, Wright TL. Hepatitis C in patients undergoing liver transplantation. Ann Intern Med 1991; 114:282-284.
30. Poterucha RJ, Lumeng L, Lee CH, Taswell HF, Wiesner RH. Diagnosis of chronic hepatitis C after liver transplantation by the detection of viral sequences with polymerase chain reaction. Hepatology 1992; 15:42-45.
31. Wright TL, Donegan E, Hsu H, Ferrell L, Lake J, Kim M, Combs C, Fennessy S, Roberts J, Asher N. Recurrent and acquired hepatitis C viral infection in liver transplant recipients. Gastroenterology 1992; 103:317-322.
32. Feray C, Samuel D, Thiers V, Gigou M, Pichon F, Bismuth H, Reynes M, Maisonneuve P, Bismuth H, Brechot C. Reinfection of liver graft by hepatitis C virus after liver transplantation. J Clin Invest 1992; 89:1361-1365.
33. König V, Bauditz J, Lobeck H, Lüsebrink R, Neuhaus P, Blumhardt G, Bechstein WO, Neuhaus R, Steffen R, Hopf U. Hepatitis C virus reinfection in allografts after orthotopic liver transplantation. Hepatology 1992; 16:1137-1143.
34. Feray C, Gigou M, Samuel D et al. The course of hepatitis C virus infection after liver transplantation. Hepatology 1994; 20:1137-1143.
35. Ferrell LD, Wright TL, Roberts J, Ascher N, Lake J. Hepatitis C viral infection in liver transplant recipients. Hepatology, 1992; 16:865-876.
36. Chazouilleres O, Kim M, Ferrel L, Robert J, Ascher N, Wilber J, Neuwald P, Pescador R, Urdea M, Wright T. Quantitation of hepatitis C virus RNA in liver transplant recipients. Gastroenterology 1994; 106:994-999.
37. Feray C, Gigou M, Samuel D et al. Influence of the genotypes of hepatitis C virus on the severity of recurrent liver disease after liver transplantation. Gastroenterology 1995 (in press).
38. Gane E, Naoumov NV, Quian KP, Mondelli M, Maertens G, Lau JYN, Williams R. Enhanced HCV replication and acceleration graft injury after liver transplantation. Hepatology 1994; 20:136 A.
39. Feray C, Samuel D, Gigou M, Reynes M, Bismuth H. An open trial of interferon alpha recombinant for hepatitis C after liver transplantation: antiviral effects and risk of rejection. Submitted to publication.

New Treatments for Chronic Hepatitis B

A. M. Di Bisceglie

INTRODUCTION

Chronic infection with the hepatitis B virus (HBV) is a common underlying cause of chronic hepatitis, cirrhosis and hepatocellular carcinoma world-wide (1). Although there is a safe and effective vaccine available against HBV infection (2), difficulties with its delivery to populations at risk suggest that the vaccine alone may take a long time to eliminate chronic liver disease due to hepatitis B.

Alpha interferon has been used as therapy for chronic hepatitis B for nearly 20 years now, experimentally at first but on a larger scale more recently (3, 4). The use of alpha interferon has provided a useful model to study the effect of antiviral therapy in chronic hepatitis B. It has been used predominantly in patients with high levels of viral replication, evidenced by the presence of hepatitis B e antigen (HBeAg) or high levels of HBV DNA in serum. Clearance of these markers is usually associated with improvement in liver disease and, at least in some cases, is followed by loss of hepatitis B surface antigen (HBsAg) from serum. Unfortunately, interferon is effective in only 30 to 40% of patients (5) and its use is limited by cost and occurrence of significant side effects (6). Clearly, alternative therapies are needed against HBV infection. Ideally, such therapies should be more effective and have fewer side effects than interferon. At present, new therapies are all experimental and include those that have been tested in man, those that have been tested in experimental animals or *in vitro* systems and those that remain only theoretical possibilities (table 1).

NUCLEOSIDE ANALOGUES

Many nucleoside analogue agents have been found to have antiviral activity *in vitro* or *in vivo*. They appear to act by inhibiting the process of reverse transcription by becoming incorporated into viral DNA which is being transcribed from RNA resulting in termination of the nascent DNA chain. The first generation of nucleoside analogues (including acyclovir, adenine arabinoside, ribavirin, azidothymidine, dideoxyinosine and dideoxycytidine) have either been found to have little effect against HBV or intolerable side effects (7-10).

Currently, there is a second generation of such agents being tested amidst great optimism;

Tabla 1. Promising new therapies for chronic hepatitis B

Second generation nucleoside analogues
Lamivudine (3TC)*
Famciclovir*
FTC
Immune modulators
Beta interferon*
Alpha thymosin*
Interferon inducers*
Viral peptides (HBcAg)*
Viral vaccines (HBsAg)*
Activated lymphocyte therapy*
Bone marrow transplantation
HBIg/monoclonal antiHBs*
Molecular biological agents
Ribozymes
Antisense oligonucleotides

* Currently being tested in humans.

they may be effective in chronic hepatitis B. One of these second generation agents, with very potent anti-viral effects against HBV, was unfortunately found to have severe and fatal side effects thought to be related to mitochondrial injury. Thus, the use fialuridine (FIAU) was associated with lactic acidosis, fulminant hepatic failure, pancreatitis, myopathy and neuropathy resulting in the death of several patients treated in an experimental protocol (11). Although this adverse experience raised the possibility that other second generation nucleoside analogues may be associated with similar toxicity none of these agents have shown evidence of similar mitochondrial toxicity to date. *In vitro* experiments suggest that fialuridine may have been singularly toxic because of its propensity to become incorporated within mitochondrial DNA.

The second generation nucleoside analogues with the most promising potential at present include lamivudine (3-TC) and famciclovir. Lamivudine has an excellent safety profile when administered for prolonged periods in patients with human immunodeficiency virus (HIV) infection. Preliminary studies suggest that it has potent antiviral action against HBV (12, 13). Thus, in a pilot study in which lamivudine was administered for 1 month in doses varying between 5 and 600 mg daily, serum levels of HBV DNA became undetectable in up to 75% of patients by the end of therapy. In a more recent study in which lamivudine was administered for a longer period (3 months), a similar beneficial effect was seen (12). Interestingly, levels of HBV DNA tended to rise promptly to pretreatment levels when the drug was stopped and relatively few patients cleared HBeAg from serum. This suggests that lamivudine might be effective in suppressing but not eliminating HBV replication. Studies currently under way with long term follow up after therapy may help to clarify this point. Famciclovir has not been tested to the same extent as lamivudine, but preliminary studies suggest that it may have a similarly powerful effect against HBV (14).

The potential advantage of using agents with direct antiviral effect such as lamivudine and famciclovir include the fact that they can be taken orally, they appear to have very few side effects even when given for prolonged periods and they may be effective in immunosuppressed hosts (for example after organ transplantation or in advanced HIV infection) where interferon seems to have little role.

NEW IMMUNOMODULATORY AGENTS

The persistence of HBV infection and hepatic injury associated with chronic hepatitis B appear to reflect a balance between viral and host factors. Thus, a vigorous cellular immune response is required for clearance of HBV infection, presumably by causing lysis of hepatocytes harboring HBV. This enhanced immune response may occur spontaneously in some patients, resulting in clearance of viral replication if it is effective or a transient exacerbation of liver disease if not (15, 16). It is likely that one of the actions of alpha interferon is to enhance immune reactivity, promoting the clearance of viral replication. Other agents that might similarly enhance the immune response have been tested as therapies for chronic hepatitis B. These include corticosteroid withdrawal and levamisole which were found to be ineffective or even dangerous (17). Alpha thymosin also has many non-specific immune enhancing effects and has been shown to be effective against HBV in a small pilot study (18). The results of a larger, randomized, placebo-controlled trial of alpha thymosin which might confirm these preliminary findings are not yet available.

Other forms of interferon have immune stimulating effects similar to alpha interferon. These include beta interferon which is most similar to alpha and even acts via the same cellular receptor as alpha interferon (19). Beta interferon has not been tested extensively against HBV infection in humans, but appears to be as effective as alpha interferon. In contrast, gamma interferon appears to have little antiviral effect against HBV and may even be associated with worsening of liver disease (20). Similarly, interleukin-2 appears to have little antiviral effect against HBV but is hepatotoxic (21).

The therapies described above appear to act by stimulating cells of the immune system to increased action. Another approach might be to provide the patient with a supply of activated cells. Examples of this include bone marrow transplantation and infusion of activated cells. Transplantation of bone marrow from donors immune to hepatitis B has occasionally been shown to result in clearance of HBV replication in recipients with chronic HBV infection. Studies are currently underway to infuse autologous ex-vivo activated lymphocytes into patients with chronic hepatitis B (22).

Another approach is to try and stimulate the immune system to respond specifically to components of the HBV itself. Certain HBV peptides have been shown to stimulate an immune response *in vitro* and attempts are underway to use these peptides to stimulate an immune response *in vivo* (23). This may be accomplished by administering the peptides directly or by introducing a retroviral vector which expresses whole viral proteins in transfected cells (24). Components of the HBV core protein have been shown to elicit the greatest HLA-restricted cellular immune response (25) and are the focus of interest in the experiments described above. It remains to be seen whether this approach will stimulate any immune response over and above that normally present in chronic HBV infection where HBcAg is continually being expressed on cell surface. An intriguing recent report of HBV clearance following the administration of hepatitis B vaccine (comprised of HBsAg) also suggests a role for specific immune stimulation (26).

Although it is clear that cell-mediated immunity is important in clearing HBV from the liver, it is not certain whether humoral immune mechanisms may also play a role. Humoral immunity is important in preventing HBV infection and is the basis for the widely-used HBV vaccine, made of HBsAg. Antibodies to HBsAg (anti-HBs) have also been used to prevent HBV infection when administered in the form of hyperimmune B immunoglobulin (HBIG). HBIG is now widely used in the prevention of recurrent HBV infection after liver transplantation (27). Monoclonal anti-HBs has been used in similar situations (28) and also in patients with common variable hypogammaglobulinemia and HBV infection. It is unlikely that HBIg or monoclonal anti-HBs would have a role in the treatment of chronic hepatitis B although this has not been widely explored.

MOLECULAR BIOLOGIC APPROACHES

Several other approaches to therapy of HBV infection have been tested in the laboratory or in experimental animals but have not yet been used in humans. These approaches take advantage of the molecular biology of HBV. Thus, antisense oligonucleotides have been shown to inhibit transcription of HBV in cells transfected with HBV (29). One of the major problems associated with the use of antisense molecules is their delivery to the required site of action. One approach currently being tested is the use of glycosylated conjugates of the oligonucleotides which may be taken up by hepatocytes via the asialoglycoprotein receptor (30).

Many oligonucleotide molecules induce local production of interferon by cells. Further experiments are required to determine whether the antiviral effect noted with antisense oligonucleotides is related to interferon induction or direct inhibition of viral transcription. Another interesting approach based on molecular biology is the use of ribozymes. Ribozymes are small RNA molecules that are able to cleave RNA. Some have important physiological actions, an example being self-cleavage of genomic RNA of the hepatitis delta virus by its own RNA. The actions of ribozymes appear to be dependent on secondary and tertiary structure of the RNA molecule. Ribozymes have been shown *in vitro* to cleave HBV RNA molecules and inhibit transcription of HBV proteins (31).

THERAPY OF NEW CATEGORIES OF PATIENTS

The development of the therapies described above has evolved based on studies showing that clearance of HBeAg and HBV DNA from serum was associated with improvement of liver disease. Thus, therapy was not aimed at eliminating HBV infection but at decreasing the level of HBV replication. Patients negative for HBeAg and HBV DNA have not been considered for therapy up to now but they remain at risk for having the hepatitis become active again and for transmitting HBV to their contacts. It is possible that with some of the newer therapies described above, they may become candidates for therapy. Because these patients are usually asymptomatic and have only a small risk of developing significant liver disease any therapy used in them would have to have minimal side effects. It is possible that use of nucleoside analogues or a stimulator of the immune system might be successful in eliminating HBV infection entirely.

Similarly, other patients who have typically been excluded from treatment with alpha interferon might become candidates for therapy including those with recurrent HBV after organ transplantation or those with advanced HIV infection. Another group of patients that have been very difficult to treat include those with recurrent episodes of exacerbation and remission of hepatitis B where chronic administration of an antiviral might sufficiently suppress HBV replication to prevent the relapses from occurring. An antiviral agent with potent activity against HBV might be used together with anticancer chemotherapy in patients with chronic HBV infection to prevent the frequent relapses which are often severe or even fatal (32).

EVALUATION OF NEW THERAPIES FOR CHRONIC HEPATITIS B

Clearly, several potential new therapeutic strategies are being developed against HBV. Ideally, they should be adequately tested for safety and efficacy in animals before being used in humans. However attaining this goal is often hampered by lack of suitable experimental models to test new therapies. Thus, the only cell culture model used is based on transfection of cloned HBV into malignant hepatocytes (33, 34). While HBV appears to undergo full cycles of replication in this model, it does lack the immune component which plays a crucial role in natural HBV infection and is thus purely a model of inhibition of viral replication and inhibition of viral protein production. Alpha interferon, for example, has little appreciable effect against HBV in this system.

There are several animal models that have been used to study the pathogenesis of hepadnaviral replication including the woodchuck (woodchuck hepatitis virus), ground squirrel (ground squirrel hepatitis virus) and pekin duck (duck hepatitis virus). Many agents have been found to have inhibitory effects against HBV replication in these animal systems. But they, too, lack similarity to human HBV infection. Indeed, the events associated with clearance of HBeAg and HBV DNA from serum are not readily found in these animal models (35, 36). Thus HBV infection is rarely eliminated and generally only temporarily suppressed. Furthermore, it is not clear how generalizable data from these animal models are to the human disease. For example, dideoxynosine was found to be a potent inhibitor of duck HBV replication but had little beneficial effect in humans (7). The chimpanzee animal model has some potential advantages in that the infecting agents (HBV) is the same that causes disease in humans. Unfortunately, very few infected chimpanzees are available for such studies and the costs associated with their use are prohibitive.

The use of animals models to study the toxicity of new therapies may also be of limited use. Thus, fialuridine was found to be associated with virtually no toxic effects in animals treated with high doses in preclinical studies (36). Nonetheless, the use of animals to study toxicity remain mandatory but in some situations it may be possible to try a new therapy in humans without conclusive evidence of beneficial effect in an experimental or animal model. The main role of these models is as a tool to screen new compounds for possible effect against HBV or to try and study the mechanism of action of new drugs.

SUMMARY AND CONCLUSIONS

Alpha interferon is at present the only therapeutic agent with proven efficacy against HBV. Studies of the molecular biology and immunology of HBV infection have led to several potential therapeutic strategies that might or even are being tested in humans with chronic hepatitis B. The development of better therapies might also expand the pool of patients possibly suitable for therapy. Experimental and animal models of HBV infection are of limited benefit in evaluating therapeutic and toxic potential of new therapies.

REFERENCES

1. Hoofnagle JH, Davis GL, Hanson RG. Chronic type B hepatitis: Clinical course. In: Viral hepatitis and delta infection. New York: Alan R Liss, 1983; 41-53.
2. Hepatitis B virus: A comprehensive strategy for eliminating transmission in the United States through universal childhood vaccination. MMWR 1991; 40:1-20.
3. Greenberg HB, Pollard RB, Lutwick LI, Gregory PB, Robinson WS, Merigan TC. Effect of human leucocyte interferon on hepatitis B virus infection in patients with chronic active hepatitis. N Engl J Med 1976; 295:517-522.
4. Perrillo RP. Treatment of chronic hepatitis B with interferon: experience in western countries. Sem Liver Dis 1989; 9:240-248.
5. Hoofnagle JH, Peters M, Mullen KD, Jones DB, Rustgi V, Di Bisceglie AM et al. Randomized, controlled trial of recombinant human alpha-interferon in patients with chronic hepatitis B. Gastroenterology 1988; 95:1318-1325.
6. Renault PF, Hoofnagle JH. Side effects of alpha interferon. Sem Liver Dis 1989; 9:273-277.
7. Fried MW, Korenman JC, Swain MG, Di Bisceglie AM, Park Y, Waggoner JG et al. A pilot study 2'3'-dideoxyinosine for treatment of chronic hepatitis B. Hepatology 1992; 16:861-864.
8. Fried MW, Fong T, Swain MG, Park Y, Beames MP, Banks SM et al. Therapy of chronic hepatitis B with a 6-month course of ribavirin. J Hepatol 1994; 21:145-150.
9. Schalm SW, Heytink RA, Van Buuren HR, de Man RA. Lymphoblastoid alpha-interferon weekly, daily and combined with acyclovir for chronic HBeAg-positive hepatitis. J Hepatol 1986, 3(Suppl 2):S189-S192.
10. Hoofnagle JH, Minuk GY, Dusheiko GM, Schafer DF, Johnson R, Straus S et al. Adenine arabinoside 5'-monophosphate treatment of chronic type B hepatitis. Hepatology 1982; 2:784-788.
11. Parker WB, Cheng YC. Mitochondrial toxicity of antiviral nucleoside analogs. J NIH Res 1994; 6:57-61.
12. Dienstag JL, Perrillo RP, Schiff ER, Bartholomew M, Vicary C, Rubin M. Double-blind, randomized, three month, dose-ranging trial of lamivudine for chronic hepatitis B. Hepatology 1994; 20:199A(Abstr).
13. Tyrrell DLJ, Mitchell MC, de Man RA, Schalm SW, Main C, Thomas HC et al. Phase II trial of lamivudine for chronic hepatitis B. Hepatology 1993; 18:112A(Abstr).
14. Tillmann HL, Trautwein C, Bode U, Oldhafer K, Boker K, Pichlmayr R et al. Treatment of hepatitis B virus reinfection after liver transplantation with famciclovir. Hepatology 1994; 20:130A(Abstr).
15. Hoofnagle JY, Dusheiko M, Seeff LB, Jones A, Waggoner JG, Bales ZB. Seroconversion from Hepatitis B e Antigen to Antibody in Chronic Type B Hepatitis. Ann Intern Med 1981; 94:744-748.
16. Dusheiko GM, Bowyer SM, Paterson A, Song E, Di Bisceglie A, Kew MC. Clinical and serological events accompanying changes in hepatitis B viral replication: case reports. Liver 1985; 5:77-83.
17. Nair PV, Tong MJ, Stevenson D, Roskamp D, Boone C. A pilot study on the effects of prednisone withdrawal on serum hepatitis B virus DNA and HBeAg in chronic active hepatitis B. Hepatology 1986; 6:1319-1324.
18. Mutchnick MG, Appelman HD, Chung HT, Aragona E, Gupta TP, Cummings GD et al. Thymosin treatment of chronic hepatitis B: A placebo-controlled pilot trial. Hepatology 1991; 14:410-415.
19. Peters M, Davis GL, Dooley JS, Hoofnagle JH. The interferon system in acute and chronic viral hepatitis. Prog Liver Dis 1986; 8:453-467.
20. Di Bisceglie AM, Rustgi VK, Kassianides C, Lisker-Melman M, Park Y, Waggoner JG et al. Therapy of chronic hepatitis B with recombinant human alpha and gamma interferon. Hepatology 1990; 11:266-270.
21. Fisher B, Keenan AM, Garra BS, Steinberg SM, White DE, Di Bisceglie AM et al. Interleukin-2 induces profound reversible cholestasis. A detailed analysis in treated patients. J Clin Oncol 1989; 17:1852-1862.
22. Graham S, Babayan RK, Lamm DL, Sawczuk I, Ross SD, Lavin PT et al. The use of ex-vivo activated memory T cells (autolymphocyte therapy) in the treatment of metastatic renal cell carcinoma: final results from a randomized, controlled, multisite study. Semin Urol 1993; 11:27-34.
23. Bertoletti A, Chisari FV, Penna A, Guilhot S, Galati L, Missale G et al. Definition of a minimal cytotoxic T-cell epitope within the hepatitis B virus nucleocapsid protein. J Virol 1993; 67:2376-2380.
24. Jolly D. Viral vector systems for gene therapy. Cancer Gen Ther 1994; 1:51-64.
25. Lee SD, Tong MJ, Wu JC, Lin HC, Tsai YT, Lo KJ. A randomised double-blind placebo-controlled trial of prednisolone therapy in HBeAg and HBV DNA positive Chinese patients with chronic active hepatitis B. J Hepatol 1991; 12:246-250.
26. Pol S, Driss F, Carnot F, Michel M, Berthelot P, Brechot C. Vaccination against hepatitis B virus: an efficient immunotherapy against hepatitis B multiplication. C R Acad Sci Paris 1993; 316:688-691.
27. Samuel D, Muller R, Alexander G, Fassati L, Ducot B, Benhamou JP et al. Liver transplantation in European patients with the hepatitis B surface antigen. N Engl J Med 1993; 329:1885-1887.
28. Fung J, Ostberg L, Shapiro R, Todo S, Demetris A, Starzl T. Human monoclonal antibody against hepatitis B surface antigen in preventing recurrent hepatitis B following liver transplantation. In: Hollinger FB, Lemon SM, Margolis HS, eds. Viral Hepatitis and Liver Disease. Baltimore: Williams and Wilkins, 1991; 651.
29. Wands JR, Zhang ZS, Brown NV, Blum HE. Effect of antisense oligodeoxynucleotides on hepatitis B viral replication and gene expression. Hepatology 1993; 18:145A(Abstr).
30. Wu GY, Wu CH. Specific inhibition of hepatitis B viral gene expression in vitro by targeted antisense oligonucleotides. J Biol Chem 1992; 267:12436-12439.

31. Weizsaecker FV, Bkum HE, Wands JR. Ribozyme mediated cleavage of hepatitis B and duck hepatitis B virus RNA. Hepatology 1992; 16:88A.
32. Lok ASF, Liang RHS, Chiu EKW, Wong K, Chan T, Todd D. Reactivation of hepatitis B virus replication in patients receiving cytotoxic therapy. Gastroenterology 1991; 100:182-188.
33. Sells MA, Chen ML, Acs G. Production of hepatitis B virus particles in HepG2 cells transfected with cloned hepatitis B virus DNA. Proc Natl Acad Sci USA 1987; 84:1005-1009.
34. Korba BE, Gerin JL. Use of a standardized cell culture assay to assess activities of nucleoside analogs against hepatitis B virus replication. Antiviral Res 1992; 19:55-70.
35. Gerin JL, Korba BE, Cote PJ, Tennant BC. A preliminary report of a controlled study of thymosin alpha-1 in the woodchuck model of hepdnavirus infection. In: Block T, ed. Innovations in antiviral development and the detection of virus infection. New York: Plenum Press, 1992; 121-123.
36. Fourel I, Hantz O, Watanabe A, Jacquet C, Chomel B, Fox JJ et al. Inhibitory effects of 2'-fluorinated arabinosyl-pyrimidine nucleosides on woodchuck hepatitis virus replication in chronically infected woodchucks. Antimicr Chemother 1995; 34:473-475.

Section 5

Prophylaxis of Hepatitis Virus Infection

Epidemiology of Hepatitis B Virus Infection in Countries with Intermediate Prevalence. Immunization in Teenagers

M. Bruguera, L. Salleras

GEOGRAPHICAL DISTRIBUTION

HBV infection is spread all over the world. According to the prevalence of hepatitis B virus (HBV) markers the world has been divided into high, intermediate and low prevalence regions. In hyperendemic regions the prevalence of HBsAg carriers is higher than 5 %, and more than 50-90 % of the population have serological evidence of prior HBV infection. Areas of intermeadiate endemicity have an HBsAg carrier prevalence of 2 to 5% with 30 to 50% of the population having serological evidence of past HBV infection. Areas of low endemicity have a prevalence of HBsAg in the general population lower than 1 %. Some areas of intermediate endemicity have a prevalence of HBsAg carriers close to that of areas of low endemicity, such as Spain and the north of Italy, and other have a prevalence close to that found in countries with high endemicity, such as Eastern Europe countries.

MODES OF TRANSMISSION

HBV is transmitted by sexual contact, both homosexual and heterosexual, by contact with infected blood (i.e., transfusion with blood not tested for HBV), use of nonsterile needles for injecting drugs or non sterilized medical or dental equipment, sharing of razors and toothbrushes, tribal scarifications, or tattoing, and by perinatal (mother to child) transmission, usually at birth.

These mechanisms have a different predominance in the three epidemiological areas in which the world has been divided. In some countries of high HBV endemicity, such as Japan, China and the Pacific islands, perinatal transmission is the most efficient mechanism of transmission, and may account for as many as 40% of the total HBsAg carriers. In other regions such as Africa, horizontal transmission from child to child is responsible for the majority of HBV infections. The exact mode of transmission has not been established, but skin contact during plays or sharing the same bed may permit the entrance of virus from skin lesions of infected children through the injured skin of susceptible children.

In low endemicity areas hepatitis B occurs predominantly in adult population, mainly transmitted by sexual contact. A lower proportion of infected people have acquired the infection through intravenous drug abuse or in relation to their occupation, such as health care workers, policemen or educators of mentally handicapped people.

In intermediate endemicity areas, transmission may occur perinatally, during childhood due to the close contact of children with their carrier parents or brothers, or during adulthood due to sexual contact with a carrier or to parenteral inoculations. The epidemiological situation may greatly vary from one region to another. In south Italy transmission occurs predominantly during childhood, while in Spain it occurs predominantly among young adults. Perinatal transmission accounts for 20% of chronic HBsAg carriers in areas of intermediate endemicity.

OUTCOME OF HBV INFECTION

Clinical expression and outcome of HBV infection are mainly related to the duration of infection and status of the immune system. Young children rarely develop overt disease following HBV infection, but many of them become chronic carriers. The earlier the infection occurs, the higher the probability of progression to chronicity. More than 90% of children infected at birth become HBV carriers, but only about 25% of those infected between the age of 1 and 7.

HBV infection in adults induces clinical hepatitis in about one third of them. Infection progresses to chronicity in less than 5% of immunocompetent patients, but in more than 30% of those with any type of immunodeficiency, such as old age, renal failure or AIDS.

CONTROL OF HEPATITIS B

Preventive Measures

Some of these measures, such as the screening of blood donors of HBsAg, availability of disposable syringes and needles, and use of properly sterilized dental and medical equipment have been very useful to limit the spread of HBV infection, but have had a limited impact on the overall prevalence of the disease. The same has occurred with the educational campaigns, addressed to recommend safe sexual practices and not to share syringes and needles among drug addicts. Although they may account for a trend to the decrease of notified cases of hepatitis B since the end of the eighties in all developed countries, the burden of HB remains too heavy.

Table 1. High risk groups for hepatitis B virus infection

Intravenous drug-users
Sexually promiscuous (homosexual male and heterosexual)
Hemodialysis patients
Family contacts of HBV carriers
Newborns to HBsAg-positive mothers
Health care personnel
Institutionalized mentally-handicapped persons
Prisoners
Hemophiliacs and multitransfused patients

High Risk Group Immunization

Since its introduction in 1982, hepatitis B vaccination was recommended by health authorities for certain risk groups (table 1). The use of this strategy in developed countries has drastically reduced the incidence of hepatitis B in some of these groups, such as health care personnel, dialysis patients, hemophiliacs, institutionalized mentally-handicapped patients, and newborns to HBsAg carrier mothers. Its limited impact on the overall incidence of the disease is due to different reasons: *a*) members of such target groups for vaccination account for less than 10% of cases with hepatitis; *b*) the groups with higher risk, such as i.v. drug-users and promiscuous homosexual males, are not easily accessible to health services, and when they are reached because of other health problems they are very often already infected; *c*) more than 30% of cases of hepatitis B occur in the «normal» population. These individuals not belonging to one of the well-known risk groups would never be vaccinated according to the traditional vaccination strategies.

Universal Hepatitis B Vaccination

Universal hepatitis B immunization of infants in areas of high or intermediate endemicity (HBsAg carrier prevalence of 2% or greater) was recommended by the 1990 WHO EPI Global Advisory Group Meeting.

This is the only sure method to achieve the goal of hepatitis B eradication. In high endemicity countries in which most infections are acquired during childhood, no alternative strategies to generalized vaccination can be proposed. Developed countries of intermediate endemicity with programs of prevention of neonatal hepatitis B through universal screening of pregnant women and passive-active immunization of children born to infected mother, can choose universal immunization of adolescents instead of that of children in certain epidemiological situations. In these countries selective immunization of adults at high risk of infection should be maintained and implemented if possible.

Rationale for Adolescent Immunization

The following arguments may justify the decision to select adolescent as the target group for hepatitis B vaccination in developed countries of intermediate endemicity:

1. Hepatitis B is a disease of young adults, mainly related to sexual contacts and intravenous drug abuse. Infection of children is infrequent. Thus, vaccinating immediatly before the age of higher risk will be more cost-effective than earlier immunization. The delay before appreciating the reduction of incidence of hepatitis B infection will be 15-25 years shorter with the adolescent immunization strategy than with infants immunization.
2. A combined DTP and HB vaccine is not yet available. Thus integration of hepatitis B vaccine in routine infants immunization would require additional injections, a procedure that could decrease the compliance of vaccination programs in countries in which pediatricians are not familiar with hepatitis B among infants.
3. There is no yet information on the duration of the protection induced by hepatitis B vaccine when given in the first year of life. The assumption of long-lasting protection of responders to this vaccine is based on a less than 10 years follow-up of adults. Immunogenicity of hepatitis B vaccine is lower in newborns and very young children than in adolescents. Thus, it is conceivable that a part of vaccinees in infancy will become unprotected when they will be exposed to HBV 20 years later.
4. A strategy of adolescents immunization can only be proposed in countries in which a health service addressed to prevent other transmissible diseases or to early detection of treatable diseases in school population is available.

EXPERIENCE IN CATALONIA

Background Information

Catalonia is a 6 millions inhabitants region in the north east of Spain. According to the number of notified cases the estimated incidence rate of overt hepatitis B is 20-30 cases per 100,000. We can estimate 4,800 to 7,200 new HB infections each year assuming that subclinical cases are 3 times more frequent than icteric cases.

Hepatitis B is a disease of young adults in Catalonia, since about 65% of cases occur at ages between 15 and 30. Cases in people below 15 are less than 10%. A likely mode of transmission is recognized in 70% of patients.

A serologic survey of HBV markers in a representative sample of general population has shown that prevalence of markers in 14 year-old children is less than 2%. In people older than 25 the prevalence is 20%, and this prevalence practically does not raise despite increasing age.

All pregnant women are systematically screened for HBsAg and three doses of hepatitis B vaccine are given in most children born to HBsAg-positive mothers. These data suggest that hepatitis B is very infrequent during childhood and most cases acquire the infection between 15 and 30 years of age.

Description of the Program

The program was launched by the Health Department of Catalonia governement in September 1991 and was addressed to all 12 year-old school boys and girls. This age was chosen to avoid coincidence with immunization for measles, mumps and rubella, which is done at 11 years of age and for tetanus which is done at age 14.

One year before starting the program a booklet explaining the importance of hepatitis B and the epidemiologic rationale for the immunization program to be initiated was distributed to health professionals involved in the program, to school directors and to local authorities. An instruction manual outlining the exact procedures to be used was distributed to health officers in charge of the vaccination program in each health district.

An information campaign specifically addressed to hepatitis B and to the vaccination program was carried out during several months. A letter of informed consent was sent to all parents before vaccination of their children.

The vaccine used is Engerix B (20 mg per dose). The first dose is given without prevaccinal screening between the months of September and December. The second dose is given one month after the first and the third between March and June. Most vaccines are given in the school by school health teams composed by one doctor and one nurse, and others are given in the vaccination centers of Basic Health Services.

Since the program was launched, 3 cohorts of children (born in 1979, 1980 and 1981) have been immunized. A registration form for each vaccinee should be filled up and send to the Public Health Directory to allow the assessement of compliance of the program and coverage rate.

Results

During the first two years 114,854 children received three doses of vaccine, 5,383 two doses and 1,369 one dose. Vaccine coverage (three doses) for the first year of program was 76.2% and for the second year 79.3%.

Reasons for non vaccination were: lack of informed consent from the parents (28%), absentism (7%), previous hepatitis B vaccination (9%) and deficiencies of the program (57%).

Compliance to vaccination was slightly higher when the vacine was given in the school (93.5%) than when given in the Basic Health Service (90.5%) (NS).

There were two cases of unsuspected untoward reactions related to the vaccine. Both cases had an urticariform reaction after injection of the first dose of vaccine. A challenge with each component of the vaccine did not induce any specific reaction.

COMMENT

Strategies for hepatitis immunization will differ from area to area according to the epidemiologic patterns of HBV infection, socioeconomic factors and characteristics of health delivery services. Spain is a country of intermediate-low endemicity with well organized school health services. Hepatitis B is mainly a disease affecting adolescents and young adults, being very infrequent among children.

The vaccination program was designed to prevent infection in most exposed population. The assessment of the two first years shows a good coverage rate. The improvement of information of parents and health care providers will improve this coverage.

Taking into account the excellent immunogenicity of hepatitis B vaccine in young people we can assume that most vaccinees are protected against hepatitis B. Thus, a decline of the incidence of hepatitis B should be appreciated in the following years.

When a combined DTP and HB vaccine will be available universal immunization of infants with this vaccine will probably be started simultaneously with adolescent HB vaccination. When the first cohort of immunized infants will reach the age of 12, the program of vaccination of adolescents will end. A booster may be given at this age if loss of protection following HB vaccination at birth is demonstrated.

Epidemiology and Prevention of Hepatitis A

F. E. André

SUMMARY

In many countries serological surveys reveal a high prevalence of antibodies to the hepatitis A virus (HAV). This is particularly the case in underdeveloped countries and among people over the age of 50 in industrialised countries. Endemicity of the infection depends on the level of environmental sanitation and prevailing socio-economic and hygienic conditions, reflecting the enteric mode of HAV transmission. Travellers originating from industrialised countries are therefore at risk when travelling to endemic regions of the world. Improving sanitary standards in developing countries are also resulting in a growing proportion of older people being susceptible to HAV infection. Since worldwide travel is increasing and infection with HAV is more severe in older age groups, protection against infection is becoming more urgent. A vaccine (Havrix™) which offers long-term protection against HAV after a 2-dose primary course of vaccination followed by a booster became commercially available in early 1992. It is an inactivated whole-virion vaccine. A new formulation of the vaccine (Havrix 1440) has been licensed recently for adults, which is also safe and results in nearly 100% seroconversion 1 month after one dose. It contains twice the amount of viral antigen present in Havrix™. A booster dose administered 6-12 months after the first dose of either formulation induces high antibody titres which have been estimated by mathematical extrapolation to provide protection against HAV for 2 decades.

INTRODUCTION

Hepatitis A is a widespread disease of global importance that results from infection of the liver by the hepatitis A virus (HAV). HAV is a picornavirus which is virtually exclusively transmitted enterically (i.e., by the faecal-oral route), through ingestion of contaminated food or water and close contact with infected cases. It is very resistant to heat, pH changes, solvents and detergents (1). Hence the virus has a high prevalence in regions of the world where the quality of water supply and sewage disposal is less than ideal. The prevalence of HAV is also linked to behavioural and socio-economic factors (2). Despite most infected persons remaining asymptomatic and recovering completely, hepatitis A still has an elevated morbidity and mortality which leads to a large economic burden on society (3, 4). Around 1.4 million cases of hepatitis A are estimated to occur annually worldwide (5). Hepatitis A was the most frequently diagnosed type of hepatitis until a decade ago in USA (6).

In many underdeveloped countries, a high level of contamination of the environment with HAV leads to ubiquitous exposure of the population from a young age. In these hyperendemic regions, almost everyone demonstrates previous infection with HAV by the presence of specific antibodies (anti-HAV). In overdeveloped countries, the prevalence of antibodies against HAV is much lower, and has been falling continuously since the end of World War II, primarily through improved water supply and sewage disposal. These factors contribute to general improvements in hygiene and have also resulted in a continuing fall in the prevalence of hepatitis A infection in a growing number of rapidly industrialising countries. The consequence is an important and ongoing rise in the number and age of individuals who have not been exposed to HAV, and who are thus at risk of infection and disease. The potential health and economic impacts of HAV infection on these growing susceptible older populations are great, for infections at a young age are usually subclinical or asymptomatic, whereas the risk of symptomatic, clinical and fulminant hepatitis A rises with age, particularly in individuals over the age of 40.

PREVENTION

Preventive measures against hepatitis A remain the most effective and attractive approach for disease control, as no specific and reliable treatment for hepatitis A has yet been successfully developed. Administration of immunoglobulins, containing antibodies against hepatitis A, was the first method shown to be effective in preventing hepatitis A (7). Until recently, this was the only specific prevention method against hepatitis A. Frequent readministration of immunoglobulins every 3-6 months is required to ensure continuous protection. This is costly, logistically complex and results in low patient compliance through endured pain and higher incidence of reactions. The latter are due to the frequently large volumes of immunoglobulin that are injected to ensure protection. A vaccine stimulating long-term active immunity against hepatitis A would simplify and improve greatly both the prevention of hepatitis A on an individual basis as well as the implementation of public health measures against the disease.

The identification of HAV in 1973 accelerated research and development on candidate vaccines against HAV (8). Subsequently many different strains have been isolated; despite the fact that nucleotide sequencing of the HAV genome has shown almost 20% genetic heterogenicity between these strains (9), it is believed that there is only one serotype, as polyclonal antibodies cross-neutralise viruses from all genotypes (10). Initial work on vaccine development showed that marmosets immunised with a formaldehyde-inactivated virus (purified from infected marmoset liver) were protected against hepatitis A (11). Subsequent work focused on the development of a live attenuated vaccine (12, 13). Passaging of HAV in cell culture induces mutations over the whole genome and attenuates the virus (14). Several candidate attenuated vaccines have been demonstrated to be safe and immunogenic in humans (15-17). The major drawback with live attenuated vaccines is that reversion of the attenuated HAV to virulence cannot be completely ruled out, as the exact mutation(s) that is(are) responsible for attenuation is(are) unknown. High infectivity titres need to be injected to obtain a «take» that stimulates a good immune response. Furthermore, the likely difficulty in gaining regulatory approval also lowers the economic attractiveness of developing a live attenuated vaccine, particularly in view of the recent introduction of an inactivated vaccine.

It is interesting that the first safe, immunogenic and efficacious commercially available vaccine against hepatitis A, manufactured by SmithKline Beecham Biologicals, resulted from focusing on in vitro culture and inactivation of HAV, as initially attempted in the 1970s by Provost and Hilleman in their search for a vaccine against hepatitis A (11).

The development, manufacture and quality control of the inactivated hepatitis A vaccine bear similarities to the production process for the inactivated polio (Salk) vaccine. The HM 175 HAV strain used for manufacture was adapted for growth in human diploid MRC 5 cells by serial passaging. The virus is harvested and extracted by freezing and thawing, after a 3-week incubation period in plates with a unicellular layer of MRC 5 cells. The HAV is purified by several steps which include sterile filtration, ultrafiltration and concentration by chromatography (18). This virus suspension is finally inactivated by treatment with formaldehyde, at a concentration of 250 µg/ml, for 15 days at 37 °C. The suspension is tested to ensure complete HAV inactivation both during and after the inactivation step (19). The inactivated virions are then adsorbed on aluminium hydroxide as adjuvant, and 2.5-phenoxyethanol is added as preservative at a concentration of 5 mg/ml. The potency of the vaccine is measured in arbitrary enzyme-linked immunosorbent assay (ELISA) units (ELU) of HAV antigen, and the vaccine is formulated either at 720 or 1440 ELU/ml.

Up to the end of 1993, > 100 clinical studies with > 50,000 subjects had been initiated, involving the administration of > 120,000 doses. The 720 ELU vaccine is safe, clinically well-tolerated and immunogenic in all age groups above one year and elicits almost 100% seroconversion (anti-HAV ≥ 20 mIU/ml) one month after primary vaccination consisting of two doses 2-4 weeks apart. In adults, a 1440 ELU dose stimulates 88.1% seroconversion (SC) when measured 15 days later, and by month 1 the SC is 98.9% with a geometric mean titre (GMT) of 466 mIU/ml. In children, a 360 ELU dose administered at months 0 and 1 results in 95.4% SC at month 1 and 100% SC at month 2. A booster dose with the appropriate vaccine, given to either children or adults at month 6 or 12, results in a dramatic rise in antibody titres. These have been calculated, using a mathematical formula that fits the observed fall in antibody titre over time, to confer protection for approximately 20 years. The validity of this extrapolating formula was shown by taking the GMTs observed one year after the booster dose to calculate the predicted GMTs at years 2 and 3. These predicted GMTs were compared with the actual GMTs measured at years 2 and 3: only a 5% difference was found. If the lowest individual anti-HAV titre one year after the booster is applied to the formula, the persistence of protective titres would last 16 years. Likewise if the lower 95% GMT confidence limit one year after the booster is used for the formula, seroconverting anti-HAV titres would persist for 25 years.

The reactogenicity of the vaccine was assessed by evaluating individual and self-assessed symptom checklists. Around 50% of healthy vaccinated adults report no symptoms at all. The vaccine is well-tolerated, inducing mainly mild, transient local soreness at the site of injection in those reporting side effects. These resolve spontaneously. No adverse events of clinical importance which could be considered to be directly related to vaccination have been reported. To date, post-marketing surveillance of > 4 million distributed vaccine doses has confirmed the excellent safety profile of this vaccine in adults and children.

CONCLUSION

The disease and economic burden inflicted by the hepatitis A virus on a global basis is sufficiently heavy to justify efforts to control or eliminate the disease or even eradicate the virus. Recently a safe and efficacious vaccine that will make this possible was introduced. This first commercially-available vaccine against hepatitis A is being licensed in a continuously growing number of countries (so far in more than 30), including most Western European countries, Australasia and Canada. The advantages offered by this inactivated whole-virion vaccine is that it is inherently safe, and uses a simple and well-known manufacturing process for its production. The safety, immunogenicity and efficacy of inactivated vaccines against hepatitis A have been demonstrated in a trial in the USA, as well as in a larger double-blind, randomised protective efficacy field trial among over 40,000 schoolchildren in Thailand (20, 21). Under the field conditions for the latter trial, a protective efficacy of over 94% was observed a year after primary vaccination prior to administration of the booster dose. No cases occurred among vaccinees after the booster dose. As additional vaccines against hepatitis A developed by other research teams become licensed, and as the number of countries in which these hepatitis A vaccines are commercially available continues to grow, the ability to initiate, organise and implement immunisation programmes across the world will enable the global control and ultimate eradication of hepatitis A, as the virus does not have a natural animal reservoir. However eradication will become a reality only if there is global commitment to achieve it, as is currently the case for poliomyelitis.

REFERENCES

1. Flehmig B, Heinricy U, Pfisterer M. Prospects for a hepatitis A virus vaccine. Prog Med Virol 1990; 37:56-71.

2. Coulepis AG, Anderson BN, Gust ID. Hepatitis A. Adv Virus Res 1987; 32:129-169.
3. Centers for Disease Control. Trends based on reporting to national notifiable diseases surveillance system, 1989. Atlanta: United States Department of Health and Human Services. MMWR CDC Surveill Summ 1992; 54:9-12.
4. Özsoyen S, Kocak N. Acute hepatic failure related to hepatitis A. Lancet 1989; I:901.
5. Institute of Medicine. The prospects for immunizing against hepatitis A virus. In: New vaccine development: establishing priorities volume II. Diseases of importance in developing countries. Washington: National Academy Press 1986; 197-206.
6. Centers for Disease Control. Centers for Disease Control hepatitis surveillance. Atlanta: United States Department of Health and Human Services. MMWR CDC Surveill Summ 1990; 53:1-35.
7. Stokes J Jr, Neefe JR. The prevention and attenuation of infectious hepatitis by gamma globulin: preliminary note. JAMA 1945; 127:144-145.
8. Feinstone SM, Kapikian AZ, Purcell RH. Hepatitis A: detection by immune electron microscopy of a virus-like antigen associated with acute illness. Science 1973; 182:1026-1028.
9. Cohen JL, Ticehurst JR, Purcell RH, Buckler-White A, Baroudy BM. Complete nucleotide sequence of wild-type hepatitis A virus: comparison with different strains of hepatitis A virus and other picornavirus. J Virol 1987; 61:50-59.
10. Lemon SM, Chao SF, Jansen RW, Binn LN, LeDuc JW. Genomic heterogeneity among human and non-human strains of hepatitis A virus. J Virol 1987; 61:735-742.
11. Provost PJ, Hilleman MR. An inactivated hepatitis A virus vaccine prepared from infected marmoset liver. Proc Soc Exp Biol Med 1978; 159:201-203.
12. Hilleman MR, Provost PJ, Buynak EB, McLean AA. Progress toward a live attenuated human hepatitis A virus vaccine. Dev Biol Stand 1983; 54:433-440.
13. Karron RA, Daemer R, Ticehurst J, D'Hondt E, Popper H, Mihalik K, Philips J, Feinstone SM, Purcell RH. Studies of prototype live hepatitis virus vaccines in primate models. J Infect Dis 1988; 157:338-345.
14. Cohen JI, Rosenblum B, Ticehurst JR, Daemer RJ, Feinstone SM, Purcell RH. Complete nucleotide sequence of an attenuated hepatitis A virus: comparison with wild-type virus. Proc Natl Acad Sci USA 1987; 84:2497-2501.
15. Midthun K, Ellerbeck E, Gershman K, Calandra G, Krah D, McCaughtry M, Nalin D, Provost P. Safety and immunogenicity of a live attenuated hepatitis A virus vaccine in seronegative volunteers. J Infect Dis 1991; 163:735-739.
16. Mao JS, Dong DX, Zhang HY, Chen NL, Zhang XY, Huang HY, Xie RY, Zhou TJ, Wan ZJ, Wang YZ, Hu Z-H, Cao YY, Li HM, Chu CM. Primary study of attenuated live hepatitis A vaccine (H2 strain) in humans. J Infect Dis 1989; 159:621-624.
17. Sjogren M; Purcell RH, McKee K, Binn L, Macarthy P, Ticehurst J, Feinstone S, Caudill J, See A, Hoke C, Bancroft W, D'Hondt E. Clinical and laboratory observations following oral or intramuscular administration of a live attenuated hepatitis A vaccine candidate. Vaccine 1992; 10(Suppl 1):135-137.
18. André FE, Hepburn A, D'Hondt E. Inactivated candidate vaccines for hepatitis A. Prog Med Virol 1990; 37:72-95.
19. Peetermans J. Production, quality control and characterization of an inactivated hepatitis A vaccine. Vaccine 1992; 10(Suppl 1):99-101.
20. Werzberger A, Mensch B, Kuter B, Brown L, Lewis J, Sitrin R, Miller W, Shouval D, Wiens B, Calandra G, Ryan J, Provost P, Nalin D. A controlled trial of a formalin-inactivated hepatitis A vaccine in healthy children. N Engl J Med 1992; 327:453-457.
21. Innis BL, Snitbhan R, Kunasol P, Laorakpongse T, Poopatanakool W, Kozik CA, Suntayakorn S, Suknuntapong T, Safary A, Tang DB, Boslego JW. Protection against hepatitis A by an inactivated hepatitis A vaccine. JAMA 1994; 271:1328-1334.

Prevention of Transfusion-Associated Hepatitis C

A. González, J. I. Esteban

THE FIRST STEPS

Transfusion-associated hepatitis occurred in about 33 percent of transfused patients prior to 1970 according to a prospective study carried out at the National Institutes of Health in the United States (1). Such as high incidence was attributed to the high volume of blood received by the patients and the regular use of commercial donors. When serological tests to detect HBsAg positive donors were available and commercial donors were not further accepted, the incidence of transfusion-associated hepatitis fell abruptly to about 10 % (2). Retrospective analysis of stored serum samples from these patients showed that only 25 percent of them were related to the hepatitis B virus (1). Few years later, when an assay for hepatitis A virus was developed, it was found that no cases were related to hepatitis A. It was at this time when the term non-A, non-B hepatitis was first established (3).

SURROGATE MARKER SCREENING

The incidence of non-A, non-B transfusion-associated hepatitis in the United States after 1970 ranged from 7 to 10 percent as estimated from two large prospective studies, the Transfusion-Transmitted Virus Study and the study from the National Institutes of Health (NIH) (4-6). The analysis of sera from both donors and recipients from these studies suggested that transfusion of blood products from donors with elevated levels of ALT or with antibodies against the core antigen of the hepatitis B virus was three to four times more likely to transmit non-A, non-B hepatitis than blood lacking those markers. Both studies predicted that exclusion of such donors might prevent up to 45% of cases of transfusion-associated hepatitis. On this basis, elevated ALT and the presence of anti-HBc in blood were considered surrogate markers for non-A, non-B infection. Although a prospective study was never conducted in the United States to confirm these findings, the American Association of Blood Banks recommended routine donor ALT and anti-HBc screening in 1986. The implementation of these measures and the effect of donor screening for AIDS-related risk factors reduced the incidence of transfusion-associated hepatitis below 5% by 1990 (7).

A DIFFERENT SCENERY ACROSS THE OCEAN

The situation in Europe and more specifically in Spain was not the same. While the incidence of transfusion-associated hepatitis in the late 1970s and early 1980s in Northern Europe was a low as 2-4%, studies from the Mediterranean area showed an incidence up to 14% (8). The Hospital Vall d'Hebron from Barcelona carried out its first prospective study on transfusion-associated hepatitis at that time and a 12.6% incidence of non-A, non-B transfusion-associated hepatitis was found (9). Implementation of surrogate marker screening in Spain remained controversial because of the associated blood donors loss that would be close to 15 percent.

The Barcelona Post-transfusion Hepatitis Study is a prospective investigation that began in August 1988 as a randomized, double-blind, controlled trial of the efficacy of surrogate marker screening to decrease the incidence of non-A, non-B transfusion-associated hepatitis. The study was prematurely halted in June 1989 after the identification of hepatitis C virus. Analysis of the 280 patients included up to that moment showed an incidence of transfusion-associated hepatitis of 9.6% (10).

HEPATITIS C VIRUS FINALLY IDENTIFIED

In 1989, Michael Houghton and his colleagues from the Chiron Corporation reported the cloning of a part of the hepatitis C virus (HCV) genome (11). The proteins derived from this clones were then used to develop an assay to detect antibodies against HCV (12). Retrospective analysis of stored sera from prospectively followed patients with transfusion-associated hepatitis using this first-generation assay were subsequently published (10, 13, 14). Seroconversion to anti-HCV in the NIH study occurred in all patiens who developed chronic disease and in only 3 of 5 patients (60%) with apparently resolving disease (13). In the Barcelona study, 24 of 27 patients (89%) seroconverted to anti-HCV positive (10). Using the subsequently developed second-generation assays seroconversion rates reached 91% of cases (14). The presence of an anti-HCV positive donor was detected in 60 to 88 percent of cases using first generation antibody tests (10, 13) and in up to 93% of cases with second generation assays (14). From these studies it was anticipated that routine screening of all donors with first generation assays could prevent 60 to 85% of cases of transfusion-associated hepatitis (10, 14).

FIRST-GENERATION ANTI-HCV SCREENING. THE BEGINNING OF A NEW ERA

In July 1989 the Barcelona Post-tranfusion Hepatitis Study was converted into a prospective open efficacy trial of the prevention of transfusion-associated hepatitis by screening donors with the first generation enzyme immunoassay. Since a controlled study was ethically unacceptable, the pre-screening cohort of 280 recipients enrolled in the study in the immediate preceding year was used as an external control group. Until May 1990, 478 recipients were enrolled in the study. As shown in table 1, non-A, non-B hepatitis developed after transfusion in 9 of the 478 study recipients (1.9%); this represented an 80% reduction in the incidence of transfusion-associated hepatitis when compared with the 9.6% baseline incidence of the historial cohort (15).

When a second generation enzyme immunoassay became available, all stored sera were restrospectively tested. In the recipients of blood unscreened for anti-HVC, all 27 patients with transfusion-associated hepatitis plus one additional patient without symptoms or signs of hepatitis seroconverted to anti-HCV. So, 28 out of 262 patients without previous evidence of HVC infection became infected, for an incidence of 10.7%. In the recipients of anti-HCV negative blood, 7 of the 9 cases of hepatitis seroconverted and became HCV RNA positive. The incidence of HCV infection in that group was 1.5%, with an efficacy in reduction the risk of transfusion-associated hepatitis C infection of 86% (table 1). A seropositive donor was detected in 4 of the 7 hepatitis cases, suggesting that anti-HCV screening with a second generation assay would have further reduced the incidence of transfusion-associated hepatitis to 1 percent, and that of HCV infection to 0.6%.

Similar results using first generation anti-HCV assays have been reported from Japan (16) and United States (17). The study from the Japanese Red Cross (16) included patients with large volume transfusions. Starting from a baseline incidence of 7.7% while donors were screened only for ALT, after anti-HCV screening and simultaneous implementation of anti-HBc screening the incidence fell to 2.1%, for a prevention of about 70% of cases of transfusion-associated hepatitis. Regarding those recipients of less than ten blood units, the final incidence was 1.9%, the same as that from the Barcelona study. Donahue et al. in United States (17) analyzed sera from transfusion recipients prospectively followed from 1985 to 1991 and found that the incidence of HCV infection fell from a 3.8% o 0.7% after routine surrogate markers and anti-

Table 1. Impact of first and second-generation anti-HCV screening in the incidence of transfusion-associated non-A, non-B hepatitis and hepatitis C virus infection

	Donor anti-HCV status unknown	First-generation anti-HCV negative donors	Second-generation anti-HCV negative donors
Transfusion-associated non-A, non-B hepatitis			
Number at risk	280	478	471
Number of cases (rate)	27 (9.6%)	9 (1.9%)	4 (0.85%)
Risk reduction (%)		80	55[a]
Hepatitis C virus infection[b]			
Number at risk[c]	262	456	448
Number of cases (rate)	28 (10.7%)	7(1.5%)	2 (0.4%)
Risk reduction (%)		86	73[a]

From the Barcelona Post-transfusion Hepatitis Study.
[a] Risk reduction as compared to first-generation anti-HCV screening.
[b] Hepatitis C virus infection as detected by second-generation anti-HCV assay.
[c] Recipients with an anti-HCV positive pre-transfusion sample were not considered at risk for HCV infection.

HCV screening, for an 89% reduction in the relative risk of HCV seroconversion. Similarly, Aach et al. (14) in the retrospective analysis of patients from the TTV study predicted an 83% reduction in the incidence of transfusion-associated hepatitis after first generation anti-HCV screening. Remarkably, the decrease in transfusion-associated hepatitis was similar in the four studies, despite the different baseline incidence.

Of particular interest is the fact that in the Barcelona study, donors were not screened for surrogate markers and therefore, the decrease in incidence of transfusion-associated hepatitis was only due to anti-HCV screening. These results suggest that surrogate marker screening would not be necessary for the prevetion of HCV infection, specially in countries with high anti-HBc prevalence where such screening would result in unacceptable donor loss. Prevention of cryptic hepatitis B virus transmission would be the only reason to maintain anti-HBc screening in those countries in which it is already performed.

SECOND-GENERATION ANTI-HCV SCREENING. THE FINAL STEP?

In 1990 second generation anti-HCV screening of donors was introduced in the Blood Bank of the Hospital Vall d'Hebron. In order to prospectively assess the reduction of risk of transfusion-associated hepatitis after such policy, the Barcelona Post-transfusion Hepatitis Study has enrolled and followed 471 blood recipients since June 1992, and compared them with the 478 recipients included in the first generation study. The patients of both studies were similar according to age, sex, number of units of blood transfused, previous transfusion and prevalence of prior HCV infection. After six months of follow-up, 4 patients out 471 (0.85%) in the study group have developed hepatitis, as compared with 9 of 478 recipients (1.9%) in the control group (table 1). Thus, second generation anti-HCV screening achieved a 55% reduction in the risk of developing transfusion-associated hepatitis. Only 2 of the 4 recipients of second generation negative blood who developed hepatitis seroconverted. Second generation anti-HCV screening reduced the incidence of HCV infection from 1.5 to 0.4%, indicating a 73% reduction in risk of developing hepatitis C infection, as compared to first generation screening.

Aach et al. (14) in their retrospective analysis of the TTV study predicted a residual incidence of HCV transfusion-associated infection of 0.3% after screening donors by a second-generation assay. Only two prospective studies reporting the incidence of transfusion-associated hepatitis C infection after second-generation anti-HCV screening have been published (18, 19). Chung et al. (18), in a study carried out in Hong-Kong involving 158 transfusion recipients of second-generation anti-HCV negative blood found a 0.6% incidence of hepatitis C infection. Huang et al. (19) had a 13.8% baseline incidence of transfusion-associated hepatitis that second-generation anti-HCV screening reduced to 2.7%, from a group of only 112 recipients. Regarding hepatitis C infection, they found an initial incidence of 8.8% and no infected patients among the recipients of anti-HCV negative blood.

ANALYSIS OF RESIDUAL CASES OF HEPATITIS. WOULD IT NEVER END?

Retrospective testing by second-generation anti-HCV of the donors implicated in the 9 hepatitis cases from the first-generation branch of the Barcelona Post-transfusion Hepatitis Study detected an infectious donor in 4 of the 7 recipients who seroconverted to anti-HCV and in none of the 3 non-seroconverters. Further analysis of these donors and those implicated in the 4 cases of hepatitis from the second-generation assay study with a third generation anti-HCV enzyme immunoassay found no additional seropositive donors. Moreover, investigation of the presence of HCV-RNA by means of nested PCR failed to find any possible anti-HCV negative infectious donor. This finding probably means that second-generation is good enough to eliminate the risk of donor-recipient transfusion-associated transmission of the hepatitis C virus. Adding up the residual hepatitis cases from the two groups, there were 5 recipients with transfusion-associated hepatitis C infection in which no infectious donor could be detected, and 4 cases of transfusion-associated non-A, non-B, non-C hepatitis.

The origin of these residuals cases is still unclear. With regard to the 5 cases of HCV infection, the intensive investigations carried out seem to exclude transmission from an infectious donor. On this basis, the possibility of having non-transfusional acquired infections, that means, nosocomial infections needs to be addressed. Although it is still under investigation, 4 of these 5 infections could probably be considered as surgical but non-transfusion related.

The non-A, non-B, non-C hepatitis cases should be discussed apart. Aach et al. (14) found a 3.6% incidence of non-A, non-B, non-C hepatitis after retrospective analysis in recipients of anti-HCV unscreened blood. This incidence was not different from that among the control subjects that did not received blood products during surgery (3%). This result suggests that these hepatitis cases could probably be non-transfusion related. In an analysis from the NIH study (7), Alter found 12 cases of transfusion-associated non-A, non-B, non-C hepatitis. These cases had the same incubation period as hepatitis C cases, but jaundice was not present, the mean peak of ALT was lower and chronic infection developed only in 25% of cases. The non-C cases from the Barcelona study had a very similar clinical behaviour. Current investigations at the NIH seem to have found a new transfusion-transmitted viral agent that may be responsible for some of these non-A, non-B, non-C hepatitis cases. Would it be the hepatitis G virus?

REFERENCES

1. Alter HJ. You'll wonder where the yellow went: a 15-year retrospective of post-transfusion hepatitis. In: Moore SB, ed. Transfusion-transmitted viral diseases. Arlington: American Association of Blood Banks, 1987; 53-86.
2. Alter HJ, Holland PV, Purcell RH, Lander JJ, Feinstone SM, Morrow AG, Scmidt PJ. Post-transfusion hepatitis after exclusion of commercial and hepatitis-B-antigen-positive donors. Ann Intern Med 1972; 77:691-699.
3. Feinstone SM, Kapikian AZ, Purcell RH, Alter HJ, Holland PV. Transfusion-associated hepatitis not due to viral hepatitis type A or B. N Engl J Med 1975; 292:767-770.
4. Aach RD, Szmuness W, Mosley JW, Hollinger FB, Kahn RA, Stevens CE, Edwards VM, Werch J. Serum alanine aminotransferase of donors in relation to the risk of non-A, non-B hepatitis in recipients. The Transfusion-Transmitted Viruses Study. N Engl J Med 1981; 304:989-994.
5. Stevens CE, Aach RD, Hollinger FB, Mosley JW, Szmuness W, Kahn R, Werch J, Edwards V. Hepatitis B virus antibody in blood donors and the occurrence of non-A, non-B hepatitis in transfusion recipients. An analysis of the Transfusion-Transmitted Viruses Study. Ann Intern Med 1984; 101:733-738.
6. Koziol DE, Holland PV, Alling DW, Melpolder JC, Solomon RE, Purcell RH, Hudson LM, Shoup FJ, Krakauer H, Alter HJ. Antibody to hepatitis B core antigen as a paradoxical marker for non-A, non-B hepatitis agents in donated blood. Ann Intern Med 1986; 104:488-495.
7. Alter HJ. Post-transfusion hepatitis in the United States. In: Nishioka K, Suzulci H, Mishiko S, Oda T, eds.: Viral hepatitis and Liver Disease. Tokyo: Springer, 1994; 551-553.
8. Genescá J, Esteban JI, Alter HJ. Blood-borne non-A, non-B hepatitis: Hepatitis C. Sem Liver Dis 1991; 11:147-164.

9. Hernández JM, Piqueras J, Carrera A, Triginer J. Posttransfusion hepatitis in Spain. A prospective study. Vox Sang 1983; 44:231-237.
10. Esteban JI, González A, Hernández JM, Viladomiu L, Sánchez C, López-Talavera JC, Lucea D, Martín-Vega C, Vidal X, Esteban R, Guardia J. Evaluation of antibodies to hepatitis C virus in a study of transfusion-associated hepatitis. N Engl J Med 1990; 323:1107-1112.
11. Choo QL, Kuo G, Weiner AJ, Overby LR, Bradley DW, Houghton M. Isolation of a cDNA clone derived from a blood borne non-A, non-B viral hepatitis genome. Science 1989; 244:359-362.
12. Kuo G, Choo QL, Alter HJ, Gitnick GL, Redeker AG, Purcell RH, Miyamura T. An assay for circulating antibodies to a major etiologic virus of human non-A, non-B hepatitis. Science 1989; 244:362-364.
13. Alter HJ, Purcell RH, Shih JW, Melpolder JC, Houghton M, Choo QL, Kuo G. Detection of antibody to hepatitis C virus in prospectively followed transfusion recipients with acute and chronic non-A, non-B hepatitis. N Engl J Med 1989; 321:1494-1500.
14. Aach RD, Stevens CE, Hollinger FB, Mosley JW, Peterson DA, Taylor PE, Johnson RG, Barbosa LH, Nemo GJ. Hepatitis C virus infection in post-transfusion hepatitis. An analysis with first- and second generation assays. N Engl J Med 1991; 325:1325-1329.
15. Esteban JI, González A, Viladomiu L, Madoz P, Enriquez J, Genescá J, Quer J, Houghton M, Shih JWK, Alter HJ, Esteban R, Guardia J. Open prospective efficacy trial of anti-HCV screening of blood donors to prevent transfusion-associated hepatitis. Hepatology 1991; 14:94A.
16. Japanese Red Cross Non-A, Non-B Hepatitis Research Group. Effect of screening for hepatitis C virus antibody and hepatitis B virus core antibody on incidence of post-transfusion hepatitis. Lancet 1991; 338:1040-1041.
17. Donahue JG, Muñoz A, Ness PM, Brown DE, Yawn DH, MacAllister HA, Reitz BA, Nelson KE. The declining risk of post-transfusion hepatitis C virus infection. N Engl J Med 1992; 327:369-373.
18. Chung HT, Lee JSK, Lok ASF. Prevetion of post-transfusion hepatitis B and C by screening for antibody to hepatitis C virus and antibody to HBcAg. Hepatology 1993; 18:1045-1049.
19. Huang YY, Yang SS, Wu CH, Shih WS, Huang CS, Chen PH, Lin YM, Shen CT, Chen DS. Impact of screening blood donors for hepatitis C antibody on posttransfusion hepatitis: a prospective study with a second-generation anti-hepatitis C virus. Transfusion 1994; 34:661-665.

Section 6

Advances in Liver Transplantation

Opportunistic Infection after Liver Transplantation

D. Mutimer

INTRODUCTION

The liver transplant recipient is especially prone to infection. End-stage chronic liver disease and fulminant hepatic failure are frequently complicated by bacterial and fungal infection (1, 2). In the absence of pharmacological immunosuppression, chronic liver disease may also be associated with reactivation of latent cytomegalovirus infection (3). Patients with advanced autoimmune liver disease, patients with rheumatological disorders, and patients with failing grafts nominated for retransplantation, may have received significant amounts of immunosuppression prior to transplantation. Such patients are clearly «at risk» for infectious complications after major upper abdominal surgery.

BACTERIAL INFECTION COMPLICATING LIVER TRANSPLANTATION

Early pulmonary bacterial infection is due to atelectasis and sputum retention, and is secondary to major abdominal surgery in the presence of malnutrition and myopathy. Nevertheless, most liver transplant recipients are successfully extubated within 24 hours of surgery. Late bacterial infection is associated with biliary complications, and most frequently involves enterococcus and aerobic gram-negative organisms. Cholangitis, biliary leaks, and biliary strictures may be a consequence of biliary ischaemia. When these complications are experienced, doppler ultrasound examination of the hepatic artery is mandatory. In the absence of arterial thrombosis, bacterial infection usually resolves with the administration of broad-spectrum antibiotics and surgical drainage. Bacterial infection complicating arterial thrombosis may be controlled by antibiotics, but is usually an indication for regrafting. Bacterial infection and antibiotics predispose to fungal infection, and early use of prophylactic antifungal therapy should be considered in this context. Bacterial infection may also be associated with reactivation of latent Herpesvirus infection.

Most liver transplant units now experience a fairly restricted range of opportunistic infections. The most commonly encountered opportunistic pathogens include cytomegalovirus and fungi. Infection with Epstein-Barr virus is clearly associated with the development of post-transplant lymphoproliferative disease. Infection with these pathogens is discussed in detail.

CYTOMEGALOVIRUS INFECTION COMPLICATING LIVER TRANSPLANTATION

Cytomegalovirus (CMV) infection frequently complicates both bone marrow and solid organ transplantation. CMV «infection» simply means laboratory evidence of infection. Conventional methods for diagnosis of infection include serology (appearance of CMV-specific IgM, and/or rise in IgG titre), viral culture (usually buffy-coat and urine), and histology (characteristic «owl's eye» inclusions, immunohistology). The reported incidence of CMV infection in liver transplant recipients ranges from 28-60% (4-9), with higher rates of infection reported when surveillance is performed prospectively. Most infection is asymptomatic, and the reported incidence of symptomatic infection (often called «CMV disease») in the same series ranges from 15-40%. Clinical manifestations of infection are principally dependent on the pre-transplant immune status of the recipient. «Infection» usually complicates the use of a CMV-seropositive organ (5, 6, 9), but «disease» is most often associated with primary CMV exposure (infection of a seronegative recipient). Other risk factors for CMV infection include a pre-transplant diagnosis of fulminant hepatic failure, and the use of antilymphocyte preparations (6, 8, 9).

Symptomatic infection is a viraemic illness, and CMV disease is nearly always associated with a «flu-like» syndrome. In addition, laboratory features and clinical symptoms of specific organ involvement may be encountered. Hepatitis, enteritis, colitis, and pneumonitis are observed. Compared with other solid-organ transplant recipients, CMV hepatitis may be more frequently encountered in liver transplant recipients. CMV pneumonitis is the scourge of bone marrow transplantation, but this complication is rarely experienced by liver recipients (present incidence in Birmingham less than 1%). CMV may be responsible for significant morbidity, but rarely causes the death of a liver transplant recipient. Asymptomatic infection is of no clinical significance, and has no sequelae.

Diagnosis

The ideal diagnostic method should be sensitive, specific (for symptomatic versus asymptomatic infection), and provide results at the time of the onset of symptoms. Surveillance methods should be positive prior to the onset of symptoms. Prospective studies have highlighted the inadequacy of conventional diagnostic methods for the surveillance and diagnosis of CMV infection (10-12). The potential of CMV viraemia (positive viral culture) for differentiating clinically important CMV infection from asymptomatic infection is recognised (11-14), but cytopathic effect is slow to develop in conventional cell culture. Many laboratories now combine viral culture with immunohistochemical detection (15), a modification which expedites diagnosis.

More recently, the polymerase chain reaction (PCR), and the «antigenaemia test» have been promoted as clinically useful diagnostic methods (16). For both techniques, blood (buffy-coat) is used as substrate. PCR is an extremely sensitive method for the detection of viral nucleic acid. A negative result excludes significant infection, but a positive result is often observed in patients with asymptomatic infection. Specificity and positive predictive value (for symptomatic infection) of the PCR may be improved by the development of quantitative assays (17-19).

«Antigenaemia» techniques involve the *in situ* immunological detection (using one or more monoclonal antibodies) of CMV antigens in buffy-coat smears. The number of antigen-positive cells correlates with the clinical expression of the infection. Therefore, when the number of CMV positive cells is high (greater than 10/50,000 cells), then symptoms are likely to be the consequence of CMV infection.

PCR and antigenaemia tests have been used for surveillance, for rapid confirmation of symptomatic infection, and for monitoring response to antiviral therapy.

Many transplant units employ no virological surveillance and do not rely on rapid diagnostic techniques. In the context of liver transplantation, most symptomatic infection can be recognised by a pattern of clinical features. When primary exposure is associated with the development of fever and neutropenia in the second month after transplantation, then CMV infection is likely, and appropriate measures (including reduction of immunosuppression) should be taken. When immunosuppression is reduced, relapse after specific therapy is rare (fig. 1). Despite theoretical merit, the use of laboratory techniques to monitor antiviral therapy is of unproven benefit. Nevertheless, the prevention of symptomatic infection has been the focus of numerous clinical studies.

Prevention of Infection (table 1)

Approaches to the prevention of symptomatic infection include:

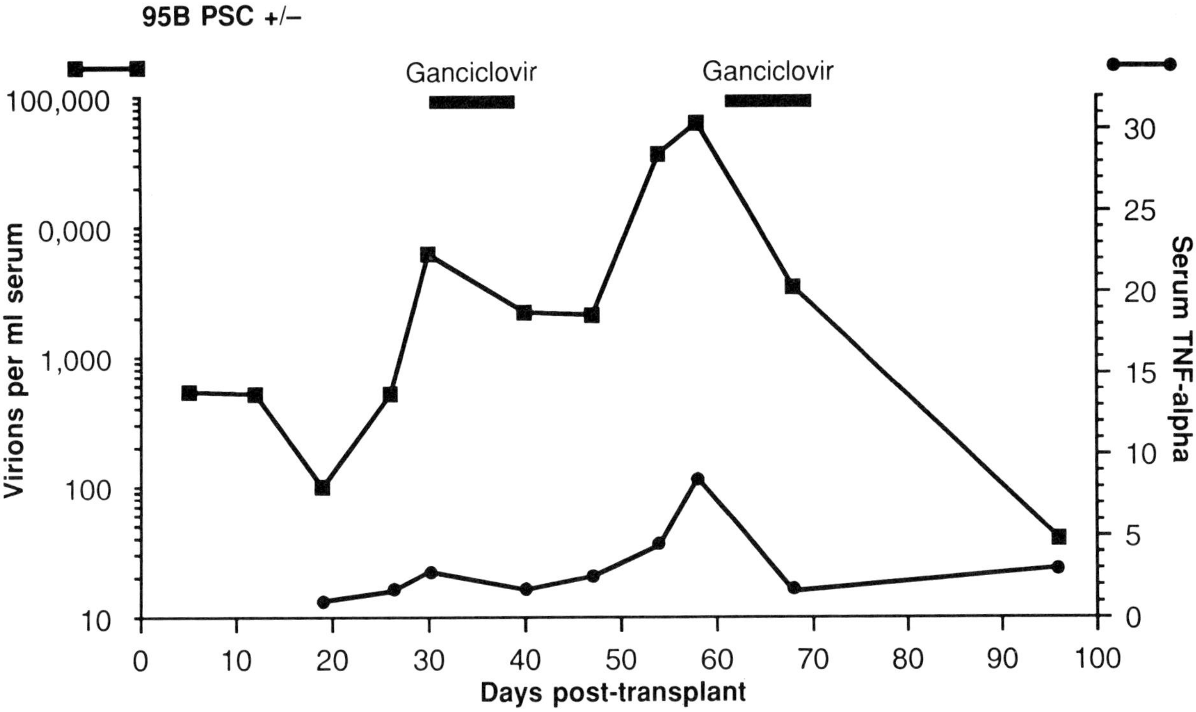

Creatinine	138	143	157	170	104
K	4.6	4.6	5.9	5	4.9
FK 506 level	20.1	18.3	14.5	10.1	6.8
FK 506 dose	12	10	8	3	2/3

Fig. 1. Management of CMV infection should include appropriate reduction in immunosuppression. Patient 95B was transplanted for end-stage primary sclerosing cholangitis (PSC). He was a seronegative recipient of a seropositive organ (+/-). CMV DNA was measured in serum using a newly developed quantitative PCR assay. Synchronous serum electrolytes (creatinine and potassium), FK506 blood levels, and FK506 dose are shown below x axis. Serum tumour necrosis factor (TNF-alpha) is also shown graphically. This patient received pre-emptive treatment with ganciclovir commencing on day 28 post-transplantation. Serum electrolytes and FK506 levels suggest that the reduction of FK506 dose was inadequate. Despite pre-emptive treatment he presented on day 57 with symptomatic infection which responded to ganciclovir. Appropriate reduction of FK506 dose was achieved. Levels of CMV fell rapidly.

1. *CMV matching.* The use of CMV seronegative liver and blood for seronegative recipients. This approach is often precluded by considerations of urgency and organ size compatibility.

Table 1. Strategies to reduce the incidence of symptomatic infection

A. *CMV matching:* seronegative liver and blood for seronegative recipients
B. *Universal prophylaxis:* anti-viral prophylaxis from the time of transplantation for seropositive recipients and for recipients of seropositive organs
C. *Diagnostic surveillance and pre-emptive therapy:* antiviral therapy for asymptomatic patients with positive surveillance cultures

2. *Universal prophylaxis.* The use of antiviral prophylaxis from the time of transplantation (or from the time of marrow recovery in the context of bone marrow transplantation). Most studies of this type have excluded the «low-risk» seronegative recipient of a seronegative liver. Passive immunoprophylaxis with high-titre anti-CMV immunoglobulin (20), high-dose acyclovir (21), ganciclovir (22), and various combinations of these three, have all been recommended.

The landmark study of this type was conducted by Balfour et al in renal transplant recipients (23). In that placebo-controlled study, high-dose acyclovir effectively reduced the incidence of CMV disease, and this reduction was also observed in patients with primary CMV exposure. Some investigators have been unable to confirm this beneficial effect in renal transplant patients (24, 25). The merit of high-dose acyclovir prophylaxis for liver transplant recipients also remains unproven (21, 26). The sequential use of IV ganciclovir, then oral acyclovir may provide more effective prophylaxis (27, 28).

3. *Diagnostic surveillance and pre-emptive therapy.* The use of pre-emptive antiviral therapy directed by the results of surveillance diagnostic methods. Implementation of this type of strategy requires the application of rapid diagnostic methods, and frequent sampling. Effective strategies for prevention of symptomatic infection in bone marrow transplant recipients have been published (29, 30). Pre-emptive ganciclovir treatment for patients with positive surveillance cultures may also prevent the subsequent development of symptomatic infection in liver transplant recipients (26).

The medical literature will be biassed by publication of studies with favorable results. Proposed strategies should be exposed to rigorous prospective testing and cost-benefit analysis. Strategies proposed and proven in the context of bone marrow transplantation may not be relevant to the management of liver transplant recipients.

Treatment of CMV Disease

The treatment of established symptomatic CMV infection should always include an appropriate reduction of immunosuppression. Infection is usually associated with neutropenia, and most clinicians suspend treatment with, or at least reduce the dose of azathioprine. When infection is life-threatening, or associated with other opportunistic infection, then immunosuppression should be stopped. A reduction of net immunosuppression also prevents relapse, and may be an essential component of those strategies which target pre-emptive therapy at «high-risk» patients (fig. 1).

Ganciclovir (2,3 DHPG) is routinely used by most Units for the treatment of symptomatic infection. A number of uncontrolled reports support its use (7, 9, 31-34). Dose adjustment is essential for patients with renal impairment. Side-effects include neutropenia (more commonly observed in the bone marrow transplant population), and a reversible rise in serum creatinine. The recommended duration of therapy is usually 14 days, but treatment may be shortened if rapid symptomatic improvement occurs as immunosuppression is reduced.

For patients with life-threatening infection (usually pneumonitis), the addition of CMV hyperimmune globulin may be beneficial (32).

In summary, liver transplantation is frequently complicated by evidence of CMV infection. Most infection is asymptomatic, and symptomatic infection is rarely life-threatening. Most symptomatic infection responds quickly and permanently to reduced immunosuppression and treatment with ganciclovir. Surveillance and prophylaxis are expensive, and have not been shown to influence graft or patient survival. No published strategy can be universally recommended. Transplant units should probably have access to, and/or develop a rapid diagnostic technique to verify established infection in febrile patients.

EPSTEIN-BARR VIRUS INFECTION COMPLICATING LIVER TRANSPLANTATION

Epstein-Barr virus (EBV), a human B lymphotropic herpes virus, infects more than 90% of the human population worldwide and persists for life in the infected host. Upon primary infection, EBV may cause infectious mononucleosis, a self-limiting lymphoproliferative disorder. EBV has also been associated with several human lymphoid malignancies including Burkitt's lymphoma, Hodgkin's disease, lymphomas in HIV-infected individuals, and post-transplant lymphoproliferative disorders (PTLD).

In immunocompetent individuals EBV-infected cells are effectively controlled by virus-specific cytotoxic T cells. Little is known about «latent» infection in healthy individuals. It is assumed that immunosuppression-mediated relaxation of T cell immunosurveillance may facilitate the outgrowth of EBV-harbouring cells, with the subsequent development of PTLD.

EBV immortalises resting B cells in vitro, converting them into permanently growing lymphoblastoid cell lines (LCL's). Every cell in the LCL contains multiple copies of the viral episome, and constitutively expresses a limited set of viral gene products (the latent proteins). Small non-coding RNA's (EBER's) are also expressed in abundance, and are a feature of all types of latent EBV infection. The immunoblastic lymphomas that develop in immunosuppressed patients display the same pattern of EBV gene expression that is observed in the LCL.

Diagnosis

Our understanding of EBV infection has paralleled developments in molecular virology. Initial work depended on serological testing (35-37), and cord blood transformation assays (37-40).

Spontaneous LCL formation from blood lymphocytes (with or without cyclosporin A) is a valuable tool which provides sufficient substrate for RFLP and Western blot analyses. Transformation assays are unsuitable for routine diagnostic work. Immunohistology and in situ DNA hybridisation permit phenotypic characterisation of EBV-infected cells (41, 42). The most recent developments for the study of EBV infection include the application of EBER RNA in situ hybridisation (43, 44) and the polymerase chain reaction (45-49).

Transformation assays suggest that immunosuppression results in outgrowth of EBV-infected cells, and that increased viral shedding from the oropharynx is matched by an increase in the number circulating EBV-infected B lymphocytes (36, 50). These assays also suggest that antiviral therapy reduces EBV shedding without concomitant reduction of lymphocyte-associated EBV (51). Transformation assays provide only semiquantitative information since EBV types do not possess equal transforming capacity.

A dot-blot DNA hybridisation assay has been used to quantitate oropharyngeal EBV shedding in renal transplant recipients (49). In patients with primary EBV exposure, EBV shedding is first detected by dot-blot hybridisation at a median time of 6 weeks post-transplantation. Using PCR and primers from a highly conserved region of the viral genome, Telenti et al. examined blood transplant recipients, patients with infectious mononucleosis, and normal controls (46). When transplant recipient blood was examined, amplified EBV sequences could be visualised by ethidium bromide staining without the need for Southern blotting. EBV detection in infectious mononucleosis blood required blotting and hybridisation, and virus could not be detected in the blood of normal control patients. These (semiquantitative) observations are consistent with the results of transformation assays, and suggest an immunosuppression-mediated outgrowth of EBV-infected cells.

The potential of EBER RNA *in situ* hybridisation to provide semiquantitative information, and the clinical relevence of that information, is highlighted by the study of Rhandawa et al (44). This study examined liver allograft biopsies by EBER in situ hybridisation, and found that the number of EBER-positive cells is associated with, and might even predict, the development of EBV-associated lymphoproliferative disease.

EBV-Related Syndromes Following Transplantation

Infiltration of the liver allograft with EBV-positive cells may be associated with graft dysfunction (EBV «hepatitis») (52-54), and with the subsequent development of PTLD (44).

EBV hepatitis is characterised histologically by the expansion of portal tracts with, and lobular infiltration by, EBV-positive immunoblasts, lymphocytes and plasma cells (52, 53). Langnas et al. reported the association of EBV hepatitis with the use of the monoclonal antibody OKT3 (53). Immunosuppression may further aggravate graft dysfunction in this setting, and antiviral therapy may be indicated (54). Infiltration of the graft with EBV-positive inflammatory cells may predict the subsequent development of lymphoproliferative disease (44).

Organ transplantation (and the consequent use of immunosuppression) is clearly associated with an increased incidence of lymphoma (55). Lymphomas comprise 22% of all malignancies developing in the transplant recipient (5% in the general population). Most lymphomas in this setting are non-Hodgkin's lymphomas, and there is a propensity for extranodal disease especially involving the central nervous system. Most post-transplant lymphomas are morphologically large cell lymphomas (or immunoblastic sarcomas). Burkitt's lymphoma is also seen following transplantation. In this setting, the characteristic chromosomal translocations (between ch8 and 2,14 or 22) are observed, but a minority are EBV-positive (in endemic areas more than 95% are EBV-positive) (56).

Post-transplant large cell lymphomas are clearly associated with EBV infection. Primary exposure to EBV infection at the time of transplantation appears to be associated with an increased risk for the development of lymphoma (and other PTLD's) (37, 49, 57-59). Risk also appears related to the total dose and duration of immunosuppression (60). Virtually every type of immunosuppressive agent has been implicated in the development of PTLD. Risk is proportional to the net state of immunosuppression, and possibly related to the temporal sequence in which agents are employed (49). There has been a tendency for the initial (i.e., at the time of introduction of an agent for clinical use) dosage regimen of immunosuppressive agents to be higher than is subsequently found necessary for the prevention of graft rejection. It is not surprising that the new immunosuppressive agent, FK506, has already been associated with reports of PTLD (61, 62). The use of antilymphocyte preparations such as anti-lymphocyte globulin (ALG) and OKT3 is strongly associated with the subsequent development of lymphoma (49, 59, 63-67). There is also a strong inverse relationship between the dose of immunosuppression and the time elapsed until the development of lymphoma (63, 64). Multiple courses (and total dose) of antilymphocyte preparations are strongly associated with the very early development of PTLD (64, 66, 67). The mean interval from transplantation to time of diagnosis of PTLD (for patients receiving OKT3) was only 44 days in one study (67).

The term «post-transplant lymphoproliferative disease» encompasses a range of B cell hyperplasias, and includes both benign polyclonal proliferation and malignant (monoclonal) lymphoma. Assessment of clonality may be of prognostic importance, and has implications (theoretical at least) for patient management.

Assessment may be morphological (i.e., monomorphic versus polymorphic proliferation) (68, 69). More sophisticated analyses include examination of immunoglobulin light and heavy chains eg in monotypic B cell proliferation more than 75% of immunoglobulin-positive cells carry the same light and heavy chains in double-stained sections (70), and the majority of cells will be either kappa or lambda light chain positive (68). Alternatively, clonality can be assessed by examination of immunoglobulin heavy chain gene rearrangements in B cell derived disease (69, 71), and by T cell receptor gene rearrangements in the uncommon EBV-positive T cell lymphomas (41). In EBV-positive proliferations, clonality can also be determined by RFLP (using the BamHI restriction enzyme) analysis of the terminal repeat region of the EBV genome (41, 72, 73).

No useful strategy exists for the treatment of EBV-associated PTLD. Most authors agree that immunosuppresion should be reduced or completely withdrawn. Some PTLD respond to reduction of immunosuppression, suggesting recovery of EBV-specific T cell control (61, 71). It has been suggested that polyclonal proliferation is more likely to respond to this manoeuvre (71, 74).

Antivirals have also been recommended for the treatment of EBV-associated disease following organ transplantation. During active EBV infection, infected cells have a high copy number of the EBV genome in a linear duplex, and fully assembled viral particles are produced for subsequent release. At this stage the virus is potentially susceptible to antiviral chemotherapy. Episomal circular EBV genome in latently infected cells is not susceptible. EBV early gene products (not produced in latent infection) include thymidine kinase, which is required for activation of acyclovir. Only EBV DNA synthesis dependent on the viral DNA polymerase is susceptible to inhibition by acyclovir. The latent circular form, which replicates in concert with the cell cycle using cellular DNA polymerase, is not selectively inhibited by this nucleoside analogue (75).

Immunosuppression increases viral shedding from the oropharynx (49, 50, 76), an effect inhibited by treatment with acyclovir (49, 51), ganciclovir (49) and interferon (39). The transforming capacity of patient blood, however, remains unaffected by antiviral therapy, and suggests no concomitant reduction in the levels of EBV infection of circulating B cells (51, 75). B cells contain EBV in a latent non-lytic form, and in this setting EBV should not be susceptible to currently available antiviral therapy. Linear forms of EBV have, however, been detected in EBV-associated lymphomas, and antivirals have been recommended for treatment (74). In view of the association of PTLD with primary EBV infection and with the use of antilymphocyte preparations, some groups recommend the prophylactic use of antivirals when seronegative patients require antilymphocyte treatment (49, 77). A role for antivirals in treatment and prophylaxis remains unproven, however, and Shapiro et al. reported 6 patients who developed lymphoproliferative disease while receiving prophylactic acyclovir (70). In summary, non-malignant lymphoproliferative disease will probably regress when immunosuppression is withdrawn. Malignant lymphoma is usually fatal (59), and no convincing argument exists for the use of antivirals in this setting. Immunosuppression should be withdrawn (with the hope that the proliferation will be T cell responsive), and conventional combination chemotherapy should be used for persistent disease.

Prevention is better than cure, and antilymphocyte preparations should be used sparingly, especially in the paediatric population.

INFECTION WITH HERPES SIMPLEX VIRUS

The association of immunosuppression with reactivation of other Herpesviruses is well recognised. Reactivation of Herpes Simplex Virus (HSV, types 1 and 2) is usually encountered in the first 2 weeks after transplantation. Lesions are usually mucocutaneous, and respond rapidly to treatment with acyclovir. Herpetic oesophagitis is an important cause of odynophagia, and is usually associated with oropharyngeal lesions. HSV hepatitis is a rare complication of solid organ transplantation (78). HSV hepatitis is often a manifestation of disseminated infection, and is frequently associated with disseminated intravascular coagulation. Unfortunately, the diagnosis is usually established by post-mortem examination.

Clinically significant HSV infection can be prevented by acyclovir prohylaxis. Infection is also prevented by prophylactic regimes designed to prevent CMV infection.

FUNGAL INFECTION COMPLICATING LIVER TRANSPLANTATION

Liver transplant recipients appear more prone to fungal infection than are other solid organ transplant recipients. Fungal infection is rarely encountered when the first-time recipient has a technically successful transplant operation and a brief ICU stay with early extubation. Clinically important fungal infection is particularly associated with the transplantation of high-risk candidates who then experience significant perioperative complications. Infection is strongly associated with death, but is almost invariably a sign that something else has «gone wrong».

A number of transplant groups have reported their experience with fungal infection. These reports usually describe, or at least include, early experience in liver transplantation. With improvements in patient selection and timing of transplantation, refinements in surgical technique and intensive care, and also reflecting a more conservative approach to immunosuppression, it seems likely that the reported incidence of fungal infection is higher than that currently experienced by established liver transplant centres. In addition, recent improvements in anti-fungal prophylaxis may have further reduced the incidence of this complication.

Candida (principally *C.albicans*) and *Aspergillus* (*fumigatus* and *flavus*) species are responsible for most episodes of fungal infection. Most reports distinguish fungal «colonisation» (isolation from a single superficial site such as the oropharynx) from deep-seated and invasive «infection». In reported experience, infection complicated 8-42% of transplants, and dissemination occured in 6-38% of all transplants (79-85). Infection with *Candida* species uncommonly (about 15% of cases) disseminates, whereas isolation of Aspergillus species is nearly always associated with disseminated infection (79, 84, 85). The median interval from transplantation to diagnosis of infection is about 2 weeks, and the majority of infections occur in the first 2 months after transplantation.

Candida albicans is a commensal organism which can be isolated from the gut and oropharynx of most recipients prior to transplantation. Infection is endogenous, and consequent upon *a*) physical breakdown of mucosal defences (ie surgery and its complications), and *b*) translocation secondary to mucosal ischaemia, in the presence of overgrowth encouraged by broad-spectrum antibiotics and immunosuppression.

Aspergillus is not commensal, and infection is secondary to environmental contamination. *Aspergillus* infection may be sporadic or may occur in clusters. Clustering of infection may be observed in association with environmental hazards such as concurrent hospital renovations, or faulty air-conditioning and ward ventilation. We have observed a remarkable seasonal variation in the incidence of Aspergillus infection (November to April)(86).

Diagnosis

Diagnosis depends on recognition of fungal hyphae in biological specimens and/or positive culture. Culture of Candida species from superficial sites has poor predictive value for dissemination. Blood cultures are insensitive for the diagnosis of dissemination, but predictive value is high. Of available diagnostic techniques, detection of free antigen in serum may have the greatest sensitivity and predictive value for the diagnosis of disseminated Candidiasis (84).

Risk Factors for Infection (table 2)

Risk factors for fungal infection are well characterised, and identify potential recipients of prophylactic therapy. Aetiology of liver failure has not been recognised as a risk factor, but patients with fulminant hepatic failure (FHF) are underrepresented in most reported series. FHF is frequently complicated by bacterial and fungal sepsis (1, 2), and our own experience strongly suggests that patients with FHF undergoing liver transplantation are at special risk of complicating fungal infection. Analyses agree that retransplantation is the major risk factor for fungal infection (79, 80, 82, 86). In addition to retransplantation, preoperative characteristics identifying patients at high risk for the subsequent development of fungal infection include: *a*) hospitalisation prior to transplantation, *b*) need for the intensive care unit (ICU) and mechanical ventilation immediately prior to transplantation, and *c*) pre-transplant serum bilirubin and albumin (79, 80, 82, 86). Intra-operative risk factors include operative time and transfusion requirements (79, 80). Post-operative factors associated with fungal infection include: *a*) duration of ICU stay and/or return to ICU, *b*) re-intubation and need for tracheostomy, *c*) need for further laparotomy, *d*) bacterial infection and prolonged antibiotic therapy, *e*) number of rejection episodes and number of steroid boluses, *f*) haemodialysis requirement, and *g*) vascular complications (79, 80). It is clear that many of these risk factors are related, and that most patients with significant fungal infection will have more than one risk factor. For instance, hepatic artery thrombosis is complicated by bacterial infection with a need for prolonged antibiotic therapy and regrafting. Death following transplantation is frequently associated with disseminated fungal infection. Diagnosis is frequently missed *ante mortem*, and often established only at postmortem examination (79, 81, 86). Dissemination is especially associated with *Aspergillus* infection (79, 83, 86), and involvement of the central nervous system is particularly common (86). *Aspergillus* infection should be suspected when a patient with pul-

Table 2. Risk factors for fungal infection: these characteristics identify potential recipients of antifungal prophylaxis

Preoperative:
Retransplantation (most important)
Need for hospitalization pre-transplant
Need for intensive care and ventilation
High bilirubin and low albumin
Intra-operative
Operative time
Transfusion requirements
Post-operative:
Duration of ICU stay or return to ICU
Pre-intubation and need for tracheostomy
Bacterial infection and antibiotic therapy
Rejection and steroids
Need for further laparotomy
Need for haemodialysis
Vascular complications

monary infiltrates develops unexplained neurological symptoms.

Treatment

Treatment of established *Aspergillus* infection is unsatisfactory, and most infected patients die despite treatment with amphotericin (79, 80, 85, 86). Wajszczuk et al. (80) reported 3 patients who developed disseminated *Aspergillus* during amphotericin treatment for *Candida* infection. Such reports suggest a limited role for amphotericin as prophylaxis against *Aspergillus* infection. A potential role for itraconazole in the treatment of *Aspergillus* infection has been suggested (85). Cyclosporin (and FK506) levels should be monitored carefully during concomitant itraconazole (and ketoconazole) therapy.

Clinically significant candidiasis is frequently responsive to treatment with amphotericin (79) or fluconazole (87). Liposomal encapsulation of amphotericin reduces nephrotoxicity, and this preparation may be preferable to the non-encapsulated form in patients with renal dysfunction. Fluconazole is not nephrotoxic, and has minimal effect on hepatic cytochrome function. It can be administered orally or intravenously, and is now employed extensively by many transplant centres. Its favourable toxicity profile, and bioavailability following oral administration, suggest a role for its use in prophylaxis for high-risk patients (88, 89).

Selective bowel decontamination (SBD) reduces *Candida* colonisation of the gut, and may reduce the incidence of significant *Candida* infection (90).

To reduce the incidence of candidiasis, we use oral non-absorbable antifungals (nystatin and amphotericin) in all transplant recipients, we encourage early enteral feeding, and fluconazole is administered at an early stage for high-risk patients. These measures appear to prevent clinically significant candidiasis. Prophylaxis and treatment of *Aspergillus* infection remain an unsolved challenge.

SUMMARY AND CONCLUSIONS

Infectious complications are an important cause of morbidity and mortality following liver transplantation. Most transplant units now observe a reduced incidence and narrower range of opportunistic infections. This is a consequence of improved patient selection and timing of transplantation, better surgical technique (fewer technical complications), and a more conservative approach to immunosuppression. In particular, a greater reluctance to use anti-lymphocyte preparations has reduced the incidence of *Herpesvirus* and fungal infection.

Infectious complications rarely cause the death of our patients. Instead, the patient who dies after liver transplantation usually succumbs to infection with multiple organisms in the setting of multiple organ system failure. In this context, such patients frequently had poor preoperative condition, and transplantation was complicated by technical problems.

REFERENCES

1. Rolando N, Harvey F, Brahm J, Philpott-Howard J, Alexander G, Gimson A, Casewell M, Fagan E, Williams R. A prospective study of bacterial infection in acute liver failure: an analysis of fifty patients. Hepatology 1990; 11:49-53.
2. Rolando N, Harvey F, Brahm J, Philpott-Howard J, Alexander G, Casewell M, Fagan E, Williams R. Fungal infection: a common, unrecognised complication of acute liver failure. J Hepatol 1991; 12:1-9.
3. Tanaka S, Toh H, Minagawa H, Mori R, Sugimachi K, Minamishima Y. Reactivation of cytomegalovirus in patients with cirrhosis: analysis of 122 cases. Hepatology 1992; 16:1409-1414.
4. Barkholt L, Ericzon B-G, Tollemar J, Malmborg A-S, Ehrnst A, Wilczek H, Andersson J. Infections in human liver recipients: different patterns early and late after transplantation. Transplant Int 1993; 6:77-84.
5. Gorensek MJ, Carey WD, Vogt D, Goormastic M. A multivariate analysis of risk factors for cytomegalovirus infection in liver-transplant recipients. Gastroenterology 1990; 98:1326-1332.
6. Paya CV, Wiesner RH, Hermans PE, Larso-Keller J, Ilstrup DM, Krom RAF, Rettke S, Smith TF. Risk factors for cytomegalovirus and severe bacterial infections following liver transplantation: a prospective multivariate time-dependent analysis. Hepatol 1993; 18:185-195.
7. Sayage LH, Gonwa TA, Goldstein RM, Husberg BS, Klintmalm GB. Cytomegalovirus infection in orthotopic liver transplantation. Transplant Int 1989; 2:96-101.
8. Singh N, Dummer S, Kusne S, Breinig MK, Armstrong JA, Makowka L, Starzl TE, Ho M. Infections with cytomegalovirus and other herpesviruses in 121 liver transplant recipients: transmission by donated

organ and the effect of OKT3 antibodies. J Infect Dis 1988; 158:124-31.

9. Stratta RJ, Shaefer MS, Markin RS, Wood P, Kennedy EM, Langnas AN, Reed EC, Woods GL, Donovan JP, Pillen TJ, Duckworth RM, Shaw BW Jr. Clinical patterns of cytomegalovirus disease after liver transplantation. Arch Surg 1989; 124:1443-1450.
10. Umana JP, Mutimer DJ, Shaw JC, McLeish PJ, Buchan A, Martin B, Neuberger JM, McMaster P. Cytomegalovirus surveillance following liver transplantation: does it allow presymptomatic diagnosis of cytomegalovirus disease? Transplant Proc 1992; 24:2643-2645.
11. Pillay D, Charman H, Burroughs AK, Smith M, Rolles K, Griffiths PD. Surveillance for CMV infection in orthotopic liver transplant recipients. Transplantation 1992; 53:1261-1265.
12. Pillay D, Ali AA, Liu SF, Kops E, Sweny P, Griffiths PD. The prognostic significance of positive CMV cultures during surveillance of renal transplant recipients. Transplantation 1993; 56103-56108.
13. Meyers JD, Ljungman P, Fisher LD. cytomegalovirus excretion as a predictor of cytomegalovirus disease after marrow transplantation: importance of Cytomegalovirus viraemia. J Infect Dis 1990; 162:373-380.
14. Van den Berg AP, Klompmaker IJ, Haagsma EB, Scholten-Sampson A, Bijleveld CMA, Schirm J, van der Giessen M, Sloof MJH, The TH. Antigenaemia in the diagnosis and monitoring of active cytomegalovirus infection after liver transplantation. J Infect Dis 1991; 164:265-270.
15. Pillay D, Griffiths PD. Diagnosis of cytomegalovirus infection: a review. Genitourinary Med 1992; 68:183-188.
16. Van der Ploeg M, van den Berg AP, Vlieger AM, van der Giessen M, van Son WJ. Direct detection of cytomegalovirus in peripheral blood leukocytes –a review of the antigenaemia assay and polymerase chain reaction. Transplantation 1992; 54:193-198.
17. Fox JC, Griffiths PD, Emery VC. Quantification of human cytomegalovirus DNA using the polymerase chain reaction. J Gen Virol 1992; 73:2405-2408.
18. Schafer P, Braun RW, Mohring K, Henco K, Kang J, Wendland T, Kuhn JE. Quantitative determination of human cytomegalovirus target sequences in peripheral blood leukocytes by nested polymerase chain reaction and temperature gradient gel electrophoresis. J Gen Virol 1993; 74:2699-2707.
19. Gerdes JC, Spees EK, Fitting K, Hiraki J, Sheehan M, Duda D, Jarvi T, Roehl C, Robertson AD. Prospective study utilizing a quantitative polymerase chain reaction for detection of cytomegalovirus DNA in the blood of renal transplant patients. Transplant Proc 1993; 25:1411-1413.
20. Saliba F, Arulnaden JL, Gugenheim J, Serves C, Samuel D, Bismuth A, Mathieu D, Bismuth H. CMV hyperimmune globulin prophylaxis after liver transplantation: a prospective randomised controlled study. Transplant Proc 1989; 21:2260-2262.
21. Mollison LC, Richards MJ, Johnson PDR, Hayes K, Munckhof WJ, Jones RM, Dabkowski PD, Angus PW. High-dose oral acyclovir reduces the incidence of cytomegalovirus infection in liver transplant recipients. J Infect Dis 1993;168:721-724.
22. Cohen AT, O'Grady JG, Sutherland S, Sallie R, Tan K-C, Williams R. Controlled trial of prophylactic versus therapeutic ganciclovir after liver transplantation in adults. J Med Virol 1993; 40:5-9.
23. Balfour HH Jr, Chace BA, Stapleton JT, Simmons RL, Fryd DS. A randomised, placebo-controlled trial of oral acyclovir for the prevention of cytomegalovirus disease in recipients of renal allografts. N Engl J Med 1989; 320:1381-1387.
24. Chitwood KK, Heim-Duthoy KL, Kasiske BL. Questionable benefit of prophylactic acyclovir in renal transplant recipients at high risk for cytomegalovirus disease. Clin Transplant 1993; 7:320-324.
25. Legendre C, Ducloux D, Ferroni A, Chkoff N, Geffrier C, Rouzioux C, Kreis H. Acyclovir in preventing cytomegalovirus infection in kidney transplant recipients: a case-controlled study. J Med Virology 1993; Suppl:118-122.
26. Singh N, Yu VL, Mieles L, Wagener MM, Miner RC, Gayowski T. High-dose acyclovir compared with short-course preemptive ganciclovir therapy to prevent cytomegalovirus disease in liver transplant recipients. Ann Intern Med 1994; 120:375-381.
27. Freise CE, Pons V, Lake J, Burke E, Ascher NL, Roberts JP. Comparison of three regimens for cytomegalovirus prophylaxis in 147 liver transplant recipients. Transplant Proc 1991; 23:1498-1450.
28. Martin M. Antiviral prophylaxis for CMV infection in liver transplantation. Transplant Proc 1993; 25:10-14.
29. Goodrich JM, Mori M, Gleaves CA, Du MOnd C, Cays M, Ebeling DF, Buhles WC, DeArmond B, Meyers JD. Early treatment with ganciclovir to prevent cytomegalovirus disease after allogeneic bone marrow transplantation. N Engl J Med 1991; 325:1601-1607.
30. Schmidt GM, Horak DA, Niland JC, Duncan SR, Forman SJ, Zaia JA. A randomised, controlled trial of prophylactic ganciclovir for cytomegalovirus pulmonary infection in recipients of allogeneic bone marrow transplants. N Engl J Med 1991; 324:1005-1011.
31. Dunn DL, Mayoral JL, Gillingham KJ, Loeffler CM, Brayman KL, Kramer MA, Erice A, Balfour HH Jr, Fletcher CV, Bolman RM III, Matas AJ, Payne WD, Sutherland DER, Najarian JS. Treatment of invasive cytomegalovirus disease in solid organ transplant recipients with ganciclovir. Transplantation 1991; 51:98-106.
32. George MJ, Snydman DR, Werner BG, Dougherty NN, Griffith J, Rohrer RH, Freeman R, Jenkins R, Lewis WD. Use of ganciclovir plus cytomegalovirus immune globulin to treat CMV pneumonia in orthotopic liver transplant recipients. Transplant Proc 1993; 25:22-44.
33. Harbison MA, De Girolami PC, Jenkins RL, Hammer SM. Ganciclovir therapy of severe cytomegalovirus infections in solid-organ transplant recipients. Transplantation 1988; 46:82-8.
34. Paya CV, Hermans PE, Smith TF, Rakela J, Wiesner RH, Krom RAF, Torres VE, Sterioff S, Wilkowske CJ. Efficacy of ganciclovir in liver and kidney transplant

recipients with severe cytomegalovirus infection. Transplantation 1988; 46:229-234.
35. Marker SC, Ascher NL, Kalis JM, Simmons RL, Najarian JS, Balfour HH Jr. EBV antibody responses and clinical illness in renal transplant recipients. Surgery 1979; 85:433-440.
36. Yao QY, Rickinson AB, Epstein MA. A re-examination of the Epstein-Barr virus carrier state in healthy seropositive individuals. Int J Cancer 1985; 35:35-42.
37. Breinig MK, Zitelli B, Starzl TE, Ho M. EBV, CMV, and other viral infections in children after liver transplantation. J Infect Dis 1987; 156:273-279.
38. Chang RS, Lewis JP, Reynolds RD, Sullivan MJ, Neuman J. Oropharyngeal excretion of EBV by patients with lymphoproliferative disorders and by recipients of renal homografts. Ann Intern Med 1978; 88:34-40.
39. Cheeseman SH, Henle W, Rubin RH, Tolkoff-Rubin NE, Cosimi B, Cantell K, Winkle S, Herrin JT, Black PH, Russell PS, Hirsch MS. Epstein-Barr virus infection in renal transplant recipients. Effects antithymocyte globulin and interferon. Ann Intern Med 1980; 93:39-42.
40. Chatterjee SN, Chang RS. A prospective study of oropharyngeal excretion of EBV in renal homograft recipients. Scand J Infect Dis 1982; 14:95-98.
41. Jones JF, Shurin S, Abramowski C, Tubbs RR, Sciotto CG, Wahl R, Sands J, Gottman D, Katz BZ, Sklar J. T-cell lymphomas containing Epstein-Barr viral DNA in patients with chronic Epstein-Barr infections. N Engl J Med 1988; 318:733-741.
42. Su IJ, Hsieh HC, Lin KH, Uen W-C, Kao C-L, Chen C-J, Cheng A-L, Kadin ME, Chen J-Y. Aggressive peripheral T-cell lymphomas containing EBV DNA: a clinicopathologic and molecular analysis. Blood 1991; 77:799-808.
43. Niedobitek G, Herbst H, Young LS, Brooks L, Masucci MG, Crocker J, Rickinson AB, Stein H. Patterns of EBV infection in non-neoplastic lymphoid tissue. Blood 1992; 79:2520-2526.
44. Rhandawa PS, Jaffe R, Demetris AJ, Nalesnik M, Starzl TE, Chen YY, Weiss LM. Expression of EBV-encoded small RNA (by the EBER-1 gene) in liver biopsy specimens from transplant recipients with post-transplantation lymphoproliferative disorders. N Engl J Med 1992; 327:1710-1714.
45. Sixbey JW, Shirley P, Chesney PJ, Buntin DM, Resnick L. Detection of a second widespread strain of EBV. Lancet 1989; ii:761-765.
46. Telenti A, Marshall WF, Smoth TF. Detection of Epstein-Barr virus by polymerase chain reaction. J Clin Microbiol 1990; 28:2187-2190.
47. Yao QY, Rowe M, Martin B, Young LS, Rickinson AB. The Epstein-Barr virus carrier state: dominance of a single growth-transforming isolate in the blood and in the oropharynx of healthy virus carriers. J Gen Virol 1991; 72:1579-1590.
48. Boyle MJ, Sewell WA, Sculley TB, Apolloni A, Turner JJ, Swanson CE, Penny R, Cooper DA. Subtypes of EBV in HIV-associated non-Hodgkin lymphoma. Blood 1991; 78:3004-3011.
49. Preiksaitis JK. Lymphoproliferative disorders in renal transplant recipients: virologic aspects. Clin Transplant 1992; 6:235-239.
50. Yao QY, Rickinson AB, Gaston JSH, Epstein MA. *In vitro* analysis of the EBV: host balance in long-term renal allograft recipients. Int J Cancer 1985;35:43-49.
51. Yao QY, Ogan P, Rowe M, Wood M, Rickinson AB. EBV-infected B cells persist in the circulation of acyclovir-treated virus carriers. Int J Cancer 1989; 43:67-71.
52. Rhandawa PS, Markin RS, Starzl TE, Demetris AJ. EBV-associated syndromes in immunosuppressed liver transplant recipients. Am J Surg Pathol 1990; 14:538-547.
53. Langnas AN, Castaldo P, Markin RS, Stratta RJ, Wood RP, Shaw BW Jr. The spectrum of EBV infection with hepatitis following liver transplantation. Transplant Proc 1991; 23:1513-1514.
54. Telenti A, Smith TF, Ludwig J, Keating MR, Krom RAF, Wiessner RH. EBV and persistent graft dysfunction after liver transplantation. Hepatology 1991; 14:282-286.
55. Penn I. Immunosuppression —a contributory factor in lymphoma formation. Clin Transplant 1992; 6:214-219.
56. Okano M, Thiele GM, Davis JR, Grierson HL, Purtillo DT. EBV and human diseases: recent advances in diagnosis. Clin Microbiol Rev 1988; 1:300-312.
57. Ho M, Miller G, Atchison W, Breinig MK, Dummer JS, Andiman W, Starzl TE, Eastman R, Griffith BP, Hardesty RL, Bahnson HT, Hakala TR, Rosenthal JT. EBV infections and DNA hybridisation studies in post-transplant lymphoma and lymphoproliferative lesions: the role of primary infection. J Infect Dis 1985;152:876-86.
58. Ho M, Jaffe R, Miller G, Breinig MK, Dummer JS, Makowka L, Atchison RW, Karrer F, Nalesnik MA, Starzl TE. The frequency of EBV infection and associated lymphoproliferative syndrome after transplantation and its manifestations in children. Transplantation 1988; 45:719-727.
59. Cockfield SM, Preiksaitis J, Harvey E, Jones C, Hebert D, Keown P, Halloran PF. Is sequential use of ALG and OKT3 in renal transplant recipients associated with an increased incidence of fulminant post-transplant lymphoproliferative disorder? Transplant Proc 1991; 23:1106-1107.
60. Legendre C, Kreis H. Effect of immunosuppression on the incidence of lymphoma formation. Clin Transplant 1992;6:220-222.
61. Frayha HH, Nazer H, Kalloghlian A, Antonius JI, Sabbah R. Lymphoproliferative disorder in a liver transplant patient on FK506. Lancet 1991; 337:296-297.
62. Nalesnik MA, Demetris AJ, Fung JJ, Starzl TE. Lymphoproliferative disorders arising under immunosuppression with FK506: initial observations in a large transplant population. Transplant Proc 1991; 23:1108-1110.
63. Swinnen LJ, Costanzo-Nordin MR, Fisher SG, O'Sullivan EJ, Johnson MR, Heroux AL, Dizikes GJ, Pifarre R, Fisher RI. Increased incidence of lymphoproli-

ferative disorder after immunosuppression with the monoclonal antibody OKT3 in cardiac transplant recipients. N Engl J Med 1990; 323:1723-1728.
64. Swinnen LJ, Costanzo-Nordin MR, Fisher SG, O'Sullivan EJ, Johnson MR, Heroux AL, Dizikes GJ, Pifarre R, Fisher RI. Increased risk of lymphoproliferative disorders following the use of OKT3 in cardiac transplantation. Clin Transplant 1992; 6:253-259.
65. Ratkovec RM, O'Connell JB, Bristow MR, Jones KW, Gay WA Jr, Rasmussen LG, Renlund DG. Post-transplant lymphoproliferative disease in cardiac transplant patients receiving OKT3 therapy. Clin Transplant 1992; 6:260-264.
66. Klintmalm GB. *De novo* lymphoma after liver transplantation. Clin Transplant 1992; 6:272-274.
67. Cockfield SM, Preiksaitis J, Jewell LD, Parfrey NA. Post-transplant lymphoproliferative disorder in renal allograft recipients. Transplantation 1993; 56:88-96.
68. Malatack JJ, Gartner JC, Urbach AH, Zitelli BJ. Orthotopic liver transplantation, EBV, cyclosporine, and lymphoproliferative disease: a growing concern. J Paediatr 1991; 118:667-675.
69. Purtillo DT. Malignant lymphomas in children with primary immunodeficiency diseases. Clin Transplant 1992; 6:223-226.
70. Shapiro RS, McClain K, Frizzera G, Gajl-Peczalska KJ, Kersey JH, Blazar BR, Arthur DC, Patton DF, Greenberg JS, Burke B, Ramsay NKC, McGlave P, Filipovich AH. EBV associated B cell lymphoproliferative disorders following bone marrow transplantation. Blood 1988; 71:1234-1243.
71. Nalesnik MA, Locker J, Jaffe R, Jaffe R, Reyes J, Cooper M, Fung J, Starzl TE. Experience with post-transplant lymphoproliferative disorders in solid organ transplant recipients. Clin Transplant 1992; 6:249-252.
72. Raab-Traub N, Flynn K. The structure of the termini of the Epstein-Barr virus as a marker of clonal proliferation. Cell 1986; 47:883-889.
73. Patton DF, Wilkowski CW, Hanson CA, Shapiro R, Gajl-Peczaska KJ, Filipovich AH, McClain KL. EBV-determined clonality in post-transplant lymphoproliferative disease. Transplantation 1990; 49:1080-1084.
74. Hanto DW. Polyclonal and monoclonal post-transplant lymphoproliferative diseases. Clin Transplant 1992; 6:227-234.
75. Straus SE. Epstein-Barr virus infections: biology, pathogenesis, and management. Ann Intern Med 1993; 118:45-58.
76. Sumaya CV, Boswell RN, Ench Y, Kisner DL, Hersh EM, Reuben JM, Mansell WA. Enhanced serological and virological findings of EBV in patients with AIDS and AIDS-related complex. J Infect Dis 1986; 154:864-870.
77. Hibberd PL, Rubin RH. Antiviral therapy —an antimalignancy strategy for transplant recipients. Clin Transplant 1992; 6:240-245.
78. Kusne S, Schwartz M, Breinig MK, Dummer JS, Lee RE, Selby R, Starzl TE, Simmons RL, Ho M. *Herpes Simplex Virus* hepatitis after solid organ transplantation in adults. J Infect Dis 1991; 163:1001-1007.
79. Castaldo P, Stratta RJ, Wood P, Markin RS, Patil KD, Shaefer MS, Langnas AN, Reed EC, Li S, Pillen TJ, Shaw BW Jr. Clinical spectrum of fungal infections after orthotopic liver transplantation. Arch Surg 1991; 126:149-156.
80. Wajszczuk CP, Dummer JS, Ho M, Van Thiel D, Starzl TE, Iwatsuki S, Shaw B Jr. Fungal infections in liver transplant recipients. Transplantation 1985; 40:347-353.
81. Colonna JO II, Winston DJ, Brill JE, Goldstein LI, Hoff MP, Hiatt JR, Quinones-Baldrich W, Ramming KP, Busuttil RW. Infectious complications in liver transplantation. Arch Surg 1988; 123:360-364.
82. Paya CV, Hermans PE, Washington II JA, Smith TF, Anhalt JP, Wiesner RH, Krom RAF. Incidence, distribution and outcome of episodes of infection in 100 orthotopic liver transplants. Mayo Clin Proc 1989; 64:555-564.
83. Ascher NL, Stock PG, Bumgardner GL, Payne WD, Najarian JS. Infection and rejection of primary hepatic transplant in 93 consecutive patients treated with triple immunosuppressive therapy. Surg Gynaecol Obstet 1988; 167:474-484.
84. Tollemar J, Ericzon B-G, Holmberg K, Andersson J. The incidence and diagnosis of invasive fungal infections in liver transplant recipients. Transplant Proc 1990; 22:242-244.
85. Rossi G, Tortorano AM, Viviani MA, Pagano A, Colledan M, Fassati LR, Ferla G, Gridelli B, Reggiani P, Doglia M, Caccamo L, Lucianetti A, Paone G, Langer M, Galmarini D. *Aspergillus fumigatus* infection in liver transplant patients. Transplant Proc 1989; 21:2268-2670.
86. Boon AP, Adams DH, Buckels J, McMaster P. Cerebral aspergillosis in liver transplantation. J Clin Pathology 1990;43:114-118.
87. Conti DJ, Tolkoff-Rubin NE, Baker GP Jr, Doran M, Cosimi AB, Delmonico F, Auchincloss H Jr, Russell PS, Rubin RH. Successful treatment of invasive fungal infection with fluconazole in organ transplant recipients. Transplantation 1989; 48:692-695.
88. Samonis G, Rolston K, Karl C, Miller P, Bodey GP. Prophylaxis of oropharyngeal Candidiasis with fluconazole. Rev Infect Dis 1990; 12:S369-373.
89. Slotman GJ, Burchard KW. Ketoconazole prevents Candida sepsis in critically ill surgical patients. Arch Surg 1987; 122:147-151.
90. Weisner RH, Hermans PE, Rakela J, Washington JA II, Perkins JD, DiCecco S, Krom R. Selective decontamination to decrease gram-negative aerobic bacterial and *Candida* colonisation and prevent infection after orthotopic liver transplantation. Transplantation 1988; 45:570-574.

Long Term Outcome after Liver Transplantation

D. Samuel, O. Farges, H. Bismuth

INTRODUCTION

With the development of liver transplantation, most transplant centers achieved a 80-90% one year patient survival. However, the aim is not only to improve the one-year survival of patients, but also the long term-survival and, moreover, the long-term quality of life of the patients. Long-term results will depend on the age of patients, original liver disease, risk of recurrence of the initial liver disease, and compliance of the patients.

SURVEILLANCE OF THE PATIENT AT LONG TERM

The long-term success of a liver transplantation in a patient is a combination of good short-term results, and of a good surveillance, taking into account the personality of each patient, and the initial liver disease. In other words, liver transplantation is not only a surgical act, and long-term success will be achieved only if all problems related to long-term immunosupression, recurrence of initial liver disease on the graft, long-term compliance, and quality of life, are taken into account.

The rythm of surveillance after one year will depend on the ability of the patient to take care of himself, home location of the patient, policy of the center (some centers are doing all the surveillance, some centers are doing only the post-transplant surveillance), and participation of the local or referring physician in this surveillance. In our own center, our policy is to take in charge all patients even for the long-term follow-up. However, to improve the long-term quality of life, we encourage both patients and their local physicians to participate actively in the surveillance. During the first two years patients are seen at our out-patient clinic every 2 to 3 months and laboratory tests performed locally and sent to us every month by the patient. After 2 years, the patient is seen at the out-patient clinic every 3-4 months and laboratory tests performed every month by the patient locally and sent to us. A doppler ultrasound of the liver is performed every year, and apart from specific protocols, a liver biopsy is performed at 1, 2, 5, and 10 years post-transplant.

We will develop here several points which should be taken into account:

The long-term survival.

The immunosuppression and its long-term consequences: the specific complications of the immunosuppression, the risk of development of cancer.

The risk of rejection.

The risk of recurrence of the initial liver disease.

The quality of life.

LONG TERM SURVIVAL

In our Center, the overall one-year survival was 85% and the 5 year-survival was 70%. The one- and five-year survival was related to the initial liver disease: 83 and 80% for patients transplanted for primary biliary cirrhosis, 92 and

85% for those transplanted for viral delta cirrhosis, 85 and 74% for those transplanted for viral B cirrhosis, 85 and 75% for those transplanted for viral C cirrhosis, 78 and 56% for those transplanted for hepatocellular carcinoma on cirrhosis, and 68 and 61% for those transplanted for fulminant hepatitis. These results reflect the discrepancy between each liver disease: the one year survival was lower in patients transplanted for fulminant hepatitis, but the main decline in survival between one and 5 years was observed in patients transplanted for hepatocellular carcinoma and at a lowest degree in patients transplanted for viral B liver cirrhosis. This lower survival in these two groups of patients indicates that the recurrence of the initial liver disease was the cause of death in some patients. As stated later in this chapter, in patients transplanted for hepatocellular carcinoma, the long-term outcome was influenced by tumor size, number of nodules and presence of vascular extension. Thus, the one- and five-year survival was 80 and 67% in patients transplanted for small hepatocellular carcinoma (less than 3 nodules of less than 3 cm, without vascular extension) and 58 and 22% in those with diffuse and large tumors (1).

IMMUNOSUPPRESSION AND ITS LONG-TERM CONSEQUENCES

There is no consensus on the nature and dosage of long-term immunosupressive treatment that patients should receive. In fact, the policy of long-term immunosuppression is different among centers. The need for immunosuppressive treatment is also different for each individual patient. It has been shown that patients can be free of immunosuppression (2, 3) without rejection. However, those patients are not well defined and we have no way to know, in advance, if a patient can be maintained without immunosuppressive treatment. It has been suggested that the presence of a chimerism between donor and recipient will predict a complete tolerance of the graft (2-4). However, this has not been confirmed in organs other than the liver (5, 6), and further studies are needed. In contrast, many patients cannot be maintained without immunosuppressive treatment. The main problem is that there is no accurate way to know which level of immunosuppresion is required for an individual patient. Thus, the immunosuppressive treatment is mainly based on a balance between rejection of the graft and toxicity of the immunosuppresive drugs. The majority of centers are reducing progressively the dose of immunosuppressive treatment taking into account the fact that the risk of rejection of the graft decreases with time. The Birmingham group advocate the discontinuation of steroids in the first post-transplant year (7). Most of their patients are free of steroids but a few proportion developed rejection and need to be retreated with steroids. This approach is particularly interesting in pediatric patients to facilitate their growth. Future protocols should evaluate the long-term benefit of this approach by the assessment of long-term graft function, renal function, immunosuppression-related complications, risk of occurrence of late rejection episodes, and chronic rejection.

Long-Term Complications of Immunosuppression

Specific complications related to the steroids. These complications include mainly diabetes mellitus, arterial hypertension, osteoporosis, and growth retardation in children.

Specific complications related to the use of cyclosporine. These complications include arterial hypertension, hirsutism and renal failure. Chronic renal failure requiring dialysis was mainly described in cardiac transplant recipients; in contrast, this complication was only observed in 3 out of 700 of our liver transplant recipients. This is probably due to lower doses used in liver transplant patients than in cardiac transplant patients.

Specific complications related to the use of FK 506. The introduction of FK 506 in the armentarium of immunosuppressive drugs is too recent to know the long-term effects of its use. Renal failure, diabetes, and arterial hypertension are the main complications.

Specific complications related to the use of azathioprine. Pancytopenia is the main reported complication. Peliosis, venooclusive disease and nodular regenerative hyperplasia have been described in few cases of liver transplant recipients.

General Complications

Development of cancer. Long-term immunosuppression increases the risk of all types of cancer and especially skin cancers and Kaposi sarcoma (8, 9). The risk of development of skin cancer increases with time, patients and physicians should be aware of this risk and any new skin lesion should be biopsied (10). The risk of lymphoma is greatly increased, mostly in the first post-transplant year (9, 11). Appearance of oligoclonal or monoclonal gammopathies may predict the risk of development of lymphoma (12).

Hepatic vessels thrombosis. Thrombosis of the hepatic artery or portal vein may occur, in some cases, several years after transplantation.

SPECIFIC LONG-TERM OUTCOMES

Viral B Liver Cirrhosis

As reported elsewhere, it is of prime importance that patients become and remain HBsAg negative to achieve a good long-term outcome of the patient and graft (13, 14). When HBsAg is negative the graft is mostly normal histologically (15). To achieve this goal, patients should receive long-term anti-HBs passive immunoprophylaxis. In our own center, this immunoprophylaxis is not discontinued and patients receive a mean of 6 injections of 10,000 IU of anti-HBsIg per year. Anti-HBs titer in serum is monitored every week and anti-HBsIg readministered when the titer is near 100 IU/l. Some centers are using a more flexible protocol, by administering anti-HBsIg every month or 2 months without measuring anti-HBs titer. The question concerning the possibility to stop the administration of anti-HBsIg remains a matter of debate. Patients with HBV recurrence will develop, in most of the cases, chronic hepatitis. There is a risk of long-term development of cirrhosis on the graft and of hepatocellular carcinoma. For this reason, patients should be monitored by serial liver biopsies, oesophagal endoscopy to detect portal hypertension, alpha foetoprotein measurement and ultrasound examination of the liver. The viral replication should be surveyed by the detection of HBV DNA is serum, and antiviral therapy has been used in some centers.

Viral C Cirrhosis

Long term outcome of patients transplanted for HCV cirrhosis is not known. It is estimated that 60% of the patients will develop chronic active hepatitis on the graft within 3 years after transplantation (16). The number of patients with chronic hepatitis on the graft at 5 or 10 years is not known, but will be probably near 80%. In our experience and in the experience of other centers, the 5-year patient survival is not different from that of other group of patients. However, the 10- and 15-year graft survival will probably be lowered due to the development of liver cirrhosis on the graft leading to retransplantation. For this reason, these patients should be monitored by serial liver biopsies, oesophageal endoscopy to detect portal hypertension, alpha foetoprotein measurement and ultrasound examination of the liver.

Hepatocellular Carcinoma

The surveillance is based upon the risk of recurrence of hepatocellular carcinoma. We perform every month, alpha foetoprotein level measurement, every 4 months a CT scan of the chest and abdomen, and an ultrasound examination of the liver. In case of recurrence, we evaluate the patient for a surgical resection of the metastasis and for antitumorous chemotherapy. As stated above, the risk of tumor recurrence is dependent of the number and size of nodules and presence of vascular involvement (1, 17, 18).

Alcoholic Cirrhosis

The risk of recidivism of alcoholism is probably low in the immediate post-transplant period. It appears that this risk is related to the duration of abstinence before transplantation and increases with the length of follow-up after transplantation (19-21). For this reason, a long-term psychological support may be beneficial for these patients.

Quality of Life

One of the main goals is to give to the patient the best quality of life. The quality of life is related to the age of the patient, the nature of the initial liver disease, and the function of the graft (22-25). Long-term results are better in young patients and children than in old patients. The quality of life is greatly improved in patients transplanted for decompensated cirrhosis with a long-lasting deteriorating course; in contrast, the quality of life is not always improved in patients transplanted for hepatocellular carcinoma on compensated cirrhosis, and is not improved in patients transplanted for fulminant hepatitis since these patients were in good health few weeks before transplantation. The outcome of the graft influence the quality of life, thus patients with normal liver tests are frequently not readmitted and have a good quality of life. Pregnancy can be successful: in our center more than 15 children were born to liver transplanted women, these children and their mothers are in good health (26).

CONCLUSION

In order to improve the long-term results of liver transplantation, it is necessary to give a good quality of life to the patients, by finding the lowest dosage of immunosuppression without occurrence of rejection and with the minimal complications related to the immunosuppression. The outcome of the graft should be improved by finding ways to reduce the rate and severity of recurrence of the initial liver disease on the graft.

REFERENCES

1. Bismuth H, Chiche L, Adam R, Castaing D, Diamond T, Dennison A. Liver resection versus transplantation for primary hepatocellular carcinoma in cirrhotic patients. Ann Surg 1993; 218:145-151.
2. Starzl TE, Demetris AJ, Trucco M et al. Systemic chimerism in human female recipients of male livers. Lancet 1992; 340:876-877.
3. Starzl TE, Demetris AJ, Trucco M et al. Chimerism and donor-specific non reactivity 27 to 29 years after kidney allotransplantation. Transplantation 1993; 55:1272-1277.
4. Starzl TE, Demetris AJ, Trucco M et al. Chimerism after liver transplantation for type IV glycogen storage disease and type 1 Gaucher's disease. N Engl J Med 1993; 328:745-749.
5. Superbielle C, Caillat-Zucman F, Legendre C et al. Peripheral microchimerism in long-term cadaveric-kidney allografts recipients. Lancet 1994; 343:1468-1469.
6. Schlitt HJ, Hundriesser J, Hisinaga M et al. Patterns of donor-type microchimerism after heart transplantation. Lancet 1994; 343:1469-1471.
7. Padbury RT, Gunson BK, Dousset B et al. Steroids withdrawal from long-term immunosuppression in liver allograft recipients. Transplantation 1993; 55:789-794.
8. Penn I. Cancers following cyclosporine therapy. Transplantation 1987; 43:32-35.
9. Bismuth H, Samuel D, Venancie PY, Menouar G, Szekely AM. Development of kaposi's sarcoma in liver transplant recipients: Characteristics, management, and outcome. Transplant Proc 1991; 23:1438-1439.
10. Hartevelt ML, Bavinck JNB, Koote AMM, Vermeer BJ, Vandenbroucke JP. Incidence of skin cancer after renal transplantation in the Netherlands. Transplantation 1990; 49:506-509.
11. Wilkinson AH, Smith JLK, Hunsicker LG et al. Increased frequency of post-transplant lymphomas in patients treated with cyclosporine, azathioprine, and prednisone. Transplantation 1989; 47:293-296.
12. Pham H, Lemoine A, Sol O, Azoulay D, Royer P, Samuel D, Charpentier C, Bismuth H, Debuire B. Monoclonal and oligoclonal gammopathies in liver recipients. Transplantation 1994; 58:253-257.
13. Demetris AJ, Todo S, Van Thiel DH et al. Evolution of hepatitis B virus liver disease after hepatic replacement practican and theoretical considerations. Am J Pathol 1990; 137:667-676.
14. Samuel D, Bismuth A, Mathieu D et al. Passive immunoprophylaxis after liver transplantation in HBsAg-positive patients. Lancet 1991; 337:813-815.
15. Samuel D, Müller R, Alexander G, Fassati L, Ducot B, Benhamou JP, Bismuth H and the investigations of the European concerted action on viral hepatitis study. Liver transplantation in European patients with the hepatitis B surface antigen. N Engl J Med 1993; 329:1842-1847.
16. Feray C, Gigou M, Samuel D et al. The course of hepatitis C virus infection after liver transplantation. Hepatology 1994; 20:1137-1143.
17. Ringe B, Wittekind C, Bechstein WO, Bunzendahl H, Pichlmayr R. The role of liver transplantation in he-

patobiliary malignancy. A retrospective analysis of 95 patients with particular regard to tumor stage and recurrence. Ann Surg 1989; 209:88-98.
18. O'Grady JG, Polson RJ, Rolles K, Calne RY, Williams R. Liver transplantation for malignant disease. Results in 93 consecutive patients. Ann Surg 1988; 207:373-379.
19. Osorio RW, Ascher NL, Avery M, Bacchetti P, Roberts JP, Lake JR. Predicting recidivism after orthotopic liver transplantation for alcoholic liver disease. Hepatology 1994; 20:105-110.
20. Lucey MR, Merion RM, Henley KS et al. Selection for and outcome of liver transplantation in alcoholic liver disease. Gastroenterology 1992; 102:1736-1741.
21. Kumar S, Stauber RE, Gavaler JS et al. Orthotopic liver transplantation for alcoholic liver disease. Hepatology 1990; 11:159-164.
22. Leyendecker B, Bartholomew U, Neuhaus R et al. Quality of life of liver transplant recipients. A pilot study. Transplantation 1993; 56:561-567.
23. Bonsel GJ, Essink-Bot ML, Klompmaker IJ, Sloof MJ. Assessment of the quality of life before and following liver transplantation. First results. Transplantation 1992; 53:796-800.
24. Nicholas JJ, Oleske D, Robinson LR et al. The quality of life after liver transplantation. Arch Phys Med Rehabil 1994; 75:431-435.
25. Tarter RE, Switala J, Arria A et al. Quality of life before and after orthotopic hepatic transplantation. Arch Int Med 1991; 151:1521-1526.
26. Ville Y, Fernández H, Samuel D, Bismuth H, Frydman R. Pregnancy in liver transplant patients: course and outcome in 19 cases. Am J Obstet Gynecol 1993; 168:896-902.

Sharing a Liver

J. B. Otte

INTRODUCTION

The impressive improvement of results in liver transplantation during the last decade has led to more than a ten-fold increase in the number of candidates. Despite parallel efforts to increase the number of organ donors, a relative shortage has developped and the gap between offer and demand is widening over the years, resulting in the death of quite a number of candidates before an appropriate organ can be found (around 8% in UNOS and Eurotransplant). The situation is even more worrying in pediatric liver transplantation where the scarcity of age and size-matched donors remains a major limiting factor everywhere around the world. Indeed, mortality from liver diseases in children is concentrated during infancy with nearly half of the deaths occurring before the age of one (1, 2). This results in a mortality rate on waiting list as high as 20% (3-6). Another consequence of organ shortage is a long waiting time which has a heavy psychological impact on the child and his/her family with worsening of the clinical condition, suffering, deterioration of overall results and increased costs for the society.

The organ shortage being more severe in children than in adults led to the development of the «reduced» or «cut-down» liver to allow children to gain access to the relatively much larger adult donors pool. The principle of the cutting down is based on the well-known segmentation of the liver; after retrieval and cooling, the liver is submitted to a partial resection on a back-table to make it smaller and fit for use in a recipient of smaller size than the donor. Most often only the left lobe (segments 2 and 3) or the left liver (segments 2, 3 and 4) is conserved for transplantation of an adult donor liver in a pediatric recipient although, conversely, the right lobe may be conserved. Beside its reduction, the graft is transplanted orthotopically in the same standard manner as a full-size graft.

The first clinical application was published by Bismuth and Houssin in 1984 (7), followed by Broelsch (8) and our group (9, 10). Our first patient to receive a cut-down liver was transplanted in August 1984 (9); to the best of our knowledge, she is currently the longest survivor worldwide after liver transplantation of a reduced graft. T. E. Starzl reported in 1990 a case he performed in 1975 where he reduced the transplant during the donor operation (11) but the recipient died 36 hours later.

When the learning phase was passed, results obtained in elective cases by experienced teams (12, 13) were not different from those obtained with full-size grafts. As an example, the 5-year patient survival rate in our series was 81% in 81 children transplanted with a full size graft for biliary atresia as well as in 71 children who received a cut-down liver (14).

During the early phase of development of the cutdown liver, ethical questions were raised because poorer results were obtained in patients who received a reduced graft on an emergency basis (15). By incorporating both pre- and post-transplantation deaths (overall survival calculated from the time the patient is listed), the Center for Clinical Medical Ethics of the University of Chicago was able to demonstrate that therapeutical strategies using either full-size grafts alone or in combination with reduced livers were in a state of equipoise, with similar overall survival (16). The reduced liver has become a standard procedure and is routinely used in many pediatric transplantation centers (17-20), even exceeding in number the full-size grafts in some centers (21).

In our own center, of the 389 liver transplants performed between 1984 and 1993, 175 were full-size grafts and 214 were reduced grafts (including 21 split grafts) (22). Surgical complications were similar in the two groups although there was a tendency to increased peroperative bleeding with cut-down livers.

In spite of its merits, reduced size liver transplantation does little more than redistribute the adult liver donor pool to the advantage of children, hereby placing adult patients at a potential disadvantage. The fact that potentially usable liver tissue is discarded when performing a reduced size liver transplantation stimulated the development of split liver graft transplantation in four centers in 1988 (23-26). In this procedure, the adult donor liver is divided on a back table into a segmental left graft (either the left lobe or the left lateral segment), usually to be transplanted into a pediatric recipient and a right lobe graft to be transplanted into an adult recipient. Split liver transplantation allows one to make maximum use of the cadaveric liver donor pool; however it is a very demanding and elaborate surgical procedure that requires extensive experience with liver anatomy, major liver resections and reduced liver grafting.

As it was the case in the early stage of development of reduced livers, ethical questions arose for the split livers because of the initial poor results obtained in critically ill patients (27) with a high retransplantation rate leading Broelsch and his associates in Chicago to conclude in 1990 (28) that the procedure was not safe enough to be pursued under elective conditions. However, because the technical feasibility had been demonstrated, further anatomical studies refined the technical aspects (29, 30) and led several centers to successfully reactivate the clinical application (31).

Between 1988 and 1993, we split 15 donor livers (32). Of the 30 split grafts, 2 were not transplanted, due either to lack of capacity or to steatosis of the graft. Two right grafts were sent to another center while we received three grafts from another center. In total then, 29 grafts were transplanted (16 lefts grafts, 13 right grafts) into 28 recipients. Eleven right grafts were transplanted into adult patients and two into children; all left split grafts were transplanted into pediatric recipients. Seven transplants were performed electively while 14 were performed in urgent (hospital-bound) and 8 in highly urgent (ICU bound) recipients. The 6-month survival rate was 71 and 67% for the left and right split grafts, respectively. Six grafts were lost as a result of death of the recipient unrelated to the splitting procedure.

The collective European experience assembled at the first European workshop on split liver transplantation (Brussels, March 19, 1993) consisted of 100 split liver grafts prepared from 50 donor livers in nine transplant centers between March 1988 and March 1993. This unique experience which is the largest worldwide has been analyzed by Jean de Ville de Goyet, custodian of the European Split Liver Registry (33). Out of the 100 split grafts, two were discarded because of the death of the recipient before implantation in one case and for logistical reasons in the other one. Eighty-nine grafts were kept in the liver splitting center while the remaining nine were shipped to another center. Fourty split procedures were performed in four major centers while the remaining 10 split procedures were performed in 5 centers. In 24 cases, the surgical teams decided to perform a liver graft division in order to transplant simultaneously two urgent patients; in 20 cases, splitting replaced a cutting down procedure and benefited 19 adults and one child who came to receive the right part of the liver which, otherwise, would have been discarded (including 3 adults with a liver cancer and 6 other patients who were rapidly deteriorating). In one case, an oversized graft implanted into a small size adult had to be reduced and the left part of it was used to transplant an urgent patient. In 5 cases, the liver was split by the most experienced teams for deliberately transplanting two elective recipients.

The 6-month actual survival rate was 65% for the 44 recipients of a left split graft and 75% for the 49 recipients of a right split graft (NS). The 6-month survival rate was 71% for the 53 pediatric recipients and 70% for the 40 adult recipients. It was 52, 73 and 85% for the 31 highly urgent, 30 urgent and 33 elective patients respectively. The 6-month survival rate was 65% for the 47 left split grafts and 63% for the 49 right split grafts. Of a total of 96 grafts, 20 were lost to a cause related to the graft itself and thirteen were lost as a result of death of the recipient that was unrelated to the graft.

It may be concluded from this collaborative study that split liver transplantation has no major disadvantages as compared to the standard technique, including the cutdown liver. Splitting the donor liver into two grafts fit for use in two recipients is the only way to maximise a limited cadaveric donor liver pool. We consider that the split liver procedure has been validated by the collective european experience, the Groningen experience (34) and by our own series. When performed in elective patients by an experienced team, it yields results similar to transplantation of a full-sized graft; neither recipient is submitted to increase hazards, and specifically not the adult recipient of the right split graft. These data should reassure teams limiting their activity to adult patients that their patients will be provided with the best possible care and should encourage their collaboration with other teams already experienced in splitting procedures.

Indeed, splitting of the liver is a lengthy procedure. Because of its complexity as well as that of the two ensuing transplants, only an ideal donor liver should be considered for splitting. On the other hand, there is evidence that cold ischemia of a liver graft preserved with University of Wisconsin solution should ideally not exceed 12-15 hours in order to reduce the incidence of late ischemic strictures of the bile ducts. Therefore, logistics should be adapted to transplant the two potential recipients in parallel. Shipping one of the two grafts to another well-trained liver transplant center is an option that should be encouraged further.

The extensive use of reduced and split liver grafts has resulted in a decrease in the mortality of pediatric patients awaiting a donor. In our own center, it decreased from 15% before 1989 to 7.5% in 1991. However these innovative techniques have not changed the outlook for the adult candidates. Moreover, the ever increasing number of adult patients on waiting lists has diminished the number of adult liver donor grafts available to pediatric recipients. The split liver has not filled the gap because it is not considered yet as an established procedure by most centers (quite wrongly in M.Slooff's opinion (34) and in our own experience (34)). As a result, the mortality of pediatric candidates, while waiting, increased again to 15-20% in 1993 and 1994.

The shortage of cadaveric organs is the main, if not the only justification to develop living related liver donation (LRLD). This procedure consists of resecting the left lateral segment or the left lobe from a healthy and voluntary donor for transplantation into a child. To the best of our information, only family members —mostly one of the parents— have been accepted as living liver donors in the world experience. Such an approach is the best (although not absolute) guarantee that the decision of the donor has been made in complete freedom and without any coercion. Further guarantees are provided by entrusting an internist who is not member of the transplantation team with the medical assessment of the health and the motivation of the potential donor («medical advocate of the donor») and a psychologist with the evaluation of the willingness to donate without any coercion and of the capacity to resist stressful situations. Beside the real impact on the organ shortage, LRLT has other potential advantages. In case of parental donation, the sharing of one haplotype might decrease the risk of rejection although this effect has not been proved yet. A major advantage is the provision of an organ of perfect quality with a short ischemic time to a child operated under elective condition, sparing both the child and his/her parents the hazards and sufferings of a long waiting time with the best chances for a low morbidity and a high hope of long life. Of course, ethical aspects have to be considered very seriously because LRLT put a healthy person at a non neglectable risk of mortality which has been evaluated to be < 1% by extrapolation of data from left liver resections for benign or malignant lesions in an otherwise normal liver. Morbidity is not uncommon either, with a high incidence of gastritis and duodenal ulcer likey related to stress in a Japanese series (35).

The first case of LRLT was performed in Brazil on 8 December 1988 (36); however, the patient died shortly thereafter. The first successful case of LRLT was performed in Brisbane, Australia, in July 1989 (37); here a child received the left liver lobe from his mother and became a long-term survivor (he later needed retransplantation for chronic rejection). In Japan, LRLT was initiated at the University of Shimane Medical School in 1989 (38); the recipient died of multiple organ failure 6 months after transplantation. The main program of LRLT in Japan was started in June 1990 at Kyoto University. The rapid expansion of LRLT to several other Japanese centers has been made possible by the intense efforts made by our Japanese colleagues who are not yet allowed to remove organs from brain-dead patients.

The University of Chicago Pritzker School of Medicine was the first to develop a prospective protocol of LRLT on the basis of a collaborative effort between clinical ethicists (led by M. Siegler) and clinical investigators (led by C. E. Broelsch, surgeon, and P. F. Whitington, pediatrician). The protocol was elaborated after a yearlong series of seminars and discussions that were open to the entire community. Very remarkable was the publication of their protocol (39) before they performed their first case on November 29, 1989. Intense activity in this field has continued since then in Chicago, even after Broelsch who had been the pioneering surgeon returned to Germany.

During recent years, several programs have been started in Western Europe and in the United States. The total number of LRLT performed worldwide was exceeding 300 cases by the end of 1994; the largest single center experience (137 cases) has been acquired in Kyoto by Ozawa and Yamaoka and their colleagues (Yamaoka, personal communication, December 20, 1994). There has been one donor fatality from pulmonary thromboembolism and this occurred in Hamburg on the 4th postoperative day (C. E. Broelsch, personal communication). In experienced centers, the overall patient survival rate is averaging 85%.

In 1991-1992, at the University of Louvain Medical School in Brussels, we took the example from the model in Chicago to conduct several seminars, bringing together clinicians involved in liver transplantation and members of the Center of Bioethical Studies. All aspects of LRLT, including psychological, legal and medical problems, were discussed in length and in depth. A protocol was developed on the basis of these reflections, and this was approved by the Ethics Committee of the Medical School and by the Board of Trustees of the University Hospital. Potential recipients are children with a chronic liver disease in a stable clinical condition, allowing for elective transplantation.

Our first case was performed on July 28, 1993, the father who donated being himself a trauma surgeon. Fourteen more cases were performed in 1994 with only one death from hepatitis two months after transplantation for an acute liver failure of unknown origin; the remaining children were transplanted for biliary atresia except for one whose liver disease was a familial cholestasis. All donors were either the father or the mother; we observed no complication of any kind except for a minor and very transient bile leak from the cut surface which healed spontaneously within few days.

Five cases of LRLT in adult recipients were reported by the group of Makuuchi at the 1994 Congress of the Transplantation Society (40). The volume of the left lateral segment or the left lobe can be quite accurately estimated by CT scan volumetric analysis. On the other hand, the minimal liver mass needed is not yet precisely known. According to the group of Kyoto (38), a ratio > 1% between liver mass and body weight of the recipient is the limit of safety, although the ratio between liver mass and body surface is probably more accurate in children. In adults, a ratio > 35% between the graft volume and the standard recipient liver volume would be appropriate according to the group of Makuuchi (40).

Clinical application of LRLT must be strictly controlled in order to avoid the stricly prohibited commerce of organs or rewarded gift which has developped in some countries suffering of poverty and underdevelopment.

The transplant professionals must also pay much care to avoid that the development of LRLT decreases the efforts to be made and made again to expand the pool of potential donors; in this regard the results obtained by our spanish colleagues in promoting cadaveric organ donation are very remarkable.

REFERENCES

1. Lloyd-Still JD. Mortality from liver disease in children. Implications for hepatic transplantation programs. Am J Dis Child 1985; 139:381-384.
2. Mowat AP. Liver disorders in children: the indications for liver replacement in parenchymal and metabolic diseases. Transplant Proc 1987; 19:3236-3241.
3. Gordon RD, Hartner CM, Casavilla A et al. The liver transplant waiting list —a single-center analysis. Transplantation 1991; 51:128-134.
4. Lynch SV, Strong RW, Ong TH, Praga Pillay S, Balderson GA. Reduced-size liver transplantation in children. Transplant Rev 1992; 6:89-101.
5. Salt A, Noble-Jamieson G, Barnes ND et al. Liver transplantation in 100 children: Cambridge and King's College Hospital series. Br Med J 1992; 304:416-421.
6. Zitelli BJ, Malatack JJ, Garnter JC et al. Evaluation of the pediatric patient for liver transplantation. Pediatrics 1986; 78:559-565.
7. Bismuth H, Houssin D. Reduced-sized orthotopic liver graft in hepatic transplantation in children. Surgery 1984; 95:367-370.
8. Broelsch CE, Emond JC, Thistlethwaite JR, Rouch DA, Whitington PF, Lichtor JL. Liver transplantation with reduced-size donor organs. Transplantation 1988; 45:519-523.
9. Otte JB, de Hemptinne B, Moulin D et al. La transplantation hépatique chez l'enfant. Chir Pediatr 1985; 26:261-273.
10. Otte JB, de Ville de Goyet J, Sokal EM et al. Size reduction of the donor liver is a safe way to alleviate the shortage of size-matched organs in pediatric liver transplantation. Ann Surg 1990; 211:146-157.
11. Starzl TE, Demetris GA. Liver transplantation —a 31 year perspective. Chicago: Year Book 1990; 39-41.
12. Otte JB, Yandza T, de Ville de Goyet J, Sokal EM et al. Liver transplantation in children: surgical alternatives. Jpn J Paediatr Surg 1990; 22:979-986.
13. Broelsch CE, Whitington PF, Emond JC. Evolution and future perspectives for reduced-size hepatic transplantation. Surg Gynecol Obstet 1990; 171:353-360.
14. Otte JB, de Ville de Goyet J, Reding R, Hausleithner V, Sokal E, Chardot C, Debande B. Sequential treatment of biliary atresia with Kasai portoenterostomy and liver transplantation: a review. Hepatology 1994; 20:41S-48S.
15. Broelsch CE, Whitington PF, Emond JC. Evolution and future perspectives for reduced-size hepatic transplantation. Surg Gynecol Obstet 1990; 171:353-360.
16. Singer PA, Lantos JD, Whitington PF, Broelsch CE, Siegler M. Equipoise and the ethics of segmental liver transplantation. Clin Res 1988; 10:539-545.
17. Houssin D, Soubrane O, Boillot O et al. Orthotopic liver transplantation with a reduced-size graft: an ideal compromise in pediatrics. Surgery 1992; 111:532-542.
18. Ryckman FC, Flake AW, Fisher RA, Tchervenkov JI, Pedersen SH, Balistreri WF. Segmental orthotopic hepatic transplantation as a means to improve patient survival and diminish waiting-list mortality. J Pediatr Surg 1991; 26:422-428.
19. Ringe B, Pichlmayr R, Burdelski M. A new technique of hepatic vein reconstruction in partial liver transplantation. Transplant Int 1988; 1:30-35.
20. Strong R, Ong Th, Wall D, Balderson G, Lynch S. A new method of segmental orthotopic liver transplantation in children. Surgery 1988; 104:104-107.
21. Yandza T, Gauthier F, Valayer J. Lessons from the first 100 liver transplantations in children at Bicêtre Hospital, 1992.
22. De Ville de Goyet J, Hausleithner V, Reding R, Lerut J, Janssen M, Otte JB. Impact of innovative techniques on the waiting list and results in pediatric liver transplantation. Transplantation 1993; 56:1130-1136.
23. Pichlmayr R, Ringe B, Gubernatis G, Hauss J, Bunzendahl H. Transplantation einer Spenderleber auf zwei empfänger (splitting-transplantation) —Eine neue methode in der weiterentwicklung der lebersegmenttransplantation. Langenbecks Arch Chir 1988; 373:127-130.
24. Bismuth H, Morino M; Castaing D et al. Emergency orthotopic liver transplantation in two patients using one donor liver. Br J Surg 1989; 76:722-724.
25. Emond JC, Whitington PF, Thistlethwaite JR et al. Transplantation of two patients with one liver. Analysis of a preliminary experience with «split-liver» grafting. Ann Surg 1990; 212:14-22.
26. Otte JB, de Ville de Goyet J, Alberti D, Balladur P, de Hemptinne B. The concept and technique of the split liver in clinical liver transplantation. Surgery 1990; 107:605-612.
27. Thistlethwaite JR, Emond JC, Woodle ES et al. Increased utilization of organ donors: transplantation of two recipients from single donor livers. Transplant Proc 1990; 22:1485-1486.
28. Broelsch CE, Whitington PF, Emond JC. Evolution and future perspectives for reduced-size hepatic transplantation. Surg Gynecol Obstet 1990; 171:353-360.
29. Couinaud C, Houssin D. Controlled partition of the liver for transplantation. Anatomical limitations. Paris: Personal edition, 1991; 1-80.
30. Rat P, Paris P, Friedman S, Favre JP Split-liver orthotopic liver transplantation: how to divide the portal pedicle. Surgery 1992; 112:522-526.
31. Houssin D, Boillot O, Soubrane O et al. Controlled liver splitting for transplantation in two recipients: technique, results and perspectives. Br J Surg 1993; 80:75-80.
32. Otte JB. It is right to develop living related liver

transplantation? Do reduced and split livers not suffice to cover the needs? Transplant Int 1995; 8:69-73.

33. De Ville de Goyet J. Review of the European experience with 100 split liver grafts: technical aspects and clinical outcome. European Split Liver Registry, 1994.
34. Slooff MJH, Reduced size liver transplantation, split liver transplantation, and living related liver transplantation in relation to the donor organ shortage. Transplant Int 1995; 8:65-68.
35. Marimoto T, Yamaoka Y, Tanaka K, Ozawa K. Quality of life among donors of liver transplants to relatives. N Engl J Med 1993; 329:363.
36. Raia S, Nery JR, Mies S. Liver transplantation from live donors. Lancet 1989; ii:497-498.
37. Strong RW, Lynch SV, Ong Th. Successful liver transplantation from a living donor to her son. N Engl J Med 1990; 322:1505-1507.
38. Osawa K. Living related donor liver transplantation. Basel: Karger, 1994.
39. Singer PA, Siegler M, Whitington PF, Lantos JD, Emond JC, Thistlethwaite JR, Broelsch CE. Ethics of liver transplantation with living donors. N Engl J Med 1989; 321:620-622.
40. Kawasaki S, Makuuchi M, Matsunami H, Hashikura Y, Ikegami T, Kawarazaki N, Takayama T. Living-related liver transplantation with a wider application. Abstract, XVth Congress of the Transplantation Society. Kyoto, Aug 28-Sept 2, 1994.

Hepatic Xenotransplantation

S. C. Robson

OVERVIEW

Xenotransplantation refers to the surgical grafting of organs from a member of one species to another, and may be classified as either concordant or discordant according to the presumptive immunological barriers to graft acceptance (1). Concordant transplants are performed between species that are relatively closely related phylogenetically, such as from baboon to human; in such species combinations, hyperacute rejection (HAR) is not observed (1-3). Discordant xenotransplantation procedures between members of distantly related species, on the other hand, such as from pig to human, invariably results in HAR in unmodified recipients (1, 4, 5). This process is comparable in part to the hyperacute rejection seen in sensitised individuals receiving incompatible allografts (2, 3).

The liver may be considered as the optimal xenograft in certain concordant models. In the light of the synthesis of donor specific coagulation factors and complement in the post-transplant setting (6, 7), the liver xenograft may also be able to protect itself from further immune damage and potentially evade T cell responses (8-11).

Despite a critical shortage of donor allografts for liver transplantation, xenotransplantation has been limited to occasional use of primate concordant organs such as described by Starzl et al. in 1993 (11) or to isolated instances of discordant graft implantation as a temporizing liver support measure as performed by Makowka (5). Although these clinical experiments failed, valuable information on the effects of xenotransplantation in humans may have been obtained which I will attempt to summarize.

Tom Starzl's two cases were men aged 35 and 62 (one of whom was HIV positive), transplanted in June, 1992, and January, 1993, respectively, for chronic hepatitis B infection and liver failure. The first patient awoke following the surgery and became ambulant surviving for 70 days; the second patient remained jaundiced and comatose with anuria. Causes of death were multifactorial including rupture of a fungal mycotic aneurysm and peritonitis (12).

Cellular and humoral (vascular) type immune rejection responses in these liver xenografts were considered to be covered by FK506, prednisone, prostaglandin E_1 and cyclophosphamide. Repeated biopsies in both instances revealed no evidence for rejection related vascular damage, although platelet sludging in the sinusoids was noted post-reperfusion; likewise there was minimal evidence of cellular type rejection processes. A major complication was the development of intrahepatic cholestasis and microsteatosis which could have been ascribed to metabolic incompatibilities (12).

Leonard Makowka's case report concerned a 26 year-old woman with autoimmune hepatitis who developed fulminant hepatic failure with cerebral oedema. She received a heterotopically placed porcine liver following plasmapheresis, cyclophosphamide, steroid and cyclosporine therapy with perfusion of the donor kidneys to deplete the circulating host blood of xenoreactive antibody and complement (already low in the light of the liver failure). As a result of several circumstances, including the administration of eleven units of fresh frozen plasma to replace clotting factors, increases in xenoreactive antibodies and complement were observed. This was associated with progressive damage to the vascular endothelium of the graft and hyperacute rejection. The patient died before human liver allotransplantation could be performed (13).

Porcine livers have been utilised in the past in clinical xenoperfusion models to allow regeneration of the host liver and more recently as a bridge to allotransplantation. Short-term perfusion may be feasible in patients with fulminant liver failure in spite of inflammatory responses and immune reactions; the metabolic activity of the porcine liver is to some extent compatible with the human subjects tested to date (14).

The use of porcine hepatocytes as a short-term metabolic support has developed in the context of a extracorporeal perfusion device using hepatocytes prepared following collagenase treatment of pig liver (15). These devices are separated from the perfused human blood by a membrane. Their use in uncontrolled studies, appears to impart some clinical benefit in prolonging survival, thus enhancing the opportunity for an allograft procedure (AASLD Postgraduate Course. A. Demetriou, 1993).

The use of non-vascularised xenografts is not associated with HAR. However, the limited success of porcine xeno- and even human allo-pancreatic islet grafting even with sophisticated immunological interventions, suggest that the use of xenogeneic tissue in this setting is premature (16). A concern with all these procedures, is the possibility of transmission of certain infections from the animal donors. These include certain parasites, brucellosis, leptospirosis, porcine herpes virus (pseudorabies) from the pig and tuberculosis, several simian retroviruses, CMV, EBV-like viruses and the alphaherpesvirinae from baboons and primates (17).

Thus, the further development of these therapeutic modalities is limited by significant practical considerations, in addition to certain ethical concerns, particularly with respect to the use of primate organs. Furthermore, the clinical use of discordant xenografts is restricted by the very real dangers of rapid graft loss because of the process of HAR and the potential short and long-term metabolic incompatibilities between widely separated species (5, 12, 18). The clinical application of xenotransplantation is therefore still limited by the the lack of sufficient published, experimental data in non-human primates and other animals. A current perspective of the problems and issues in this field will now be discussed.

HYPERACUTE AND DELAYED XENOGRAFT REJECTION

HAR is associated with co-deposition of recipient complement (C) and xenoreactive natural antibodies (XNA) on the endothelial cells (EC) of the donor organ (4, 5, 7). This process is extremely rapid and can result in graft destruction and infarction within just 10-15 min in small animal models (a discordant xenograft from guinea pig to rat, for instance), or in approximately 1-2 hours if for example, a pig heart is transplanted to a baboon or a rhesus monkey (5, 19).

The process of HAR appears to involve EC activation (5). Experimental models suggest that following transplantation and the establishment of blood flow from the recipient to the transplanted organ, recipient xenoreactive natural antibodies attach to donor endothelial cells (20). Natural antibodies are in significant measure IgM, and thus fix complement very efficiently. The combination of the recipient's natural antibodies plus the activated complement leads to activation of the endothelial cells lining the vessels of the donor organ (21). This EC activation is a central event that leads to the complications of vascular occlusion and organ infarction associated with xenograft rejection (5). There are fundamental pathophysiological differences between the transplantation of an immediately-vascularized organ, such as heart, kidney, liver or pancreas where the grafted endothelium is immediately exposed to the recipient's circulating blood and thus to XNA and C, and the transplantation of neovascularized tissues, such as in the case of pancreatic islets, in which blood vessels from the host grow over days into the transplanted tissues. In the immediately-vascularized organ, the endothelium of the transplanted vasculature persists in very large measure as donor type, and thus remains foreign to the recipient. Furthermore, if endothelial cells are damaged, it is not clear whether they would be preferentially and rapidly replaced by other donor xenogeneic EC or by host EC (5, 19).

In the very few minutes that it takes for an organ to be destroyed in HAR in some discordant species combinations, there is no time for gene up-regulation and synthesis of new proteins. In contrast, in delayed discordant xenograft rejection (DXR), which takes place if the recipient is treated prophylactically in one or another way to remove complement and ameliorate the initial events, the rejection process may take place over a matter of hours, or even days, permitting EC gene up-regulation and its consequences. Given present day treatments with cobra venom factor, DXR in a guinea pig to rat transplant can occur in many hours or a few days, as compared with HAR that takes 10-15 min; in the pig to primate transplant, DXR takes place after several days or even weeks (22). The events that occur when EC are stimulated can be divided into those that occur very rapidly and do not require protein synthesis, and those that do require protein synthesis and take longer to manifest. These have been referred to as EC stimulation and EC activation, respectively (23, 24). To avoid the problem of using the term «stimulation» both for the action of stimuli that lead to activation of the EC, and for a part of that activation response, Bach et al have used the terms «Type I» and «Type II» activation, and grouped both types of responses as «EC activation» (4, 5). It is likely that HAR involves the consequences of events that constitute type I EC activation, whereas DXR likely involves the consequences of type II EC activation as well.

HETEROGENEITY OF ENDOTHELIAL CELLS

Although vascular EC share common features and functions, it is now clear that there is significant functional, structural and anatomical heterogeneity of these cells. In a manner also analogous to the studies of the lymphocyte, studies conducted *in vitro* may not be comparable to those conducted in the context of blood flow and in the vascular bed per se. The successful cell culture of several types of EC has provided further evidence for remarkable differences in the specific biochemical functioning and antigenic determinants of these cells (25). In addition to these organ specific endothelial cell antigens, there are both allo and xeno-specific endothelial cell antigens and there appear to be differential abilities of EC to act as antigen presenting cells *in vitro* (26).

In certain vascular beds, notably the spleen and hepatic sinusoids, the EC monolayer is discontinuous with large fenestrations and the basement membrane is rudimentary to permit filtration of high Mr solutes (chylomicrons, immune complexes) or even cells (25). This observation suggests that there are likely to be differing EC responses to xenotransplantation of hearts and livers for example.

ENDOTHELIAL CELL ACTIVATION

Quiescent EC perform several functions. First, because they are tightly juxtaposed, each touching its neighbours, they maintain a barrier that keeps cells and proteins of blood in the intravascular space and prevents leakage into the extracellular fluids of the organ. Second, the EC have on their surface a number of molecules that help maintain anticoagulation and perform other functions. Two of the most important of these are heparan sulfate, a proteoglycan, and thrombomodulin, both of which are lost from the surface of the EC with EC activation (27, 28-30) (fig. 1). Heparan sulfate consists of a protein core with glycosaminoglycan chains attached to it. Antithrombin III (ATIII) binds to appropriately substituted residues on the glycosaminoglycan chains. When ATIII attaches to the heparan sulfate, it is activated and becomes a very powerful anticoagulant, interfering with the action of thrombin, a key component of the coagulation cascade, as well as other factors (27). Also associated with the heparan sulfate are superoxide dismutases (SOD), which break down oxygen radicals (O_2^-) that are produced, for instance, by activated neutrophils that attach to the activated EC (28, 31). More recent data suggests that interacting leukocytes

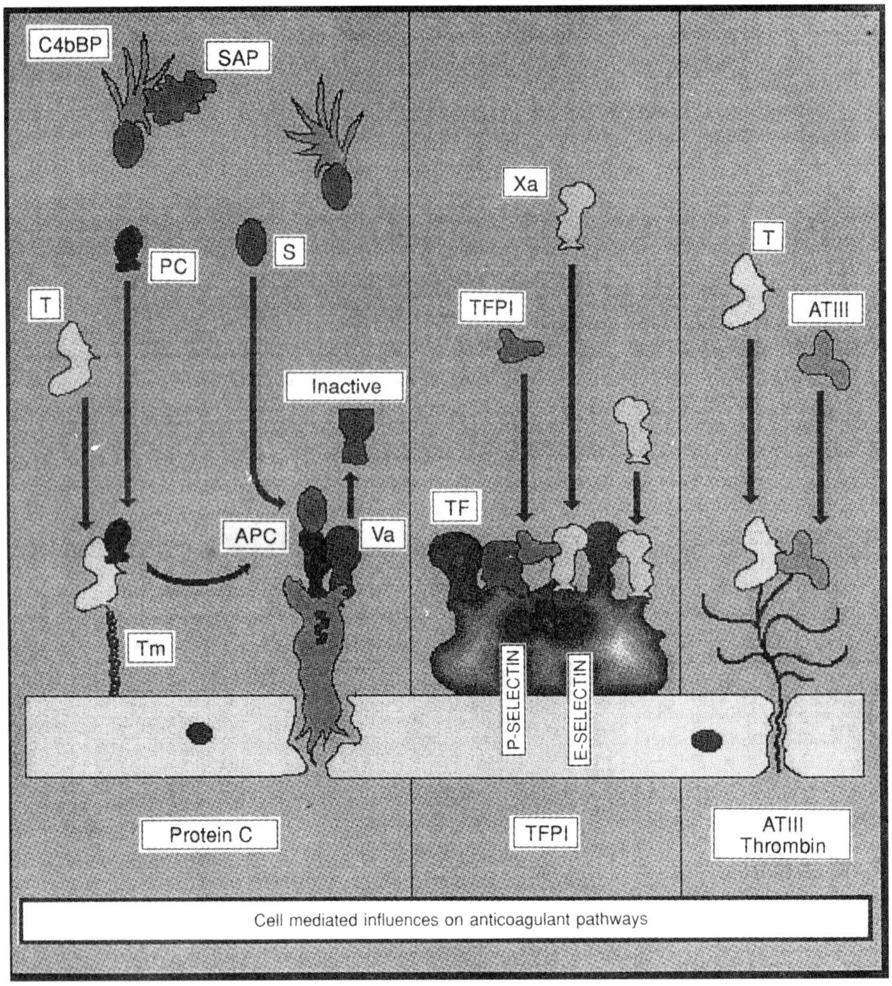

Fig. 1. Endothelial cell anticoagulant proteins: protein C and S, tissue factor pathway inhibitor (TFPI) and antithrombin III. Protein C is activated by thrombin bound to thrombomodulin which is depicted as a elongated multi-domain protein on the endothelial cell surface. The activated protein C interacts with uncomplexed protein S and the new complex is bound by platelets or endothelial cells where the complex is responsible for the inactivation of factor Va. Only free protein S is an active anticoagulatory protein and the circulating protein S may be complexed to C4bBP, an inhibitory protein of the classical complement pathways. TFPI has three inhibitor domains, one of which interacts with factor Xa and inhibits it. The resultant complex of Xa-TFPI interacts with the Tf-VIIa complex and results in reversible inhibition of its catalytical function. On the right hand side of the monocyte membrane, factors Xa and Va are preparing to bind prothrombin to form the prothrombinase complex. The balance of these opposing processes on the cell surface is influenced by the circulating and endothelial associated TFPI and its activation by factor Xa. Finally the antithrombin activity may be localised on either thrombomodulin or on the heparin-like proteoglycans, depicted as an arboreal structure on the endothelial cell. Interestingly, antithrombin III when complexed to heparin is also capable of inhibiting the Tf-VIIa complex but not free VIIa (not shown). TF: tissue factor; TFPI: tissue factor pathway inhibitor; T: thrombin; C4bBP: C4b binding protein; SAP: serum amyloid P; PC: protein C; APC: activated protein C; S: protein S; TM: thrombomodulin; ATIII: antithrombin. Factor is deleted before the Roman numerals for convenience.

and platelets also release proteases, endoglycosidases and heparanases which actively metabolise these proteoglycans in association with phospholipase C (27). In certain models of discordant graft rejection, approximately 50% of labelled heparan sulphate is lost within 5 minutes of reperfusion. Through interactions with antigen presenting cells, these heparan sulphate fragments and the native molecule either upregulate or downregulate cellular immune responses and influence cell migration (27).

Thrombomodulin, present on the surface of quiescent EC, binds thrombin. As a consequence of that interaction, protein C (PC), which is present in blood, is converted to activated protein C (APC). Together with protein S, another component of blood, APC interferes in the coagulation cascade by splitting clotting factors Va and VIIIa, and thus interfering with thrombosis, i.e., having an anticoagulant effect (28-31) (fig. 1).

XENOREACTIVE NATURAL ANTIBODIES (XNA)

In the context of future clinical xenotransplantation, it is important to note that humans and Old World primates lack a gene encoding a1,3 galactosyl transferase which causes terminal glycosylation of many proteins, including those expressed by EC, leucocytes and RBC of other species (32). Moreover, humans possess high concentrations of anti-Gal IgG (1% of circulating IgG). Their presence in plasma constitutes a major barrier to the use of discordant xenografts (32).

HAR in other species combinations also involves circulating XNA which develop in early neonatal life. These Ig, possibly produced by CD5+ B cells are often polyspecific and may arise as an early humoral defense to gut microorganisms, analogous to the development of isohemagglutinin Ig by cross-reaction with bacterial carbohydrates (33).

In some discordant models, such as primate rejection of a pig xenograft, XNA play a key role in initiating HAR since their depletion appears to prevent C activation and abrogates HAR allowing prolongation of xenograft survival for variable periods. In other discordant models, such as rat anti-guinea pig responses described above, depletion of XNA alone does not appear to prevent HAR. Such grafts may undergo HAR as a result of direct activation of the alternate pathway of complement (34).

COMPLEMENT (C) AND TYPE I EC ACTIVATION

Certain *in vivo* data suggest that C activation is critical to the pathogenesis of HAR and may, as reviewed by Dalmasso (7), result from either the classical or alternate pathways of activation. In the guinea pig to rat model, activation of the alternative pathway of C is the main factor leading to HAR. C activation has multiple effects on EC, resulting in various responses collectively termed EC stimulation or type I EC activation (23, 24). Such responses occur within seconds to minutes and given their rapidity, do not involve gene activation or protein synthesis. The activated complement components, C3a and C5a are the classical anaphylatoxins of acute inflammation and increase vascular permeability. In this context, C5a is needed for the cleavage of heparan sulfate which tightly tethers anti-thrombin III (AT-III) (35) from the EC. C5a also results in activation of xanthine oxidase, which generates reactive oxygen intermediates, which in association with the loss of superoxide dismutase associated with the proteoglycan may potentiate EC injury (36, 37).

The C3bi fragment which interacts with EC promotes adhesion of PMN and monocytes via CR3 (38). Generation of the membrane attack complex causes the exposure of a prothrombinase complex (39). All these pathways are further integrated by the interaction of C5b-C9, the membrane attack complex, with platelets, inducing not only the secretion of fibrinogen, other coagulation factors, ADP and serotonin but also platelet activation, adhesion and aggregation (40). This process occurs not only on the xenogeneic platelets carried over with the graft (where the situation is analogous to the xenogeneic EC activation of complement) but also on the circulating host platelets as an «innocent bystander response». Thus, C activation can result in direct damage to EC and of great importance, the activation of coagulation upon the EC and platelet surface inducing HAR (6, 40).

PAF AND OTHER INFLAMMATORY MEDIATORS IN HAR

Normally, EC provide a barrier to the egress of protein and cells from blood vessels and are non-adherent for platelets or PMN. However, when EC *in vitro* are stimulated by various agents, including XNA, C3a and C5a, and histamine, thrombin and leukotrienes, their functional properties change significantly (23, 41). The extent to which such EC responses occur *in vivo*, and if so, the extent to which they are responsible for the markedly increased vascular permeability, thrombosis and other pathologic hallmarks of HAR remains speculative. Additional studies of the generation of inflammatory mediators and their importance to discordant xenograft rejection considered the role of PAF and eicosanoids. Work in this field was initiated by Makowka et al. (41). PAF-antagonists (CV-3988), also prolong xenograft survival to a maximum of 7.5 hours in small animal models. At rejection after several hours, small numbers of monocytes and NK cells, but no PMN, are seen (42).

THROMBOREGULATION

Fibrin deposition and platelet aggregation in vascularised solid organ grafts are most likely to be a consequence of the immune and inflammatory responses observed during the complex process of rejection (6). Some products of the coagulation pathway, such as fibrin, participate in immunologically-mediated tissue damage and degradation products of fibrin may modify the function of cells of the immune system (43, 44). In a reciprocal fashion, immune stimulation and complement activation are crucial to several key events in blood coagulation which include thrombin generation and platelet aggregation and adhesion (40, 45) (fig. 2).

Furthermore, in the case of xenografts, potential incompatibilities in the necessary mix of donor EC associated coagulation inhibitory factors (for example the tissue factor pathway inhibitor) could lead to significant generation of procoagulant activity in vivo in a manner analogous to the complement decay acceleration factor (fig. 1).

Alternatively, grafted vessel subendothelial components (such as von Willebrand factor) could act to spontaneously promote platelet activation responses (40) (fig. 2).

Functional tissue factor is not normally present on endothelial cells but is found associated with the subendothelial matrix. Upon EC activation, there is an increase in tissue factor associated with the matrix as well as new expression on the surface of the activated cells (46).

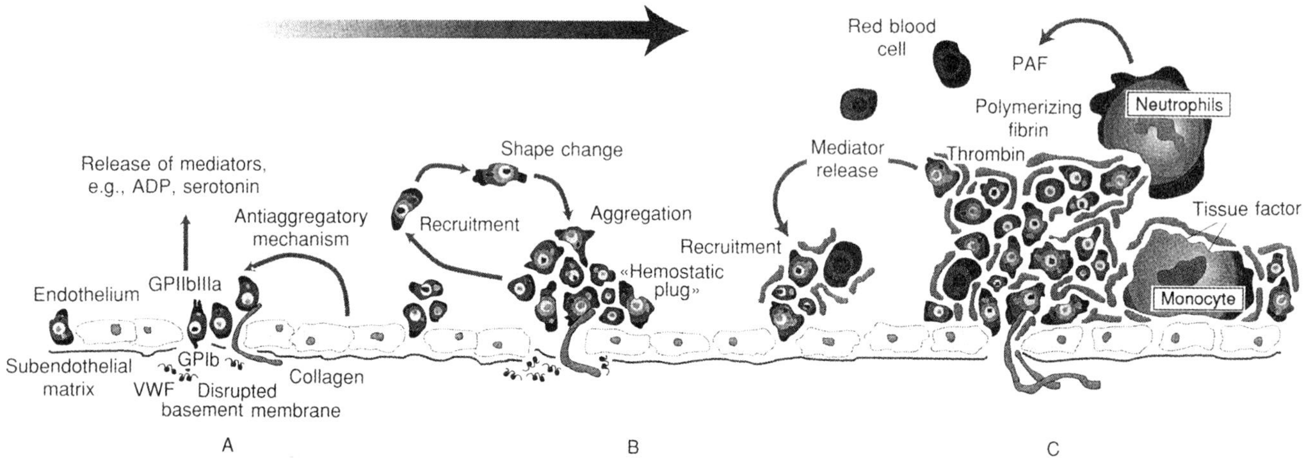

Fig. 2. Diagrammatic representation of platelet reactivity in xenograft rejection. A) Platelets circulate in the blood in an inactive state. Following endothelial cell activation or injury, platelets adhere to and spread on the subendothelial matrix initially by the interaction of GPIb and von Willebrand factor (VWF) which is facilitated by shear stress. It is feasible that xenogeneic VWF may have increased affinity for GPIb in the apparent absence of stress or vascular injury. The activation of platelets with increased expression of P-selectin and GPIIbIIIa is accompanied by mediator release, further recruitment and the promotion of the coagulation process. This process can be antagonised by the endothelial cell antiaggregatory mechanisms which include the ADPase systems, the synthesis of the prostacycline PGI2 and nitric oxide or endothelial cell derived relaxing factor (EDRF). B) Recruitment is accompanied by platelet activation with the shape changes and aggregation associated with this process. Platelet aggregates co-localize with the initial adherent platelets to form the early haemostatic plugs of platelet deposition. C)Thrombosis is a multicellular process. Both bound neutrophils and monocytes may participate in the inflammatory process(release of cytokines) and platelet activation (platelet activating factor) associated with the vascular injury. Monocytes in particular, promote the local process of thrombogenesis by the expression of TF. Red blood cells modulate platelet activation and are also incorporated into the clot. The endothelial surface loses its barrier function and extravasation begins.

The membrane assembly of the prothrombinase complex, including factors Xa, Va and prothrombin (PT), is dependent upon the association with factor Va, which then accelerates the conversion of prothrombin to thrombin. Thrombin then cleaves the fibrinopeptides A and B from the intact fibrinogen protein to form fibrin monomers, which associate and are cross-linked by factor XIIIa to form polymeric fibrin (47).

Activated monocytes, which also express tissue factor, may interact with the endothelium and platelets by cell surface adhesion molecules and also create loci for the initiation of coagulation (28, 48). Neutrophils are considered to have both a negative or positive overall influence on platelet hemostatic function; this negative action occurs despite the release of platelet activating factor (PAF) by activated cells (49). Neutrophil generated superoxides and radicals are also capable of activating platelets (50). Erythrocytes promote platelet aggregation by the co-expression of adhesion receptors, such as for thrombospondin, a large adhesion molecule, and by modulating the eicosanoid formation by platelets (40).

Platelet adhesion to the subendothelium by specific interactions further promotes the haemostatic mechanism. The assembly of coagulation factors on the platelet surface is facilitated by several events. *a*) There is expression of specific receptors for coagulation factor V, which are upregulated as a consequence of platelet activation. *b*) The platelet membrane aminophospholipids are exposed as a result of microparticle formation, which enhance the binding and assembly of the prothrombinase complex. *c*) Platelets contain in their alpha granules high concentrations of fibrinogen and other coagulation proteins which, when expressed on the cell surface or secreted into the extracellular environment, promote local fibrin deposition (40, 45).

The endothelial cell is crucial for the co-ordination of these processes; in turn, the degradation products of fibrin(ogen) generated during these reactions impact on the EC (51). There are three major EC mediated (anticoagulatory) systems in the blood that modulate the cell mediated events that initiate and control coagulation and which are influenced by EC activation responses. These include: *a*) the vitamin-K dependent factors, proteins C and S ; *b*) the tissue factor pathway inhibitor, and *c*) ATIII, the activity of which is potently enhanced by heparin (28) (fig. 1).

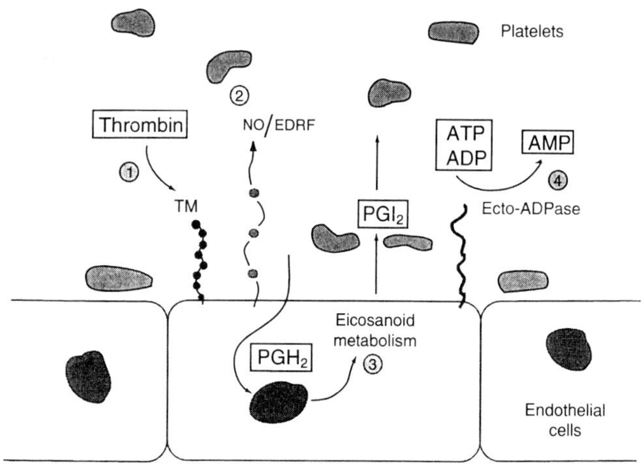

Fig. 3. Endothelial cell platelet anti-aggregatory mechanisms. Thrombomodulin expressed by the vascular endothelium is capable indirectly of abrogating platelet responses to thrombin. Endothelial cells also inhibit platelet aggregation by several mechanisms which include the release of prostacyclin (PGI_2), the generation of nitric oxide (NO) and the action of the ecto-ADPases, which efficiently degrade platelet derived ADP, thus inhibiting amplification pathways which result in platelet plug formation.

In addition to specific inhibitors of coagulation, endothelial cells also influence the process of fibrinolysis by the regulated secretion of plasminogen activators and their specific inhibitors. Endothelial cells also release thrombospondin, a large adhesion molecule which modulates plasmin generation and hence fibrinolysis (52).

Endothelial cells can also inhibit platelet aggregation by at least three mechanisms. These include the release of prostacyclin, the generation of nitric oxide and the action of the ecto-ADPase, which efficiently binds and degrades platelet derived ADP to AMP, thus inhibiting amplification pathways which result in platelet plug formation (53) (fig. 3). Finally, thrombomodulin expressed by the vascular endothelium is also capable of indirectly abrogating platelet responses to thrombin by virtue of high capacity binding by thrombomodulin of thrombin (28).

Recent data from our laboratories has demonstrated the ability of porcine EC in the absence of soluble complement factors to downregulate human blood mononuclear cell procoagulant activity despite expression of immunologically active tissue factor in vitro. The explanation appears to be the expression of both anticoagulatory factors including tissue factor pathway inhibitor and the expression of factor VII/VIIa receptors unrelated to tissue factor. In a similar fashion, EC ecto-ADPases are responsible for profound xenogeneic platelet inhibition in vitro. EC activation by recombinant human cytokines appears to reduce these inhibitory potentials. The mechanisms for this are under further evaluation.

THERAPEUTIC INTERVENTIONS

In part, our knowledge regarding precise mechanisms is based on the effects of various drugs, or other manipulations, aimed at prolonging xenograft survival and mirrors the situation observed in the development of clinical allotransplantation. The information gained from such studies, however, is difficult to interpret due to the pleiotropic effects that many manipulations and/or drugs have. Immunosuppressive agents, for instance, which are known to be effective in terms of suppressing T lymphocytes and B lymphocytes, may also block endothelial cell activation, or some components thereof. Mycophenolate mofetil (RS61443) inhibits smooth muscle proliferation (a component of certain forms of microvascular injury) while blocking antibody production and T cell responses. Physical depletion of natural antibodies, while clearly lowering the levels of those antibodies, in most protocols likely lowers complement factors and, in the case of physical removal as by plasmapheresis, lowers coagulation factors and other molecules as well (4, 5, 19).

Given the importance of XNA and complement in initiating vascular rejection, many investigators have focused on methods that would inhibit one or both of these factors for the hoped-for lifetime of the graft. If successful, the inhibition of recipient complement by membrane-associated inhibitors of complement placed in the ECs of the donor organ by transgenic or other methodology might achieve this for complement (54, 55). Alternatively, soluble complement receptors may have therapeutic benefit and less toxic side effects than the cobra venom factor used in the experimental setting (7, 56).

There are also potential approaches that would achieve long-term depletion for XNA; two examples include: *a*) B cells producing the XNA might be selectively eliminated by immunotoxins attached to antibodies recognizing the idiotypes that characterize the XNA, or *b*) tolerance to the xenoantigens recognized by XNA and elicited antibodies might be achieved. However, these approaches to lower XNA and elicited antibodies are far from reality at this time (57, 58).

It may not however, be necessary to remove XNA and compromise the complement system for the life-time of the graft to prevent vascular rejection (57, 58). Based on findings in allotransplantation across the ABO barrier (59), it may transpire that if XNA and complement are depleted for a limited time after the transplant is in place, that at a later time it may be possible to let XNA, C and possibly other factors return to pretransplant levels without evoking EC activation to the extent that rejection occurs. Bach et al have referred to the potential survival of a graft under such circumstances as «accommodation» (58). In brief, the factors which could lead to this include possible changes in the antibodies that return after depletion, including the possibility that non-complement fixing antibodies block the target sites on the EC, and/or that the targets themselves change, thus protecting them from XNA binding (58).

GENE THERAPY

One of the potential advantages of the use of animal when compared to human organs for clinical transplantation would be the greater potential for the genetic alteration of animal donors so that their tissues would theoretically elicit weaker immune responses. There are basically two ways that genetic engineering can be used to generate designated donor animals. First, transgenic technology can be used to insert new genes into animals, sometimes controlling the expression of these genes by incorporating specific promoters. Second, the technique of homologous recombination can be used to replace normal genes with new ones that may be unable to be expressed or expressed in an altered form. The first technique is already in use in large animals while the second is available only for mice at this time. Other modalities which are currently under study in our laboratories involve the generation of somatic recombinant EC with transient expression models to study the potential of expressing human anticoagulant proteins in porcine EC by the use of adenoviral vectors (59).

Further work will be directed at the expression of certain immunomodulatory factors in xenogeneic endothelium (60, 61). Should research indicate that several adhesion molecules or cytokines and their receptor combinations do not function across a particular species combination, but immune responses remain intact because of remaining compensatory interactions, then obviously alterations in the remaining interactions will be more useful than efforts to modify interactions that are inoperative (62-65). Similarly, a better knowledge of the specific mechanisms of xenograft destruction may suggest other more specific genetic and other manipulations to diminish these responses and to induce tolerance (62).

CONCLUSIONS

This short paper has attempted to summarise the currently available data on clinical xenotransplantation of the liver but has focussed primarily on the description of the various pathological processes of organ rejection that now prevent clinical application of this procedure. Increasing interest in this field will open up several new avenues for investigation. These developments may lead to new treatment modalities for allograft damage, acute or chronic rejection, non-transplant related diseases and even the clinical application of xenotransplantation.

REFERENCES

1. Calne RY. Organ transplantation between widely disparate species. Transplant Proc 1970; 2:550-553.
2. Auchincloss H. Xenografting: A review. Transplant Rev 1990; 4:14-27.
3. Auchincloss H Jr. Xenogeneic transplantation. A review. Transplantation 1988; 46:1-20.
4. Bach FH, Blakely ML, Van der Werf W, Vanhove B, Stuhlmeier KM, Hancock WW, de Martin R, Winkler H. Discordant xenografting: A working model of problems and issues. Xeno 1993; 1:8-16.
5. Bach FH, Robson SC, Ferran C, Winkler H, Millan MT, Stuhlmeier, Vanhove B, Blakely ML, van der Werf WJ, Hofer E, de Martin R, Hancock WW. Endothelial cell activation and thromboregulation during xenograft rejection. Immunol Rev (in press).
6. Hunt BJ, Rosenberg RD. The essential role of haemostasis in hyperacute rejection. Xeno 1993; 1:16-20.
7. Dalmasso AP. The complement system in xenotransplantation. Immunopharmacology 1992; 24:149-160.
8. Moses R D, Auchincloss H Jr. Mechanisms of cellular xenograft rejection. In: Cooper DKC, Kemp E, Reemstma K, White DJG, eds. Xenotransplantation: The Transplantation of Organs Between Species. Berlin: Springer, 1991; 101-120.
9. Moses RD, Winn HJ, Auchincloss H Jr. Evidence that multiple defects in cell-surface molecule interactions across species differences are responsible for diminished xenogeneic T cell responses. Transplantation 1992; 53:203-209.
10. Nakamura K, Murase N, Becich MJ, Furuya T, Todo S, Fung JJ, Starzl TE, Demetris AJ. Liver allograft rejection in sensitized recipients —observations in a clinically relevant small animal model. Am J Pathol 1993; 142:1383-1391.
11. Starzl TE, Fung JJ, Tzakis A. Baboon to human liver transplantation. Lancet 1993; 341:65-71.
12. Starzl TE, Tzakis A, Fung JJ, Toda S, Marino IR, Demetris AJ. Human liver xenotransplantation. Xeno 1993; 1:4-7.
13. Makowka L, Cramer DV, Hoffman A, Sher L, Podesta L. Pig liver xenografts as a temporary bridge for human allografting. Xeno 1993; 1:27-29.
14. Burdick JF, Fair JH. Xenoperfusion:the pig liver as a bridge. Xeno 1994; 2:3-5.
15. Rozga J, Williams F, Ro MS, Neuzil D, Giorgio T, Demetriou AA. Development of a bioartificial liver: properties and function of hollow-fibre module innoculated with liver cells. Hepatology 1993; 17:258-271.
16. Lenschow DJ, Zeng Y,Thistlethwaite J R, Montag A, Brady W, Gibson M G, Linsley PS, and Bluestone JA. Long-term survival of xenogeneic pancreatic islet grafts induced by CTLA4Ig. Science 1992; 257:789-792.
17. Michaels MA, Simmons RL. Xenozoonoses: possible xenotransplant associated infections. Xeno 1994; 3:47-51.
18. Bach FH. Xenotransplantation: A view to the future. Transplant Proc 1993; 25:25-29.
19. Bach FH, Dalmasso G, Platt JL. Xenotransplantation: A current perspective. Transplant Rev. 1992; 6:1-20.
20. Vanhove B, Bach FH. Human xenoreactive natural

antibodies: avidity and targets on porcine endothelial cells. Transplantation 1993; 56:1251-1253.
21. Lesnikoski BA, Shaffer DA, Van der Werf WJ, Hancock WW, Bach FH. Endothelial and host mononuclear cell activation and cytokine expression during rejection of pig-to-baboon discordant xenografts. Transplant Proc (in press).
22. Hancock WW, Blakely ML, Vanderwerf W, Bach FH. Rejection of guinea pig cardiac xenografts post-cobra venom factor therapy is associated with infiltration by mononuclear cells secreting interferon-gamma and diffuse endothelial activation. Transplant Proc 1993; 25:2932-2935.
23. Cotran RS, Pober JS. Endothelial activation and inflammation. Prog Immunol 1989; 8:747-754.
24. Pober JS, Cotran RS. The role of endothelial cells in inflammation. Transplantation 1991; 50:537-544.
25. Zetter BR. Endothelial heterogeneity: Influence of vessel size, organ localization, and species specificity on the properties of cultured endothelial cells. In: Ryan US, ed. Endothelial Cells, vol II. Boca Raton: CRC Press, 1988; 63-80.
26. Savage CO, Hughes CC, McIntyre BW, Picard JK, Pober JS. Human CD4+ T cells proliferate to HLA-DR+ allogeneic vascular endothelium. Identification of accessory interactions. Transplantation 1993; 56(1):128-134.
27. Ihrcke NS, Wrenshall LE, Platt JL. Role of heparan sulfate in immune system-blood vessel interactions. Immunol Today 1993; 14:500-505.
28. Esmon CT. Cell mediated events that control blood coagulation and vascular injury. Annu Rev Cell Biol 1993; 9:1-26.
29. Bevilacqua MP and Gimbrone, Jr MA. Modulation of endothelial cell procoagulant and fibrinolytic activities by inflammatory mediators. In: Ryan US, ed. Endothelial Cells, vol II. Boca Raton: CRC Press, 1988; 107-118.
30. Parkinson JF, Grinnell BW, Moore RE, Hoskins J, Valhos CJ, Bang NU. Stable expression of a secretable deletion mutant of recombinant human thrombomodulin in mammalian cells. J Biol Chem 1990; 265:12602-12610.
31. Balla, G, Jacob HS, Balla J, Rosenberg M, Nath K, Apple F, Eaton JW, Vercellotti GM. Ferritin: a cytoprotective antioxidant stratagem of endothelium. J Biol Chem 1992; 267:18148-18153.
32. Galili U. Interaction of the natural anti-Gal antibody with alpha-galactosyl epitopes —a major obstacle for xenotransplantation in humans. Immunology Today 1993; 14:480-482.
33. Springer GF, Horton RF. Blood group isoantibody stimulation in man by feeding blood group active bacteria. J Clin Invest 1969; 48:1280-1285.
34. Miyagawa S, Hirose H, Shirakura R, Naka Y, Nakata S, Kawashima Y, Seya T, Matsumoto M, Uenaka A, Kitamura H. The mechanism of discordant xenograft rejection. Transplantation 1988; 46:825-830.
35. Platt JL, Vercellotti GM, Lindman BJ, Oegama TR, Bach FH, Dalmasso AP. Release of heparan sulphate from endothelial cells: Implications for pathogenesis of hyperacute rejection. J Exp Med 1990; 171:1363-1368.
36. Platt JL, Lindman BJ, Chen H, Spitalnik SL, Bach FH. Endothelial cell antigens recognized by xenoreactive human natural antibodies. Transplantation 1990; 50:817-822.
37. Friedl HP, Till GO, Ryan US, Ward PA. Mediator-induced activation of xanthine oxidase in endothelial cells. FASEB J 1989; 3:2512-2518.
38. Vercellotti GM, Platt JL, Bach FH, Dalmasso AP. Enhanced neutrophil adhesion to xenogeneic endothelium via C3bi. J Immunol 1991; 146:730-736.
39. Hamilton KK, Hattori R, Esmon CT, Sims PJ. Complement proteins C5b-C9 induce vesiculation of the endothelial plasma membrane and expose catalytic surface for assembly of the prothrombinase enzyme complex. J Biol Chem 1990; 265:3809-3814.
40. Robson SC, Kopp C, Lesnikoski BA. Platelets and xenograft rejection. Xeno 1994; 2:38-46.
41. Makowka L, Chapman FA, Cramer DV, Qian S, Sun H, Starzl TE. Platelet-activating factor and hyperacute rejection. The effect of a platelet-activating factor antagonist, SRI 63-441, on rejection of xenografts and allografts in sensitised hosts. Transplantation 1990; 50:359-365.
42. Coughlan AF, Berndt MC, Dunlop LC, Hancock WW. In vivo studies of P-selectin and platelet activating factor during endotoxemia, accelerated allograft rejection, and discordant xenograft rejection. Transplant Proc 1993; 25:2930-2931.
43. Mosesson MW. The roles of fibrinogen and fibrin in hemostasis and thrombosis. Sem Hematol 1992; 29:177-188.
44. Robson SC, Saunders R, de Jager C, Purves L, Kirsch RE. Fibrin and fibrinogen degradation products with an intact D-domain C-terminal gamma chain inhibit an early step in accessory cell dependent lymphocyte mitogenesis. Blood 1993; 81:3006-3014.
45. Sims PJ, Wiedmer T. The response of human platelets to activated components of the complement system. Immunol Today 1991; 12:338-342.
46. Bach RR. Initiation of coagulation by tissue factor. Crit Rev Biochem Mol Biol 1988; 23:339-368.
47. Furie B, Furie BC. Molecular and cellular biology of blood coagulation. N Engl J Med 1992; 326:800-806.
48. Edwards RL, Rickles FR. The role of leukocytes in the activation of blood coagulation. Semin Hematol 1992; 29: 202-212.
49. Zhou WG, Javors MA, Olson MS. Platelet activating factor as an intercellular signal in neutrophil-dependent platelet activation. J Immunol 1992; 149:1763-1769.
50. Practico D, Iuliano L, Alessandri C, Camastra C, Violi F. Polymorphonuclear leukocyte-derived O2-reactive species activate primed platelets in human whole blood. Am J Physiol 1993; 264:1582-1587.
51. Ge M, Tang G, Ryan TJ, Malik AB. Fibrinogen degradation product D induces endothelial cell detachment by activation of cell-mediated fibrinolysis. J Clin Invest 1993; 90:2508-2516.

52. Anonick PK, Yoo JK, Webb DJ, Gonias SL. Characterisation of the antiplasmin activity of human thrombospondin-1 in solution. Biochem J 1993; 289:903-909.
53. Marcus AJ, Safier LB. Thromboregulation: multicellular modulation of platelet reactivity in hemostasis and thrombosis. FASEB J 1993; 7:516-522.
54. Dalmasso AP, Vercellotti GM, Platt JL, Bach FH. Inhibition of complement-mediated endothelial cell cytotoxicity by decay accelerating factor: potential for prevention of xenograft hyperacute rejection. Transplantation 1991; 52:530-538.
55. White DJ, Oglesby T, Liszewski MK.Expression of human decay accelerating factor or membrane cofactor protein genes on mouse cells inhibits lysis by human complement. Transplant Proc 1992; 24(2):474-476.
56. Hebell T, Ahearn JM, Fearon DT. Suppression of the immune response by a soluble complement receptor of B lymphocytes. Science 1991; 254:102-106.
57. Bach FH, Platt JL, Cooper D. Accommodation: the role of natural antibody and complement in discordant xenograft rejection. In: Cooper D, Kemp E, Reemtsma K, White DJG, eds. Xenotransplantation —the transplantation of organs and tissues between species. Heidelberg: Springer, 1991; 81-100.
58. Bach FH, Turman MA, Vercellotti GM, Platt JL, Dalmasso AP. Accommodation: A working paradigm for progressing toward clinical discordant xenografting. Transplant Proc 1991; 23:205.
59. Alexandre GPJ, Latinne D, Gianello P, Squifflet JP. Preformed cytotoxic antibodies and ABO-incompatible grafts. Clin Transplant 1991; 5:583-594.
59. Gerard, RD, Meidell RS. Adenovirus mediated gene transfer. Trends Cardiovasc Med 1993; 3(5):171-177.
60. Inverardi L, Socci C, Pardi R. Leukocyte adhesion molecules in graft recognition and rejection. Xeno 1993; 1:35-39.
61. Inverardi L, Samaja M, Motterlini R, Mangili F, Bender JR, Pardi R. Early recognition of a discordant xenogeneic organ by human circulating lymphocytes. J Immunol 1992; 149:1416-1423.
62. Latinne D, Gianello P, Smith CV, Nickelett V, Kawai T, Beadle M, Haug C, Sykes M, Lebowitz E, Bazin H, Colvin R, Cosimi AB, and Sachs DH. Xenotransplantation from pig to cynomolgus monkey: approach toward tolerance induction. Transplant Proc 1993; 25:336-338.
63. Colvin RB. Pathogenesis of vascular rejection. Transplant Proc 1991; 23:2052-2055.
64. Albelda SM, Smith CW, Ward PA. Adhesion molecules and inflammatory injury. FASEB J 1994; 8:504-512.
65. Butcher EC. Leukocyte-endothelial cell recognition: three (or more) steps to specificity and diversity. Cell 1991; 67:1033-1036.

Section 7

Treatment of Alcoholic Liver Disease

Early Diagnosis and Control of Alcohol Abuse

M. Salaspuro

INTRODUCTION

Early diagnosis of alcoholic liver injury is crucial for the attempts to retard the progression of the disease and improve prognosis. In the early stages of alcoholic liver disease it is not possible to make the diagnosis solely on the basis of clinical features. At this stage the symptoms and signs are unspecific such as nausea, anorexia, weight loss, diarrhea, weakness and indefinite gastric pains. Up to 30% of patients with early alcoholic liver disease are practically symptom-free and are admitted for further examinations because of an occasional hepatomegaly or an abnormal laboratory test. More specific symptoms such as jaundice, ascites or variceal bleeding are indicative for a more severe liver injury, i.e.,cirrhosis or alcoholic hepatitis. However, severe forms of fatty liver may also be associated with similar severe complications.

Three basic requirements in the diagnostics of alcohol-related liver diseases are as follows: *a*) to differentiate the alcohol-related liver disease from nonalcoholic liver diseases; *b*) to determine the type of the alcoholic liver disease (fatty liver, alcoholic hepatitis, cirrhosis), and *c*) to detect a possible alcohol-related liver injury in a patient admitted to hospital because of some other alcohol-related disease, trauma, pancreatitis or withdrawal treatment.

DRINKING HISTORY

Heavy alcohol consumption for months or years before hospital admission are highly indicative of alcohol-related liver disease. Problem drinkers have a tendency to ignore or hide their drinking. Furthermore, they may try consciously or subconsciously to deny the existence of alcohol problems. Heavy alcohol consumption, however, is frequently associated with guilty and a variety of social problems, the presence of which can be specified by using Cage- (1) or Malmö-MAST questionnaires (2). The questions focusing on the quantity and pattern of alcohol consumption or on alcohol problems should be part of the routine history taking, in which also other living habits such as smoking, nutrition and exercise should be elucidated. It should be emphasized, that even in the most careful interviews, individuals underestimate their alcohol consumption —the more, the larger the problem is.

In order to improve the obtention of alcohol history in outpatient units and among g-i inpatients a standard questionnaire should be a routine. Such a questionnaire could for instance be the WHO core screening instrument termed AUDIT (3), which consists of ten simple questions focusing on the amount and pattern of alcohol consumption (3 questions), alcohol dependence and black-outs (4 questions), negative reactions to alcohol (1 question) and alcohol problems (2 questions). The sensitivity of AUDIT in the detection of hazardous alcohol consumption (over 40 g for men and over 20 g for women, daily) has been reported to be 80%, with a 89% specificity.

CLINICAL FINDINGS

Characteristic clinical features of recent alcohol consumption include the smell of alcohol, intoxication, facial flushing, tremor and sweating. Spider naevi, acne rosacea, palmar erythema, parotid enlargement, gynaecomastia, testicular atrophy, finger clubbing and Dupuytren's contracture are unspecific signs of chronic liver disease. However, they are frequently found in chronic alcoholics without significant liver injury. Scars, bruises and old fractures can equally be considered as signs of alcohol abuse.

On the basis of clinical features it is not possible to differentiate the various types of alcoholic liver diseases from each other or from endstage nonalcoholic liver diseases. Accordingly, a patient presenting with signs of severe liver failure —ascites, jaundice, variceal bleeding— may have alcoholic hepatitis, cirrhosis, massive fatty liver or nonalcoholic liver disease.

LABORATORY TESTS

Laboratory tests are used to facilitate the recognition of chronic heavy drinking (4, 5), differentiate alcoholic from nonalcoholic liver disease and assess the severity of liver injury. Biological marker of alcohol abuse is an abnormal blood or urinary test, which most often results from the excessive release of cellular contents or products either to blood or urine. With respect to alcohol abuse, biological markers may be valuable both in the early diagnosis as well as in the treatment of alcohol problems. Laboratory signs of excessive and harmful alcohol consumption can be divided into two main groups: trait markers and state markers.

Trait markers, which can also be called vulnerability markers, are hoped to be able to identify people who may be vulnerable to developing alcoholism. These tests should be positive even before the person has consumed alcohol and that positivity should persist during the development of alcoholism as well as during abstinence. Most of the studies on trait markers involve children of alcoholics. These markers include for instance dopamine D_2 receptor gene, dopamine beta-hydroxylase, platelet adenylate cyclase, and platelet monoamine oxidase. The present knowledge about the true value of trait markers is still rather preliminary.

State markers reflect the physiological and/or pathological changes occurring in the body after alcohol use or abuse. The aim of state markers is to detect, at an early stage, levels of alcohol consumption that are likely to be harmful in the long run. This allows intervention and treatment before severe pathological changes or negative social consequences associated with alcohol abuse have appeared. State markers play an important role in the follow-up of abstinence and may be the earliest indicators of relapses occurring during treatment. Consequently, their use in the studies on treatment evaluation is nowadays considered essential. They may further function as a reinforcing feed-back mechanism during treatment of alcoholics, who thus have a possibility to follow the positive effects of abstinence on these tests.

In clinical practice two types of state markers are needed. The first type of markers are used in the detection of recent drinking, for instance a positive urinary ethanol in the follow-up of abstinence in patients with alcoholic liver disease. The second group of markers are used in the screening of general population. They are less sensitive and react only to long lasting heavy drinking, for instance gamma-glutamyl transferase (GGT). The ideal test should be sensitive, specific, simple, noninvasive, and inexpensive. We have to admit that so far none of the available tests fulfils all criteria of an ideal marker (5, 6-8).

Ethanol

Simple and specific evidence for recent alcohol use is obtained by the detection of alcohol in blood, breath, urine, sweat, or saliva. The test has been recommended as a routine in emergency admissions of ambulatory patients. In addition regular, determination of urinary alcohol concentration has been successfully used to assess the reliability of the self-reports on alcohol consumption by patients (9-11).

Detection of alcohol, however, does not allow the distinction between acute and chronic alcohol use, unless it can be related to increased tolerance towards alcohol. Thus, according to the diagnostic criteria proposed by the National Council on Alcoholism in 1972 (12) the following are first level signs of alcoholism: *a*) a blood ethanol concentration above 1 g/l in a routine examination; *b*) 1.5 g/l in a patient showing no signs of clinical intoxication, or *c*) 3 g/l at any time.

Gamma-Glutamyl Transferase (GGT)

Gamma-glutamyl transferase is a well characterized enzyme that is released mainly from the liver to the blood during chronic excessive alcohol consumption. It should be emphasized that the activity of serum GGT may increase after chronic alcohol consumption already before the development of alcohol-related liver injury. At present the test is the most commonly used single laboratory marker for the detection of alcohol abuse. Chronic heavy alcohol consumption has been shown to lead to an increased serum GGT activity in a variable percentage of alcohol abusing patients (29-90%) in a number of studies performed during the last 2 decades (5, 6). The rather large variation in the results depends on the patient populations used in different reports. It is well established that a large majority of chronic alcoholics who have been hospitalized for withdrawal treatment show an elevated serum GGT level during the first week after the admission. Accordingly, the sensitivity of serum GGT in the detection of active alcoholism is good, but because of a self-evident diagnosis not so much needed. On the other hand it should be remembered that the sensitivity of the test is not 100%, i.e., some chronic alcoholics may have totally normal liver enzyme tests including GGT even though they have been known to be drinking heavily for weeks or months before the testing.

In the screening of heavy drinkers from the general population, serum GGT, however, is far less sensitive and should always be supplemented with questionnaires focused on the quantity and frequency of alcohol consumption as well as on the alcohol-related social or other problems. GGT has been reported to detect correctly heavy drinking in only 37.5% of young adult alcoholics with a specificity of 90.2% (13). Furthermore, serum GGT is almost insensitive in the detection of heavy drinking among young university students (14). Information about the correlation of GGT to alcohol consumption is controversial, as some investigators have found a significant but low correlation between these two parameters, whereas others have not. On the other hand, serum GGT correlates rather well (r = 0.55-0.66) with reported alcohol consumption in treated alcoholics and accordingly it suits well for the detection of relapses (10, 15).

An acute intoxicating dose of alcohol does not increase serum GGT activity. Neither is GGT activity influenced by drinking of 60 g of ethanol daily for three weeks (16). Accordingly, elevated serum GGT value most often indicates long-lasting and heavy-alcoholic-drinking. The probability that the patient has more than six drinks per day increases from 20 to 50% when GGT exceeds 60 IU/l (17). It has been reported, that in drinking debauches lasting less than 2 weeks, GGT stays within the normal limits. In debauches lasting 2-6 weeks GGT may exceed the upper limit of normal, and debauches of more than 6 weeks may increase serum GGT values considerably (18). The half-life of increased serum GGT is about 26 days and, consequently, in patients with very high initial GGT values, elevated levels can be found even after an abstinence period longer than one month. During abstinence of only a week, GGT decreases in almost all alcoholics. Accordingly, a decrease in GGT during total abstinence lasting not more than 7 days is indicative for an «alcoholic» origin of elevated GGT with a sensitivity of 90% (19).

The worst drawback concerning the use of GGT as a screening test of alcohol abuse is its poor specificity in population samples containing mostly nonalcoholics. In a random sample of middle-aged Swedish males 16% had elevated serum GGT; in 75% of these the main reason was excessive alcohol consumption, and in 2% it was a nonalcoholic liver disease (20). In another study on apparently healthy men, however, only 50% of elevated GGT values were due to alcohol (21). In hospital samples the prevalence of non-alcoholic origins of increased GGT is also high, and the diagnostic value of GGT in the detection of alcohol problems has therefore been questioned (22). In addition to alcohol abuse, elevated serum GGT is found in many non-alcoholic diseases. Serum GGT increases in all type of liver diseases and high levels are seen in obstructive jaundice. Highly overlapping elevations of both serum and hepatic GGT are seen in alcoholic fatty liver, alcoholic hepatitis, alcohol-induced liver fibrosis, and alcoholic cirrhosis. In relation to alcohol abuse the most important injury is perhaps pancreatitis. Non-alcoholic diseases with occasional GGT elevations are: heart attacks, heart failure, nephrotic syndrome, renal transplant rejection, diabetes mellitus (up to 57% with those with vascular complications), overweight by more than 30%, hyperlipidaemia type IV, hepatic spread of cancers, and severe trauma (4, 18). Drugs inducing the hepatic microsomal system may increase serum GGT levels. The most important drugs of this group are antiepileptics (phenytoin, phenobarbital), anticoagulants (warfarin), and barbiturates (23).

Mean Corpuscular Volume (MCV)

The association between macrocytosis (increased size of red cells) and alcoholism was found as early as the 1930s. As a marker of excessive alcohol consumption it has been used since 1974. The mechanism behind alcohol-induced macrocytosis is unknown, but has been related to the direct toxicity of ethanol on erythroblasts. In various patient populations, increased MCV values are found in 26-94% of alcoholic patients (17, 24, 25). Increased MCV value has been shown to correlate weakly with the total amount of alcohol consumed and the length of the drinking period. The probability that a patient uses over six drinks per day increases from 20 to 60%, when MCV increases from 90 to 100 fl (17).

As a biological marker of alcohol abuse, increased MCV is less sensitive but more specific than GGT. Macrocytosis is independent on the severity of the liver injury. Increased MCV values may be found in about 20% of patients with non-alcoholic liver disease, but in these cases MCV does not exceed 100 fl (25). The incidence of macrocytosis among patients in general practice has been reported to be 2.4% (26). Of those with macrocytosis, 80.2% of men and 34.1% of women were alcohol abusers. Other causes of increased MCV include vitamin B_{12} and folate deficiency, liver disease, reticulocytosis, antiepileptic drugs, age, smoking and menopause. Patient history and clinical findings such as marital problems, smoking, and, at least among men, elevated blood pressure should remind the physician of the possibility of alcohol abuse. Due to the long survival of red cells, MCV normalizes slowly (within months) during abstinence. In some studies MCV has been shown to correlate better with the admitted alcohol consumption than GGT. Most importantly, MCV is inexpensive and readily available in most hospital laboratories.

Carbohydrate Deficient Transferrin (CDT)

CDT is an abnormal variant of human transferrin, which is deficient in sialic acid, neutral galactose and N-acetylglucosamine. This variant transferrin is found in increased amounts in the serum of persons abusing alcohol (27, 28). In studies dealing with dependent alcoholics the sensitivity of the test to detect alcoholism has ranged from 61 to 91%. The sensitivity may be lowest among patients with alcohol-related liver injury (29). In comparison to conventional biological markers of alcohol abuse the major advantage of CDT is its high specificity (> 95%), with primary biliary cirrhosis being the only major disease group producing high CDT values in approximately 30-40% of the cases (29, 30).

The half-life of elevated CDT level is suitable for a marker (around 2 weeks). Serum CDT levels are higher in women than in men, and no correlation is found between serum CDT and GGT, liver transaminases, or MCV. In patients with alcoholic liver disease CDT is a better marker of abstention than GGT or MCV (31). In addition to its higher specificity, serum CDT may be more informative than GGT and liver transaminases (aspartate aminotransferase = ASAT, alanine aminotransferase = ALAT) also with respect to its sensitivity. During controlled heavy drinking of 60 g ethanol per day for three weeks, a statistically significant increase in the mean CDT but not in GGT and ASAT levels could be observed (16). However, only in two out of the ten volunteers did CDT exceed the upper normal limit. This finding as well as studies on the screening of heavy drinkers from general populations indicate that the sensitivity of CDT to detect early alcohol problems may be limited. Among 77 non-alcoholic heavy drinkers the sensitivity of CDT was 28.6% and specificity 91.8% (32). In the same study the best conventional marker, GGT, detected correctly 35.1% of heavy drinkers with a specificity of 86.9%. Unsatisfactorily low sensitivities in the detection of heavy drinking have been reported also in other screening studies focused on normal populations, drunken drivers, young problem drinkers, and university students (33, 34).

Unavailability of a simple method to determine CDT concentration has so far limited the general use of the test. Recent release of a commercially available kit (CDT RIA, Pharmacia AB, Sweden) will hopefully solve this problem, although the relatively high price and the somewhat poorer sensitivity of the test kit as compared to the original method may still limit the use of the test. Another method for CDT determination using isoelectric focusing and Western blotting has recently been reported to have somewhat higher accuracy than the Pharmacia kit (35).

CONTROL OF ALCOHOL ABUSE

The treatment of choice of alcoholic liver diseases is a strict control of drinking or abstinence. In this process the role of the physician, who is primarily responsible for the patient's care, is essential. At first the physician should give to her/his patient information about the biochemical, histological and other evidence of the alcohol-related liver injury. This should be followed by the encouragement of the patient to abstain from alcohol. If the patient do not accept total abstinence, an agreement between the patient and the physician about the length of the abstinence should be done. The fact that the progression of the liver injury can be stopped only by abstinence should be emphasized. The information should also include the dismal effects of continued drinking on the liver injury including complications such as variceal bleeding, ascites and liver coma.

There is a lot of evidence of the effectiveness of a brief intervention in about 50% of the patients with heavy drinking or alcohol problems (36, 37). However, patients should also be provided with all possible information on the local and regional treatment facilities. This also includes self-help groups such as Alcoholics Anonymous. The follow-up of the patient at the outpatient clinic once a week at least in the beginning is important. These visits should include laboratory tests both for the control of abstinence as well as for the motivation of the patient for further attempts to reduce his drinking. If these visits are combined with supervised treatment with disulfiram the treatment result can be markedly improved (38). Although there is a wide range of different treatment forms both in outpatient and inpatient settings, none of them has been shown to produce markedly better results than a brief intervention combined with careful follow-up carried out by the patient's own physician.

REFERENCES

1. Mayfield D, McLeod G, Hall P. The CAGE questionnaire: Validation of a new alcoholism screening instrument. Am J Psych 1974; 131:1121-1123.
2. Kristenson H, Trell E. Indicators of alcohol consumption: Comparisons between a questionnaire (Mm-MAST), interviews and serum gamma-glutamyl transferase (GGT) in a health survey of middle-aged males. Br J Addict 1982; 77:297-304.
3. Anderson P. Management of drinking problems. WHO Regional Publications, European Series, no. 32, 1990; 1-168.
4. Salaspuro M. Characteristics of laboratory markers in alcohol-related organ damage. Scand J Gastroenterol 1989; 24:769-780.
5. Salaspuro M, Roine R. Alcohol. In: Noe DA, Rock RC, eds. Laboratory Medicine. The Selection and Interpretation of Clinical Laboratory Studies. Baltimore: Williams & Wilkins, 1994; 554-564.
6. Salaspuro M. Conventional and coming laboratory markers of alcoholism and heavy drinking. Alcohol: Clin Exp Res 1986; 10(6):5S-12S.
7. Rosman AS. Utility and evaluation of biochemical markers of alcohol consumption. J Substance Abuse 1992; 4:277-297.
8. Mihas AA, Tavassoli M. Laboratory markers of ethanol intake and abuse; a critical appraisal. Am J Med Sci 1992; 303: 415-428.
9. Staun-Olsen P, Thomsen AC. Serum ethanol estimations in the control of alcohol abstinence in patients with liver disease. Scand J Gastroenterol 1979; 14:785-789.
10. Orrego H, Blake JE, Israel Y. Relationship between gamma-glutamyl transpeptidase and mean urinary alcohol levels in alcoholics while drinking and after alcohol withdrawal. Alcohol Clin Exp Res 1985; 9:10-13.
11. Caballeria J, Torres M, Camps J, Parés A, Reixach M, Rodés M. Urine ethanol assessment: a helpful method for controlling abstinence in alcoholic liver disease. Alcohol Alcohol 1988; 23:403-407.

12. National Council on Alcoholism, The Criteria Committee. Criteria for the diagnosis of alcoholism. Ann Intern Med 1972; 77:249-258.
13. Chan AWK, Welte FW, Whitney RB. Identification of alcoholism in young adults by blood chemistries. Alcohol 1987; 4:175-179.
14. Nyström M, Peräsalo J, Pikkarainen J, Salaspuro M. Conventional laboratory tests as indicators of heavy drinking in young university students. Scand J Prim Care 1993; 54:528-533.
15. Keso L, Salaspuro M. Comparative value of self-report and blood tests in assessing outcome amongst alcoholics. Br J Addict 1993; 85:209-215.
16. Salmela K, Laitinen K, Nyström M, Salaspuro M. Carbohydrate-deficient transferrin during 3 week's heavy alcohol consumption. Alcohol Clin Exp Res 1994; 18: 228-230.
17. Chick J, Kreitman N, Plant M. Mean cell volume and gamma-glutamyl-transpeptidase as markers of drinking in working men. Lancet 1981; i:1249-1251.
18. Wadstein J, Skude G. Serum ethanol, hepatic enzymes and length of debauch in chronic alcoholics. Acta Med Scand 1979; 205:317-318.
19. Weill J, Schellenberg F, Le Goff A-M, Benard J-Y. The decrease of low serum gamma glutamyl transferase during short-term abstinence. Alcohol Alcohol 1988; 5:1-3.
20. Kristenson H, Trell E, Fex G, Hood B. Serum gamma-glutamyltransferase: Statistical Distribution in a middle-aged male population and evaluation of alcohol habits in individuals with elevated levels. Prev Med 1980; 9:108-119.
21. Penn R, Worthington LJ, Clarke CA, Whitfield AGW. Gamma-glutamyl-transpeptidase and alcohol intake. Lancet 1981; i:894.
22. Penn R, Worthington DJ. Is serum gammaglutamyltransferase a misleading test? Br Med J 1983; 286:531-535.
23. Whitfield JB, Moss DW, Neale G, Orme M, Breckeridge A. Changes in plasma-gammaglutamyltranspeptidase activity associated with alterations in drug metabolism in man. Br Med J 1973; 274:316-318.
24. Wu A, Chanarin I, Levi AJ. Macrocytosis of chronic alcoholism. Lancet 1974; i:829-830.
25. Morgan MY, Camilo ME, Luck W, Sherlock S, Hoffbrand AV. Macrocytosis in alcohol-related liver disease: its value for screening. Clin Lab Haematol 1981; 3:35-44.
26. Seppä K. Laippala P, Saarni M. Macrocytosis as a consequence of alcohol abuse among patients in general practice. Alcohol Clin Exp Res 1991; 15:871-876.
27. Stibler H, Allgulander C, Borg S, Kjellin KG. Abnormal microheterogeneity of transferrin in serum and cerebrospinal fluid in alcoholism. Acta Med Scand 1978; 204:49-56.
28. Stibler H. Carbohydrate-deficient transferrin in serum: a new marker of potentially harmful alcohol consumption reviewed. Clin Chem 1991; 37:2029-2037.
29. Bell H, Tallaksen C, Sjåheim T, Weberg R, Raknerud N, Örjasaeter H, Tyr K, Haug, E. Serum carbohydrate-deficient transferrin as a marker of alcohol consumption in patients with chronic liver diseases. Alcohol Clin Exp Res 1993; 17:246-252.
30. Behrens UJ, Worner TM, Braly LF, Schaffner F, Lieber CS. Carbohydrate deficient transferrin, a marker for chronic alcohol consumption in different ethnic populations. Alcohol Clin Exp Res 1988; 12:427-432.
31. Behrens UJ, Worner TM, Lieber CS. Changes in carbohydrate-deficient transferrin levels after alcohol withdrawal. Alcohol Clin Exp Res 1988; 12:539-544.
32. Sillanaukee P, Seppä K, Löf K, Koivula T. CDT by anion-exchange chromatography followed by RIA as a marker of heavy drinking among men. Alcohol Clin Exp Res 1993; 17:230-233.
33. Nielssen O, Huseby NE, Höer G, Brenn T, Schirmer H, Förde OH. New alcohol markers —how useful are they in population studies: The Svalbard study. Alcoholism Clin Exp Res 1992; 16:82-86.
34. Nyström M, Peräsalo J, Salaspuro, M. Carbohydrate-deficient transferrin (CDT) in serum as a possible indicator of heavy drinking in young university students. Alcohol Clin Exp Res 1992; 16:93-97.
35. Xin Y, Lasker JM, Rosman AS, Lieber CS. Isoelectric focusing/western blotting: A novel and practical method for quantitation of carbohydrate-deficient transferrin in alcoholics. Alcohol Clin Exp Res 1992; 5:814-821.
36. Kristenson H, Öhlin H, Hultén-Nosslin M-B, Trell E, Hood B. Identification and intervention of heavy drinking in middle-aged men: Results and follow-up of 24-60 months of long-term study with randomized controls. Alcohol Clin Exp Res 1983; 7:203-209.
37. Chick J, Lloyd G, Crombie E. Counselling problem drinkers in medical wards: a controlled study. Br Med J 1985; 290:965-967.
38. Azrin NH, Sissons R, Myer SR. Alcoholism treatment by disulfiram and community reinforcement therapy. J Behav Ther Exp Psych 1982; 13:105-112.

Antioxidant Drugs and Colchicine in the Treatment of Alcoholic Liver Disease

H. K. Seitz, G. Pöschl

INTRODUCTION

The pathogenesis of alcoholic liver disease is complex and far from clear. During the last three decades a variety of mechanisms involved in the development of alcoholic liver disease have been elucidated. Among those are toxic effects of ethanol and acetaldehyde. Such toxicity may result in functional impairment of the hepatocyte leading to morphological alterations and cell death as well as to an enhanced active and/or reactive fibrogenesis which eventually leads to cirrhosis. In addition, a variety of electrophilic free radicals may appear during ethanol oxidation and/or during the enhanced metabolism of a great number of xenobiotics by an induced microsomal cytochrome P-450 2E1 ethanol oxidizing pathway (1).

It has been shown that during ethanol oxidation a variety of electrophilic intermediates are produced which are capable to react with cell macromolecules leading to lipid peroxidation. Among those are oxygen- and carbon-centered radicals (2-8) (fig. 1). Furthermore, chronic ethanol consumption does not only result in increased generation of reactive oxygen species but also in a severe alteration and reduction of the antioxidant defense system which includes, among others, hepatic glutathion, vitamin E, selenium and related compounds (1, 9-11). On the basis of these pathogenetic aspects it is not surprising that antioxidative drugs have been attempted in the treatment of alcoholic liver disease. Among these drugs (+)-cyanidanol-3 (catechin) and silymarin have been investigated experimentally in detail and a number of clinical trials have been performed. Because of the autoimmune hemolytic anemia as a side effect (+)-cyanidanol-3 has been withdrawn from the market, at least in Germany. In addition, colchicine, a drug primarily introduced to treat acute attack of gout and familial Mediterranean fever has also some interesting effects on hepatic secretion processes, immunology, and fibrogenesis (12-17).

ANTIOXIDANT DRUGS

(+)-Cyanidanol-3

This compound is a naturally occuring flavonoid with antioxidant and membrane stabilizing properties and the ability to scavenge free radicals (18-19). On the basis of this, (+)-cyanidanol-3 has been used to treat alcoholic liver disease. Most of the studies in which (+)-cyanidanol-3 was given in a dosage between 1.5-3 g per day over 0.5 to 12 months did not show any significant beneficial effect of the drug (20-26, for review see 27). In one study by Palmas, 31 patients with compensated cirrhosis of the liver, mostly of alcoholic origin, were treated over 5 months with 3 g (+)-cyanidanol-3. The treated group showed some improvement in laboratory values after the third month (23). The results of this trial have to be interpreted with caution

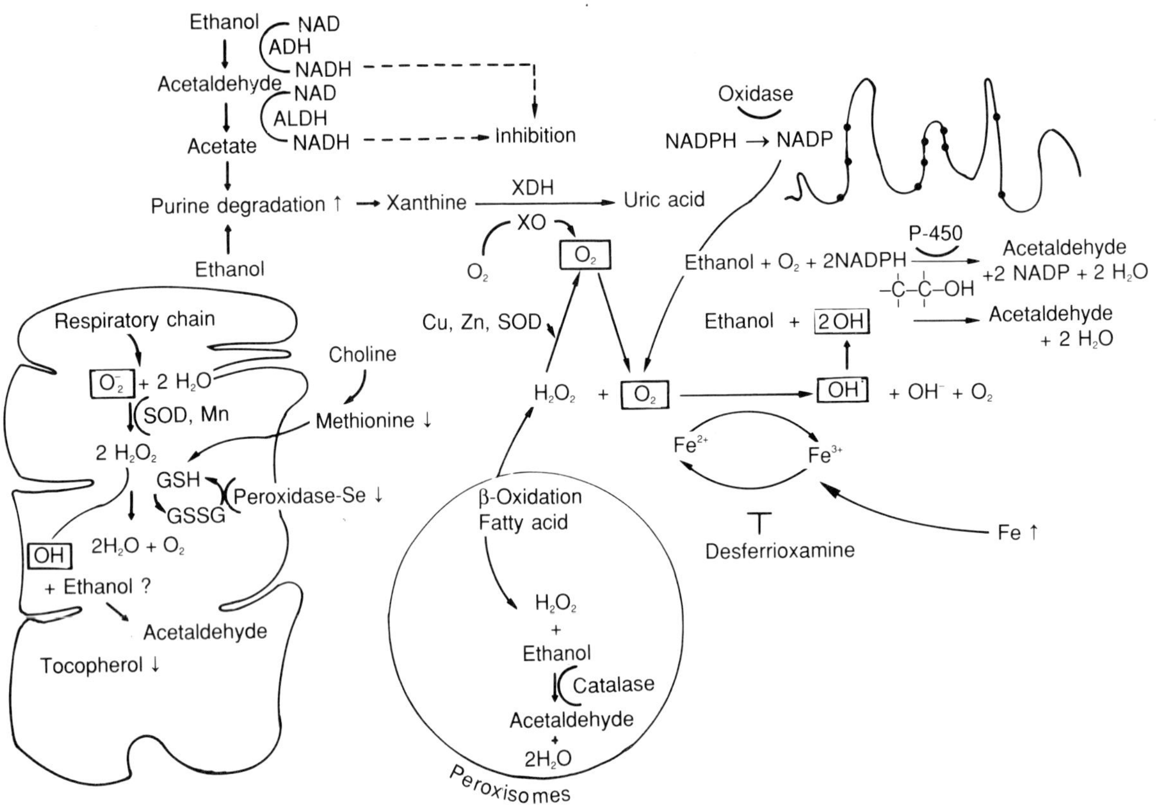

Fig. 1. Ethanol metabolism and radical formation in the hepatocyte.

since the drinking behaviour was not monitored during the study.

It has to be pointed out that (+)-cyanidanol-3 has a positive effect on the rat liver (27). However, such an effect could not be reproduced in humans, which could be due to the fact that the doses used in animal experiments were approximately 5-10 times higher. An increase in dosage may be difficult in humans since side effects of the drug such as allergic hyperthermia and autoimmune hemolytic anemia may increase with increasing dosage (20, 22). To solve this problem a derivative with better pharmokinetic characteristics has been used. Thus, 3-palmitoyl-(+)catechin was used and had again no significant beneficial clinical, biochemical and histological effect in patients with biopsy-proven alcoholic liver disease (28).

Silymarin

The hepatoprotective properties of silymarin which consists of silybinin, silychristin and silydianin has been claimed for many years. The effect of silymarin and its main constituent silybinin on experimentally-induced liver toxity has been investigated intensively. Although in animal studies using galactosamine, CCl_4, paracetamol, phalloidin, GSH depleting agents and ischemia a beneficial effect of silymarin could be documented (29-32), the mechanism of action of this drug is not completely clarified.

It has been clearly shown that silymarin is a scavenger of oxygen radicals including OH and HOCl (33, 34), but not of O_2– and possibly not of H_2O_2, although some controversy exists. Furthermore, it has been claimed that silybinin is a weak iron chelator (33). Several studies have clearly identified silybinin as a protective agent against lipid peroxidation (35, 36). In one study silymarin protected against paracetamol-induced lipid peroxidation and liver damage possibly by its antioxidant properties acting as free radical scavenger (29). It was interesting to note that glycogen was restored much faster under silymarin. In another experimental study, silymarin prevented membrane alterations in acute CCl_4 liver damage —again through its antioxidant properties by modifying the plasma membrane phospolipid content (30).

The fact that silymarin possesses membrane stabilizing properties has been recognized for a long time and therefore silymarin was used in *Amanita phalloides* poisoning to prevent the uptake of the toxin by hepatocytes. Thus, silymarin intravenously administered is a well established drug in the treatment of *Amanita phalloides* poisoning.

In addition, silymarin also increases protein biosynthesis by stimulating r-RNA polymerase leading to an unspecific increase of hepatic proteins (37). Furthermore, silybin decreases ethanol metabolism in rats and it was thought that this effect is due to an inhibition of the ethanol metabolizing oxidizing system (MEOS). It was proposed that this inhibition of MEOS by silybin is also related to its antioxidant properties acting as a scavenger of free radicals (38).

On the basis of these experimental data obtained in cultures and in the rat model, silymarin was also used in patients with various types of liver diseases. Salmi and Sarna performed a prospective randomized double-blind trial over 4 weeks with 420 mg silymarin daily versus placebo in 97 patients who had persistent elevation of serum transaminases. The majority of those patients drank alcohol regularly and liver biopsies were performed in all patients. The silymarin group showed a significantly greater decrease in serum transaminase activities. Eleven out of 15 patients who were re-biopsied had an improvement of liver histology under the drug. However, drinking behaviour of the patients during the trial was not monitored (39). Salvagnini et al. treated 122 alcoholic patients with either 420 mg silymarin or placebo for 6 weeks and found an improvement of serum aspartate transaminase activity in the treated group (27). Velussi et al. investigated the effect of 600 mg silymarin on diabetes caused by alcoholic liver cirrhosis for 6 months. In silymarin treated patients mean level of fasting blood glucose, glycosylated hemoglobin, daily insulin requirements, fasting insulinemia, blood malonaldehyde and basal as well as glucagon stimulated C-peptide were all significantly lower than in untreated patients and lower than at baseline (40). These results indicated that silymarin reduces lipid peroxidation of liver cell membranes also in cirrhotic diabetes patients and increases the sensitivity of the insulin receptor among others.

Only one long-term double-blind controlled trial in patients with cirrhosis of the liver has been performed. Ferenci et al. randomized 170 cirrhotic patients (61% with alcohol abuse) with either 420 mg silymarin per day or placebo over 2 years. The 4-year survival rate of the patients of the verum group was 58% compared to 39% in the placebo group ($p = 0.04$). A detailed analysis of the study showed that only patients with alcoholic cirrhosis and patients with Child A classification had a significant benefit from silymarin treatment (41). Again drinking history was not recorded in this study which makes it very difficult to draw conclusions.

Meanwhile another 2-year study with silymarin is on its way in which alcohol intake and compliance is well documented. Thus, hopefully, within the next 2 years we shall have further additional information about the effect of this interesting drug on liver function and outcome in patients with alcoholic cirrhosis.

Vitamin E and Selenium

Both tocopherol and selenium belong to the antioxidant defense system and both compounds are decreased in alcoholism and alcoholic liver disease. Selenium is an essential component of the tetramere glutathion peroxidase and of the monomere phospholipid hydroxyperoxyd-glutathionperoxidase and they act as repair system for peroxidized membrane phospholipid fatty acids. Because of these facts both compounds have been used in a clinical trial (42). 56 patients with alcoholic hepatitis and cirrhosis of the liver (Child B and C) received either 600 mg α-tocopherol, 200 μg selenium and 12 mg zinc daily or placebo. In the antioxidant group a significant improvement of serum bilirubin, ammonia and malondialdehyde was observed. Mortality of the control group was 40% as compared to 6.5% in the antioxidant group, a difference statistically significant. Again neither compliance nor alcohol intake was recorded and therefore the results have to be questioned.

Thioctic Acid (α-lipoic acid)

Thioctic acid has antioxidant properties in addition to its antiinflammatory effect due to its action on prostaglandin cyclo-oxygigenase. Furthermore, thioctic acid is a cofactor in pyruvate dehydrogenase and a-ketoglutarate dehydrogenase and might therefore prevent changes in citric acid cycle activity which accompanies ethanol oxidation in the liver. One randomized double-blind trial of 300 mg thioctic acid versus placebo in 40 patients with precirrhotic alcoholic liver disease over 6 months did not show any beneficial effect of the drug (43).

Colchicine

Colchicine has been introduced as therapeutic agent for the treatment of gout and familial Mediterranean fever. Colchicine inhibits granulocyte migration and interferes with the degradation of polymorphonuclear leucocytes (PMN). Since PMN's accumulation in the liver is one characteristic feature of alcoholic hepatitis and since PMN derived cytokines possibly mediate some clinical symptoms in alcoholic hepatitis, colchicine was tried as a therapeutic agent. In addition, colchicine has other properties which may be beneficial in alcoholic liver disease including inhibition of fibrogenesis (12, 17). Colchicine reduces collagen synthesis and increases collagenase activity. Theoretically the drug is able to inhibit or prevent or even reverse fibrosis. Since colchicine affects the microtubular system in the hepatocytes, it interferes with transport and secretion of macromolecules such as procollagens (13, 14). In CCl_4-treated rats colchicine reduced the degree of fibrosis and improved liver function (44). Furthermore, colchicine also partially prevented the toxic effect of D-galactosamine on rat liver. Since lipid peroxidation may be a prerequisite for galactosamine-induced hepatic damage, the protection by colchicine may be related to its capacity to inhibit lipid peroxidation (45).

Since colchicine inhibits microsomal ethanol oxidation (MEOS) by approximately 30% in the rat, it could theoretically prevent the production of free radicals generated via this pathway (46).

Clinically, several trials have been performed with colchicine as therapeutic agent. Akriviadis et al. performed a randomized placebo controlled trial in 72 patients with severe alcohol hepatitis given either 1 mg of colchicine daily or placebo for 30 days. The mortality was 19% vs. 17% which was not statistically significant (47). Similar negative data were collected by Trinchet et al. in a randomized placebo controlled trial in 67 patients with biopsy-proven alcoholic hepatitis. Repeated biopsies were taken during the trial and alcoholic drinking behaviour was recorded. No significant effect was observed in clinical, laboratory or histological variables between the two groups. However, an improvement of biopsy scores at 3 months was greater in the colchicine treated group (48).

Since colchicine, as already pointed out, has antifibrotic effects in the rat model, it was also used in cirrhosis. A double blind controlled trial of 43 cirrhotic patients was published 1979 by Kershenobich et al. (49). After treatment up to 4 years the colchicine group (1 mg per day) showed greater clinical improvement and a reduction of fibrosis. However, mortality was not statistically significant between the two groups (49). Later the same investigators reported an extended trial including 100 patients with cirrhosis, 45 of them had alcoholic cirrhosis, 41 had posthepatitic cirrhosis and 14 had cirrhosis of various causes (50). All patients except of one were classified as Child A or B. The patients were followed up over 14 years and sequential liver biopsies were performed. The overall mean survival time in the colchicine group was 11 years and in the control group 3.5 years ($p = 0.001$). The cumulative 5-year survival rate was 75% in the colchicine group and 34% in the placebo group. The corresponding 10-year survival rates were 56 and 20%. In 9 out of 30 patients having received colchicine histological improvement was seen. No histological improvement was seen in 14 patients of the control group who had two or more biopsies. Although these data seem impressive at first glance, a variety of problems exists in this study: there were a number of differences in the two groups including the presence of esophageal varices and laboratory values influencing the Child classification such as serum albumin. In addition, alcohol consumption during the trial was not recorded and compliance was not monitored. Thus, at the present time certainly more trials are necessary to evaluate the effect of colchicine especially on alcoholic cirrhosis before recommending its use.

Summary and Conclusions

In animal experiments it has been convincingly shown that chronic alcohol consumption leads to the generation of free radicals either during ethanol metabolism itself or by influencing the intermediary metabolism of other compounds. In addition, chronic alcohol ingestion also leads to an alteration of the antioxidant defense system in the liver and other tissues including a reduction of tocopherol, selenium and glutathion. On the basis of these experimental finding, antioxidants have been used in the treatment of alcoholic liver disease. However, none of the drugs used in the treatment of alcoholic liver disease worked convincingly. For two drugs still more data need to become available before discharging them: Colchicine and silymarin. For the latter one, the German randomized placebo-controlled double-blind multicenter trial will hopefully answer the question in the near future.

REFERENCES

1. Lieber CS. Alcohol and the Liver: 1994 update. Gastroenterology 1994; 106:1085-1105.
2. McCay PB, Reinke RL, Rau JM. Hydroxyl Radicals are Generated by Hepatic Microsomes During NADPH Oxidation: Relation to Alcohol Metabolism. FASB J. 1991; 5:A1614.
3. Cederbaum AI. Oxygen Radical Generation by Microsomes: Role of Iron and Implication for Alcohol Metabolism and Toxicity. Free Radic Biol Med 1989; 7:559-564.
4. Reinke LA, Lao EK, Dubose CM, McCay PB. Reactive Free Radical Generation in vivo in Heart and Liver of Ethanol-fed Rats: Correlation with Radical Formation in vitro. Proc Natl Acad Sci USA 1987; 84:9223-9227.
5. Albano E, Tomasi A, Goria-Gatti L, Poli G, Dianzani MU. Spin Trapping of Ethanol Derived Free Radicals in Rat Liver Microsomes. Adv Biosci 1988; 71:17-24.
6. Albano E, Tomasi A, Goria-Gatti L, Dianzani MU. Spin Trapping of Free Radical Species Produced during the Microsomal Metabolism of Ethanol. Chem Biol Interact 1988; 65:223-227.
7. Knecht KT, Bradford BV, Mason P, Thurman RG. In Vivo Formation of a Free Radical Metabolite of Ethanol. Mol Pharmacol 1990; 838:26-31.
8. Shaw S. Lipid Peroxidation, Iron Mobilization and Radical Generation Induced by Alcohol. Free Radic Biol Med 1989; 7:541-544.
9. Ward RJ, Peters TJ. The antioxidant status of patients with either alcohol-induced liver damage or myopathy. Alcohol Alcohol 1992; 27:359-365.
10. Zidenberg-Cherr S, Olin KL, Villanueva J, Tang A, Phinney SD, Halsted CH, Keen CL. Ethanol Induced Changes in Hepatic Free Radical Defense Mechanisms and Fatty Acid Composition in the Miniature Pig. Hepatology 1991; 13:1185-1191.
11. Nordmann R. Alcohol and Antioxidant Systems. Alcohol Alcohol 1994; 29:513-522.
12. Rojkind M, Mourelle M, Kershenobich D. Antiinflammatory and Antifibrogenic Activities of Colchicine: Treatment of Liver Cirrhosis. In: Myelofibrosis and the Biology of Connective Tissue. New York: Alan R Liss, 1984; 475-489.
13. Kaufmann S, Tuma DJ, Sorrell MF, Vanderhoof JA. Increasing Inhibition of Hepatic Protein Secretion by Colchicine During Development. Am J Physiol 1984; 247:G311-G318.
14. Stein O, Sanger L, Stein Y. Colchicine Induced Inhibition of Lipoprotein and Protein Secretion into the Serum and Lack of Interference with Secretion of Biliary Phospholipids and Cholesterol by Rat Liver in vivo. J Cell Biol 1974; 62:90-103.
15. Walker PR, Withfield JF. Colchicine Prevents the Translation of mRNA Molecules Transcribed Immediately after Proliferative Activation of Hepatocytes in Regenerating Liver. J Cellular Physiol 1984; 118:179-185.
16. Mourelle M, Rojkind M, Rubalcava B. Colchicine Improved the Alterations in the Liver Adenylate Cyclase System of Cirrhotic Rats. Toxicology 1981; 21:213-222.
17. Tanner MS, Jackson D, Mowat AP. Hepatic Collagen Synthesis in a Rat Model of Cirrhosis and its Modification by Colchicine. J Pathol 1981; 135:179-187.
18. Das NP, Sothy SP. Studies on Flavonoid Metabolism. Biliary and Urinary Excretion of Metabolites of (+)-(U-14C)catechin. J Biochem, 1971; 125:417-423.
19. Lang I, Nekam K, Deak G,Muzes G, Gonzales CR, Kadar J, Perl A, Gergely P, Feher J. Effect of (+)cyanidanol-3 on Cellular Immune Reactions and on Superoxide Dismutase Activity in Vitro. Free Radic Res Comm, 1987; 4:51-60.
20. Colman JC, Morgan MY, Scheuer PJ, Sherlocks S. Treatment of Alcohol Related Liver Disease with (+)-cyanidanol-3: a Randomized Double Blind Trial. Gut 1980; 21:965-969.
21. Abonyi M, Kisfaludy S, Szalay F. Therapeutic Effects of (+)-Cyanidanol-3 in Toxic Alcoholic Liver Disease and in Chronic Active Hepatitis. Acta Physiol Hung 1984; 64:455-460.
22. World MJ, Aps EJ, Shaw GK, Thomson AD. (+)-Cyanidanol-3 for Alcoholic Liver Disease: Results of a Six Month Clinical Trial. Alcohol Alcohol. 1984; 19:23-29.
23. Palmas S. Treatment of Alcoholic Cirrhosis with (+)-Cyanidanol-3; In: Conn HO, Wood C, eds. Internatio-

nal Workshop on (+)-Cyanidanol-3 in Diseases of the Liver. 1981; 167-171.
24. Sánchez-Tapias JM, Fiol B, Rodés J. (+)-Cyanidanol-3 in Mild Alcoholic Hepatitis. In: Conn HO, Wood C, eds. International Workshop on (+)-Cyanidanol-3 in Diseases of the Liver. 1981; 173-175.
25. Henning H. Influence of (+)-Cyanidanol-3 on Chronic Alcoholic Liver Injury. In: Conn HO, Wood C, eds. International Workshop on (+)-Cyanidanol-3 in Diseases of the Liver. 1981; 177-179.
26. Ugarte G, Bunout D, Iturriaga H. Effect of (+)-Cyanidanol-3 on Alcoholic Liver Disease With or Without Overt Hepatic Failure. In: Conn HO, Wood C, eds. International Workshop on (+)-Cyanidanol-3 in Diseases of the Liver. 1981; 181-183.
27. Morgan M. Alcoholic Liver Disease: Natural History, Diagnosis, Clinical Feature, Evaluation, Management, Prognosis and Prevention. In: McIntyre N, Benhamou JP, Bircher J, Rizzetto M, Rodés J, eds. Oxford Textbook of Clinical Hepatology. Oxford: Oxford University Press, 1991; vol 2, 815-855.
28. World MJ, Ryle PR, Aps EJ, Shaw GK, Thomson AD. Palmitoyl-catechin for Alcoholic Liver Disease: Results of a Three-month Clinical Trial. Alcohol Alcohol 1987; 22:331-340.
29. Muriel P, Garcipina T, Perez-Alvarez V, Mourelle M. Silymarin Protects against Paracetamol-induced Lipid Peroxidation and Liver Damage. J Appl Toxicology 1992; 12:439-442.
30. Muriel P, Mourelle M. Prevention by Silymarin of Membrane Alterations in Acute CCl_4 Liver Damage. J Appl Toxicology 1990; 10:275-279.
31. Chuan-Ging W, Chamuleau RAFM, Bosch KS, Frederiks WM. Protective Effect of Silymarin on Rat Liver Injury Induced by Ischemia. Virchows Arch B Cell Pathol 1993; 64:259-263.
32. Carini R, Comoglio A, Albano E, Poli G. Lipid Peroxidation and Irreversible Damage in the Rat Hepatocyte Model. Biochem Pharmacol 1992; 43:2111-2115.
33. Mira L, Silva M, Manso CF. Scavenging of Reactive Oxygen Species by Silybinin Dehemisuccinate. Biochem Pharmacol 1994; 48:753-759.
34. Pascual C, Gonzales R, Armesto J, Muriel P. Effect of Silymarin and Silybinin on Oxygen Radicals. Drug Dev Res 1993; 29:73-77.
35. Bosisio E, Benelli C, Pirola O. Effect of the Flavanolignants of *Silybum marianum L.* on Lipid Peroxidation in Rat Liver Microsomes and Freshly Isolated Hepatocytes. Pharmacol Res 1992; 25, n.° 2.
36. Bindoli A, Cavallini L, Siliprandi N. Inhibitory Action of Silymarin of Lipid Peroxide Formation in Rat Liver Mitochondria and Microsomes. Biochem Pharmacol 1977; 26:2405-2409.
37. Sonnenbichler J, Zetl J. Influence of Silybinin on the Synthesis of Ribosomal-RNA, mRNA and tRNA in Rat Livers in vivo. Hoppe Seylers Z Physiol Chem 1984; 365:555-566.
38. Valenzuela A, Bustamate JC, Videla C, Guerra R. Effect of Silybin Dihemisuccinate on the Ethanol Metabolizing Systems of the Rat Liver. Cell Biochem Funct 1989; 7:173-178.
39. Salmi HA, Sarna S. Effect of Silymarin on Chemical, Functional, and Morphological Alterations of the Liver. A Double Blind Controlled Study. Scand J Gastr 1982; 17:517-521.
40. Velussi M, Cernigoi AM, Viezolli L, Dapas F, Caffau C, Zilli M. Silymarin Reduces Hyperinsulinemia, Malondialdehyde Levels, and Daily Insulin Need in Cirrhotic Diabetes Patients. Current Ther Res 1993; 53:533-545.
41. Ferenci P, Dragosics B, Dittrich H, Frank H, Benda L, Lochs H, Meryn S, Base W, Schneider B. Randomized Controlled Trial of Silymarin in Patients with Cirrhosis of the Liver. J Hepatol 1989; 9:105-113.
42. Wenzel G, Kuklinski B, Rühlmann C, Ehrhardt D. Alcohol Toxic Hepatitis - A Free Radical Associated Disease. Decreased Mortality by Adjuvant Antioxidant Therapy. Inn Med 1993; 48:490-496.
43. Marshall AW, Graul RS, Morgan MY, Sherlock S. Treatment of Alcoholic Liver Disease with Thioctid Acid: a Six Month Randomized Double-Blind Trial. Gut 1982; 23:1088-1093.
44. Rojkind M, Kershenobich D. Effect of Colchicine on Collagen, Albumin and Transferrin Synthesis by Cirrhotic Rat Liver Slices. Biochim Biophys Acta 1975; 378:415-423.
45. Mourelle M, Meza M. Colchicine Prevents D-Galactosamine Induced Hepatitis. J Hepatol 1989; 8:165-172.
46. Seitz HK, Busenkell R, Simanowski UA, Boesche J, Kommerell B and Rojkind M. Effect of Colchicine on in Vivo and in Vitro Ethanol Metabolism in the Rat. Gastroenterol 1987; 25:270-273.
47. Akriviadis EA, Steindel H, Pincto PC, Fong TL, Kanel G, Reynolds TB, Gupta S. Failure of Colchicine to Improve Short-term Survival in Patients with Alcoholic Hepatitis. Gastroenterol 1990; 99:811-818.
48. Trinchet JC, Beaugrand M, Callard P, Hartmann DJ, Gotheil C, Nusgens BV, Lapiere CM, Ferrier JP. Treatment of Alcoholic Hepatitis with Colchicine. Results of a Randomized Double Blind Trial. Gastroenterol Clin Biol 1989; 13:551-555.
49. Kershenobich D, Uribe M, Suarez GI, Mata JM, Perz-Tamayo R, Rojkind M. Treatment of Cirrhosis with Colchicine. A Double Blind Randomized Trial. Gastroenterol 1979; 77:532-536.
50. Kershenobich D, Vargas F, Garcia-Tsao G, Perez-Tamayo R, Gent M, Rojkind M. Colchicine in the Treatment of Cirrhosis of the Liver. N Engl J Med 1988; 318:1709-1713.

Corticosteroid Therapy in Patients with Severe Alcoholic Hepatitis

P. Mathurin, S. Rueff, M. J. Ramond, T. Poynard

RANDOMIZED CONTROLLED TRIALS (RCTs) ASSESSING THE EFFICACY OF NON STEROID TREATMENT IN PATIENTS WITH ALCOHOLIC HEPATITIS

The prognosis of severe alcoholic hepatitis is poor. In the past three decades, multiple terapies have been studied in an attempt to improve the poor survival in these patients. Therapies that have been evaluated include hypernutrition, androgenic steroids, propylthiouracil, colchicine, insuline, and glucagon. None of these treatments has been associated with reduction of short or long-term mortality (1).

RCTs OF CORTICOSTEROIDS IN ALCOHOLIC HEPATITIS: RATIONAL BASIS FOR CORTICOSTEROID THERAPY IN PATIENTS WITH ALCOHOLIC HEPATITIS

It has been suggested that altered immunologic responses may have a role in the initiation and perpetuation of alcoholic hepatitis. Acetaldehyde forms adducts with macromolecules in the hepatocyte which probably serve as neoantigens eliciting an immune response. Furthermore, there is evidence that cytokines (for example TNF alpha or interleukins 8 or 6) may play a role in the pathogenesis of alcoholic hepatitis (2-5). These findings provide further rationale for evaluation of corticosteroids in alcoholic hepatitis.

OVERVIEW OF CORTICOSTEROIDS RCTs IN ALCOHOLIC HEPATITIS

The results of randomized trials were conflicting (6-18). Two previous meta-analysis had evaluated the treatment effect of corticosteroids in short-term mortality of alcoholic hepatitis (19-20) The authors had concluded for the benefit of corticosteroids, especially in severe forms. Since these 2 previous meta-analysis, we have published another randomized trial of corticosteroid in severe biopsy-proved alcoholic hepatitis which had demonstrated the benefit of short-term mortality of 40 mg prednisolone per day during 28 days. In this study 2 months survival of the corticoid group was significantly higher than survival of placebo group (88 ± 5% vs. 45 ± 8%, p = 0.001). The survival advantage for prednisolone persisted after stratification according to the presence of encephalopathy, and after adjustement for prognostic factors in a proportional-hazards model incluiding the modification of prognostic factors between admission and randomization.

In this chapter we want to present the results of two studies. The first is a new meta-analysis including the last published randomized trial (Mathurin et al., AFEF, Nantes 1995, submitted for publication). The second is a new study including patients of the previous randomized trial and 61 new patients prospectively treated by methylprednisolone (21, submitted for publication). The original data of these two studies are submitted elsewhere for publication, and therefore only summary of previously presented data will be discussed here. The other details will be given during the oral presentation of the international meeting on therapy in liver diseases in Barcelona, Spain.

A NEW META-ANALYSIS OF CORTICOSTEROIDS RCTs IN ALCOHOLIC HEPATITIS: GASTROINTESTINAL BLEEDING AND RENAL INSUFFICIENCY, TWO FACTORS OF CONFUSION IN ANALYSIS OF CORTICOSTEROID THERAPY IN ALCOHOLIC HEPATITIS

To be included in this meta-analysis, an RCT had to fulfill the following criteria: it had to be published as an article, clearly randomized, and have included patients with alcoholic hepatitis. All included trials except that by Lesesne et al. were placebo controlled. Trials published as abstracts or letters, not clearly randomized, using combinations of drugs, were excluded. All analysis were performed according to the intention-to-treat method. No randomized patient was excluded. For all end points patients will truncated data were considered as failures, whatever the cause. For each evaluated endpoint the following strategy was used: *a*) assessment of heterogeneity between results observed in the control groups; *b*) assessment of drug efficacy vs. placebo by Peto and Der Simonian and Laird methods. The sensitivity of this meta-analysis was analysed after exclusion of trials including mild forms. Comparisons were made using the Der Simonian and Laird and Peto et al. methods. 12 RCTs satisfied our inclusion criteria. Overview of the previous randomized trials are summarised in table 1. In the present meta-analysis 12 RCTs were included: 304 patients treated by corticosteroids, and 304 patients treated by placebo. We have excluded one study because the authors had used a regimen wich is effective in reversing acute rejection in liver or renal transplants; they had prescribed 1 g of methyl-prednisolone only for three days. Another trial had three groups (placebo, prednisolone, oxandrolone), and patients receivingo xandrolone were excluded in this analysis. We used mortality reported within 60 days of randomization. Five trials reported a statistically significant reduction in mortality among patients receiving corticosteroids, whereas seven trials reported no statistical significant reduction of mortality (table 1). Overall, the percent reduction of mortality due to corticosteroids was 17% (CI: 7-26%, $p < 0.01$) in patients treated by corticosteroids. It had been previously reported that corticosteroids were more efficient in patients with encephalopathy. Then, we stratified trials by presence or absence of encephalopathy. In subgroup of patients with encephalopathy the percent reduction of mortality due to corticosteroids was 27% (CI: 11-44%; $p < 0.0001$); among subgroup of patients without encephalopaty there was no difference of mortality according to corticosteroid treatment (1%). In RCTs which excluded patients with gastrointestinal bleeding the percent of reduction of mortality due to corticosteroids was 26% (CI: 16-36%, $p < 0.01$); in RCTs without exclusion of patients with gastrointestinal bleeding there was not significant reduction of mortality (1%). In RCTs which excluded patients with renal insufficiency there was a significant reduction of mortality 35% (CI: 33-47%, $p < 0.01$); in RCTs without exclusion criteria of patients with renal insufficiency there was no significant reduction of mortality (14%; CI: – 2 to 30%, $p = 0.10$). Because individual data were not available, the independent prognostic values of these factors were not assessed.

Table 1. RCTs corticosteroid therapy in patients with alcoholic hepatitis included in the meta-analysis

Author	Number of patients	Authors conclusions on the efficacy
Helman (1971)	37	Significant; p < 0.01
Depew (1979)	28	Not significant
Lesesne (1978)	17	Significant; p < 0.01
Blitzer (1977)	28	Not significant
Shumaker (1978)	27	Not significant
Porter (1971)	20	Not significant
Campra (1973)	46	Not significant
Maddrey (1978)	55	Significant; p = 0.1
Mendehall (1984)	178	Not significant
Carithers (1989)	66	Significant; p = 0.006
Bories (1987)	45	Not significant
Ramond (1992)	61	Significant; p = 0.001

LONG TERM SURVIVAL AND PROGNOSTIC FACTORS IN PATIENTS WITH SEVERE BIOPSY-PROVED ALCOHOLIC HEPATITIS TREATED BY PREDNISOLONE: RANDOMIZED TRIAL, NEW COHORT AND SIMULATION (21)

The aims of this study were: *a*) to confirm the efficacy of corticosteroids in severe alcoholic hepatitis on short-term survival in more patients; *b*) to assess long-term survival (two years); *c*) to identify patients who better benefit of prednisolone. A prognostic model (22) has been used to confirm the efficacy of corticosteroids in the new group of patients which were not randomized. We analyze 6, 12 and 24 month-survival of 183 patients. Sixty-one were randomized in a previous trial: 32 treated (group I), 29 non treated (group II); 61 prospectively treated since the end of this trial (group III); 61 simulated (group IV) with a prognostic model. Clinical, biological and 6 histological features (balloonning degeneration, acidophilic necrosis, Mallory bodies, polymorphonuclear infiltrate, cholestasis, severity of the hepatitis) were assessed.

In group III survival at 6 months (Kaplan-Meier, m ± se, 84 ± 6%) was similar than survival previously observed in the randomized treated group I (73 ± 6%, log-rank, ns). At 12 month survival was 69 ± 6% in group I, 71 ± 8% in group III, that is significantly higher than in non treated control group (II = 41 ± 9%, $p = 0.01$) and in simulated group (IV = 44%, $p = 0.05$). Treatment effect persisted after adjustement by prognostic factors (Cox model). At 24 month survivals were not significantly different: group I = 46 ± 10% vs. group II = 41 ± 9%; group III = 59% ± 7% vs. group IV = 33%. Patients with a marked polymorphonuclear infiltrate had 1 year-survival (76 ± 6%) significantly higher than patients without (53 ± 9%, $p < 0.07$). Patients with serum polymorphonuclear count above 6,000/m^3 had 1 year-survival (76 ± 6%), significantly higher than the others (52 ± 10%, $p = 0.03$). Those prognostic values persisted after adjustement (Cox model) by other prognostic factors: $p < 0.06$ and $p < 0.02$.

In conclusion, this study incluiding a larger number of patients confirms that prednisolone reduces 1 year-mortality. Peripheral leucocyte count and polymorphonuclear infiltrate are independent prognostic factors useful to identify patients who better benefit from treatment with prednisolone.

GENERAL CONCLUSIONS

These two studies confirm that corticosteroids reduce mortality at least at one year in patients with severe alcoholic hepatitis. Factors associated with a better response to corticosteroids were: absence of gastrointestinal bleeding, absence of renal failure, presence of encephalopathy, increased blood neutrophilia, and marked liver neutrophil infiltrate.

REFERENCES

1. Morgan MY. Alcoholic liver disease: natural history, diagnosis, clinical features, evaluation, management, prognosis and prevention. In: McIntyre N, Benhamou J, Bircher J, Rizetto M, Rodes J, eds. Oxford Textbook of Clinical Hepatology. Oxford: Oxford University Press, 1991; 815-855.
2. Sheron N, Bird G, Koskinas J, Portmann B, Ceska M, Lindley I, Williams R. Circulating and tissue levels of the neutrophil chemotaxin IL 8 are elevated in severe acute alcoholic hepatitis, and tissue level correlate with neutrophil infiltration. Hepatology 1993; 18:41-46.
3. Hill DB, Marsano LS, McClain CJ. Increased Plasma IL8 concentrations in alcoholic hepatitis. Hepatology 1993; 18:576-580.
4. Shiratori Y, Takada H, Hikiba Y, Nakata R, Okano K, Komatsu Y et al. Production of chemotactic factor, IL8, from hepatocytes exposed to ethanol. Hepatology 1993; 18:1477-1482.
5. Ölinger W, Dinges HP, Zatloukal K, Mair S, Gollowitsch F, Denk H. Immunohistochemical detection of tumor necrosis factor-alpha, other cytokines and adhesion molecules in human livers with alcoholic hepatitis. Virchows Arch A Pathol Anat 1993; 423:169-176.
6. Ramond MJ, Poynard T, Rueff B, Mathurin P, Theodore C, Chaput JC, Benhamou JP. A randomized trial of prednisolone in patients with severe alcoholic hepatitis. N Engl J Med 1992; 326:507-512.
7. Mendenhall CL, Anderson S, Garcia-Pont P, Goldberg S, Kiernan T, Seeff LB, Sorrell M, Tamburro C, Weesner R, Zetterman R, Chedid A, Chen T, Rabin L and The Veterans Administration Cooperative Study on Alcoholic Hepatitis. Short-term and long-term survival in patients with alcoholic hepatitis treated with oxandrolone and prednisolone. N Engl J Med 1984; 311:1464-1470.
8. Carithers RL, Herlong F, Diehl AM, Shaw EW, Combes

B, Fallon HJ, Maddrey WC. Methylprednisolone therapy in patients with severe alcoholic hepatitis. A randomized multicenter trial. Ann Int Med 1989; 110:685-690.

9. Porter HP, Simon FR, Pope CE, Volwiler W, Fenster F. Corticosteroid therapy in severe alcoholic hepatitis. A double-blind drug trial. N Engl J Med 1971; 284:1350-1355.
10. Maddrey WC, Boinott JK, Bedine MS, Weber FL, Mezey E, White RI. Corticosteroid therapy of alcoholic hepatitis. Gastroenterology 1978; 75:193-199.
11. Theodossi A, Eddleston WF, Williams R. Controlled trial of methyl-prednisolone in severe acute alcoholic hepatitis. Gut 1982; 23:75-79.
12. Bories P, Guedj JY, Mirouze D, Yousfi A, Michel H. Traitement de l'hépatite alcoolique aigüé par la prednisolone. Presse Med 1987; 16:769-772.
13. Campra JL, Hamlin EM, Kirshbaum RI, Olivier M, Redeker AG, Reynolds TB. Prednisolone therapy of acute alcoholic hepatitis. Ann Intern Med 1973; 79:625-631.
14. Depew W, Boyer T, Omata M, Redeker A, Reynolds T. Double-blind controlled trial of prednisolone therapy in patients with severe acute alcoholic hepatitis and spontaneous encephalopathy. Gastroenterology 1980; 78:524-529.
15. Shumaker JB, Resnick RH, Galambos JT, Makopour H, Iber FL. A controlled trial of 6 methylprednisolone in acute alcoholic hepatitis. Am J Gastroenterol 1978; 69:443-449.
16. Blitzer BL, Mutchnick MG, Joshi PH, Philips MM, Fessel JM, Conn HO. Adrenocorticosteroid therapy in alcoholic hepatitis: a prospective double-blind randomized trial study. Dig Dis Sci 1977; 22:477-484.
17. Helman RA, Temko MH, Nye SW, Fallon HJ. Alcoholic hepatitis natural history and evaluation of prednisolone therapy. Ann Intern Med 1971; 74:311-321.
18. Lesesne HR, Bozymski EM, Fallon HJ. Treatment of alcoholic hepatitis with encephalopathy. Comparison of prednisolone with caloric supplements. Gastroenterology 1974; 74:169-173.
19. Imperiale TF, McCullough AJ. Do corticosteroids reduce mortality from alcoholic hepatitis? A meta-analysis of the randomized trials. Ann Intern Med 1990; 113:299-307.
20. Daures JP, Peray P, Bories P, Blanc P, Youfsi A, Michel H, Gremy F. Place de la corticothérapie dans le traitement des hépatites alcooliques aigües. Résultats d'une métaanalyse. Gastroenterol Clin Biol 1991; 15:223-228.
21. Mathurin P, Duchatelle V, Ramond MJ, Degott C, Bedossa P, Erlinger S, Benhamou JP, Rueff B, Poynard T. Long term survival and prognostic factors in patients with severe biopsy proved alcoholic hepatitis treated by prednisolone: Randomized trial, New cohort and simulation American Association for the Study of Liver Diseases. Chicago, Oct 1994.
22. Poynard T, Barthelemy P, Fratte S, Boudjema K, Doffoel M, Vanlemmens C, Miguet JP, Mantion G, Messner M, Launois B, Naveau S, Chaput JC for a Multi-Center Group. Evaluation of efficacy of liver transplantation in alcoholic cirrhosis by a case-control study and simulated controls. Lancet 1994; 344:502-507.

Nutritional Therapy of Alcoholic Liver Disease

S. Schenker, A. M. Hoyumpa

INTRODUCTION

This brief review addresses the role of nutritional therapy in the management of patients with alcoholic liver disease. The interaction of poor nutrition and alcohol-induced liver disease has a long history. Indeed, malnutrition was originally proposed as the *main* cause of liver disease accompanying excessive alcohol intake. This premise, which was based on studies in rodents with fatty liver induced by choline deficiency (1), has now been supplanted by the primacy of ethanol in the causation of significant alcohol-induced liver damage as a result of the elegant metabolic studies in non-human primates (2). Nevertheless, the contributory effects of poor nutrition continue to be of interest. This interest is fueled by reports of high prevalence of malnutrition, especially of protein-calorie type, in hospitalized patients with alcoholic liver disease (3), and the development of similar histologic findings (fat, Mallory's hyaline, pericentral sclerosis and fibrosis) in patients with impaired nutrition due to prior intestinal bypass surgery for morbid obesity and patients with obesity/diabetes who manifest nonalcoholic steatonecrosis (4, 5). In addition, there is recent evidence in the constant intragastric alcohol infusion rat model of alcohol-induced liver injury that administration of unsaturated fat as corn oil promotes the development of the hepatic lesion (6), again pointing to the importance of diet. Not only in the area of pathogenesis, but also as regards prognosis (7) and therapy (8), the role of nutrition has continued to attract interest. This is not surprising as until recently (9) no specific therapy for this disorder had been validated. A number of reviews on this general subject has been published (8, 10, 11). This analysis draws importantly on these papers as well as on our own recent review of this subject (8). It is an update of this larger review (8).

INCIDENCE AND SEVERITY OF MALNUTRITION IN PATIENTS WITH ALCOHOLIC LIVER DISEASE

There are two main variables in defining the incidence and degree of malnutrition in patients with alcohol-induced hepatic dysfunction —selection of patients and manner in which nutrition is assessed. As to the former, it has been clearly shown that patients of low socioeconomic status with alcoholic liver disease ill enough to warrant admission to municipal or Veterans Administration hospitals almost uniformly exhibit evidence of some malnutrition (3). In general, this consisted of some combination of low body weight, decreased lean body mass, failure to react to skin testing (i.e., marasmus) and of kwashiorkor, defined as decreased serum albumin, transferrin, lymphocytopenia and decreased response to skin testing. Moreover, the severity of alcoholic liver disease assessed clinically and the degree of protein caloric malnutrition correlated well (7). By contrast, in patients well enough not to warrant hospitalization, the incidence and severity of malnutrition were much lower (about two-thirds) (12). Interestingly, malnutrition is not

Table 1. Factors modifying routine nutritional assessment

Nutritional parameters	Protein calorie malnutrition	Excess alcohol	Liver disease
Ideal body weight	×	-	×
Triceps skin-fold thickness	×	-	±[a]
Midarm muscle circumference	×	-	±[a]
Hand dynamometry	×	-	-
Serum albumin	×	-	×
Serum transferrin	×	-	×
Total lymphocyte count	×[b]	×	×
Skin tests[c]	×[b]	×	×
Creatinine-height index	×	-	±

Modified with permission from McCullough et al (13) and Nompleggi et al (11).
[a] Less likely to be abnormal with volume overload as fluid does not accumulate in arm.
[b] Especially with low protein malnutrition.
[c] Delayed hypersensitivity.

exclusively seen with alcoholic liver disease in that it occurs also in patients with other severe hepatic dysfunction (12).

In addition to patient selection, identification of malnutrition in these individuals is methodologically difficult. This is because both liver disease *per se* and alcoholism may mimic abnormal nutritional assessment (11, 13). As is shown in table 1, there are a number of methods for determining nutritional status. These can be categorized into anthropometric (triceps, skin-fold thickness, mid-arm muscle circumference), body weight, serum indices (albumin, transferrin), immunologic indices (lymphocyte count, skin tests), and urinary indices (creatinine/height ratio) (11). Unfortunately, some of the tests (i.e., triceps thickness) exhibit variability depending on examiner training and/or accuracy of specimen collection (i.e., creatinine/height ratio) (14, 15). As indicated above, liver disease *per se* and alcoholism can each confound the interpretation of some of these tests. For instance, body weight is difficult to determine with concomitant presence of ascites and edema due to liver disease, serum albumin levels are also altered with severe hepatic dysfunction and delayed hypersensitivity skin testing may be altered by alcoholism (13). Thus, interpretation of data requires special care. For instance, emphasis on the upper extremity muscle mass and body fat by triceps skin-fold thickness may avoid some of the problems due to fluid accumulation in more dependent body parts (11). Muscle strength can be assessed by hand dynamometry as one functional parameter. Other techniques for more precise definition of body cell mass involve more complex isotopic tools (16). These difficulties in assessing nutritional status in patients with alcoholic liver disease are best overcome by using multiple tests. Despite these caveats, it is generally agreed that protein-calorie malnutrition is a common finding in patients with clinically significant alcoholic liver disease (3).

In addition to protein-calorie malnutrition, patients with alcoholic liver disease may have vitamin deficiencies (11). The most common and clinically best appreciated is a deficiency of folate which is reflected in macrocytosis. In about a quarter of the patients surveyed there may be low serum thiamine, pyridoxine, riboflavin and nicotinic acid. Thiamine deficiency observed in alcoholics, and possibly in genetically susceptible individuals, may manifest as peripheral neuropathy, Wernicke's and possibly Korsakoff's encephalopathy. A deficit of pyridoxins may explain the relatively low SGPT activity in these patients. A decrease in plasma vitamin A also has been described and may manifest as a decrease in peripheral (night) vision (17). This may be enhanced by depletion of zinc.

MECHANISMS OF MALNUTRITION IN ALCOHOLIC LIVER DISEASE

There are many reasons for malnutrition in these patients (table 2) (18). Perhaps the most important is decreased intake of nutrients. In many large series of patients with alcoholic liver disease, calories derived from alcohol, so called «empty calories», constituted about 50%

Table 2. Basis for malnutrition in alcoholic liver disease

Empty calories from ethanol
Anorexia and poor nutrient intake
Maldigestion
Malabsorption
Impaired nutrient storage
Abnormal food metabolism
Combination of above

of total calories ingested (3, 8). The term «empty calories» refers to the observations that alcohol, which has 7.1 kcal/g, is not utilized properly by the body as a nutrient (10). Thus, its intake is not associated with normal (expected) weight gain (19). This may be due to the metabolism of ethanol via the microsomal oxidizing system without concomitant energy production, an increase in sympathetic body metabolism consuming more energy or consumption of energy (as ATP) during alcohol degradation (10). Interestingly, this effect of alcohol seems to be related to fat intake, implying an interaction of alcohol and fat processing (20). Moreover, calories derived from protein were only about 6-10% of the total (8). Meaningful (nonalcoholic) caloric intake decreased in parallel with increasing severity of alcoholic liver disease. The reasons for decreased intake of calories are many and include alcohol intake *per se*, presence of liver disease and use of funds to purchase alcohol rather than nutrients. Perhaps most importantly, these patients exhibit anorexia even when provided with proper calories (13). Hypozincemia may contribute, at least partly, to anorexia in patients with cirrhosis (21), as the taste and smell acuity may be impaired in patients with acute or chronic liver disease (21, 22) and zinc supplementation improved the sense of taste and smell (23). These observations have important implications for inhospital therapy as supplemental food often has to be given to these individuals enterally by nasogastric tube.

In addition to poor intake, there may be significant problems in the processing of ingested food. This may occur at the digestive phase (i.e., decrease in bile salts due to cholestasis) or impaired fat degradation due to a lower lipase on the basis of alcoholic chronic pancreatitis (18, 24). Perhaps more importantly it may be due to malabsorption due to chronic ethanol abuse and/or accompanying malnutrition (18). The mechanisms are complex and involve changes in gut mucosa and its enzymes (i.e., lactase), altered permeability, changes in motility and possibly gut edema due to a low albumin and any increase in portal hypertension.

It has also been suggested that tumor necrosis factor (cachexin) may contribute to the cachexia in alcoholic patients and the increased levels of tumor necrosis factor may be associated with increased mortality (24).

Moreover, the storage and metabolic processing of various nutrients may be altered both by excessive alcohol intake and liver disease resulting from it. As to storage, with decreased parenchymal cell mass due to increasing replacement of fat and fibrous tissue, there is less storage of glycogen and various vitamins (26).

Probably more important is altered metabolism of carbohydrates, protein, vitamins and trace metals. Ethanol is almost exclusively metabolized in the liver and is the preferential fuel. It displaces and depresses the normal oxidation of carbohydrate, fat and protein (27). The decrease in fatty acid oxidation shunts these lipids towards esterification and increases triglyceride stores in the liver. Decreased secretion of triglycerides and a high fat diet contribute to this (28). The interplay among these nutrients is complex, but fairly predictable. With low glycogen stores in the liver and, especially in fasting or with decreased carbohydrate intake, lower hepatic gluconeogenesis and hypoglycemia may ensue due to a higher NAD/NADH ratio derived from alcohol metabolism (29). This, in turn, draws on other body fuels, i.e., fat and muscle protein for energy and typically results in a lower respiratory quotient due to greater fat utilization and muscle wasting, respectively (30).

Amino acid homeostasis can be altered both by ethanol and by liver disease due to it, especially with its acute complications such as gastrointestinal bleeding and infection. Alcohol *per se* may impair protein synthesis and inhibits protein secretion from liver, as one mechanism of hepatic enlargement due to protein retention (31, 32). Nitrogen balance in patients with alcoholic liver disease has suffered from methodologic controversy (13). The most sophisticated techniques, however, suggest increased nitrogen catabolism in these individuals, especially with more severe disease (33).

Deficiencies in protein calorie malnutrition and altered carbohydrate and fat processing is also often complicated by decreases in key vitamins and zinc. Probably the most important mechanism is decreased intake of vitamins from food sources. It should be especially noted that alcoholic beverages generally have a low vi-

Table 3. Nutrients in alcoholic beverages

				Vitamins								Minerals			
	Kcal (g)	Prot (g)	CHO (g)	A (IU)	B_1 (mg)	B_2 (mg)	B_6 (mg)	Fol (μg)	B_{12} (μg)	Panth (mg)	C (mg)	Zinc (mg)	Mn (mg)	Fe (mg)	Mg (ng)
Beer (12 oz)	146	0.9	13.2	0	0.02	0.09	0.18	21	0.06	–	0	0.06	0.04	0.11	23
Wine/table (3.5 oz)	72	0.2	1.4	0	0	0.02	0.03	1	0.01	0.03	0	0.01	0.15	0.42	10
Whiskey 86 proof (1.5 oz)	105	0	0.1	0	0	0	0	0	0	0	0	0.02	0.006	0.01	0
Gin 90 proof (1.5 oz)	110	0	0	0	0	0	0	0	0	0	0	0	0	0	0
Vodka 80 proof (1.5 oz)	97	0	0	0	0	0	0	0	0	0	0	0	0	0	0

Adapted from Bowes & Church. Food Values of Portions Commonly Used, 16th ed. In: Pennington JAT, Hagerstown: JB Lippincott, 1994; 3-5.

tamin content (table 3). However, there appear to be additional problems. Thus, thiamine and folate absorption may be decreased following alcohol intake, although the data for thiamine in man require confirmation (34). Also, alcohol may inhibit the enterohepatic circulation of folate, and acetaldehyde may complex with circulating plasma folate resulting in its rapid oxidation (35). Acetaldehyde may also displace pyridoxal 5-phosphate from its protein binding sites in liver, permitting its degradation by alkaline phosphatase (36). In liver disease, degradation of pyridoxal 5-phosphate is enhanced, presumably via alkaline phosphatase (37). Moreover, alcohol is known to enhance the conversion of vitamin A in liver to its derivatives, some apparently being toxic (33). This results in a lower the parent vitamin in serum and liver and implies that there is a narrow therapeutic window for vitamin A administration in alcoholics. It is evident that alcohol intake and liver disease may result in complex effects on the homeostasis of various key vitamins.

In patients with alcoholic liver disease, zinc deficiency, as a result of decreased intake, malabsorption and increased urinary loss, has been well documented and has been related to impaired night vision, acrodermatitis, hypogonadism, altered immune function, mental changes and diarrhea (38).

Table 4. Mechanisms of malnutrition effects on alcoholic liver disease

Impaired hepatic metabolic defenses vs. alcohol (i.e., decreased glutathione, low vitamin E vs. oxidative stress; decreased methionine vs. membrane phospholipids)
Impaired immune response (i.e., infection)
Impaired hepatic regeneration (i.e., zinc and pyridoxal defficiency, amino acid loss)
Increased surgical morbidity (i.e., poor wound healing)

POSSIBLE MECHANISMS OF MALNUTRITION EFFECTS ON ALCOHOLIC LIVER DISEASE

The theoretical mechanisms by which malnutrition can modify alcoholic liver disease are depicted in table 4. First, nutrients may buttress some «defense» mechanisms against the effects of excess alcohol. Thus, provision of key amino acids (i.e., cysteine) is essential to maintenance of glutathione which, in turn, may protect the liver against ethanol-induced peroxidative stress (6, 39). The role of oxidative stress as a consequence of ethanol, has been especially emphasized with chronic liver disease and development of fibrosis (40-42). Moreover, provision of methionine or its precursors may be important to the maintenance of S-adenosylmethionine and, in turn, phospholipids for membrane integrity (43). Thus, a deficit in protein may augment alcohol-induced liver disease. In addition, the reduced levels of vitamin E and other antioxidants in alcoholics with or without liver disease may play a role in the pathogenesis of alcohol-induced liver injury (42).

Second, poor nutrition may impair immune response (both humoral and cell-mediated) in alcoholics and may augment the chance of concomitant infection. An example of this is depression of opsonic activity in ascitic fluid and likely greater frequency of spontaneous bacterial peritonitis in patients with protein depletion (44).

Third, a variety of nutrients (i.e., amino acids, zinc and pyridoxal 5-phosphate) contribute to hepatic regeneration after injury (8, 45). It is likely that this repair process may suffer with combined alcohol-induced liver damage and poor nutrition.

Finally, the morbidity of surgical procedures, including hepatic transplantation, is likely to be increased in patients with alcoholic liver disease and malnutrition, likely as a result of poorer wound healing and sepsis (46, 47).

NUTRITION THERAPY

Nutritional supplementation should include vitamins, calories to provide 1.2 times the required resting energy expenditure (≥ 30 kcal/kg body weight) and protein (1.0 to 1.5 g/kg body weight) to prevent catabolism. Nutritional therapy of alcoholic liver disease in the modern era can be divided into *general* dietary supplements and *special* diets. The latter will be discussed only very briefly in this text as it has been covered extensively in our prior review and is the subject of another chapter in this book.

Two approaches to assessing the value of improved *general nutrition* (i.e., protein calories) in patients with alcoholic liver disease have been used. In one, the prognosis of patients with this hepatic dysfunction and varying degrees of malnutrition was determined. The mortality at 1, 6 and 12 months of follow up correlated well with the severity of protein-calorie malnutrition (7). Moreover, when patients whose nutritional status improved over 30 days were compared with those in whom it did not, a similar morbidity divergence was also noted (7). Also, in several other series, one post-surgical, good nutrition seemed to correlate with better prognosis (46, 47). These composite surveys *suggest* that good nutrition may decrease the morbidity of alcoholic liver disease. Unfortunately, the data are not rigorous. In some studies there is the confounding variable of underlying liver disease *per se*, which may be the determinant of prognosis. In others there is patient drop out and variable medications. Most are retrospective in nature.

Another group of studies has attempted to define the role of nutrition in this patient population in controlled prospective studies. Some 20 such studies have been carried out (8, 48). These are analyzed in detail in two recent reviews (8, 11). The studies vary considerably among themselves in patient selection as to severity of liver disease and mortality, in patient number, nature of supplemental food given and its route of administration (enteral or parenteral) and the end points (i.e., liver tests, histology, nutritional status, mortality) assessed. There were, of course, a number of similarities —small number of patients studied and short duration, a month or less, of follow up. The conclusions reached were that: *a*) *voluntary* food intake was low, *b*) nutritional status was improved in the group provided extra calories, and *c*) conventional liver tests improved somewhat in most studies when dietary supplementation was given. Moreover, no significant side effects in terms of precipitation of encephalopathy or fluid overload were noted. Liver morphology was improved modestly in the two studies where this was determined. On the other hand, there were only two studies which demonstrated an improved short-term survival (49, 50). To be sure, in several studies (51, 52) there was no mortality in the controls, hence, such a comparison was not possible. Moreover, one can calculate that with the small number of patients enrolled in each study, it would not be feasible to detect improved survival of 50% from an average control mortality of about 25% (8). Since these studies looked at a composite of patients, one might anticipate that a more selected group, with significantly decreased nutritional status, but still capable of clinical response might benefit in terms of better survival from supplemental nutrition. Indeed, such a study has recently been reported and it showed that in a moderately malnourished group, but not in those severely malnourished, nutritional support improved survival significantly (53). Presumably the very severely malnourished group was incapable of salvage despite better nutrition. Thus, overall, it appears that a general nutritional supplementation with high protein calorie diet given enterally to malnourished patients with alcoholic liver disease may be modestly beneficial, especially in selected groups. It certainly appears to do no harm. Such therapy should include not only protein but also folate, pyridoxal and thiamine. Vitamin A replacement has to be cautious because of the narrow therapeutic index of vitamin A regards the diseased liver in alcoholics (33). The effects of alcohol and of liver disease on β-carotene, as a possible surrogate (precursor) for vitamin A, are under study (54-56). The administration of vitamin E, which is reduced in alcoholic liver disease, has not been fully evaluated. However, studies in mice (57) showed that the use of vitamin E incorporated into liposomes for a more efficient delivery to the liver drastically reduced the mortality from acute CCL_4 liver injury; whether alcoholic liver disease is similarly benefitted remains to be seen. The role of dietary fat, especially unsaturated, as a possible precipitant of hepatitic oxidative stress has been emphasized on the basis of experimental studies (58). It will require investigation in primates.

In the area of *special nutrients*, three supplements have been tried, branched-chain amino acids, S-adenosyl methionine and, lately, polyunsaturated lecithin. The hypothesis behind the use of branched chain amino acids is the low ratio of these substances to aromatic amino acids in chronic liver disease and the view of some that this may be responsible, at least in part, for the development of hepatic encephalopathy. While these special mixtures may be beneficial in some individuals unable to handle a conventional nitrogen load without adverse effects, in the control studies cited earlier (8) hepatic encephalopathy did not develop despite the use of conventional amino acid supplements. Thus, branched chain amino acids, in our view, should be offered only to those unable to handle the usual protein load. A similar conclusion was reached by others (11).

As to S-adenosyl methione, there are sound theoretical and some experimental reasons for its use (43, 59, 60). Important in methylation and a precursor of glutathione, it may improve cell glutathione, nucleic acid and protein synthesis, and promote membrane integrity. Studies in baboons exposed chronically to ethanol showed a modest beneficial effect of this supplement (43). It appears to be non-toxic. Studies in patients are needed.

Of most recent interest is the topic of polyunsaturated lecithin. Based primarily on studies in baboons with alcoholic liver disease, it would appear that this dietary supplement may delay/prevent the progression of hepatic fibrosis, presumably, at least in part, by activating collagenase (61, 62). Trials of this agent in patients are ongoing. Indeed, polyunsaturated phosphatidylcholine, which stabilizes membranes, showed a trend toward better survival in patients with acute alcoholic liver disease (63).

In summary, malnutrition, which is a concomitant of alcoholic liver disease, varies in severity, frequency and specific nutritional deficiencies, depending on the methods used to assess the nutritional state, the rigor with which the methods are applied, and the patient population studied. It is not surprising that hospitalized patients with alcoholic liver disease are more often malnourished and to a greater degree than their non-hospitalized counterparts. The malnutrition involves protein/calorie deficit, as well as deficiencies in vitamins and minerals, with attendant physical, metabolic, immunologic and other consequences. There are several underlying mechanisms of malnutrition in these patients. These include the consumption of «empty calories», inadequate food intake (due to anorexia, poor eating habits, lack of access to food), a maldigestion, malabsorption, curtailed storage of glycogen and vitamins in the liver due to reduced parenchymal mass, altered metabolism of such essential foodstuffs as carbohydrates, proteins, vitamins and minerals. Catabolism is further aided by complications such as infection and gastrointestinal bleeding in these patients. In an individual patient more than one mechanism may be in operation.

With malnutrition further metabolic events transpire that cause more hepatic damage. For instance, in alcoholic patients inadequate cysteine leads to reduced stores of glutathione which is cytoprotective, thus permitting more oxidative stress, and eventually chronic liver injury and fibrosis. Moreover, immune function is disturbed, the processes of regeneration and repair are impaired and consequently the patient is at risk for increased surgical morbidity and mortality from sepsis and poor wound healing.

In terms of management, studies, although different in designs and materials suggest that a general nutritional supplementation in terms of protein, calories and B complex vitamins, is beneficial. Mixtures enriched with branch-chain amino acids should be reserved for patients with severe refractory encephalopathy. For most patients standard, amino acid supplements given enterally will suffice. Compounds like S-adenosyl methionine, polyunsaturated lecithin, and polyunsaturated phosphatidyl choline, although potentially useful, based on animal studies, still required initial or additional clinical studies.

REFERENCES

1. Best CH, Hartroft WS, Lucas CC, Ridout JH. Liver Damage Produced by Feeding Alcohol or Sugar and Its Prevention by Choline. Br Med J 1949; 2:1001-1006.
2. Lieber CS, DeCarli LM, Gang H, Walker G, Rubin E. Hepatic Effects of Long Term Ethanol Consumption in Primates. In: Goldsmith EI, Moor-Jankowski J, eds. Medical Primatology, Pt. III. Basel: Karger, 1972; 270-278.
3. Mendenhall CL, Anderson S, Weesner RE, Goldberg SJ, Crolic KA. Protein-Calorie Malnutrition Associated With Alcoholic Hepatitis. VA Cooperative Study Group on Alcoholic Hepatitis. Am J Med 1984; 76:211-222.
4. Galambos JT. Jejunoileal Bypass and Nutritional Liver Injury. Arch Pathol Lab Med 1976; 100:229-231.
5. Itoh S, Matsuo S, Ichinoe A, Yamaba Y, Miyazawa M. Nonalcoholic Steatohepatitis and Cirrhosis With Mallory's Hyaline. With Ultrastructural Study in One Case. Dig Dis Sci 1982; 27:341-346.
6. Tsukamoto H, Goal K, French SW. Insights Into the Pathogenesis of Alcoholic Liver Necrosis and Fibrosis: Status Report. Hepatology 1990; 12:599-608.
7. Mendenhall CL, Tosch T, Weesner RE, Garcia-Pont P, Goldberg SJ, Kiernan T, Seeff LB, Sorrell M, Tamburro C, zetterman R, Chedid A, Chen T, Rabin L. VA Cooperative Study on Alcoholic Hepatitis II: Prognostic Significance of Protein-Calorie Malnutrition. Am J Clin Nutr 1986; 43:213-218.
8. Schenker S, Halff GA. Nutritional Therapy in Alcoholic Liver Disease. Semin Liver Dis 1993; 13:196-209.
9. Carithers RL, Herlong HF, Diehl AM, Shaw EW, Combes B, Fallon HJ, Maddrey WC. Methy Prednisolone Therapy in Patients With Severe Alcoholic Hepatitis: A Randomized Multicenter Trial. Ann Intern Med 1989; 110:685-690.
10. Lieber CS. Herman Award Lecture, 1993: A Personal Perspective on Alcohol, Nutrition, and the Liver. Am J Clin Nutr 1993; 58:430-442.
11. Nompleggi DJ, Bonkovsky HL. Nutritional Supplementation in Chronic Liver Disease: An Analytical Review. Hepatology 1994; 19:518-533.
12. Morgan MY. Enteral Nutrition in Chronic Liver Disease. Acta Chir Scand 1981; 507(Suppl):81-90.
13. McCullough AJ, Mullen KD, Smanik EJ, Tabbaa M, Szauter K. Nutritional Therapy and Liver Disease. Gastroenterol Clin North Am 1989; 18:619-643.
14. Morgan DB, Hill GL, Burkinshaw L. The Assessment of Weight Loss From a Single Measurement of Body Weight: The Problems and Limitations. Am J Clin Nutr 1980; 33:2101-2105.
15. Moran L, Custer P, Murphy G, Grant J. Nutritional Assessment of Lean Body Mass. JPEN 1980; 4:595 (Abstr).
16. Heymsfield SB, Waki M, Reinus J. Are Patients With Chronic Liver Disease Hypermetabolic? Hepatology 1990; 11:502-505.
17. Bonjour JP. Vitamins and Alcoholism. Int J Vitamin Nutr Res 1981; 51:166-177.
18. Mezey E. Interaction Between Alcohol and Nutrition in the Pathogenesis of Alcoholic Liver Disease. Semin Liver Dis 1991; 11:340-348.
19. Pirola RC, Lieber CS. The Energy Cost of the Metabolism of Drugs, including Ethanol. Pharmacology 1972; 7:185-196.
20. Lieber CS. Perspectives: Do Alcohol Calories Count? Am J Clin Nutr 1991; 54:976-982.
21. Burch RE, Sackin DA, Ursick JA, Jeetton MM, Sullivan JF. Decreased Taste and Small Acuity in Cirrhosis. Arch Intern Med 1978; 138:743-746.
22. Smith FR, Henkin RI, Dell RB. Disordered Gustatary Acuity in Liver Disease. Gastroenterology 1976; 70:568-571.
23. Weismann K, Christensen E, Dreyer V. Zinc Supplementation in Alcoholic Cirrhosis. Acta Med Scand 1979; 205:361-366.
24. Perlow W, Baraona E, Lieber CS. Symptomatic Intestinal Disaccharidase Deficiency in Alcoholics. Gastroenterology 1977; 77:680-684.
25. Felver FE, Mezey E, McGuire M, Mitchell MC, Herlong HF, Veech GA, Veech RL. Plasma Tumor Necrosis Factor α Predicts Decreased Long-Term Survival in Severe Alcoholic Hepatitis. Alcohol Clin Exp Res 1990; 14:255-259.
26. Baker H, Frank O, Ziffer H, Goldfarb S, Leevy C, Sobotka H. Effect of Hepatic Disease on Liver B-Complex vitamin Titres. Am J Clin Nutr 1964; 14:1-6.
27. Shelmet JJ, Reichard GA, Skutches CL, Hoeldtke RD, Owen OE, Boden G. Ethanol Causes Acute Inhibition of Carbohydrate, Fat, and Protein Oxidation and Insulin Resistance. J Clin Invest 1988; 81:1137-1145.
28. Lieber CS, Spritz N. Effects of Prolonged Ethanol Intake in Man: Role of Dietary Adipose and Endogenous by Synthesized Fatty Acids in the Pathogenesis of Alcoholic Fatty Liver. J Clin Invest 1986; 45:1400-1411.
29. Forsander OA. Influence of the Metabolism of Ethanol on the Pyruvate-Lactate Ratio of Rat Liver Slices. Biochem J 1986; 98:244-247.
30. Owen OE, Trapp VE, Reichard GA Jr, Mozzoli MA, Moctezuma J, Paul P, Skutches CL, Boden G. Nature and Quality of Fuels Consumed in Patients With Alcoholic Cirrhosis. J Clin Invest 1983; 72:1821-1832.
31. Chapman S, Ward JC, Cooksley WG. Effect of Etha-

nol and Dietary Protein Concentration on Whole Body Protein Synthesis in Rats. Nutr Rep Int 1979; 329-334.

32. Lieber CS. Biochemical and Molecular Basis of Alcohol-Induced Injury to Liver and Other Tissues. N Engl J Med 1988; 319:1639-1650.
33. Prijatmoko DWI, Strauss BJG, Lambert JR, Sievert W, Stroud DB, Wahlguist ML, Katz B, Colman J, Jones P, Korman MG. Early Detection of Protein Depletion in Alcoholic Cirrhosis: Role of Body Composition Analyses. Gastroenterology 1993; 105:1839-1845.
34. Feinman L, Lieber CS. Nutrition. Medical Problems of Alcoholism. In: Lieber CS, ed. Medical and Nutritional Complications of Alcoholism: Mechanisms and Management. New York: Plenum Medical, 1992; 515-530.
35. Shaw S, Jayatillike E, Herbert V, Colman N. Cleavage of Folates During Ethanol Metabolism. Role of Xanthine Oxidase-Generated Superoxide Dismutase. Biochem J 1989; 257:277-280.
36. Lumeng L. The Role of Acetaldehyde in Mediating the Deleterious Effect of Ethanol on Pyridoxal 5' phosphate Metabolism. J Clin Invest 1978; 62:286-293.
37. Mitchell D, Wagner C, Stone WJ, Wilkinson GR, Schenker S. Abnormal Regulation of Plasma Pyridoxal 5'-Phosphate in Patients With Liver Disease. Gastroenterology 1976; 71:1043-1049.
38. McClain CJ, Antonow DR, Cohen DA, Shedlofsky SI. Zinc Metabolism in Alcoholic Liver Disease. Alcohol Clin Exp Res 1986; 10:582-589.
39. Fernandez-Checa JC, Garcia-Ruiz C, Ookhtens M, Kaplowitz N. Impaired Uptake of Glutathione by Hepatic Mitochondria From Chronic Ethanol-Fed Rats. Tracer Kinetic Studies *in vitro* and *in vivo* and Susceptibility to Oxidant Stress. J Clin Invest 1991; 87:397-405.
40. Matsuoka M, Tsukamoto H. Stimulation of Hepatic Lipocyte Collagen Production by Kupffer Cell-Derived Transforming Growth Factor-B: Implication for a Pathogenetic Role in Alcoholic Liver Fibrogenesis. Hepatology 1990; 11:599-605.
41. Kamimura S, Gaal K, Britton RS, Bacon BR, Triadaflopoulos G, Tsukamoto H. Increased 4-hydroxynonenal levels in experimental alcoholic liver disease: Association of Lipid Peroxidation With Liver Fibrogenesis. Hepatology 1992; 16:448-453.
42. Bjornboe A, Bjornboe G-EA. Antioxidant Status and Alcohol-Related Diseases. Alcohol Alcoholism 1993; 28:111-116.
43. Lieber CS, Casini A, DeCarli LM, Kim C-I, Lowe N, Sasaki R, Leo MA. S-Adenosyl-L-methionine. Attenuates Alcohol-Induced Liver Injury in the Baboon. Hepatology 1990; 11:165-172.
44. Llach J, Rimola A, Navasa M, Ginès P, Salmerón JM, Ginès A, Arroyo V, Rodés J. Incidence and Predictive Factors of First Episode of Spontaneous Bacterial Peritonitis in Cirrhosis With Ascites: Relevance of Ascitic Fluid Protein Concentration. Hepatology 1992; 16:724-727.
45. Diehl AM. Nutrition, Hormones, Metabolism and Liver Regeneration. Semin Liver Dis 1991; 11:315-320.
46. Shaw BW, Wood RP, Gordon RD, Iwatsuki S, Gillquist WP, Starzl TE. Influence of Selected Patient Variables and Operative Blood Loss on Six Month Survival Following Liver Transplantation. Semin Liver Dis 1985; 5:385-393.
47. Garrison RN, Cryer HM, Howard DA, Polk HC. Clarification of Risk Factors From Abdominal Operations in Patients With Hepatic Cirrhosis. Ann Surg 1984; 199:648-655.
48. Morgan TR, Mendenhall CL. Nutritional Therapy for Alcoholic Hepatitis: Are We There Yet? Hepatology 1992; 16:845-848.
49. Nasrallah SM, Galambos JT. Amino acid Therapy of Alcoholic Hepatitis. Lancet 1980; 2:1276-1277.
50. Cabré E, González-Huix F, Abad-Lacruz A, Esteve M. Acero D, Fernández-Banares F, Xiol X, Gassull MA. Effect of Total Enteral Nutrition on the Short-Term Outcome of Severely Malnourished Cirrhotics. Gastroenterology 1990; 98:715-720.
51. Diehl AM, Boitnott JK, Herlong HF, Potter JJ, Van Duyn MA, Chandler E, Mezey E. Effect of Parenteral Amino Acid Supplementation in Alcoholic Hepatitis. Hepatology 1985; 5:57-63.
52. Bonkovsky HL, Fiellin DA, Smith GS, Slaker DP, Simon D, Galambos JT. A Randomized, Controlled Trial of Treatment of Alcoholic Hepatitis With Parenteral Nutrition and Oxandrolone. I. Short-Term Effects on Liver Function. Am J Gastroenterol 1991; 86:1200-1208.
53. Mendenhall CL, Moritz TE, Roselle GA, Morgan TR, Nemchausky BA, Tamburro CH, Schiff ER, McClain CJ, Marsana LS, Allen JI, Samanta A, Weesner RE, Henderson W, Gartside P, Chen TS, French SW, Chedid A, Veterans Affairs Cooperative Study Group 275. A Study of Oral Nutritional Support With Oxandrolone in Malnourished Patients With Alcoholic Hepatitis: Results of a Department of Veterans Affairs Cooperative Study. Hepatology 1993; 17:564-576.
54. Leo MA, Kim CI, Lowe N, Lieber CS. Interaction of Ethanol With β-Carotene: Delayed Blood Clearance and Enhanced Hepatotoxicity. Hepatology 1992; 15:883-891.
55. Leo MA, Rosman A, Lieber CS. Differential Depletion of Carotenoids and Tocopherol in Liver Diseases. Hepatology 1993; 17:977-986.
56. Ahmed S, Leo AM, Lieber CS. Interactions Between Alcohol and ß-Carotene in Patients With Alcoholic Liver Disease. Am J Clin Nutr 1994; 60:430-436.
57. Yao T, Esposti SD, Huang L, Arnon R, Spangenberger A, Zern MA. Inhibition of Carbon Tetrachloride-Induced Liver Injury by Liposomes Containing Vitamin E. Am J Physiol (Gastrointest Liver Physiol) 1994; 267:G476-484.
58. Nanji AA, Sadrzadeh SMH, Dannenberg AJ. Liver Microsomal Fatty Acid Composition in Ethanol-Fed Rats: Effect of Different Dietary Fats and Relationship to Liver Injury. Alcohol Clin Exp Res 1994; 18:1024-1028.

59. Harowitz JH, Rypins EB, Henderson JM, Heymsfield SB, Moffitt SD, Bain RP, Chawla RK, Bleier JC, Rudman D. Evidence for Impairment of Transsulfuration Pathway in Cirrhosis. Gastroenterology 1981; 81:668-675.
60. Duce AM, Ortiz P, Cabrero C, Mato JM. S-Adenosyl Methionine Synthetase and Phospholipid Methyltransferase Are Inhibited in Human Cirrhosis. Hepatology 1988; 8:65-68.
61. Lieber CS, DeCarli LM, Mak KM, Kim C-I, Leo MA. Attenuation of Alcohol-Induced Hepatic Fibrosis by Polyunsaturated Lecithin. Hepatology 1990; 12:1390-1398.
62. Li J, Kim C-I, Leo MA, Mak KM, Rojkind M, Lieber CS. Polyunsaturated Lecithin Prevents Acetaldehyde-Mediated Hepatic Collagen Accumulation by Stimulating Collagenase Activity in Cultured Lipocytes. Hepatology 1992; 15:373-381.
63. Panos MZ, Polson R, Johnson R et al. Polyunsaturated Phosphatidyl Choline for Acute Alcoholic Hepatitis: A Double Blind, Randomized, Placebo-Controlled Trial. Eur J Gastroenterol Hepatol 1990; 2:351-355.

Biochemistry and Molecular Biology of S-Adenosylmethionine. Synthesis and Metabolism in Liver Disease

J. M. Mato, L. Álvarez, G. Varela, P. Ortiz, M. A. Pajares

«Zeus had Prometheus chained and sent an eagle to eat his immortal liver which constantly replenished itself» (*Theogony*, Hesiod, BC 700).

INTRODUCTION

The purpose of this review is to study the abnormalities in the regulation of S-adenosyl-L-methionine (SAM) synthesis and metabolism that lead to hypermethioninemia, impaired transmethylation reactions and depletion of reduced glutathione (GSH) in liver disease. In addition, the effect of exogenous SAM on methionine metabolism and GSH synthesis will be evaluated. Recent emphasis has been placed on the study of the effect of SAM treatment on the development of human liver cirrhosis.

In mammals, dietary methionine is converted into SAM by the enzyme SAM-synthetase (fig. 1). SAM serves as the donor of methyl groups in an army of transmethylation reactions (i.e., phospholipid-, DNA- and protein-methylation) which are essential to maintain cellular structure and function. Moreover, SAM is the methyl donor for all detoxifying methylation reactions. The common product to all transmethylation reactions is S-adenosyl-L-homocysteine (SAH), a potent competitive inhibitor of methylation. Of all the enzymes that use SAM, glycine methyltransferase is the most abundant and accounts for about 1% of liver cytosolic protein. This enzyme catalyses the synthesis of sarcosine from SAM and glycine, which in turns is rapidly converted again to glycine. The function of this enzyme, which is not inhibited by SAM, is to remove excess methyl groups and thus, it seems as a means of regulating SAM/SAH ratio. SAH concentration is maintained low by being further converted into adenosine and homocysteine. Homocysteine is rapidly removed to be converted in either cystathionine and its derivatives (cysteine, GSH, taurine, inorganic sulphate) by the transsulphuration pathway, or used again for the resynthesis of methionine. The transsulphuration pathway is liver specific, since mainly this tissue expresses cystathionase, the enzyme that converts cystathionine into ketobutyrate and cysteine (fig. 1). Homocysteine methylation, to form methionine, is necessary for folate cycling and choline metabolism.

Glutathione is synthesized exclusively intracellularly in its reduced form (GSH). The liver is the major organ for GSH synthesis and excretion into circulation and bile. This thiol is the predominant low molecular cellular antioxidant and functions as a multipotential metabolite. GSH is translocated from cytosol, where its synthesis takes place, to mitochondria and nucleus and serves as an antioxidant reducer and for detoxifying electrophilic compounds.

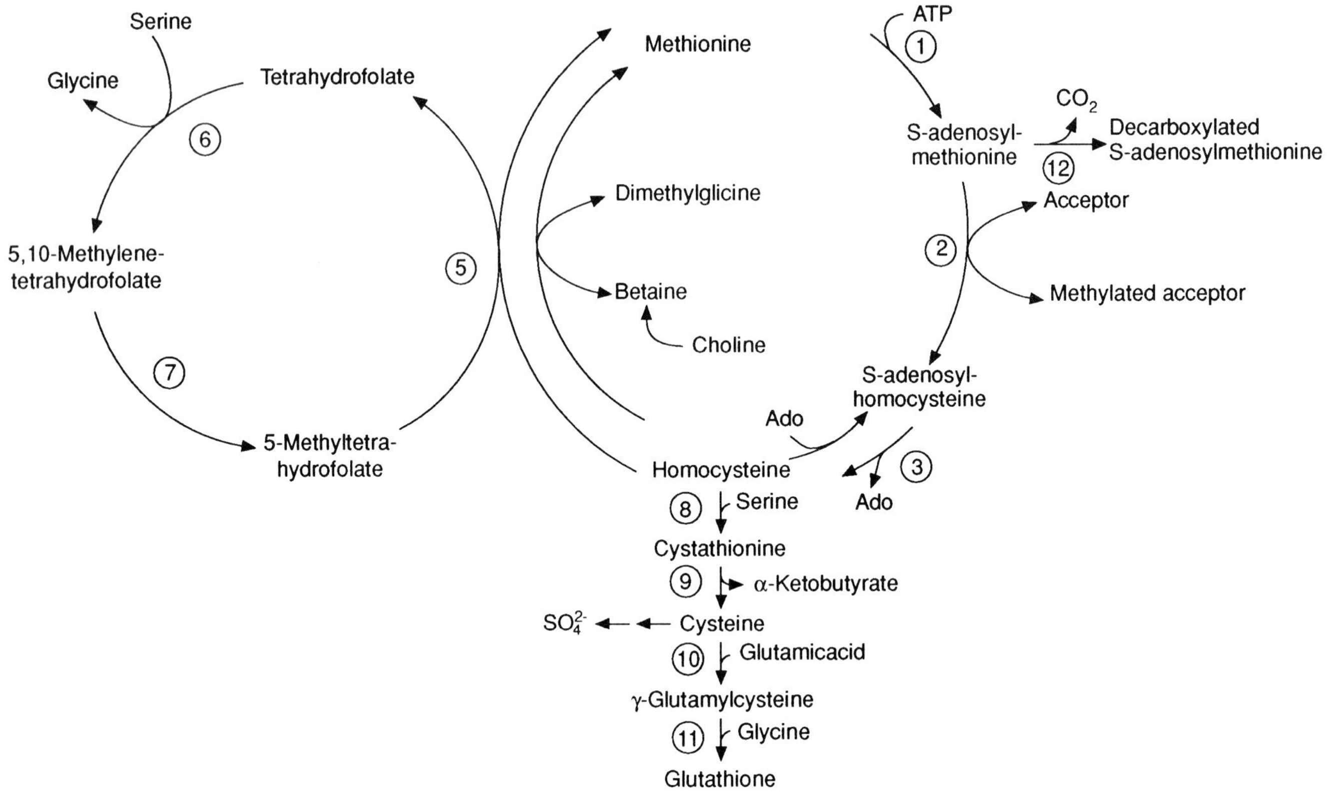

Fig. 1. Relevant reactons of liver methionine metabolism and related metabolic pathways. ①, S-adenosyl-L-methionine synthetase, also called methionine-adenosyltransferase; ②, transmethylation reactions; ③, S-adenosyl-L-homocysteine hydrolase; ④, betaine-homocysteine methyltransferase; ⑤, 5-methyltetrahydrofolate-homocysteine methyltransferase, also called methionine synthase; ⑥, serine oxidase; ⑦, 5,10-methylene-tetrahydrofolate reductase; ⑧, cystathionine *b*-synthase; ⑨, *g*-cystathionase; ⑩, *g*-glutamylcysteine synthetase; ⑪, glutathione synthetase; ⑫, *S*-adenosyl-L-methionine decarboxylase.

Among other functions, GSH participates in reductive processes that are essential for the synthesis and degradation of proteins, protection of cells against reactive oxygen compounds and free radicals, and regulation of the redox state of a number of biological macromolecules. GSH can also act as a coenzyme for several enzymatic reactions and is considered to be a storage and transport form of cysteine. Extracellular GSH is hydrolyzed on the outer surface of cells and the constitutent amino acids, including cysteine, enter cells and are used, among other metabolic pathways, for GSH synthesis. GSH depletion is associated with a reduction in the number of mitochondria, mitochondrial swelling and degeneration with rupture of membrane architecture and increased density.

SAM reduces the synthesis of 5-methyltetrahydrofolate (1), inhibits betaine-homocysteine methyltransferase activity and increases the synthesis of cystathionine by stimulation of cystathionine β-synthase (2). SAM therefore affects the liver distribution of homocysteine between remethylation and cystathionine synthesis by favouring the transsulphuration pathway (figura 1). Recently, CHO cells, which do not express β-cystathionase, have been stably transfected with rat liver cDNA SAM synthetase. In these cells both the concentration of SAM and GSH are markedly increased. The above results indicate that SAM regulates the intracellular concentration of GSH by acting at three different levels: *a*) by being a precursor of GSH synthesis; *b*) by favouring the transsulphuration pathway, and *c*) by a mechanism, independent of the later two, that involves the regulation of the synthesis and/or utilization of GSH.

Liver cirrhosis in rats can be induced by the administration of CCl_4 for several weeks (3). CCl_4 is a substrate for P-450 where it is converted to CCl_3 radicals, which generate CCl_3OO radicals by reacting with molecular oxygen. Since CCl_3OO radicals react with membranes and induce lipid peroxidation, membrane damage by free radical chain reaction has been proposed as the major cause of hepatocellular injury by CCl_4, the initial event being probably mitochondrial membrane injury (4). Hepatic steatosis occurs 2/3 weeks after CCl_4 administration. At this time liver SAM-synthetase activity is normal, but SAM concentration is lower and SAH levels are elevated. This leads to a marked reduction of the SAM/SAH ratio from about 3 in control animals to 1 in CCl_4 treated rats (table 1). This alteration in the methylation ratio of the liver has drastic consequences on DNA-methylation, phospholipid methylation and, supposedly, in many other transmethylation reactions. In this context, it is interesting to note that impaired liver phospholipid methylation has been described in human cirrhosis (5) and more recently in baboon cirrhosis(6) and during hypoxia in rats (7). A decrease in the hepatic SAM/SAH ratio has also been described in response to ethanol in rats, and reduced liver SAM levels after ethanol ingestion have been detected in rats (8) and baboons (6).

CCl_4-induced liver steatosis also has a profound effect on the levels of plasma sulphur amino acids. Thus, in CCl_4 treated rats plasma methionine is lower, homocysteine increases 20-fold and cystathionine levels are normal (table 2). Interestingly, elevated levels of plasma homocysteine (homocysteinemia) are believed to cause coronary artery disease (9).

As previously mentioned, SAM serves as donor of methyl groups for all detoxifying methylation reactions. A variety of methyltransferases, designated according to the functional group that serves as substrate as hydroxyl- amine- and thiol-methyltransferases, are view as a means of blunting the pharmacological activity of very toxic compounds by introducing a less polar, less reactive, methyl group. A loss in the methylation capacity of the hepatocyte, as that seen after the administration of CCl_4 or ethanol, might hinder the detoxifying capacity of the liver and provoke mitochondrial and plasma membrane damage.

In CCl_4-induced liver steatosis, hepatic SAM-synthetase activity and GSH concentration were normal. In contrast, when liver cirrhosis was produced by CCl_4 (about 9 weeks after the beginning of CCl_4 administration) hepatic SAM-synthetase was markedly diminished (about 50% of controls) and GSH levels depleted (3). A reduction of hepatic SAM synthetase has been demonstrated both in human cirrhosis —independently of its etiology— and in different animal models of liver disease. Similarly, hepatic GSH levels have been demonstrated to be reduced both in humans and in various models of liver disease (10). Moreover, patients with liver damage often have elevated levels of circulating methionine, a delayed clearance of this amino acid after its systemic administration and a reduced excretion of inorganic sulphate (11). Patients with alcoholic cirrhosis also have plasma cysteine deficiency when maintained on an elemental diet which provides sufficient quantities of essential nutrients, including methionine and cofactors, but lacks certain non-essential nutrients such as cysteine or choline (12).

These findings support a model where liver injury sets up two series of events within the hepatocyte. First, an early stimulus to catabolize

Table 1. S-Adenosylmethionine (SAM) and S-adenosylhomocysteine (SAH) hepatic concentrations in rats treated for 3 weeks with carbon tetrachloride (CCl_4)

Group	SAM (nmol/g)	SAH (nmol/g)	SAM/SAH
Control	102.2 ± 4.89	29.4 ± 3.83	3.47 ± 0.09
CCl_4	65.3* ± 5.27	69.5* ± 14.6	0.94* ± 0.05
CCl_4 + SAM	96.6** ± 6.1	63.3* ± 14.4	1.52*, ** ± 0.10

Results are expressed as means ± SEM for six animals per group.
* Denotes significantly different ($p < 0.05$) compared to the control group.
** Denotes statistical differences ($p < 0.05$) between CCl_4 vs. CCl_4 + SAM groups.

Table 2. Serum homocysteine (Hcy), methionine (Met) and cysthationine (Cys) concentrations in rats treated for 3 weeks with carbon tetrachloride (CCl_4)

Group	Hcy (μM)	Met (μM)	Cys (μM)
Control	0.42 ± 0.07	31.25 ± 2.37	1.42 ± 0.12
CCl_4	9.44* ± 1.08	20.87* ± 1.76	1.56 ± 0.14
CCl_4 + SAM	1.29** ± 0.28	24.76 ± 1.27	1.38 ± 0.08

Results are expressed as means ± SEM for six independent assays per group.
* Denotes statistical differences ($p < 0.01$) compared to control group.
** Denotes values significantly different ($p < 0.05$) due to the effect of SAM compared to CCl_4-treated rats.

methionine consequent on a need to maintain hepatic GSH levels to eliminate free radicals. This increased consumption of methionine, in response to stress by oxidants, leads to a reduction of the plasma concentration of this amino acid, a reduction of hepatic SAM and an elevation of liver SAH and plasma homocysteine. This results in an alteration of the methylation ratio with the resulting inhibition of transmethylation reactions and the consequent hampering effect on the function, structure and detoxifying capacity of the cell. Second, a decline of hepatic SAM synthesis leading to an impaired methionine clearance, reduced excretion of inorganic sulphate and depletion of GSH, resulting in the concomitant loss of the free radical scavenging capacity of the cell.

The biochemical basis for the reduced methylation ratio in the liver in response to CCl_4 or ethanol are uncertain but might be secondary to the incapacity of the cell to eliminate the excess of homocysteine produced as a result of oxidative stress. The mechanism of the reduction of hepatic SAM synthesis after CCl_4 administration has been worked out in certain detail.

Human and rat liver SAM-synthetase have been cloned and sequenced (13). The deduced amino acid sequence corresponds to proteins with Mr of 43647 and 43697 for the human and rat liver enzymes respectively. cDNA clones for human and rat liver SAM-synthetase detect, by Northern analysis, one single mRNA species in both human and rat liver but did not hybridize with RNA from other tissues of human or rat origin (14). A cDNA clone for rat kidney SAM-synthetase has been shown to detect two mRNA species in kidney, brain and testis, but did not hybridize with liver (14). These results indicate the existence of two different genes for SAM synthetase in mammals, one expressed specifically in the liver and a second gene expressed in extra-hepatic tissues.

The cloning and initial characterization of the rat liver-specific SAM-synthetase gene promoter may provide insights into the mechanisms that regulate the expression of this enzyme. In fact, DNA sequence analysis of 1,500 base pair 5' of the transcriptional start site has revealed the presence of several putative regulatory elements. These include potential hormonal responsive elements (HREs), AP-1 recognition motifs, NF1 binding sites and features related to consensus binding sites for liver-enriched transcription factors (HNF-1, HNF-3 and HNF-4). The latter three could be implicated in the tissue-specific enzyme expression.

Human and rat liver cytosol contain two different forms of SAM-synthetase which are called α (Mr 200 kDa) and β (Mr 110 kDa) (15). Expression of rat liver SAM-synthetase cDNA into *Escherichia coli* also yields two enzymatic forms with the same size than those seen with rat liver cytosol (16). These results indicate that the high-Mr form is a tetramer and the low-Mr form a dimer of the same 43.7 kDa subunit. Moreover, these results also indicate that post-transductional signals are not required to acquire these oligomeric structures. Both SAM-synthetase forms have been purified to homogeneity from rat liver cytosol. The purified enzymes can be bound to a thiopropyl-Sepharose 6B column (a covalent chromatography that uses as binding sites sulphydryl groups of proteins) and eluted with GSH (17). After this treatment, the high-Mr form shows a Michaelian kinetics with a Km for methionine of 125 μM. However, before this treatment or after GSH removal, the tetramer presents a sigmoidal kinetics for methionine which can be decomposed into two components, the main one with a Km for methionine of 970 μM and a second one of 36 μM. The Low-Mr enzyme, which has a Km for methionine of 700 μM did not change its kinetic properties after thiopropyl-sepharose 6B chromatography.

Further evidence about the importance of sulphydryl groups to maintain the structure and activity of SAM-synthetase has been obtained using GSSG and GSH/GSSG buffers (18). Whereas both forms of the enzyme are inhibited by GSSG, GSH alone has no effect on the enzyme activity although protects from the inhibitory effect of GSSG. Moreover, at a given GSH/GSSG ratio, SAM synthetase activity increased by rising the concentration of GSH. Inhibition of the enzyme activity by GSSG correlated with the dissociation of both SAM-synthetases to a monomer. Since no incorporation of $[^{35}S]$GSSG has been observed with either of the enzyme forms, the available data obtained in the presence of GSSG seems to suggest that oxidation leads to the formation of an intrasubunit disulphide bond. Finally, modification with N-ethylmaleimide (a sulphydryl agent) of rat liver SAM-synthetase has revealed the presence of two accessible sulphydryl groups in the native enzyme that are important in maintaining the structure and activity of the enzyme. One of these residues has been identified as Cys-150 of the protein sequence and is at the ATP binding domain of the enzyme (19). In summary, these results suggest that SAM-synthetase activity is modulated by reduction-oxidation of specific cysteine residues. Reduction of these cysteine residues is also required to maintain the oligomeric structure of the enzyme.

In keeping with this hypothesis, *in vivo* inhibition of GSH synthesis in rats by the administration of buthionine sulfoximine (BSO, a specific inhibitor of GSH-synthase) leads to a rapid reduction of hepatic SAM-synthetase activity which could be prevented by the simultaneous administration of monoethyl glutathione ester (a membrane permeable derivative of GSH which after being taken up by the cell is rapidly hydrolysed to form GSH) (20). Rat liver SAM-synthetase mRNA levels, however, remain unchanged after the administration of buthionine sulfoximine. Similarly, SAM-synthetase mRNA levels of hepatic samples from human and CCl_4-induced liver cirrhosis are similar to those measured in normal liver samples (3, 14). These experiments indicate, that the reduction of hepatic SAM-synthetase activity observed in liver disease is not due to a reduced transcription of the SAM-synthetase gene, but rather to an inhibition/inactivation of the enzyme. Interestingly, in human liver cirrhosis is the high-Mr/high-affinity form of the enzyme which is markedly reduced as compared to samples from subjects with normal liver function (21). Why this occurs is unknown but it might reflect a higher susceptibility of the high-Mr form of the enzyme to oxidative agents.

It has been recently shown that rat liver SAM-synthetase gene expression is reduced under conditions of hypoxia (7). This leads to an abnormal metabolism of SAM and impaired GSH synthesis which are similar, in several respects, to those observed during liver injury induced by ethanol or CCl_4. The mechanisms involved in the expression of the SAM-synthetase gene and its regulated response by oxygen remain unknown but it is certainly a field to be developed in the near future.

Hypoxic stress can strongly modify the expression of certain genes including erythropoietin, proto-oncogene *c-jun* and glutathione peroxidase. The antioxidant enzymes superoxide dismutase, catalase and glutathione peroxidase decrease during hypoxia. The regulation of glutathione peroxidase gene expression by oxygen has been worked out in certain detail and the available data indicate that this enzyme is regulated at the transcriptional level (22). Hypoxic stress therefore markedly impairs the scavenging capacity of the cell, just as it occurs during oxidative stress.

Evidence has been obtained during the last years suggesting that various forms of liver injury and necrosis are caused by oxidative stress and the subsequent formation of free radicals. It has been proposed that free radicals injure hepatocyte membranes through a number of mechanisms including lipid peroxidation. Free radicals have been shown, using both *in vitro* and *in vivo* models, to modify and damage lipids, proteins, DNA and carbohydrates. When the amount of free radicals generated exceeds the scavenging capacity of the hepatocyte, through systems such as catalase, superoxide dismutase and glutathione peroxidase, significant cell damage can occur. Liver injury not only demands a higher free radical scavenging capacity from the hepatocyte, but impairs its methylation capacity as well as its ability to synthesyze GSH. Therefore, a successful therapeutic approach to this pathogenic mechanism should, ideally, maintain undamaged liver methionine metabolism and safeguard, or better increase, the free radical scavenging capacity of the liver. The observation that in human liver cirrhosis the severity of the disease correlates with the intensity of methionine intolerance agrees with this model (23).

As previously seen, SAM increases liver GSH concentration by acting at three different levels: is a precursor of GSH synthesis, favours the transsuphuration pathway and regulates the synthesis/degradation of GSH. Thus, it has been of interest to examine the effect of exogenous SAM on liver injury in various models of oxidative stress.

SAM has been shown to reduce the hepatotoxic effect of galactosamine, ethanol, paracetamol (acetaminophen), thioacetamide and CCl_4 both *in vitro* and *in vivo* models. In the presence of exogenous SAM, mortality in response to paracetamol or galactosamine is reduced in experimental models and the onset of liver fibrosis is delayed for several weeks (3, 24-26). Similarly, the extent of liver damage induced by the chronic administration of ethanol to baboons and rats is reduced by SAM (6). CCl_4-induced liver DNA hypomethylation is also prevented by the administration of SAM. Maintenance of methylation reactions might be essential to prevent mitochondrial membrane damage as well as the functional integrity of other cellular membranes. In this respect it has been demonstrated that SAM, but not N-acetylcysteine (another GSH precursor) reduces ethanol-induced liver mitochondrial GSH depletion (26). Similarly, SAM has been shown to be more effective than N-acetylcysteine in preventing the hepatotoxic effect of paracetamol in mice (27) and liver injury induced by ischemia and reperfusion (28). Transient ischemia followed by reperfusion occurs during liver transplantation and radical surgical resections. Different observations indicate that superoxide radicals and related metabolites are generated during ischemia and/or reperfusion, and that these changes may impair the function of the reperfused tissue.

Although these and other observations suggest that the therapeutic potential of SAM dwells in its methylation capacity, this does not mean that the hepatoprotective effect of SAM is provided only through its ability to donate methyl groups. SAM has been shown to effectively reduce liver GSH depletion induced by various agents both *in vitro* and *in vivo* models, and the inhibition of GSH synthesis with buthionine sulfoximine blocks the protective effect of SAM on paracetamol-induced liver injury in mice (27). These results indicate that SAM exerts its hepatoprotective action both by maintaining the methylation capacity of the cell and by preventing GSH depletion.

SAM has also proven to be effective in increasing the hepatic GSH content in patients with liver injury of alcoholic and non-alcoholic origin (29). The positive effect of SAM on the free radical scavenging capacity of the injured human liver points to this molecule as a successful therapeutic agent. Ideally, a hepatoprotective molecule should meet the following three criteria: *a*) should not have side effects and should act, directly or indirectly, as a free radical scavenger; *b*) the ability to target the liver preferentially with high concentrations of the agent, and *c*) this molecule should be able to mediate its protective effect in a short period of time.

SAM has been extensively shown to be nontoxic in humans and to have no side effects (30). As previously mentioned, SAM acts as a free radical scavenger, both in humans and *in vitro* and *in vivo* models of liver disease, by increasing the hepatic GSH concentration. Moreover, SAM enhances the methylation capacity of the hepatocyte, an important effect to maintain the structure, function and detoxifying capacity of the cell. SAM is made and consumed mainly by the liver. However, when administered exogenously its biodisponibility is small although the p-toluene-sulphonate salt of SAM has been shown to be taken up by the hepatocytes from the bloodstream (31). Liposomes provide a mechanism to target compounds to the liver *in vivo*. Could SAM be targeted to the liver selectively and efficiently by its encapsulation into liposomes? Increasing the biodisponibility of SAM should be an area of future research interest. Finally, SAM has been shown to mediate its hepatoprotective effect in a short period of time. Thus, it has been shown to protect paracetamol induced mortality when administered together or even several hours later than the hepatotoxic agent (27).

Different studies have shown that SAM is effective in the symptomatic treatment of intrahepatic cholestasis of liver disease and of pregnancy (32). Moreover, SAM has also been reported to improve liver function in various chronic liver diseases including alcoholic and non-alcoholic liver cirrhosis (33). The possible beneficial effects of SAM treatment on the appearance and management of clinical complications in chronic liver diseases, such as bleeding from oesophageal varices or brain damage secondary to liver dysfunction, remain to be determined.

In addition to SAM, other molecules that enhance the free radical scavenging capacity of the liver might be successful therapeutic agents. Among these are, N-acetylcysteine, glutathione esters (GSH is not permeable through the cell membrane) and vitamin E. The first two are both GSH precursors and vitamin E is viewed as the most potent antioxidant agent present in membranes (34). N-acetylcysteine, if administered on time, prevents liver injury induced by paracetamol in humans and *in vivo* models, an effect that is inhibited by buthionine sulfoximine (27, 35). Glutathione esters have also been found to protect liver injury induced by various agents including paracetamol and buthionine sulfoximine in *in vivo* models (20, 36). Vitamin E has been shown to inhibit CCl_4-induced liver injury in rats (37) and the killing of cultured hepatocytes by tert-butyl hydroperoxide in cultured hepatocytes (38). Could the simultaneous administration of two or more of these agents provide additional protection against liver injury? SAM and vitamin E act at different, yet complementary levels. Whereas SAM is a water soluble molecule that serves as donor of methyl groups for all detoxifying methylation reactions and a GSH precursor, vitamin E is a lipophilic molecule present in membranes where exerts its antioxidant activity.

Future progress in the molecular mechanisms involved in the expression of the SAM-synthetase gene as well as of the genes of the antioxidant enzymes superoxide dismutase, catalase and glutathione peroxidase may lead to potential therapies aimed at increasing the expression of these genes in response to liver injury.

REFERENCES

1. Kutzbach C Stokstad ELR. Feedback inhibition of methylene -tetrahydrofolate reductase in rat liver by S-adenosyl-L-methionine. BBA 1967; 139:217-220.
2. Finkelstein JD, Martin JJ. Methionine metabolism in mammals: distribution of homocysteine between competing pathways. J Biol Chem 1984; 259:9508-9513.
3. Corrales F, Giménez A. Álvarez L, Caballería J, Pajares MA, Andreu H, Parés A, Mato JM, Rodés JS. Adenosylmethionine Treatment Prevents Carbon Tetrachloride-induced S-adenosylmethionine Synthetase Inactivation and Attenuates Liver Injury. Hepatology 1992; 16:1022-1027.
4. Rao KS, Glende EA, Recnagel RO Effect of drug pretreatment in carbon tetrachloride induced lipid peroxidadtion in rat liver microsomal lipids. Exp Molec Pathol 1970; 12:324-331.
5. Martín-Duce A, Ortiz P, Cabrero C, Mato JM. S-Adenosyl-L-methionine synthetase and phopholipid methyltransferase are inhibited in human cirrhosis. Hepatology 1988; 8:65-68.
6. Lieber CS, Casini A, De Carli LM, Lowe N, Sasaki R, Leo MA. S-Adenosyl-L-methionine attenuates alcohol-induced liver injury in the baboon. Hepatology 1990; 11:165-172.
7. Chawla RK, Jones DP. Abnormal metabolism of S-adenosyl-L-methionine in hypoxic rat liver. Similarities to its abnormal metabolism in alcoholic cirrhosis. BBA 1994; 1199:45-51.
8. Trimble KC, Molloy A, Scott JM, Weir DG. The effect of ethanol on one-carbon metabolism: increase methionine catabolism and lipotrope methyl group wastage. In: Mato JM, Lieber CS, Kaplowitz N, Caballero A, eds. Methionine metabolism: molecular mechanism and clinical implications. Madrid: CSIC Press, 1992; 46-58.
9. Clarke R, Daly L, Naughten E, Calahane S, Fowler B, Graham I. Hyperhomocysteinemia: an independent risk factor for vascular disease. N Engl J Med 1991; 324:1149-1155.
10. Mato JM, Álvarez L, Corrales F, Pajares MA. S-Adenosylmethionine and the liver. In: Arias IM, Boyer JL, Fausto N, Jakoby WB, Schachter DA, Shafritz DA, eds. The Liver: Biology and Pathobiology, 3rd ed. New York: Raven Press, 1994; 27:461-470.
11. Corrales F, Álvarez L, Pajares MA, Ortiz P, Mato JM. Impairment of methionine metabolism in liver disease. Drug Investigation 1992; 4(Suppl 4):8-13.
12. Marchesini G, Bianchi GP, Vilstrup H, Chechia GA, Patrono D, Zoli M. Plasma clearances of branched-chain amino acids in control subjets and in patients with cirrhosis. J Hepatol 1987; 4:108-117.
13. Álvarez L, Asunción M, Corrales F, Pajares MA, Mato JM. Analysis of the 5'non-coding region of rat liver S-adenosylmethionine synthetase mRNA and comparison of the M_r deduced from the cDNA sequence and the purified enzyme. FEBS Lett 1991; 290:142-146.
14. Álvarez L, Corrales F, Martín-Duce A, Mato JM. Charactization of a full-length cDNA encoding human liver S-adenosyl-methionine synthetase: tissue-specific gene expresion and mRNA levels in hepatopathies. Biochem J 1993; 293:481-486.
15. Cabrero C, Puerta J, Alemany S. Purification and comparison of two forms of S-adenosyl-L-methionine synthetase from rat liver. Eur J Biochem 1987; 170:299-304.
16. Álvarez L, Mingorance J, Pajares MA, Mato JM. Expression of rat liver S-adenosylmethionine synthetase in Escherichia coli results in two active oligomeric forms. Biochem J 1994; 301:557-561.
17. Pajares MA, Durán C, Corrales F, Pliego M, Mato JM. Modulation of rat liver S-adenosylmethionine synthetase activity by glutathione. J Biol Chem 1992; 267:17598-17605.
18. Pajares MA, Corrales F, Durán C, Mato JM, Álvarez L. How is rat liver S-adenosylmethionine synthetase regulated? FEBS Lett 1992; 309:1-4.
19. Pajares MA, Corrales F, Ochoa P, Mato JM. The role

of cysteine 150 in the structure and activity of rat liver S-adenosyl-L-methionine synthetase. Biochem J 1991; 274:225-229.

20. Corrales F, Ochoa P, Rivas C, Martín-Lomas M, Mato J, Pajares MA. Inhibition of glutathione synthesis in the liver leads to S-adenosyl-L-methionine synthetase reduction. Hepatology 1991; 14:528-533.
21. Cabrero C, Martín-Duce A, Ortiz P, Alemany S, Mato JM. Specific loss of the high molecular weight form of S-adenosyl-L-methionine synthetase in human liver cirrhosis. Hepatology 1988; 8:1530-1534.
22. Cowan OB, Weisel RD, Williams WG, Mickle OAG. The regulation of glutathione peroxidase gene expression by oxygen tension in cultured human cardiomyocytes. J Mol Cell Cardiol 1992; 24:423-433.
23. Marchesini G, Bugianesi E, Bianchi G, Fabbri A, Marchi E, Zoli M, Pisi E. Defective methionine metabolism in cirrhosis: relation to severity of liver disease. Hepatology 1992; 16:149-155.
24. Stramentinoli G, Gulano M, Ideo G. Protective role of S-adenosyl-L-methionine on liver injury induced by D-galactosamine in rats. Biochem Pharmacol 1978; 27:1431-1433.
25. Stramentinoli G, Pezzoli C, Galli-Kienle M. Protective role of S-adenosyl-methionine against acetaminophen induced mortality and hepatotoxicity in mice. Biochem Pharmacol 1979; 28:3567-3571.
26. García Ruiz C, Morles A, Colell A, Ballesta A, Rodés J, Kaplowitz N, Fernández-Checa JC. Feeding S-adenosyl-L-metthionine attenuates both ethanol-induced depletion of mitochondrial glutathione and mitochondrial dysfunction in periportal and perivenous hepatocites. Hepatology (in press).
27. Bray GP, Tredger JH, Williams R. S-Adenosylmethionine protects against acetaminophen hepatotoxicity in two mouse models. Hepatology 1992; 15:297-301.
28. Dunne JB, Davenport M, Williams R, Tredger JM. Evidence that S-adenosylmethionine and N-acetylcysteine reduce injury from sequential cold and warm ischemia in the isolated perfused rat liver. Transplantation 1994; 57:1161-1168.
29. Vendemiale G, Altamore E, Trizio T, Le Grazie C, Di-Padova C, Salerno MT, Carrieri V, Albano O. Effects of oral S-adenosyl-L-methionine on hepatic glutathione in patients with liver disease. Scand J Gastroenterol 1989; 24:407-415.
30. Friedel HA, Goa KL, Benfield P. S-Adenosyl-L-methionine: A review of its pharmacological properties and therapeutic potential in liver dysfunction and affective disorders in re-lation to its physiological role in cell metabolism. Drugs 1989; 38:389-416.
31. Giulidori P, Galli-Kienle M, Catto E, Stramentinoli G. Transmethylation, transsulfuration, and aminopropylation reactions of S-adenosyl-L-methionine *in vivo*. J Biol Chem 1984; 259:1-7.
32. Giudici GA, Le Grazie C, Di Padova C. The use of ademethionine (SAMe) in the treatment of cholestatic liver disorders. Meta-analysis of clinical trials. In: Mato JM, Lieber CS, Kaplowitz N, Caballero A, eds. Methionine metabolism: molecular mechanism and clinical implications. Madrid: CSIC Press, 1992; 67-79.
33. Frezza M, Surrenti C, Manzillo G, Fiaccadori F, Bortolini M, Di Padova C. Oral S-adenosylmethionine in the symptomatic treatment of intrahepatic cholestasis: a double-blind, placebo controlled study. Gastroenterology 1990; 99:211-215.
34. Mckay PB. Vitamin E: interactions with free radicals and ascorbate. Annu Rev Nutr 1985; 5:323-340.
35. Prescott LF. Paracetamol overdosage: pharmacological considerations and clinical management. Drugs 1983; 25:290-314.
36. Martesson J, Meister A. Mitochondrial damage in muscle occurs after marked depletion of glutathione and is prevented by giving glutathione monoester. Proc Natl Acad Sci USA 1989; 86:471-475.
37. Yao T, Degli Esposti S, Huang L, Arnon R, Spangenbergen A, Zern MA. Inhibition of carbon tetrachloride-induced liver injury by liposomes containing vitamin E. Hepatology (in press).
38. Glascott PA, Gilfor E, Farber JL. Effects of vitamin E on the killing of cultured hepatocytes by tert-butyl hydroperoxide. Mol Pharmacol 1992; 41:1155-1162.

Prevention and Therapy with S-Adenosyl-L-Methionine and Polyenylphosphatidylcholine

C. S. Lieber

INTERACTION OF ETHANOL WITH CHOLINE, METHIONINE AND S-ADENOSYL-L-METHIONINE

For several decades, protein, methionine and choline deficiencies have been implicated in the pathogenesis of liver injury. In growing rats, deficiences in dietary protein and lipotropic factors (choline and methionine) can produce a fatty liver (1) and it has been reported that ethanol increases choline requirements in the rat (2), possibly by enhancing choline oxidation (3). Primates, however, are far less susceptible to protein and lipotropic deficiency than rodents (4). Clinically, choline treatment of patients suffering from alcoholic liver injury has been found to be ineffective in the face of continued alcohol abuse (5-8). Human liver contains very little choline oxidase activity, which may explain the species differences with regard to choline deficiency. In humans, choline deficiency (and thus a need for choline supplementation) has been documented in only very limited circumstances of extremely restricted diets (9).

Moreover, in baboons fed ethanol, fatty liver as well as fibrosis (including cirrhosis) developed (10), with striking ultrastructural changes (11), despite an amount of choline given at twice the dose recommended for the baboon by Foy et al. (12). Nevertheless, since the possibility existed that massive choline supplementation might have a favorable effect on the process, this was the subject of an experimental study in baboons. They were given either normal or choline-supplemented diets, each with or without ethanol. They were pair-fed for 3 to 4 years liquid diets with 50 % of total energy as ethanol or isocaloric carbohydrate. Ten animals were given the regular diets, whereas in eight the choline content was increased 5-fold. With both ethanol-containing diets, ethanol intake was comparable and resulted in hepatic steatosis and striking mitochondrial lesions, with increases in serum bilirubin and AST, ALT and glutamate dehydrogenase (GDH) activities. In addition, of the five animals fed alcohol with the regular diet, one progressed to incomplete cirrhosis and two others developed perivenular and associated perisinusoidal fibrosis. Similarly, in the four baboons fed alcohol with choline supplementation, incomplete cirrhosis developed in one and perivenular fibrosis in two. Collagen deposition was demonstrated by immunoperoxidase with a specific antibody against procollagen type III. Those animals also displayed proliferation of myofibroblasts in the perivenular area and transformation of fat-storing cells to transitional cells in the perisinusoidal space, with associated enhanced collagen fiber deposition. Thus, in baboons, choline supplementation failed to prevent alcohol-induced steatosis and fibrosis. All parameters remained normal in the eight baboons fed the regular control diet. However, in the choline-supplemented controls, serum bilirubin, AST and GDH activities increased moderately and serum albumin decreased. Occasional fat droplets appeared in hepatocytes with mitochondrial changes (enlargement and alterations of the cristae) and an abundance of «myelin» figures in the cytoplasm, indicating that choline supplementation had exerted moderate hepatotoxicity (13). It was concluded that massive choline supplementation does not prevent alcoholic liver injury but that, in fact, it may be hepatotoxic.

Liberal supplementation with methionine (10) also failed to prevent alcohol induced liver injury, including cirrhosis, from developing in baboons. In man as well, methionine supplementation had been contemplated for the treatment of liver diseases, especially the alcoholic variety, but some difficulties have been encountered. Indeed, excess methionine was shown to have some adverse effects (14) including a decrease in hepatic ATP (15). Furthermore, whereas in some patients with alcoholic liver disease, circulating methionine levels are normal (16), in others, elevated levels have been reported (17-19). Moreover, Kinsell et al. (20) have observed a delay in the clearance of plasma methionine after its systemic administration to patients with liver damage. Similarly, Horowitz et al. (21) reported that the blood clearance of methionine after an oral load of this amino acid was slowed in such subjetcs. Since about half of the methionine is metabolized by the liver, the above observations suggest impaired hepatic metabolism of this amino acid in patients with alocholic liver disease. Indeed, Duce et al. (22) reported decreases of S-adenosyl-L-methionine (SAMe) synthetase activities in cirrhotic livers. Furthermore chronic alcohol consumption was found to be associated with enhanced methionine utilization and depletion (23). As a consequence, one can anticipate SAMe depletion as well as its decreased availability. Therefore, the baboon model of alcohol-induced liver injury was used to verify the latter hypothesis and to explore the possibility that SAMe repletion might oppose some of the adverse effects of alcohol on the liver (24). This study revealed that, in the baboon, chronic ethanol consumption is associated with a significant depletion of hepatic SAMe and that SAMe supplementation attenuates ethanol-induced liver injury as shown by a less striking glutathione depletion, lesser increases in plasma AST and GDH activities (fig. 1), fewer ethanol-induced megamitochondria, and a lesser increase in mitochondrial mass (as determined by hepatic succinate dehydrogenase activity).

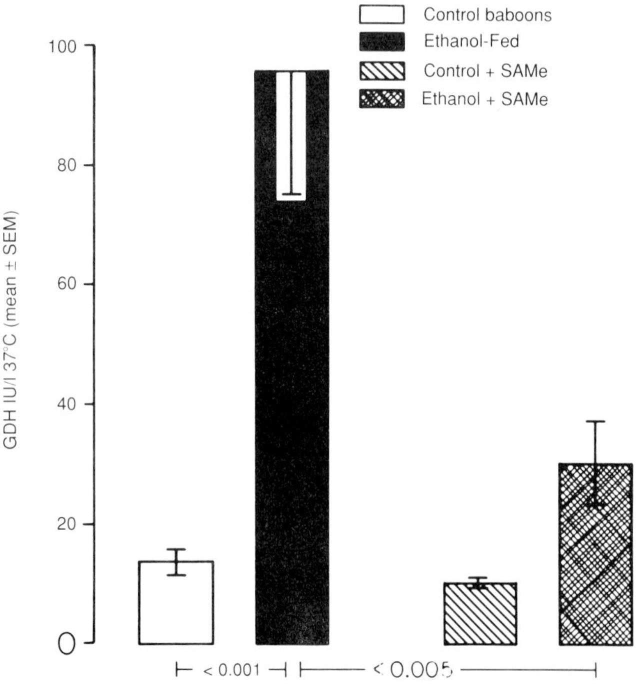

Fig. 1. Effect of SAMe ont he ethanol-induced of plasma-glutamic dehydrogenase activity (24).

Contrasting with the protective effects listed above, SAMe had no obvious action on lipid accumulation. These observations are at variance with some previous studies in rodent showing the prevention of fat accumulation in the liver by SAMe (25). The difference in results may be due to a difference in species and also in the mode of SAMe administration: whereas Feo et al. (25) dealt with the effect of intramuscular SAMe, the drug was administered orally in the study of Lieber et al. (24) in the baboon. Futhermore, SAMe was used as a powder rather than acid-resistant tablets. This could have reduced the bioavailability of SAMe, since it has been reported that intraduodenal administration improves the bioavailability of the drug (26). The significant hepatic SAMe depletion after long term ethanol consumption in primates (24) is due, in part, to increased GSH utilization se-

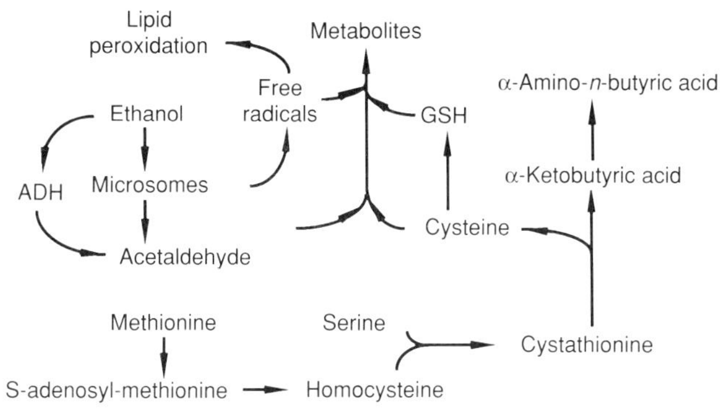

Fig. 2. Hypothetical link between accelerated acetaldehyde production, increased free radical generation by the «induced» microsomes, enhanced lipid peroxidation, and increased α-amino-*n*-butyric acid production (95).

condary to enhanced free radical and acetaldehyde generation by the induced MEOS (figure 2) as well as GSH leakage (27). Under these conditions, increased GSH turnover may ensue, as evidenced by a rise in α-amino-*n*-butyric acid (28, 29) (figs. 2 and 3). However, SAMe synthase activity may become rate limiting, especially since it is decreased in cirrhosis (22). As a consequence, methionine supplementation may be ineffective in alcoholic liver disease and SAMe depletion ensues.

Potentially, SAMe depletion may have a number of adverse effects. SAMe is the principal methylating agent in various vital transmethylation reactions which have been known to be important to nucleic acid and protein synthesis for some time. Hirata et al. (30) and Hirata and Axelrod (31) have also demostrated the importance of methylation to cell membrane function, with a role of phospholipid methylation in membrane fluidity and the transport of metabolites and transmission of signals across membranes. Thus, decreased SAMe, by being detrimental for methyltransferase activity, may thereby promote the membrane injury which has been documented in alcohol-induced liver damage (32). Not only is SAMe the methyl donor in almost all transmethylation reactions, buy it also plays a key role in the synthesis of polyamines and provides one of the sources of cysteine needed for glutathione production. Alcohol-induced depletion of glutathione has been shown to be particularly striking in primates (33), as confirmed more recently (24).

In rats, chronic alcohol feeding was found to result in decreased methionine formation via the n-5 tetrahydrofolate pathway, an effect compensated for through an adaptive increase in betainehomocysteine methytransferase activity, which maintains hepatic SAMe levels (34). This adaptive process may be particulary operative in the rodents and much less so in prima-

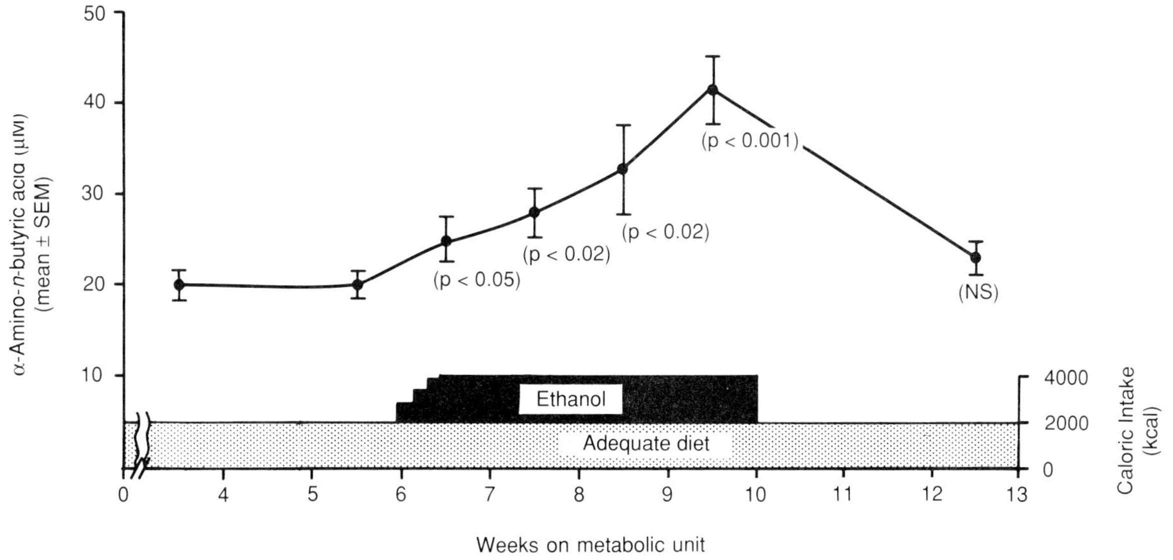

Fig. 3. Effect of ethanol consumption on plasma α-amino-*n*-butyric acid (mean ± SEM); consumption of ethanol (4 g/kg/day) in addition to and adequate diet in 3 human volunteers resulted in doubling of plasma α-amino-*n*-butyric acid after 2 to 4 weeks, which was reversed after cassation of dringking (29).

tes. Indeed, as already mentioned, rodents contain higher levels of choline oxidase than primates and therefore can produce significantly greater amounts of betaine, which may be one of the reason why rodents are less susceptible to alcohol induced liver injury than primates (35) *(vide supra)*. Thus, replenishment of methionine, and especially its activated form SAMe, may be particularly indicated in the primate when subjected to an alcoholic insult.

Compared to methionine, administration of SAMe has the advantage of bypassing the deficit in SAMe synthesis from methionine referred to above. Indeed, this deficit is due to a decrease in enzyme activity, not in the substrate and therefore cannot simply be corrected by excess methionine. Replenishment of the hepatocyte with SAMe is feasible through ingestion of the compound; it has ben shown that blood levels of SAMe are increased after oral administration in rodents (36) and in man (37). Although it has been claimed that the liver does not take up SAMe from the bloodstream (38), other results have indicated uptake of SAMe by isolated hepatocytes either at pharmacologic (39) or physiologic (40, 41) extracellular leveles. The liver SAMe transport system appears to be saturable (40, 42). Results in baboons (24) also clearly indicate hepatic uptake of exogenous SAMe as evidenced by the appearance of a peak corresponding to the (+) isomer, which is absent from the normal liver, but present to a certain extent in the liver of the animals fed the exogenous SAMe provided in the diet. Furthermore, in these baboons, the ethanol- induced hepatic SAMe depletion was partially corrected with oral SAMe administration. In addition to uptake of extracellular SAMe, extracellular methionine appears to play a major role in the synthesis of newly acquired intracellular SAMe (41). Thus, orally administered SAMe may play a precursor role for intracellular SAMe, both as unchanged SAMe and also by the methionine it provides. Since the SAMe transport system does not appear to be saturated under physiological conditions, it is likely that SAMe levels in biological compartments regulate, at least in part, the rate of transport across membranes. Indeed, hepatic levels of SAMe are increased with increasing extracellular levels (41) and the intracellular concentrations reached are above or close to the K_m for SAMe of both phospholipid methyltransferase (42, 43) and catechol-o-methyltransferase (44). Furthermore, the effective utilization of SAMe both for transmethylation and transsulfuration has been demonstrated *in vivo* (45).

Thus, the therapeutic use of SAMe is a rare example of replenishment of a naturally occurring molecule which has been depleted by liver disease, resulting in a beneficial effect. The exact role of SAMe in the treatment of liver disorders has been in part clarified by recent studies showing that this molecule is beneficial in intrahepatic cholestasis, as reviewed in detail by Osman et al. (46). Treatment with a stable salt of SAMe resulted in both improvement of standard liver function test and reduction in symptoms such as itch. Consequently, SAMe may become useful for managing pruritus associated with cholestatic liver disease. It has also been successfully used in severe cholestasis of pregnancy, where it has the advantage of few, if any, untoward effects. Recurrent intrahepatic cholestasis and severe jaundice caused by androgens or estrogens are also conditions in which treatment with SAMe appears to be helpful, perhaps because of changes in membrane phospholipid composition. Experimentally, SAMe prevented total parenteral nutrition-induced cholestasis in the rat (47). Potentially beneficial clinical effects of SAMe include enhanced bile salt conjugation with taurine in patients with liver cirrhosis (48). Other observations indicate that administration of exogenous SAMe prevents the glutathione depletion observed in the liver of patients affected by liver disease (49). Loguercio et al. (50) also measured glutathionine and cysteine concentrations in erythrocytes of alcoholics with (20 subjects) and without (20 subjects) liver cirrhosis. Glutathione levels were decreased, whereas those of cysteine were increased in all patients. Parenteral treatment with SAMe corrected the erythrocyte thiol alterations. Furthermore, in patients given SAMe, long-term treatment doubles the plasma concentration of the secondary sulphur-containing amino acid cystine and taurine, which were on average low-normal at baseline, without any change in the concentration of methionine, of neutral amino acids, and of polyamines. No changes in plasma amino acids were observed in the control group (51). In experimental animals, SAMe was shown to prevent and reverse erythrocyte membrane alterations in cirrhosis (52). It also exerted a protective effect against liver damage induced by biliary obstruction in rats (53), prevented carbon tetrachloride-induced SAMe synthetase inactivation and associated liver injury (54) and improved the histologic picture in the liver of rats treated with CCl_4 and ethanol for one month (55). Betaine administration was reported to have the capacity to elevate hepatic SAMe and to prevent the ethanol-induced fatty liver in rats (56).

Lack of methionine may also result from a deficit in methylation of homocysteine to methionine, mainly by the folate and vitamin B_{12}-dependent enzyme methionine synthase. Since in most alcoholics a disturbed folate metabolism is present (attributable to multiple mechanims, including an inadequate diet), elevated plasma homocysteine levels in alcoholics could have been anticipated and have now indeed been noted in a group of alcoholics (57). Since hyperhomocysteinemia has been associated with premature vascular disease (58) the increased plasma homocysteine in alcoholics could contribute to the increased incidence of stroke found in these patients. Furthermore, the SAMe dependant methylation of specific DNA cytosine bases to form 5-methylcytosine may block gene expression, and abnormalities in DNA methylation contribute to the loss of the normal controls on proto-oncogene expression (59-61). Indeed, a methyl-deficient diet has been linked to early stages of colorectal neoplasia (62). These observations illustrate the need to correct underlying malnutrition in the alcoholic, which may exist irrespective of the social and medical situation of the patient (63). Nutrition support was successful in decreasing nutrition-associated complications in patients with alcoholic liver disease (64). The rationale for the various modalities of nutritional intervention has also been reviewed (65). It is now clear, however, that the mere nutritional repletion may not suffice, and that «supernutrients» may be needed, such as SAMe and possibly polyunsaturated phospholipids *(vide infra)*.

In summary, in chronic liver diseases, a marked reduction in the rate of synthesis and utilization of SAMe has been described as a consequence of a decrease in the activity of the enzyme SAMe-synthetase. Exogenous SAMe may overcome this metabolic block and concomitantly reverse, at least in part, cholestatic and ethanol-related liver injury. The metabolism of exogenous SAMe appears to follow the known pathways of endogenous SAMe metabolism, and the initial data suggest that the process is largely unaffected in patients with chronic liver disease. Furthermore, studies in non-human primates also clearly indicate hepatic uptake of ingested SAMe. Moreover, it has been shown that blood levels of SAMe are increased after oral administration in rodents and man.

ATTENUATION OF ALCOHOL-INDUCED HEPATIC FIBROSIS BY POLYUNSATURATED LECITHIN

In primates, chronic ethanol consumption results in a decrease of liver phospholipids and of phosphatidylcholine (PC); both can be corrected by PC supplementation (66). The total phospholipid content of the mitochondrial membranes is decreased, with a significant reduction in the levels of PC (67) and associated striking morphologic changes with a corresponding functional counterpart, namely diminished mitochondrial oxidation due mainly to decreased cytochrome oxidase activity (11). The latter appears to result from alterations in the phospholipid composition of the mitochondrial membranes. Indeed, *in vitro* cytochrome oxidase activity could be restored with phospholipids extracted from normal mitochondria or synthetic ones, with PC being the most active (67).

The mechanism whereby chronic ethanol consumption alters phospholipids has not been clarified but may be related, at least in part, to decreased phospholipid methyltransferase (PEMT) activity described in cirrhotic livers (22). That this is not simply secondary to the cirrhosis, but may in fact be a primary defect related to alcohol, is suggested by the observation that the enzyme activity is already decreased prior to the development of cirrhosis (68) (fig. 4). Another mechanism whereby ethanol may affect phospholipids is via formation of phosphatidylethanol, with possible impact on signal transduction, as shown in isolated rat hepatocytes (69).

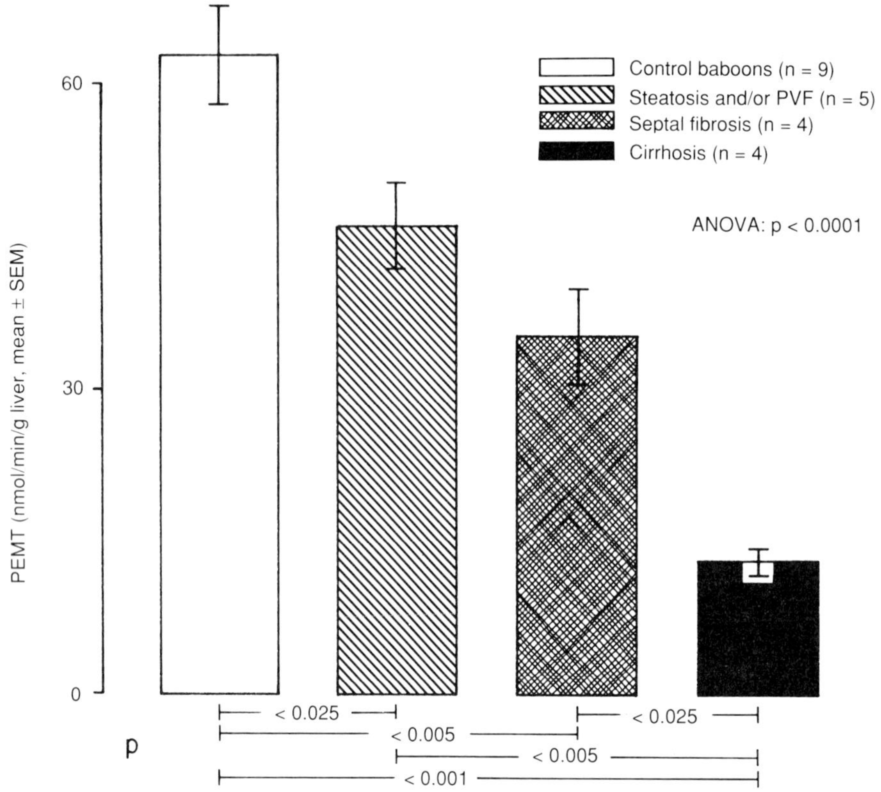

Fig. 4. Phospholipid methyltransferase (PEMT) activity at various stages of alcoholic liver disease. In 9 baboons fed the control diet and in 13 animals fed alcohol, there was a progressive decrease in PEMT activity with increasingly severe injury. The greatest reduction was observed in cirrhosis, but there was already a significant reduction at precirrhotic stages, including perivenular fibrosis (PVF) (68). ANOVA: analysis of variance.

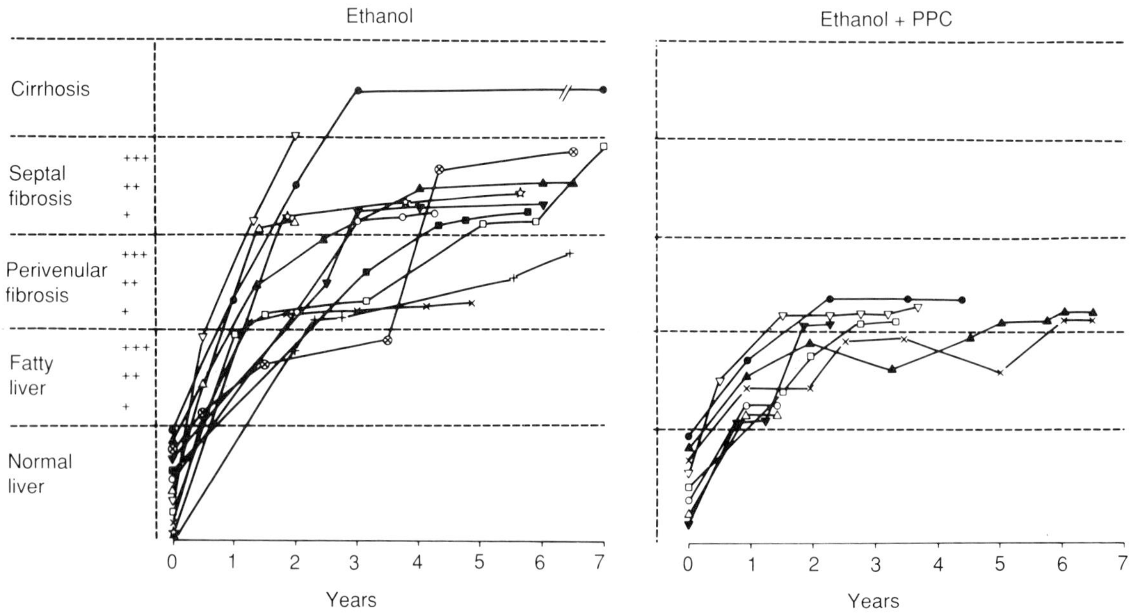

Fig. 5. Sequential development of alcoholic liver injury in baboons fed ethanol with an adequate diet (left panel) and prevention of septal fibrosis and cirrhosis by supplementation with polyunsaturated phospahtidylcholine (PPC) (right panel). Liver morphology in animals pair-fed control diets (with or without PPC) remained normal (not shown) (66).

A third mechanism is increased lipid peroxidation, as reflected by increased F_2 isoprostanes (70) which could explain the associated decrease of arachidonic acid in phospholipids (66).

In alcoholic patients, reduction in phospholipid methyltransferase activity together with the decreased activity of SAMe synthetase *(vide supra)* may promete the membrane injury which has been documented experimentally in alcohol-induced liver damage (32). The question then arose whether such deficiency could be attenuated, at least in part, by bypassing the enzyme defects through phospholipid supplementation. This was tested by feeding baboons alcohol in a diet supplemented with polyunsaturated lecithin. Administration of phospholipid preparations rich in polyunsaturated phosphatidylcholine (PPC) (71) or virtually pure PPC (66) (fig. 5) was found, in the non-human primate, to fully prevent alcohol-induced fibrosis and cirrhosis. PPC contains choline, but, as discussed before, it was found that choline, in amounts present in PPC, has no protective action against the fibrogenic effects of ethanol in the baboon (13). PPC is rich in linoleic acid, but this fatty acid *per se* is probably not responsible for the protective effect because the basic diet was supplemented with linoleate and contained large amounts of corn oil that is rich in linoleic acid. Furthermore, this fatty acid has been incriminated as a permissive rather than as a protective factor in alcoholic liver injury (72). Thus, the polyunsaturated phospholipids themselves appear to be responsible for protection, perhaps because of their high bioavailability and selective incorporation into liver membranes (73). Furthermore, PPC directly affects collagen metabolism.

Whereas there is still some discussion about the relative contributions of hepatocytes and lipocytes in the production of collagen in the liver, lipocytes are «activated» after chronic alcohol consumption (figs. 6 and 7) and appear to play a major role (74-75). Normal lipocytes, when isolated and cultured on plastic surfaces, undergo spontaneous transformation into myofibroblast-like cells, thereby mimicking *in vitro* the «activation» that prevails *in vivo* after chronic alcohol consumption (76). These cells in culture produce collagen (76). When acetaldehyde is added to these cells, they respond with a further increase in collagen accumulation (76), with enhanced mRNA for collagen (77). Other aldehydes (such as malonaldehyde) are produced from lipid peroxidation and they may also stimulate collagen production. Acetaldehyde stimulates collagen synthesis in cultured myofibroblasts as well (78) and a similar effect was observed with lactate. These cells were shown to proliferate in the perivenular zones of the liver after chronic alcohol consumption (79);

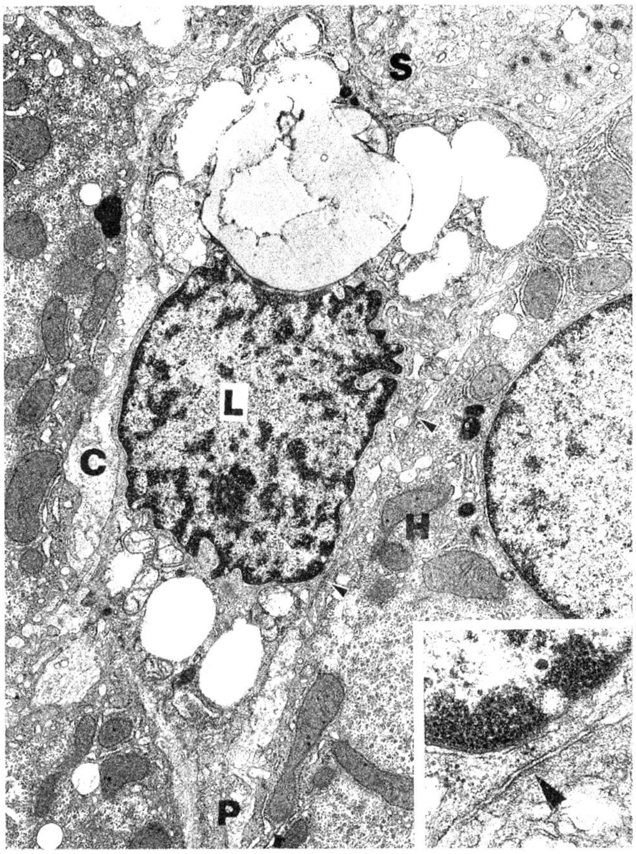

Fig. 6. Lipocyte from a patient with fatty liver. The lipocyte (L) contains lipid droplets of variable sizes with a total lipid volume density of more than 20% of the cell. The rough endoplasmic reticulum is randomly distributed in the cytoplasm as short, narrowed cisternae. The Golgi apparatus is relatively inconspicuous. At the cell periphery and in the cell process (P), there are small aggregates of filaments, dense bodies, and pinocytic vesicles. Cell contacts with increased fila mentous density of adjoining plasma membranes (arrowheads) are visible between the lipocytes and neighboring hepatocytes (H). Collagen fibers (C) are present in the extracellular space. Inset: cell contacts at higher mangification. S, sinusoid (13,000; inset, X50,000) (75).

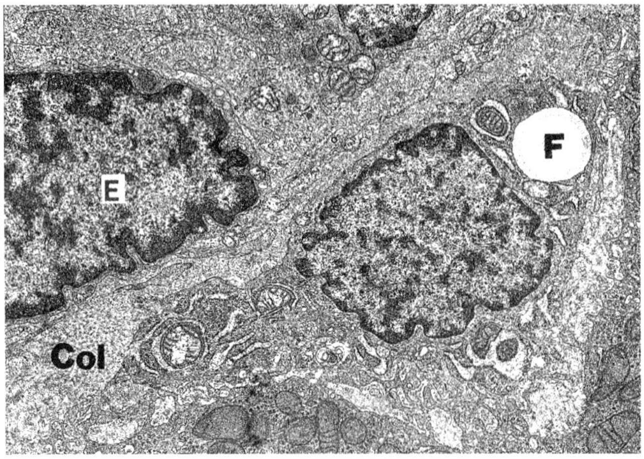

Fig. 7. Transitional cell (or «activated» lipocyte) in the Disse space in a cirrhotic liver. This myofibroblast-like cell contains a small lipid droplet (F) with a total lipid volume density of less than 20% of the cell volume. The rough endoplasmic reticulum appears conspicuous. Note that the cell profile appears smaller compared to that of the lipocyte in figure 6. In the extracellular space, an abundant amount of collgen fibers (Col) is present. E: endothelial cell nucleus (X13,000) (75).

they are similar to «activated» lipocytes, although they can be differentiated by ultrastructural and cytochemical characteristics (80). The normal liver contains a negligible number of «activated» lipocytes, whereas after chronic alcohol consumption, most lipocytes (more than 80%) are transformed. The protection afforded by PC against fibrosis (fig. 5) was associated with a lesser transformation of lipocytes to transitional cells *in vivo* (48% vs. 81%). Thus, to the extent that the transformation of lipocytes in alcohol fed animals was responsible for the fibrosis, the lesser transformation after PC may be one of the reasons for the decreased fibrosis.

Fibrosis and the associated collagen accumulation does not result simply from enhanced collagen production, but rather from an imbalance between collagen production and breakdown. Breakdown was assessed in cultured rat lipocytes by measuring collagenase activity with different phospholipids, including various species of PC. It was reported before that a mixture of PCs affected the breakdown, but not the synthesis of collagen under those conditions (81). The PC preparation used contained 18:2-18:2 PC (DLPC), 16:0-18:2 PC (PLPC) and other minor PC species. We now found that pure DLPC (table 1) stimulates collagenase activity *in vitro*. Increased collagenase activity can be expected to oppose collagen accumulation and the development of fibrosis by promoting the breakdown of collagen. The increase in collagenase activity was observed both in the absence and the presence of acetaldehyde, the metabolite of ethanol, which has been incriminated in many of its effects (82). The specificity of the DLPC effect was illustrated by the fact that the other main component of the administered PC, namely PLPC, or other unsaturated or saturated PCs such as dioleoyl-PC, diarachidonoyl-PC, distearoyl-PC, dilauroyl-PC, or another polyunsaturated phospholipid (dilinoleoylphosphatidylethanolamine), or polyunsaturated free fatty acids (linoleic, arachidonic) had no effect on collagenase activity. A similar lack of effect had also been found before with dilauroyl-PC (81). Choline was inactive *in vitro* (table 1), as it had also been found to be ineffective *in vivo (vide infra)*. Taken together, these findings suggest that DLPC is the active agent responsible, at least in part, for the protection afforded by PPC against the development of fibrosis and its ultimate stage of cirrhosis, most likely because of stimulation of collagen breakdown. Collagenase activity is generally increased during the early stage of liver injury (83). Our previous studies revealed that fibrosis coincides with the stage at which collagen breakdown slackens and stops keeping pace with increased production (84). Therefore these findings suggest that studies on collagenase activity associated with hepatic injury may be relevant to the elucidation of the pathogenesis of liver fibrosis and its treatment and prevention.

PPC could of course also act in some other ways. Phospholipids rich in essential fatty acids have a high bioavailability. More than 50% of orally administered PC is made biologically available for the organism either by intact absorption (lesser extent) or by reacylation of absorbed lysophosphatidylcholine (greater extent) (85). Pharmacokinetic studies in man using $^{3}H/^{14}C$-labeled phosphatidylcholine showed the absorption to exceed 90% (86). Similar observations were made in animals (87-89). Indeed, although much of the PC in the diet is degraded by pancreatic phospholipase A_2 (90), the products (l-acyl-lysophosphatidylcholine and fatty

Table 1. Collagenase activity in media of lipocytes (% of control): rat lipocytes were incubated with or without acetaldehyde, and collagenase activity was measured as described in Lieber et al. (66) ($p < 0.001$ vs. control)

	Without acetaldehyde			With acetaldehyde		
Additions to media	*n*	$\bar{X}$	SEM	*n*	$\bar{X}$	SEM
Control	10	100%	2.8	10	99.3	5.5
Phosphatidylcholine (10 μM)						
Dilinoleoyl (18:2-18:2)	12	160.1	15.7	13	177.2	16.7
Palmitoyl-linoleoyl (16:0-18:2)	14	99	8.7	14	96.8	8.9
Diarachidonoyl (20:4-20:4)	5	89.5	7.7	4	104.5	12.8
Dioleoyl (18:1-18:1)	5	91.5	6.3	4	99.3	4.8
Dilauroyl (12:0-12:0)	15	91.8	9.5	15	94.4	5.5
Distearoyl (18:0-18:0)	6	104.3	8.3	6	87.9	11.9
Phosphatidyl ethanolamine (dilinoleoyl) (10 μM)	7	117.4	5.6	7	113.1	8.4
Linoleic acid (20 μM)	14	90.1	10.2	14	90.0	6.6
Arachidonic acid (20 μM)	5	114.8	9.1	5	103.9	8.25
Choline (10 μM)	7	97.8	6.3	7	113.4	5.6

acids) are absorbed in the jejunum (91). Animal studies show that PCs recovered in intestinal lymph after feeding fat enriched with single fatty acids are highly enriched in both *sn*-1 and *sn*-2 positions with the same acyl groups that were fed (92). Thus, it can be anticipated that during absorption of a diet enriched with 18:2 fatty acids, new PCs will be formed from dietary 18:2-lysoPC that will have an 18:2-18:2 composition. Various authors (73, 93, 94) reported PC accumulation in the liver during the first 24 to 48 hr after administration. It was also found in this study that, although the baseline value of DLPC is low, there was a significant increase of DLPC in the liver of the supplemented baboons. Thus, PC supplementation results in increased hepatic DLPC which may be the active compound. Activity may require the presence of both 18:2 fatty acids or, alternatively, only one 18:2 in PC may suffice *in vivo*. Indeed, all 18:2 PCs were present in the liver in significantly increased amounts in baboons fed 18:2-18:2PC (66, 95).

PC has been used before empirically in nonalcoholic liver diseases; beneficial histologic effects have been reported in the recovery from kwashiorkor (96), in HBsAG-positive patients with cirrhosis (97) and in patients with chronic active hepatitis in terms of inflammatory parameters (98). PC was also used for the treatment of alcoholic hepatitis (98) and alcoholic fatty liver (99), but not as yet for the prevention or treatment of hepatic fibrosis or cirrhosis. In view of the lack of toxicity of PC, demonstrated when it was used for these other indications, and its effectiveness in the prevention of alcoholic fibrosis and cirrhosis in the baboon, demonstrated with a virtually pure PC preparation (66) and a less pure extract before (71), PC or, if possible DLPC, both natural compounds, should now be tried for the control of alcoholic fibrosis and cirrhosis in humans. Since DLPC promotes the breakdown of collagen, there is a reasonable hope that this treatment may affect not only the progression of the disease, but may also reverse preexisting fibrosis, as demonstrated for CCl_4 induced cirrhosis in the rat (100). For the same reason, it may be useful for the management of fibrosis of non alcoholic etiologies as well. Indeed, fibrosis is a common end stage for most chronic liver diseases.

In summary, PC protects against alcohol-induced fibrosis and cirrhosis and prevents the associated hepatic PC depletion by increasing 18:2 containing PC species; it also attenuates the transformation of lipocytes into collagen-producing transitional cells. Furthermore, it increases collagen breakdown, as shown in cultured lipocytes enriched with pure DLPC (18:2-18:2 PC), the main PC species present in the extract, which may be the active ingredient. In view of its inocuity and experimental effectiveness, therapeutic assessment is now warranted. Indeed, ongoing randomized, double blind, multicentered studies are now addressing this issue in man.

CONCLUSION

Although the hepatotoxicity of alcohol is now well established, replenishment of nutritional deficiencies, when present, is still valuable in the treatment of alcoholic liver disease. It is now recognized, however, that this approach is insufficient and that a more direct interference with the adverse effects of ethanol is warranted, some of which may be accomplished with SAMe and/or PPC, two natural compounds that can be viewed as «supernutrients».

REFERENCES

1. Best CH, Hartroft WS, Lucas CC, Ridout JH. Liver damager produced by feeding alcohol or sugar and its prevention by cholinc. Br Med J 1949; 2:1001-1006.
2. Klatskin G, Hrehl WA, Coon HO. The effect of alcohol on the choline requirement. I. Changes in the rat's liver following prolonged ingestion of alcohol. J Exp Med 1954; 100:605-614.
3. Thompson JA, Reitz RC. Studies on the acute and chronic effects of ethanol ingestion on choline oxidation. Ann N York Acad Sci 1976; 273:194-204.
4. Hoffbauer FW, Zaki FG. Choline deficiency in baboon and rat compared. Arch Pathology 1965; 79:364-369.
5. Olson RE. Modern Nutrition in Health and Disease. In: Wohl MG, Goodhart WS, eds. Philadelphia: Lea and Febiger, PA, 1964; 1037-1050.
6. Phillips GB, Davidson CS. Acute hepatic insufficiency of the chronic alcoholic. Arch Internal Med 1954; 94:585-603.
7. Post JJ, Benton B, Breakstone R, Hoffman J. The effects of diet and choline on fatty infiltration of the human liver. Gastroenterology 1952; 20:403-410.
8. Volwiler W, Jones CM, Mallory TB. Criteria for the measurement of results of treatment in fatty cirrhosis. Gastroenterology 1948; 11:164-182.
9. Chawla RK, Wolf DC, Kutner MH, Bonkovsky HL. Choline may be an essential nutrient in malnourished patients with cirrhosis. Gastroenterology 1989; 97:1514-1520.
10. Lieber CS, DeCarli LM. An experimental model of alcohol feeding and liver injury in the baboon. J Med Primatol 1974; 3:153-163.
11. Arai M, Leo MA, Nakano M, Gordon ER, Lieber CS. Biochemical and morphological alterations of baboon hepatic mitochondria after chronic ethanol consumption. Hepatology 1984; 4:165-174.
12. Foy H, Kondi A, Mbaya V. Effect of riboflavine deficiency on bone marrow function and protein metabolism in baboon. Br J Nutr 1964; 18:307-318.
13. Lieber CS, Leo MA, Mak KM, DeCarli LM, Sato S. Choline fails to prevent liver fibrosis in ethanol-fed baboons but causes toxicity. Hepatology 1985; 5:561-572.
14. Finkelstein JD, Martin JJ. Methionine metabolism in mammals. Adaptation to methionine excess. J Biol Chem 1986; 261:1582-1587.
15. Hardwick DF, Applegarth DA, Cockcroft DM, Ross PM, Coder RJ. Pathogenesis of methionine-induced toxicity. Metabolism 1970; 19:381-391.
16. Iob V, Coon WW, Sloan M. Free amino acids in liver, plasma and muscle of patients with cirrhosis of the liver. J Surg Res 1967; 7:41-43.
17. Iber FL, Rosen H, Stanley MA, Levenson SM, Chalmers TC. The plasma amino acids in patients with liver failure. J Lab Clin Med 1957; 50:417-425.
18. Fischer JE, Yoshimura N, Aguirre A, James JH, Cummings MG, Abel RN, Deindoerfer F. Plasma amino acids in patients with hepatic encephalopathy. Am J Surg 1974; 127:40-47.
19. Montanari A, Simoni I, Vallisa D, Trifiro A, Colla R, Abbiati R, Borghi L, Novarini A. Free amino acids in plasma and skeletal muscle of patients with liver cirrhosis. Hepatology 1988; 8:1034-1039.
20. Kinsell L, Harper HA, Barton HC et al. Rate of disappearance from plasma of intravenously administered methionine in patients with liver damage. Science 1947; 106:589-594.
21. Horowitz JH, Rypins EB, Henderson JM, Heymsfield SB, Moffitt SD, Bain RP, Chawla RK, Bleier JC, Rudman D. Evidence for impairment of transsulfuration pathway in cirrhosis. Gastroenterology 1981; 81:668-675.
22. Duce AM, Ortiz P, Cabrero C, Mato JM. S-adenosyl-L-methionine synthetase and phospholipid methyltransferase are inhibited in human cirrhosis. Hepatology 1988; 8:65-68.
23. Finkelstein JD, Cello JP, Kyle WE. Ethanol-induced changes in methionine metabolism in rat liver. Biochem Biophysics Res Commun 1974; 61:475-481.
24. Lieber CS, Casini A, DeCarli LM, Kim C, Lowe N, Sasaki R, Leo MA: S-adenosyl-L-methionine attenuates alcohol-induced liver injury in the baboon. Hepatology 1990; 11:165-172.
25. Feo F, Pascale R, Garcea R, Daino L, Piris L, Frassetto S, Ruggiu ME, Di Padova C, Stramentinoli G. Effect of the variations of S-adenosyl-L-methionine liver content on fat accumulation and ethanol metabolism in ethanol-intoxicated rats. Toxicol Appl Pharmacol 1986; 83:331-341.
26. Stramentinoli G. Pharmacologic aspects of S-adenosyl-L-methionine: pharmacokinetics and pharmacodynamics. Am J Med 1987; 83:35-42.
27. Speisky H, MacDonald A, Giles G, Orrego H, Israel Y. Increased loss and decreased synthesis of hepatic glutathione after acute ethanol administration. Biochem J 1985; 225:565.
28. Lieber CS. Alcohol, liver injury and protein metabolism. Pharmacol Biochem Behav 1980; 13:17-30.
29. Shaw S, Lieber CS. Plasma amino acid abnormalities in the alcoholic: Respective role of alcohol, nutrition and liver injury. Gastroenterology 1978; 74:677-682.

30. Hirata F, Viveros OH, Diliberto EJ Jr., Alexrod J. Identification and properties of two methyltransferases in conversion of phosphatidylethanolamine to phosphatidylcholine. Proc Natl Acad Sci USA 1978; 75:1718-1721.
31. Hirata F, Axelrod J. Phospholipid methylation and biological signal transmission. Science 1980; 209:1082-1090.
32. Yamada S, Mak KM, Lieber CS. Chronic ethanol consumption alters rat liver plasma membranes and potentiates release of alkaline phosphatase. Gastroenterology 1985; 88:1799-1806.
33. Shaw S, Jayatilleke E, Ross WA, Gordon ER, Lieber CS. Ethanol induced lipid peroxidation: potentiation by long-term alcohol feeding and attenuation by methionine. J Lab Clin Med 1981; 98:417-425.
34. Barak AJ, Beckenhauer HC, Tuma DJ, Donohue TM, Jr. Adaptive increase in betaine-homocysteine methyltransferase activity maintains hepatic S-adenosyl-L-methionine levels in ethanol-treated rats. IRCS Med Sci Biochem 1984; 12:866-867.
35. Hoffbauer FW, Zaki FG. Choline deficiency in baboon rat compared. Arch Pathology 1965; 79:364-369.
36. Stramentinoli G, Gualano M, Galli-Kienle M. Intestinal absorption of S-adenosyl-L-methionine. J Pharmacol Exp Ther 1979; 209:323-326.
37. Bombardieri G, Pappalardo G, Bernardi L, Barra D, Di Palma A, Castrini G. Intestinal absorption of S-adenosyl-L-methionine in humans. Int J Clin Pharmacol Ther Toxicol 1983; 21:186-188.
38. Hoffman DR, Marion DW, Cornatzer WE, Duerra JA. S-adenosylmethionine and S-adenosylhomocysteine metabolism in isolated rat liver. J Biol Chem 1980; 255:10822-10827.
39. Travers J, Varela I, Mato JM. Effect to exogenous S-adenosyl-L-methionine on phosphatidylcholine synthesis by isolated rat hepatocytes. Biochem Pharmacol 1984; 33:1562-1564.
40. Pezzoli C, Stramentinoli G, Galli-Kienele M, Plaff E. Uptake and metabolism of S-adenosyl-L-methionine by isolated rat hepatocytes. Biochem Biophys Res Commun 1978; 85:1031-1038.
41. Engstrom MA, Benevenga NJ. Rates of oxidation of the methionine and S-adenosylmethionine methyl carbons in isolated rat hepatocytes. J Nutr 1987; 117:1820-1826.
42. Zappia V, Galletti P, Porcelli M. Uptake of adenosylmethionine and related sulfur compounds by isolated rat liver. FEBS Lett 1978; 90:331-335.
43. Audubert F, Vance D. Pitfalls and problems in studies on the methylation of phosphatidylethanolamine. J Biol Chem 1983; 258:10695-10701.
44. Quiram DR, Weinshilboum RM. Catechol-O-methyltransferase in rat erythrocyte and three other tissues: comparison of biochemical properties after removal of inhibitory calcium. J Neurochem 1976; 27:1197-1203.
45. Giulidori P, Stramentinoli G. A radioenzymatic method for S-adenosyl-L-methionine determination in biological fluids. Anal Biochem 1984; 137:217-220.
46. Osman E, Owen JS, Burroughs AK. S-adenosyl-L-methionine —a new therapeutic agent in liver disease? Liment Pharmacol Ther 1993; 7:21-28.
47. Belli DC, Fournier LA, Lepage G, Yousef I, Roy CC. S-adenosyl-L-methionine prevents total parenteral nutrition-induced cholestasis in the rat. J Hepatology 1994; 21:18-23.
48. Angelico M, Gandin C, Nistri A, Baiocchi L, Capocaccia L. Oral S-adenosyl-L-methionine (SAMe) administration enhances bile salt conjugation with taurine in patients with liver cirrhosis. Scand J Clin Invest 1994; 54:459-464.
49. Vendemiale G, Altomare E, Trizio T, Le Grazie C, Di Padova C, Salerno MT, Carrieri V, Albano O. Effects of oral S-adenosyl-L-methionine on hepatic glutathione in patients with liver disease. Scand J Gastroenterol 1989; 24:407-415.
50. Loguercio C, Nardi G, Argenzio F, Aurilio C, Petrone E, Grella A, Del Vecchio Blanco C, Coltorti M. Effect of S-adenosyl-L-methionine administration on red blood cell cysteine adn glutathione levels in alcoholic patients with and without liver disease. Alcohol Alcohol 1994; 29:597-604.
51. Marchesini G, Bugianesi E, Bianchi G, Fabbri A, Marchi E, Zoli M, Pisi E. Effect of S-adenosyl-L-methionine administration on plasma levels of sulphur-containing amino acids in patients with liver cirrhosis. Clin Nutr 1992; 11:303-308.
52. Muriel P. S-adenosyl-L-methionine and reversed erythrocyte membrane alterations in cirrhosis. J Appl Toxicol 1993; 13:179-182.
53. Muriel P, Suárez OR, González P, Zuñiga M. Protective effect of S-adenosyl-L-methionine on liver damage induced by biliary obstruction in rats: a histological, ultrastructural and biochemical approach. J Hepatol 1994; 21:95-102.
54. Corrales F, Giménez A, Álvarez L, Caballería J, Pajares MA, Andreu H, Parés A, Mato JM, Rodés J. S-adenosylmethionine treatment prevents carbon tetrachloride-induced S-adenosylmethionine synthetase inactivation and attenuates liver injury. Hepatology 1992; 16:1022-1027.
55. Cutrin C, Meniño MJ, Otero X, Míguez J, Pérez-Becerra E, Barrio E. Effect of nifedipine and S-adenosylmethionine in the liver of rats treated with CCl_4 and ethanol for one month. Life Sci 1992; 51:113-118.
56. Barak A, Beckenhauer HC, Junnila M, Tuma DJ. Dietary betaine promotes generation of hepatic S-adenosylmethionine and protects the liver from ethanol-induced fatty infiltration. Alcohol Clin Exp Res 1993; 17:552-555.
57. Hultberg B, Berglund M, Andersson A, Frank A. Elevated Plasma Homocysteine in Alcoholics. Alcohol Clin Exp Res 1993, 17:687-689.
58. Stampfer MJ, Malinow MR, Willett WC, A prospective study of plasma homocysteine and risk of myocardial infarction in US physicians. JAMA 1992; 268:877-881.

59. Holliday R. The inheritance of epigenetic defects. Science 1987; 283:163-170.
60. Nyce J, Weinhouse S, Magee PN. 5-Methylcytosine depletion during tumor development: an extension of the miscoding concept. Br J Cancer 1983; 48:463-475.
61. Hoffman RM. Altered methionine metabolism, DNA methylation and oncogene expression in carcinogenesis. Biochim Biophys Acta 1984; 738:49-87.
62. Giovannucci E, Stampfer MJ, Colditz GA, Rimm EB, Trichopoulos D, Rosner BA, Speizer FE, Willett WC. Folate, methionine, and alcohol intake and risk of colorectal adenoma. J Natl Cancer Inst 1993; 85:875-884.
63. Koehn V, Burnand B, Niquille M, Paccaud F, Magnenat P, Yersin B. Prevalence of Malnutrition in Alcoholics and Non alcoholic Medical Inpatients: A Comparative Anthropometric Study. JPEN 1993; 17:35-40.
64. Hirsch S, Bunout D, de la Maza P, Iturriaga H, Petermann M, Icazar G, Gattas V, Ugarte G. Controlled Trial on Nutrition Supplementation in Outpatients With Symptomatic Alcohol Cirrhosis. JPEN 1993; 17:119-124.
65. Lieber CS. Herman Award Lecture, 1993: A Personal Perspective on Alcohol, Nutrition, and the Liver. Am J Clin Nutr 1993; 58:430-442.
66. Lieber CS, Robins S, Li J, DeCarli LM, Mak KM, Fasulo JM, Leo MA. Phosphatidylcholine protects against fibrosis and cirrhosis in the baboon. Gastroenterology 1994; 106:152-159.
67. Arai M, Gordon ER, Lieber CS. Decreased cytochrome oxidase activity in hepatic mitochondria after chronic ethanol consumption and the possible role of decreased cytochrome aa_3 content and changes in phospholipids. Biochim Biophys Acta 1984; 797:320-327.
68. Lieber CS, Robins SJ, Leo MA. Hepatic phosphatidylethanolamine methyltransferase activity is decreased by ethanol and increased by phosphatidylcholine. Alcohol Clin Exp Res 1994; 18:592-595.
69. Hoek JB, Thomas AP, Rooney TA, Higashi K, Rubin E. Ehtanol and signal transduction in the liver. Fed Am Soc Exp Bio J 1992; 6:2386-2396.
70. Aleynik SI, Leo MA, Ma X, Aleynik MK, Lieber CS. Polyenylphosphatidylcholine (PPC) prevents hepatic lipid peroxidation induced by CCl_4 in rats and by alcohol in baboons. Gastroenterology 1995 (in press).
71. Lieber CS, DeCarli LM, Mak KM, Kim C-I, Leo MA. Attenuation of alcohol-induced hepatic fibrosis by polyunsaturated lecithin. Hepatology 1990; 12:1390-1398.
72. Nanji AA, French SW. Dietary linoeic acid is required for development of experimentally induced alcoholic liver injury. Life Sci 1989; 44:223.
73. Lekim D, Graf E. Tierexperimentelle Studien zur Pharmakokinetik der «essentiellen» Phospholipide (EPL). Drug Res-Arzneimittelforschung 1976; 26:1772-1782.
74. Mak KM, Leo MA, Lieber CS. Alcoholic liver injury in baboons: transformation of lipocytes to transitional cells. Gastroenterology 1984; 87:188-200.
75. Mak KM, Lieber CS. Lipocytes and transitional cells in alcoholic liver disease: a morphometric study. Hepatology 1988; 8:1027-1033.
76. Moshage H, Casini A, Lieber CS. Acetaldehyde stimulates collagen production in cultured rat liver fat-storing cells but not in hepatocytes. Hepatology 1990; 12:511-518.
77. Casini A, Cunningham M, Rojkind M, Lieber CS. Acetaldehyde increases procollagen type I and fibronectin gene transcription in cultured rat fat-storing cells through a protein synthesis-dependent mechanism. Hepatology 1991; 13:758-765.
78. Savolainen E-R, Leo MA, Timple R, Lieber CS. Acetaldehyde and lactate stimulate collagen synthesis of cultured baboon liver myofibroblasts. Gastroenterology 1984; 87:777-787.
79. Nakano M, Lieber CS. Ultrastructure of initial stages of perivenular fibrosis in alcohol-fed baboons. Am J Pathol 1982; 106:145-155.
80. Takase S, Leo MA, Nouchi T, Lieber CS. Desmin distinguishes cultured fat-storing cells from myofibroblasts, smooth muscle cells and fibroblasts in the rat. J Hepatol 1988; 6:267-276.
81. Li J-J, Kim C-I, Leo MA, Mak KM, Rojkind M, Lieber CS. Polyunsaturated lecithin prevents acetaldehyde-mediated hepatic collagen accumulation by stimulating collagenase activity in cultured lipocytes. Hepatology 1992; 15:373-381.
82. Lieber CS. Medical and Nutritional Complications of Alcoholism: Mechanisms and Management. New York: Plenum Press, 1992; 579.
83. Maruyama K, Feinman L, Okazaki I, Lieber CS. Direct measurement of neutral collagenase activity in homogenates from baboon and human liver. Biochim Biophys Acta 1981; 658:124-131.
84. Maruyama K, Feinman L, Fainako M, Okazaki I, Lieber CS. Mammalian collagenase increases in early alcoholic liver diseases and decreases with cirrhosis. Life Sci 1982; 30:1379-1384.
85. Fox JM. Polyene phospahtidylcholine: pharmacokinetics after oral administration —a review. In: Avogaro P, Macini M, Ricci G, Paoletti R, eds. Phospholipids and atherosclerosis. New York: Raven Press, 1983.
86. Zierenberg O, Grundy SM. Intestinal absorption of polyenylphosphatidylcholine in man. J Lipid Res 1982; 23:1136-1142.
87. Parthasarathy S. Subbaiah PV, Ganguly J. The mechanism of intestinal absorption of phosphatidylcholine in rats. Biochem J 1974; 140:503-508.
88. Rodgers JB, O'Brien RJ, Balint JA. The absorption and subsequent utilization of lecithin by the rat jejunum. Am J Dig Dis 1975; 20:208-211.
89. Lekim D, Bezing H. The incorporation of essential phospholipids into the organs of intact and galactosamine intoxicated rats. Drug Res 1974; 24:1217-1221.
90. Arnesjö B, Nilsson Å, Barrowman J, Borgström B.

Intestinal digestion and absorption of cholesterol and lecithin in the human: Intubation studies with a fat-soluble reference substance. Scand J Gastroenterol 1969; 4:653-665.
91. Nilsson AKE. Intestinal absorption of lectihin and lysolecthin by lymph fistula rats. Biochim Biophys Acta 1968; 152:379-390.
92. Patton GM, Clark SB, Fasulo JM, Robins SJ. Utilization of individual lecithins in intestinal lipoprotein formation in the rat. J Clin Invest 1984; 73:231-240.
93. Holz J, Wagner H. Uber den Einbau von intraduodenal appliziertem $^{14}C/^{32}P$-Polyenephosphatidylcholin in die Leber von Ratten und seine Ausscheidung durch die Galle. Z Naturforsch 1971; 26:1151-1158.
94. Lekim D, Betzing H, Stoffel W. Incorporation of complete phospholipid molecules in cellular membranes of rat liver after uptake from blood serum. Hoppe-Seyler's Z Physiol Chem 1972; 353S:929-946.
95. Lieber CS. Alcohol and the liver: 1994 Update. Gastroenterology 1994; 106:1085-1105.
96. Alliet J, Comlan G, Courdier D. Steatosis of the human hepatocyte: an ultrastructure study —the reparative effects of polyenic fatty acid phosphatidylcholines. L'Ouest Med 1976; 29:85-104.
97. Fassati P, Horejsi J, Fassati M, Spizek J, Jezkova Z. Essential choline phospholipids and their effect on HBsAG and selected biochemical tests in cirrhosis of the liver. Casopis Lekaru Ceskych 1981; 120:56-60.
98. Bird GLA, Panos MZ, Polson R, Johnson R, Portman B, Neuberger J, Williams R. Activity of polyunsaturated phosphatidylcholine in HBsAG negative chronic active hepatitis and acute alcoholic hepatitis. Zeitschrift fur Gastroenterologie 1991; 29:(Suppl 2):21-24.
99. Schüller-Pérez A, González-San Martín F. Kontrollierte Studie mit mehrfach ungesättigtem Phosphatidylcholin im Vergleich zu Plazebo bei alkoholischer Lebersteatose. medizinische Welt 1985; 36:517-521.
100. Ma X, DeCarli LM, Lieber CS. Polyenylphosphatidylcholine attenuates non-alcoholic hepatic fibrosis. Gastroenterology 1994; 106:936.

Section 8

Treatment of Biliary Diseases and Hepatocellular Carcinoma

Gallstone Disease and Laparoscopic Surgery

A. M. Lacy

Laparoscopic techniques are not new. The first laparoscopy was performed in 1901. Only 19 years before this date, Langenbuch (1) introduced the cholecystectomy. This technique was the mainstay of treatment of gallstone disease for the next 105 years. In the late 1980s, a combination of modern high technology and surgical innovation: «high tech surgery», gave birth to laparoscopic cholecystectomy (LC). However, after the first LCs performed by Mühe and Mouret, this surgical approach has rapidly become the procedure of choice for most patients with symptomatic gallbladder disease. The explosion of laparoscopic techniques in general surgery has produced an important change in surgery, some authors have described these changes as *biliary perestroika* (2). As surgeons learn the technique, safety improves and contraindications to the new procedure decrease. A remarkable aspect of LC is how the radically new procedure gained acceptance. The advent of video endoscopy has facilitated the much-heralded and often-criticized use of laparoscopy in the practice of general surgery. Social, principally word-of-mouth, and economic pressures have influenced a number of minimal access operative procedures. Evidently these pressures can exert both negative as well as positive influences on any appraisal of a new technique. This procedure had attracted little attention until 1989 (3, 4). The early results suggest that there is a steep learning curve for LC associated with an increased risk of injury to the common bile duct (5). In September 1992, the National Institutes of Health (NIH) in the United States sponsored a consensus conference in Bethesda, Maryland, on «Gallstones and Laparoscopic Cholecystectomy» (6). A panel of 14 surgeons and physicians with a special interest in hepatobiliary disease were brought together in an attempt to develop a consensus on the current optimal approach to gallstone disease. Reported benefits of laparoscopic surgery specifically related to cholecystectomy; more rapid return to gastrointestinal tract function, shorter postoperative stay, decreased cost, less postoperative pain and disability, better cosmesis, and more rapid return to work (7-11)

INDICATIONS FOR LAPAROSCOPIC CHOLECYSTECTOMY

The primary and capital surgical indication for cholecystectomy is symptomatic gallstone disease; nevertheless, therapeutic choices of cholelithiasis are multiple. The various treatments can be classified into two categories: to eliminate the gallstones only or to eliminate both the gallstones and the gallbladder. The present treatments to eliminate the stones are: oral bile acid therapy (chenodeoxycolic acid), extracorporeal shock-wave lithotripsy, solvent dissolution (methyl tert-butyl ether) and mechanical disruption and extraction by percutaneous route. Two techniques are available to remove the gallbladder: open cholecystectomy or laparoscopic cholecystectomy.

LC has modified important concepts in general surgery. The rapid adoption of laparoscopic techniques by some surgeons could suggest some impulsiveness by some authors. However, the role of laparoscopic surgery requires a critical examination of the risk-benefit ratio. This new technology must be analyzed by well-trained surgeons experienced in laparoscopic techniques. In order to evaluate the available data on LC, the Office of Medical Applications of Research and the National Institute of Diabetes and Digestive and Kidney Diseases of the National Institutes of Health convened a consensus development conference on September 1992. The planning committee represented by surgeons, endoscopists, hepatologists, gastroenterologists, radiologists, epidemiologists, and representatives of the general public, accorded several conclusions in relation to LC: *a*) most patients with asymptomatic gallstones should not be treated; *b*) LC provides a safe and effective treatment and, it appears to be the treatment of choice; *c*) LC provides distinct advantages over open cholecystectomy (pain, cost savings, etc.) and, some disadvantages (common bile duct injury rate, new training for «traditional surgeons», etc.); *d*) conversion to open technique reflects sound surgical judgment and should not be considered a complication of LC (12).

INDICATIONS FOR CONVERSION

In experienced hands, the incidence of conversion from LC to open cholecystectomy is about 5% (5, 13). Decision to convert should always be based upon the ability to discern safely the anatomy and dissect the relevant structures (14). The most frequent causes for conversion are: extensive local inflammation and inadequate visualization of the anatomical landmarks, adhesions from previous surgery and, recognition of a complication during laparoscopy (bile duct and bowel injury, severe stone spillage, and bleeding). Other reasons for conversion are unexpected pathologic findings, such as carcinoma (see absolute contraindications).

MORBIDITY OF LAPAROSCOPIC CHOLECYSTECTOMY

LC has been bannered as a less morbidity and less costly alternative to open cholecystectomy. The overall morbidity of the laparoscopic approach seems to be reduced, although the incidence of major ductal injury may be increased according to some reports. Early experience showed an increased rate of common bile duct injury with LC (15-18). Recently, large prospective studies have delineated the overall morbidity and mortality at 2-6% and 0.1-0.5%, respectively (5, 11, 13, 18, 19).

Inexperience with the technique seems to be a common denominator in most of these patients. Causes of death resulting from inexperience include trocar injury to major vessels, carbon dioxide insufflation into major blood vessels, and sudden tension pneumothorax. However, Steiner recently published the surgical rates and operative mortality in LC with a 33 percent decrease in overall operative mortality per procedure contrasting with open cholecystectomy (20).

In addition, the complication rate of about 5%, including very minor problems, is favorable compared to minilaparotomy for cholecystectomy (21). The most common complications of LC are umbilical wound infection and bleeding from the trocar, cystic artery or liver bed. Bleeding after LC can occur for much the same reasons as during open cholecystectomy.

Another important complication is bile leakage that may occur at either intraoperative or postoperative period. The most frequent intraoperative cause is gallbladder perforation or bile duct injury. Postoperative bile leakage may result from an unrecognized ductal injury or even in the absence of ductal lesion. Cystic duct leakage after LC can be established from the mechanism of titanium clip dislodgment (22, 23).

The most significant complication of this LC is bile duct injury. Fortunately, the initial experience reported by Meyers and fellow members of the Southern Surgeons Club (5), has been improved upon. The classic pattern of laparoscopic injury appears to be misidentification of the common duct for the cystic duct, resection of a portion of the common and hepatic ducts, and associated right hepatic artery injury (24). Injuries to the common bile duct are the most devastating complications of LC. They tend to occur with greater frequency early in the course of a surgeon's experience (5, 24, 25). In most cases, the injury requires an endoscopic retrograde cholangiopancreatography (ERCP) for the diagnosis and classification of type of injury. The ERCP has a high success rate in the treatment of biliary problems after LC. The most easily resolved complication is the presence of retained biliary stones, that can be treated by an ERCP plus endoscopic sphincterotomy. Endoscopic sphincterotomy is also the treatment of choice in patients with bilioma or biliary leaks from the cystic duct stump. In larger leaks nasobiliary tube can be used to decompress the bile duct with the advantage that one can repeat the cholangiogram (26). The endoscopic approach is also useful if other techniques are needed such as dilatation, stents, as well as for a complete evaluation to establish the surgical indication.

Complication rates in the broad general surgical community where LC has been overwhelmingly implemented may be of a different magnitude. A national or institutional survey was therefore conducted to estimate broadly the frequency and therapy of major operative complications of LC (18).

CONTROVERSIES IN LAPAROSCOPIC CHOLECYSTECTOMY

Some concern exists about the controversies of the LC in performing appropriate treatment regarding some preoperative and intraoperative circumstances.

Contraindications of LC

When initially introduced, several contraindications to LC were described. These included, for example, choledocholithiasis, pancreatitis, and acute cholecystitis. A number of contraindications have been proposed in the evaluation of a candidate for LC. These contraindications were, at the beginning, formal and absolute; although when the surgeon gains experience and confidence with more sophisticated equipment, some authors have believed the importance of evaluating «What are the contraindications for LC?» (27). At present, LC is applicable over 95% of cases including patients with previous upper abdominal surgery (27), acute cholecystitis (9, 27-33), morbid obesity (34, 35), *situs inversus* (36), pregnancy (37, 38), pediatric patients (39, 40), liver cirrhosis (41, 42), porcelain gallbladder (43), and common bile duct stones (44-46).

It is much better for a surgeon to consider an absolute contraindication when the structures in the triangle of Cabot cannot be identified, than to continue with the operation with no clear anatomy and, to cause a nonrepairable injury. In summary, the obscured anatomy due to bleeding, inflammation or any other circumstances, should be an indication for conversion to conventional surgery.

Another important contraindication is the carcinoma of the gallbladder. In the laparoscopy procedure, the port sites can also be contaminated by exfoliated tumor cells during the laparoscopic resection. This unacceptable complication has already been reported after laparoscopy (47). It is not known what factors may contribute to this possible neoplastic contamination, but several mechanisms have been proposed, such as exfoliation induced by tumor manipulation or local ischemia at the ports. We are very careful to avoid touching the tumor during resection and this is the reason indicating conversion to open surgery in suspected cases of gallbladder carcinoma.

Indications and Utility of Cholangiography during LC

Many surgeons, indeed before the introduction of laparoscopic techniques, considered intraoperative cholangiography (IOC) to be an essential component of LC to reduce the risk of injury and to recognize the injury if it occurs (48). However, the potential disadvantages of routine IOC include increased operating time and false-positive findings leading to unnecessary efforts to clear the common duct stones (49). In a recent paper about the controversy regarding the need for IOC, they conclude that the routine use of IOC is strongly advocated (50). It is our policy to perform IOC in all patients undergoing LC. The value of routine cholangiography is not only to determine the presence of common bile duct stones but also to provide a «road map» of the ductal anatomy (51). In a recent review of the last 100 subsequent LC cases operated on in the Department of Surgery of our hospital, the cystic duct was canulated in 98 patients. Technical reasons for failed laparoscopic cholangiography were two cases with a small and scarred cystic duct. The author advocates routine cholangiography during LC because the benefits are clarification of anatomy, detection of common bile duct stones and experience when the cholangiogram is needed and essential.

Endoscopic and Laparoscopic Management of Common Bile Duct Stones

The optimal approach to patients with suspected choledocholithiasis undergoing LC remains uncertain (52). On the other hand, the use of ERCP has experienced a high rate of negative findings with the subsequent morbidity or even mortality (53). In the laparoscopic era the management of cholelithiasis and suspected choledocholithiasis is in accordance with the evolution of this new technique and the local expertise of the surgeons and endoscopists. In the conventional surgery era the ERCP and possible endoscopic sphincterotomy (EE) were restricted to patients with cholangitis, pancreatitis or high-risk patients. The evolution and revolution of the laparoscopic techniques have provided other alternatives to the conventional management.

At the beginning of the use of LC all surgeons recommend ERCP in every patient with some suspition of choledocholithiasis. However, in a recently published SAGES opinion survey with 447 respondents, ERCP was performed in 5.5% of LC patients (54). The management of common bile duct stones is in relation to the clinical state of the patient and, the time of the diagnosis. We believe that preoperative ERCP and EE should be indicated in elderly patients or patients with cholangitis or severe jaundice. The treatment and management could be different if the diagnosis of common bile duct stones is performed preoperatively, during the operation or postoperatively.

The incidence of unsuspected duct stones is 4-5 percent when operative cholangiograms are obtained in every operation. On the other hand, operative cholangiograms are falsely positive in 2 to 4% of patients. When a common bile duct stone is encountered at cholangiography, two options are available to the surgeon: delayed or immediate management. Delayed treatment includes observation in the follow-up period or postoperative ERCP. Immediate management includes common bile duct exploration by laparoscopic or conventional approach (55). In the past, if a common duct stone was suspected or identified during open procedures, the common bile duct was explored. Based on this axiom, the author does not find any reason to change the policy of treatment of ductal calculi in the laparoscopic era. In conclusion, if the IOC detects duct stones we try to apply two techniques for the laparoscopic clearance: the indirect approach through the cystic duct (56) or the direct approach by laparoscopic choledochotomy (57). If neither of these techniques is feasible, the surgeon converts to open common bile duct exploration. We do not recommend the adoption of new techniques such as ERCP + EE performed during the operation (58) or electrohydraulic lithotripsy (59). Patients with suspected and unsuspected common duct stones will not be left to the postoperative period to be removed with ERCP.

A different clinical situation is when ductal calculi are suspected preoperatively. The optimal management is still controversial. Several studies have addressed this problem, but no controlled trials have been published. Although some authors have reported great success with either preoperative or postoperative ERCP for the treatment of common duct stones (59-61), many of these accomplished endoscopists agreed that a single-stage treatment of biliary lithiasis, seems to be the ultimate goal as an interventional approach to this disease process (57). The laparoscopic techniques to clear the common bile duct have been described, but most are technically difficult and expertise related (45, 62-64). In contrast, endoscopic treatment of ductal calculi has been established and is well-known but this procedure is associated with some morbidity and mortality (53). The laparoscopic management of common duct stones should depend on the surgeon's skill (65). However, the advantages of single or double approaches has yet to be proven, since it is likely that a bias existed when selecting patients included in those uncontrolled series. Furthermore, some concern exists about the accuracy of the laparoscopic surgery in the management of common bile duct stones. In order to answer all these questions Cuschieri and the European Society of Endoscopic Surgeons have designed a prospective randomized multi-institutional trial comparing single stage laparoscopic management versus management of endoscopic stone extraction followed by LC, of which we are a collaborating group.

REFERENCES

1. Langenbuch C. Ein fall von extirpation der gallenblase wegen chronischer cholelitiasis. Heilung Berl Klin Wchnschr 1882; 19:725-727.
2. Ligoury C, Vitale G. Biliary perestroika. Am J Surg 1990; 160:237-238.
3. Dubois F, Berthelot G, Levard H. Cholecystectomy par celioscopie. Presse Med 1989; 18:980-982.
4. Reddick EJ, Olsen DO. Laparoscopic laser cholecystectomy. A comparison with mini-lap cholecystectomy. Surg Endosc 1989; 3 (3):131-133.
5. The Southern Surgeons Club. A prospective analysis of 1518 laparoscopic cholecystectomies. N Engl J Med 1991; 324:1073-1078.
6. NIH. Consensus conference stament on gallstones and laparoscopic cholecystectomy. Am J Surg 1993; 165:390-398.
7. Berci G, Sackier JM. Los Angeles experience with laparoscopic cholecystectomy. Am J Surg 1991; 213:3-12.
8. Cuschieri A, Dubois F, Mouiel J et al. The European experience with laparoscopic cholecystectomy. Am J Surg 1991; 161:385-387.
9. Flowers JL, Bailey RW, Scovill WA, Zucker KA. Laparoscopic management of acute cholecystitis: the Baltimore experience with laparoscopic management of acute cholecystitis. Am J Surg 1991; 161:388-392.
10. Arregui M, Davis C, Arkush A, Nagan R. In selected patients outpatient laparoscopic cholecystectomy is safe and significantly reduces hospitalization charges. Surg Laparosc Endosc 1991; 1:240-245.
11. Peters J, Ellison E, Innes J et al. Safety and efficacy of laparoscopic cholecystectomy. Ann Surg 1991; 213:3-12.
12. Greene F. Minimal access surgery and the «golden period» for conversion. Surg Endosc 1995; 9:11.
13. Vincent-Hamelin E, Pallarés A, Felipe J et al. National survey on laparoscopic cholecystectomy in Spain. Surg Endosc 1994; 770-776.
14. Fink A. Laparoscopic cholecystectomy: do preoperative factors predict the need to convert to open. (Invited commentary.) Surg Endosc 1994; 8:879-880.
15. Hunter J. Avoidance of bile duct injury during laparoscopic cholecystectomy. Am J Surg 1991; 162:71-76.
16. Gadacz T, Talamini M. Traditional versus laparoscopic cholecystectomy. Am J Surg 1991; 161:404-407.
17. Rossi R, Schirmer W, Braasch J et al. Laparoscopic bile duct injuries: risk factors, recognition, and repair. Arch Surg 1992.
18. Deziel D, Millikan K, Economou S, Doolas A, Ko S, Airan M. Complications of laparoscopic cholecystectomy: a national survey of 4, 292 hospitals and analysis of 77, 604 cases. Am J Surg 1993; 165:9-14.
19. Airan M, Appel M, Berci G et al. Retrospective and prospective multi-institutional laparoscopic cholecystectomy study organized by the Society of American Gastrointestinal Endoscopic Surgeons. Surg Endosc 1992; 6:169-176.
20. Steiner C, Bass E, Mark E, Talamini M, Pitt H, Steinberg E. Surgical rates and operative mortality for open and laparoscopic cholecystectomy in Maryland. N Engl J Med 1994; 330:403-408.
21. Barkun J, Barkun A, Sampalis J et al. Randomised controlled trial of laparoscopic versus mini cholecystectomy. Lancet 1992; 340:1116-1119.
22. Nathanson LK, Easter D, Cushieri A. Ligation of the cystic duct pedicle during laparoscopic cholecystectomy. Am J Surg 1991; 161:350-354.
23. Woods M, Shellito J, Santoscoy G et al. Cystic duct leaks in laparoscopic cholecystectomy. Am J Surg 1994; 168:560-565.
24. Davidof A, Pappas T, Murray E et al. Mechanism of major injury during laparoscopic cholecystectomy. Ann Surg 1992; 215:196-202.
25. Moossa AR, Easter DW, Van SE, Casola G, D'Agostino H. Laparoscopic injuries to the bile duct. A cause for concern. Ann Surg 1992; 215 (3):203-208.
26. Davis P, Ringers J, Rauws E. Bile duct injury after laparoscopic cholecystectomy: The value of endoscopic retrograde cholangiopancreatography. Gut 1993; 34:1255-1260.
27. Fraze R, Roberts J, Symmonds R et al. What are the contraindications for laparoscopic cholecystectomy? Am J Surg 1992; 164:491-495.
28. Cooperman AM. Laparoscopic cholecystectomy for severe acute, embedded and gangrenous cholecystitis. J Laparosc Surg 1990; 1:37-40.
29. Jacobs M, Verdeja J, Goldstein H. Laparoscopic cholecystectomy in acute cholecystitis. J Laparoendosc Surg 1991; 1:175-177.
30. Reddick R, Olsen D, Spaw A et al Safe performance of difficult laparoscopic cholecystectomies. Am J Surg 1991; 161:377-381.
31. Wilson RG, Macintyre IMC, King PM, Nixon SJ, Saunders JH, Varma JS. Laparoscopic cholecystectomy: a safe and effective treatment for severe acute cholecystitis. Br Med J 1992; 305:394-396.
32. Franklin MJ, Vancaillie TG, Daniel C. Is laparoscopic cholecystectomy applicable to patients with acute cholecystitis? J Laparoendosc Surg 1992; 2(3):159-163.
33. Zucker K, Flowers J, Bailey R, Graham S, Buell J, Imbembo A. Laparoscopic management of acute cholecystitis. Am J Surg 1993; 165:508-514.
34. Collet D, Edye M, Magne E, Perissat J. Laparoscopic cholecystectomy in the obese patient. Surg Endosc 1992; 6:186-188.

35. Schrimer B, Dix J, Edge S, Hyser M, Hanks J, Aguilar M. Laparoscopic cholecystectomy in the obese patient. Ann Surg 1992; 216:146-152.
36. Huang S, Chau G, Lui W. Laparoscopic cholecystectomy for colelithiasis in a patient with *situs inversus totalis*. Surg Endosc 1992; 24:802-803.
37. Hart R, Tamadon A, Fitzgibons R, Fleming A. Open laparoscopis cholecystectomy in pregnancy. Surg Laparosc Endosc 1993; 3(1):13-16.
38. Edelman D. Alternative laparoscopic technique for cholecystectomy during pregnancy. Surg Endosc 1994; 8:794-796.
39. Stigmann H, Laberge J, Croitoru D et al. Laparoscopic cholecystectomy: atreatment option for gallbladder disease in children. J Pediatr Surg 1991; 26:1181-1183.
40. Davidof A, Branum G, Murray E et al. The technique of laparoscopic cholecystectomy in children. Ann Surg 1992; 215:186-191.
41. Yerdel M, Tsuge H, Mimura H, Sakagami K, Mori M, Orita K. Laparoscopic cholecystectomy in cirrhotic patients: expandin indications. Surg Laparosc Endosc 1993; 3:180-183.
42. Lacy A, Balaguer C, Andrade E et al. Laparoscopic cholecystectomy in cirrhotic patients: Is an indication or contraindication? Surg Endosc 1995 (in press).
43. Welch N, Fitzgibbons R, Hinder R. Beware of the porcelain gallbladder during laparoscopic cholecystectomy. Surg Endosc 1991; 1:202-205.
44. Stoker ME, Leveillee RJ, McCann JCJ, Maini BS. Laparoscopic common bile duct exploration. J Laparosc Surg 1991; 1:287-293.
45. Phillips E, Carroll B, Pearlstein A, Dayshovsky L, Fallas M. Laparoscopic choledochoscopy and extraction of common duct stones. Wordl J Surg 1993; 17:22-28.
46. Voyles C, Sanders D, Hogan R. Common bile duct evaluation in the era of laparoscopic cholecystectomy. 1,050 cases later. World J Surg 1994; 219:744-752.
47. Pezet D, Fondrinier E, Rotman N. Parietal seeding of carcinoma of the gallbladder after laparoscopic cholecystectomy. Br J Surg 1992; 79:230.
48. Adams D, Borowicz M, Wooton F, Cunningham J. Bile duct complications after laparoscopic cholecystectomy. Surg Endosc 1993; 7:79-83.
49. Barkun J, Fried G, Barkun A et al. Cholecystectomy without operative cholangiography. Implications for common bile dict injury and retained common bile duct stones. Ann Surg 1993; 218:371-379.
50. Cuschieri A, Shimi S, Banting S, Nathanson L, Pietrabissa A. Intraoperative cholangiography during laparoscopic cholecystectomy. Poutine vs. selective policy. Surg Endosc 1994; 8:302-305.
51. Zucker K, Bayley R. Laparoscopic management of acute cholecystitis. In: Zucker K, ed. Surgical Laparoscopy Update. Saint Louis: Quality Medical, 1993; 109-143.
52. McEntee G, Grace P, Bouchier-Hayes D. Laparoscopic cholecystectomy and the common bile duct. Br J Surg 1991; 78:385-386.
53. Neoptolemos JP, Carr-Locke DL, Fossard DP. Prospective randomized study of peroperative endoscopy sphincterotomy versus surgery alone for common duct stones. Br Med J 1987; 294:470-474.
54. Brodish R, Fink A. ERCP, cholangiography, and laparoscopic cholecystectomy. Surg Endosc 1993; 7 (3-8).
55. Petelin J. Laparoscopic approach to common duct pathology. Surg Laparosc Endosc 1991; 1:33-41.
56. Hunter JG. Laparoscopic transcystic common bile duct exploration. Am J Surg 1992; 163:53-56.
57. Petelin J. Laparoscopic approach to common duct pathology. Am J Surg 1993; 165:487-491.
58. De Paula A. Sphincterotomie transcystique. In: Mouiel J, ed. Actualites Digestives Medicochirurgicales, serie 16. Paris: Masson, 1995 (in press).
59. Arregui M, Davis C, Arkush A, Nagan R. Laparoscopic cholecystectomy combined with endoscopic esfinterotomy and stone extraction or laparoscopic choledochoscopy and electrohydraulic lithotripsy for management of cholelithiasis with choledocholithiasis. Surg Endosc 1992; 6:10-15.
60. Cotton P. Endoscopic management of bile duct stones (apples and oranges). Gut 1984; 25:587-597.
61. Carr-Locke D. Acute gallstone pancreatitis and endoscopic therapy. Endoscopy 1990; 22:180-183.
62. Shapiro S, Grundest W. Laparoscopic exploration of the common bile duct: experience in 16 selected patients. J Laparosc Endosc 1991; 1:333-341.
63. Sackier JM, Berci G, Paz-Partlow M. Laparoscopic transcystic choledocholithotomy as an adjunt to laparoscopic cholecystectomy. Am J Surg 1991; 57:323-326.
64. Carroll BJ, Phillips EH, Daykhovsky Lea. Laparoscopic choledochoscopy: an effective approach to the common duct. J Laparosc Surg 1992; 2:15-21.
65. Berci G, Morgenstern L. Laparoscopic management of common bile duct stones. A multi-institutional SAGES study. Surg Endosc 1994; 8:1168-1175.

Endoscopic Treatment of Biliary Disease

D. L. Carr-Locke

CHOLEDOCHOLITHIASIS

Endoscopic treatment of choledocholithiasis has gained widespread acceptance since the first independent reports of endoscopic sphincterotomy (ES) by Kawai (1) and Classen in 1974 (2). Endoscopic sphincterotomy was initially considered justifiable only in elderly post-cholecystectomy patients with recurrent or retained common bile duct (CBD) stones who were at high risk of serious complications from conventional surgical CBD exploration. With improved efficacy, demand, and training in therapeutic biliary endoscopic techniques, however, there has been an expanding role for the endoscopic management of choledocholithiasis. Endoscopic removal of CBD stones is preferable to surgery: *a*) in patients who have undergone previous cholecystectomy, *b*) in the high-risk surgical patient when the gallbladder is still present, *c*) in patients with severe acute cholangitis, *d*) in selected patients with acute biliary pancreatitis, and *e*) in special circumstances for the average risk surgical patient with suspected choledocholithiasis prior to laparoscopic cholecystectomy.

Endoscopic Sphincterotomy and Stone Extraction

Once choledocholithiasis has been documented, sphincterotomy (ES) is usually required to facilitate stone removal (fig. 1). For small stones, however, it may be possible to perform extraction with a basket through the intact papilla without the need for initial ES (fig. 2). In experienced hands, access to the bile duct can be achieved in more than 95% of patients with the aid of a variety of accessory cannulas, papillotomes and guidewires (4, 5). In the 5% or less where selective cannulation fails, access to the CBD can often be obtained with the use of a precut papillotomy (6) or, rarely, combined percutaneous endoscopic techniques (7).

Many stones, particularly those under 1 cm diameter, will pass spontaneously after stan-

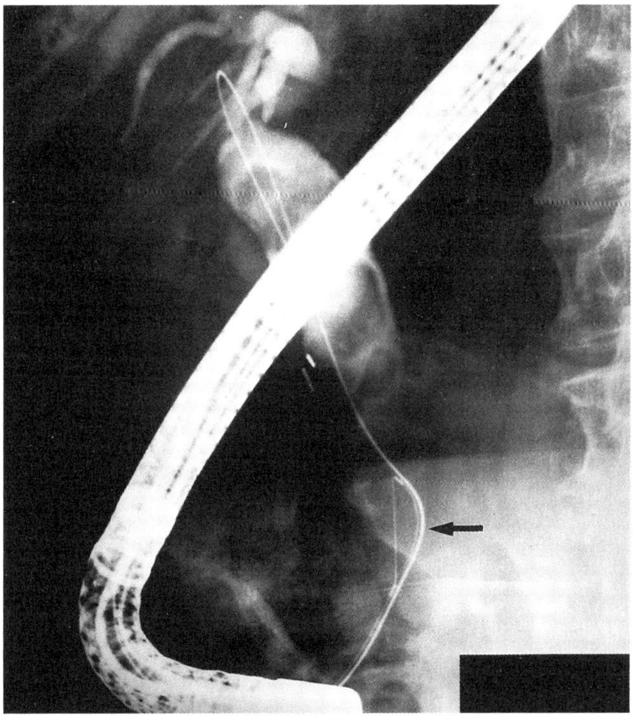

Fig. 1. Endoscopic sphincterotomy with a papillotome (arrow). Multiple large calculi are seen in an enlarged bile duct.

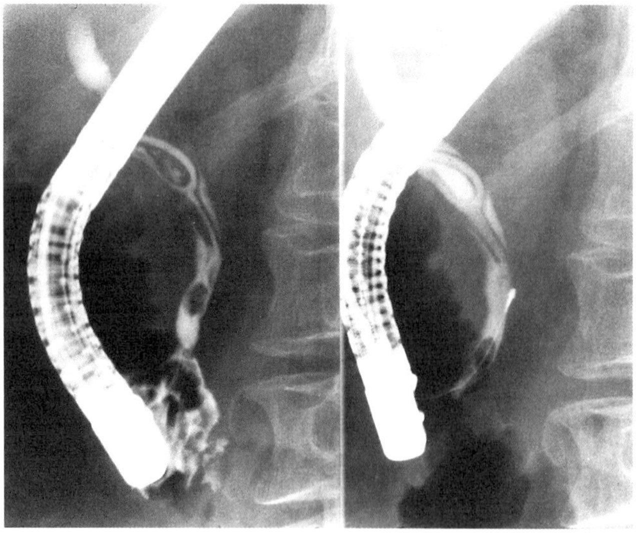

Fig. 2. Large stone in the distal end of the common bile duct (left). The stone is trapped with a basket (right).

dard ES (8-10). Nevertheless, most experts will attempt stone extraction from the CBD immediately following ES as this will reduce the incidence of retained stones and complications. A Dormia-type basket is a popular device for entrapping and removing stones (fig. 3). Care and good judgement must be utilized to avoid impaling the basket wires into the stone surface as this can result in basket impaction. Stone extraction can alternatively be accomplished with a balloon catheter which avoids the possibility of instrumental impaction. The balloon is particularly useful in individuals with small diameter common bile ducts or when multiple stones are present. Overall duct clearance can be expected in 90 to 95% of those undergoing successful sphincterotomy, resulting in an overall therapeutic success rate of endoscopic stone clearance approximating 80-95%, with the highest success rates noted as experience increases (11-16). Patients are usually hospitalized overnight for routine observation and discharged the following day if complications are not encountered although there is an increasing trend towards outpatient management.

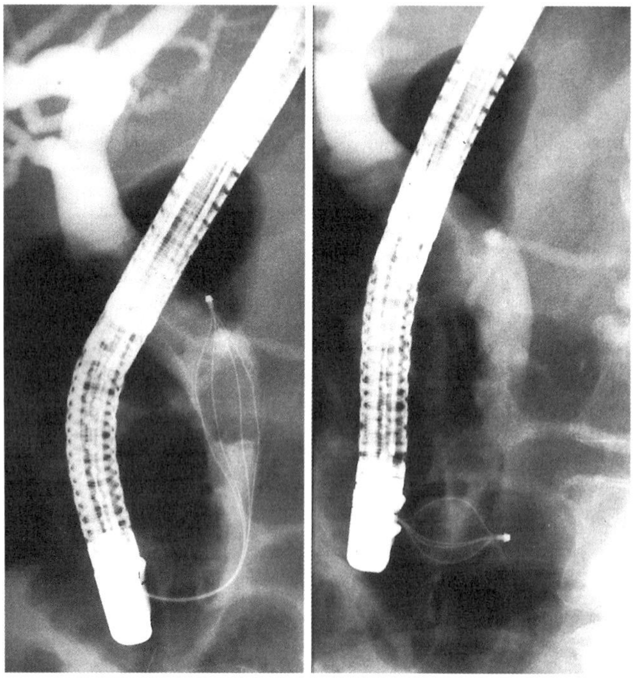

Fig. 3. Removal of a large stone using a Dormia-type basket.

Complications

Early complications encountered with ES of 8 to 10% are remarkably similar among various centers despite great differences in procedure indications and patient selection. The major complications include hemorrhage in 2-3%, acute pancreatitis in 1-6%, cholangitis in 1-3%, and retroduodenal perforation in less than 1% (11, 14, 16-35). The overall mortality from the procedure approximates 0.5 to 1.0% (11, 14, 16-18) with a 30-day mortality of 3 to 16% (15, 18, 20) that is a reflection of the severity of underlying illness at the time of the procedure. There has been debate concerning an increased complication rate in patients with small diameter bile ducts and, curiously, the morbidity of ES in pre-laparoscopic cholecystectomy patients seems less than other populations.

Long-term complications from follow-up studies for up to 11 years after sphincterotomy have documented a 10-15% incidence of subsequent biliary complications (36, 37) such as recurrent stones, sphincter stenosis, and cholangitis. This compares favorably to surgical common bile duct exploration and drainage procedures (38, 39). The majority of these can be managed through additional endoscopic therapy.

Difficult Bile Duct Stones

The most difficult circumstances encountered during endoscopic stone removal are the re-

Table 1. Difficult Bile Duct Stones

Stones greater than 20 mm
Intrahepatic stones
Multiple stones
Impacted stones
Stone proximal to a biliary stricture
Tortuous bile duct
Disproportionate size of the bile duct-stone
Duodenal diverticulum
Billroth II reconstruction
Surgical duodenotomy

sult of technical difficulties with achieving deep biliary cannulation or performing ES sometimes due to inaccessibility of the papilla and related to aberrant anatomy or unfavorable duodenal or papillary structures such as a periampullary diverticulum, or prior surgery such as a Billroth II or Roux-en-Y reconstruction. Adjuvant techniques include needle-knife sphincterotomy with either a stent or nasobiliary drain used as a guide for cutting (40) or use of specially designed reverse direction accessories.

Once ES is successfully performed a variety of factors may hinder stone extraction including a disproportionately narrow lower bile duct segment, a large stone of greater than 15mm, intrahepatic stones, a stone located proximal to a stricture, or a large number of stones (table 1). Stone consistency and shape may also adversely influence extraction success. Additional techniques that have been developed to reduce stone size prior to endoscopic removal include mechanical lithotripsy (fig. 4) (41-45), intracorporeal lithotripsy with laser (46-49) or electrohydraulic probes (51-54), extracorporeal shock wave lithotripsy (ESWL) (56-59) and chemical dissolution (60-66). These techniques allow removal of 80 to 94% of difficult bile duct stones which are refractory to standard extraction techniques.

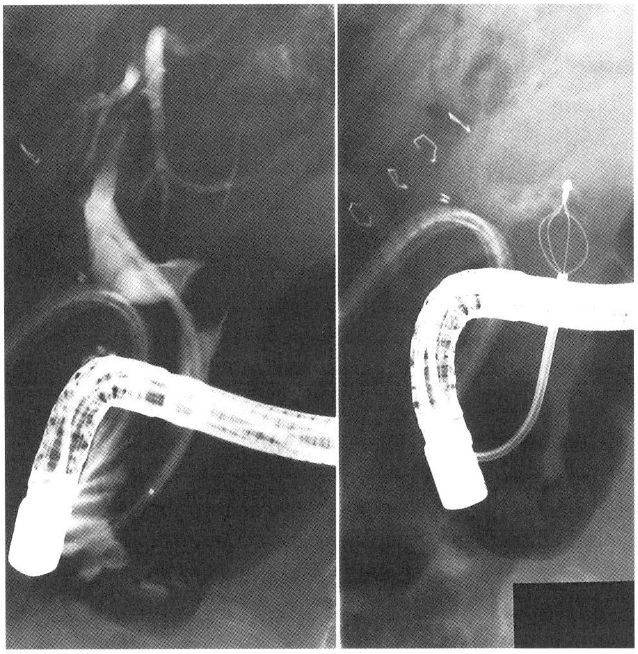

Fig. 4. Mechanical lithotripsy to remove a large stone from the common bile duct.

Nasobiliary Tube and Biliary Endoprosthesis

In the 5% or less of situations where stone extraction is incomplete or impossible a nasobiliary tube (fig. 5) (67) should be inserted to provide biliary decompression and prevent stone impaction in the distal CBD. This serves as a temporizing therapy allowing for improvement

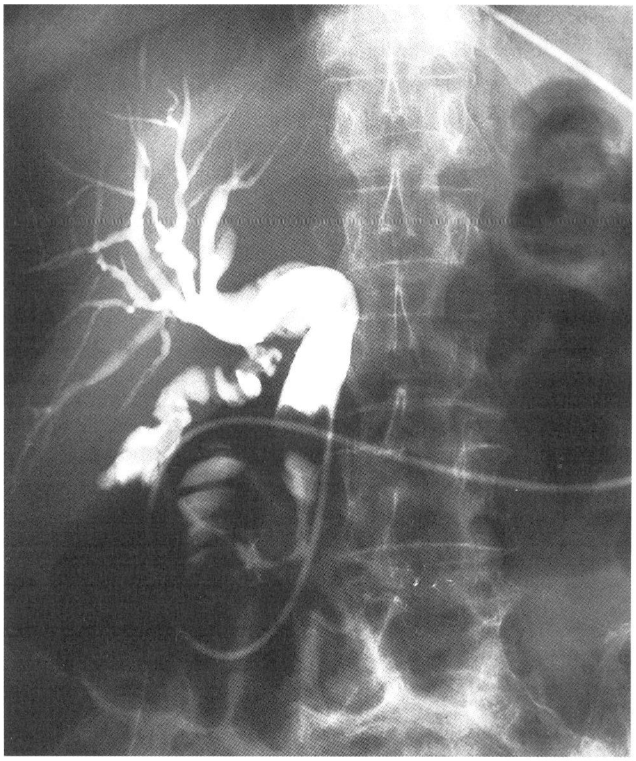

Fig. 5. Large calculus in the distal end of the common bile duct. A nasobiliary tube is left in place to decompress the biliary tract.

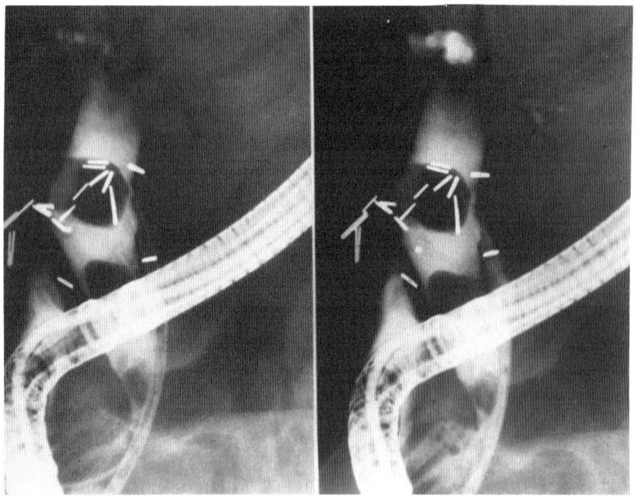

Fig. 6. Biliary endoprosthesis in a common bile duct with several large calculi.

in the patient's clinical condition until complete stone clearance is achieved either via additional endoscopic maneuvers or subsequent surgery. This is of major importance in biliary ductal obstruction where incomplete duct clearance and poor biliary drainage can lead to the development of cholangitis. The alternative therapy of temporary biliary endoprosthesis placement (fig. 6) has become popular (68, 69). In the poor surgical risk patient, an acceptable non-surgical alternative is ES and long-term placement of a biliary endoprosthesis (70-73). Stent patency is not of major clinical importance in this situation, as the sphincterotomy typically provides an adequate conduit for bile flow around the prosthesis which serves principally to prevent stone impaction (71-74).

Post-Cholecystectomy with T-Tube *in Situ*

Bile duct stones detected on T-tube cholangiography of less than 10 mm diameter may pass spontaneously or with hydrostatic pressure from flushing or perfusing the T-tube. However, the majority of these stones will require additional mechanical manipulation. Increased morbidity and mortality with secondary bile duct explorations has stimulated the development of alternative techniques including hydraulic T-tube irrigation with or without pharmacologic relaxation of the sphincter of Oddi with glucagon or nitrates (75), T-tube infusion of cholesterol solvents (75), T-tube tract choledochosopy and lithotripsy (76) or percutaneous extraction of stones through a mature T-tube track (75, 77-80). Alternatively, early endoscopic removal (fig. 2) can be safely and effectively applied after stone detection without the need for T-tube maturation allowing timely discharge from hospital. The results from 8 endoscopic series totalling 337 patients indicates an overall endoscopic success rate of 90% with a morbidity of 7% and mortality of 0.6% (80-87). The choice between these two techniques of similar efficacy and safety depends upon local expertise, as direct comparisons have not been made in controlled trials.

Pregnancy

Symptomatic choledocholithiasis during pregnancy poses a diagnostic and therapeutic challenge. Endoscopic treatment can be performed provided certain precautions are taken to minimize fetal exposure to radiation (88-90). During endoscopic retrograde cholangiopancreatography (ERCP), the fetus is shielded with an abdominal lead apron, no radiographs are taken, and dosimetry should be performed to estimate the amount of radiation exposure to the fetus. These patients should undergo elective cholecystectomy upon completion of pregnancy to prevent recurrence.

Post-Cholecystectomy without T-Tube

The incidence of retained common bile duct stones remains at approximately 2-5% following conventional and laparoscopic cholecystectomy with an incidence as high as 5-15% following common duct exploration (91). Endoscopic sphincterotomy remains the treatment of choice for the elderly patient presenting days to years after cholecystectomy (92) as these individuals are at high risk for further abdominal surgery (93, 94). ES is also recommended in the young, fit post-cholecystectomy individual. Long-term follow up will be necessary in this group of individuals as the post-ES follow-up data largely reflect results of endoscopic procedures performed in elderly patients although there is no compelling reason to suspect that the results will differ.

Selected Patients with Gallbladder *in Situ*

In the elderly, a deliberate decision is often made to leave the gallbladder in situ following ES and CBD stone removal (fig. 7). The short and long-term results and complications of ES in patients with a gallbladder do not differ from those in the post-cholecystectomy patient. These patients, in view of their shorter life expectancy, can be managed expectantly unless symptoms dictate otherwise. Careful follow-up for 5 to 10 years in these patients with intact gallbladders indicates that approximately 10% will develop gallbladder symptoms or complications sufficient to warrant cholecystectomy, the majority of which occur in the first year (95-100). This risk for developing gallbladder symptoms is similar to that of patients with asymptomatic cholelithiasis (101). Non-filling of the gallbladder with radiographic contrast at ERCP (102) or with radiotracer by nuclear scintigraphy (103) may confer a higher likelihood for developing symptoms, although results from other series do not concur (95, 98). These results suggest that the low risk of subsequent gallbladder complications after ES and bile duct clearance, when patients are kept under supervision, outweighs the known higher mortality for cholecystectomy in the elderly and militates against routine cholecystectomy in this group. Few physicians would recommend this approach in the fit patient under age 60 where the expectation for long-term survival and therefore development of symptoms necessitating cholecystectomy is great. The risk of elective cholecystectomy is probably smaller than the risk of subsequently developing gallbladder symptoms in this group and therefore elective cholecystectomy would seem most appropriate in this group.

The place of preoperative ES in young, good surgical risk patients with suspected choledocholithiasis has been examined in two prospective, randomized controlled trials (104, 105) with the conclusion that no advantage is conferred by initial endoscopic bile duct clearance prior to cholecystectomy. High risk surgical patients were excluded from these studies and both were conducted in the era of open cholecystectomy.

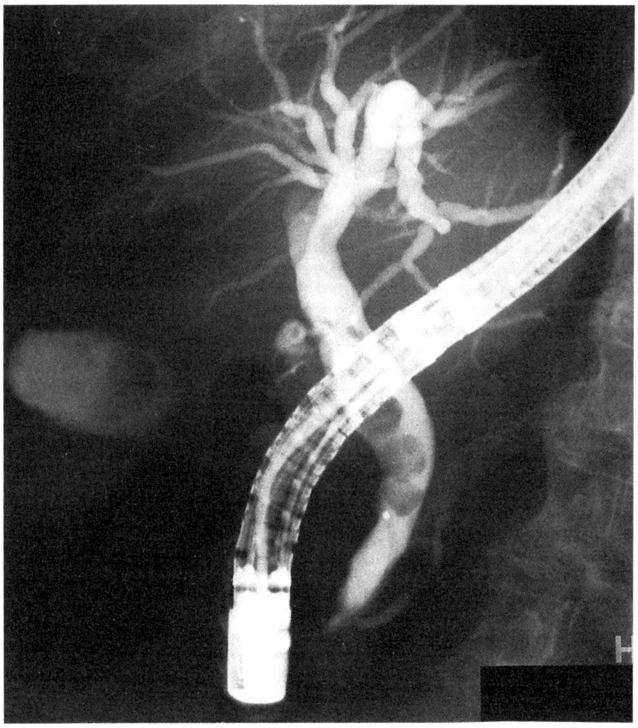

Fig. 7. Endoscopic stone removal after sphincterotomy.

Laparoscopic Cholecystectomy

Laparoscopic cholecystectomy has now replaced open cholecystectomy as the procedure of choice for gallbladder removal in the vast majority of individuals with symptomatic cholelithiasis (106, 107). Optimal management of patients with suspected common bile duct stones has yet to be determined in those undergoing laparoscopic cholecystectomy. The approach to CBD stones in the laparoscopic cholecystectomy patient is quite varied with an expanding array of available treatment options as improvements occur in endoscopic, surgical, and percutaneous procedures. Laparoscopic transcystic cholangiography (108, 109) and choledochoscopy with stone extraction (110) can be performed at the time of laparoscopic cholecystectomy but is not yet practiced widely. A need for endoscopic management has evolved, with ERCP playing a central role in pre-operative and post-operative CBD stone detection and removal.

We and others (111) have found it useful to stratify patients pre-operatively into low, intermediate, and high likelihood for CBD stones

Table 2. Cholangiography stratification for «risk» of choledocholithiasis

High likelihood = pre-operative ERC
Bilirubin > 2 mg%
Alkaline phosphatase > 150 U/l
Presence/recent history of jaundice/pancreatitis
Dilated CBD/stone on sonography
Intermediate likelihood = IOC
Bilirubin 1.5-2.0 mg%
Alkaline phosphatase 110-150 U/l
Transaminases > 2 × Normal
Remote jaundice/pancreatitis
Low likelihood = No ERC/IOC
Normal liver function tests
No ductal dilatation
No jaundice/pancreatitis

ERC: endoscopic retrograde cholangiography; IOC, intraoperative cholangiograpy.

(table 2) based on established clinical and biochemical indicators (112-114). In the absence of clinical or biochemical indicators («low likelihood» category), CBD stones will be present in only 2-3% of individuals, a yield which would likely be offset by the risks of the ERCP itself (115). Small asymptomatic stones may be of minor clinical relevance as their natural history is not known and conceivably many, if not most, of these calculi would pass spontaneously without ever coming to clinical attention. To date, we have favored selective cholangiography for patients with risk factors for choledocholithiasis. Our approach is summarized in figure 8 (115-121) and our experience in our first prospective series of 750 consecutive laparoscopic cholecystectomies is summarized in table 3.

Gallstone Pancreatitis

Acute pancreatitis due to impaction of gallstones in the ampulla of Vater was first reported by Opie in 1901 (122). From this observation derived the «obstructive theory» to explain the mechanisms responsible for gallstone pancreatitis. Stone impaction in the common channel of the pancreatic and common bile duct is postulated to result in obstruction of the two systems and resultant reflux of bile into the pancreatic duct (123). In support of the (transient) obstructive theory, gallstones can be recovered from the feces of 85-95% of patients (124, 125), and the incidence of common bile duct stones is as high as 80% in those undergoing urgent operative or endoscopic intervention compared to a 5-30% incidence when the procedure is delayed (125-127). There are now well-established criteria for assessing severity of pancreatitis (128). The use of early surgical therapy in cases of acute gallstone pancreatitis has been challenged due to the high operative morbidity and mortality (129-132). An endoscopic approach to gallstone pancreatitis offers the theoretical advantage of immediate relief of ampullary obs-

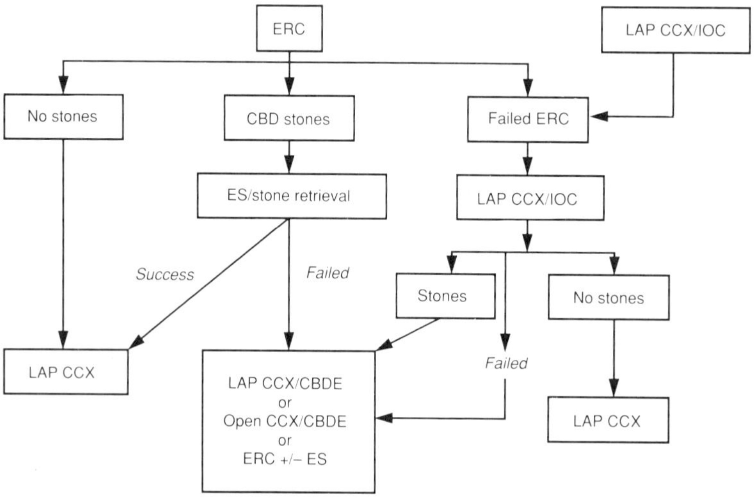

Fig. 8. Approach to patients with symptomatic gallstone disease. ERC: endoscopic retrograde cholangiography; CBD: common bile duct; LAP CCX: laparoscopic cholecystectomy; ES: sphinterectomy.

Table 3. ERCP in 750 laparoscopic cholecystectomies at Brigham & Women's Hospital (1990-1992)

Pre-operative ERCP	36	(4.8%)
Normal	23	(64%)
Stones	9	(25%)
Mirizzi's Syndrome	1	(2.8%)
Aberrant anatomy	2	(5.6%)
Failed ERC	1	(2.8%)
Intra-operative cholangiography	45	(6.0%)
Successful	39	(87%)
Stones	2	(5.1%)
Not attempted	705	(94%)
Post-operative ERCP	26	(3.5%)
Stones	11	(42%)
Bile leak	7	(27%)
Ductal injury	2	(8%)
Papillary stenosis	3	(11.5%)
Normal	3	(11.5%)
Total ERCP involvement	62	(8.3%)

truction and ductal clearance without the risks of general anesthesia or the surgical procedure (133-135). Two randomized studies (136, 137) have demonstrated that ERCP and endoscopic stone extraction can be safely performed in the setting of acute biliary pancreatitis and that urgent ERCP and ES can be performed with good rationale in those patients with severe or progressive pancreatitis due to the resultant reduction in major local peri-pancreatic complications and the increasingly recognized coexistence of acute cholangitis potentially translating into a reduced mortality. The role of endoscopic sphincterotomy in lieu of cholecystectomy for the high risk patient with cholelithiasis or microlithiasis and gallstone pancreatitis in the absence of choledocholithiasis requires further evaluation (138-140).

Cholangitis

The most common cause of suppurative cholangitis is obstruction of the biliary system by a common bile duct stone leading to raised intrabiliary pressure and cholangiovenous reflux (141). The majority of patients with calculous cholangitis will present with mild disease and Charcot's triad. They typically respond rapidly to conservative therapy consisting of intravenous fluids and antibiotics. For these individuals further treatment should be based on their fitness for surgery. The poor risk surgical patient should undergo ES and stone extraction leaving the gallbladder *in situ*. The younger good operative risk patient should undergo definitive treatment with the option of either ES followed by laparoscopic cholecystectomy or conventional cholecystectomy and CBDE.

Reynolds and Dargan in 1959 described a particularly lethal form of acute suppurative cholangitis in which shock and mental confusion were additional clinical features (142). Emergency ERCP is the treatment of choice for these individuals with severe cholangitis at presentation, as well as those individuals not responding within 24 hours to conservative treatment. Emergency surgery should be reserved for those in whom endoscopic therapy fails, as conventional surgical treatment is associated with a morbidity and mortality of 10-50% depending upon the severity of illness and the presence of comorbid illnesses (143). Endoscopic decompression can be performed successfully in 85-95% of cases (figs. 4 and 5), with a lower morbidity and mortality compared to percutaneous transhepatic (144-146) or surgical drainage (147-153). In the only prospective, randomized, controlled trial published to date (153), the hospital mortality rate was significantly lower in the endoscopically treated group (10%) compared to those treated surgically (32%).

MANAGING COMPLICATIONS OF LAPAROSCOPIC CHOLECYSTECTOMY

The recent apparent increase in post-cholecystectomy bile duct injuries (154) has provided an increasing area for endoscopic intervention in the treatment of bile leaks, bile duct lacerations, ligations, transections and strictures. Retained bile duct stones and their consequences and other less common conditions, such as papillary stenosis, complete the range of potential post-operative interactions between endoscopist and surgeon.

Choledocholithiasis

For patients presenting from a few weeks to many years after cholecystectomy with bile duct stones, few would now question the use of endoscopic management techniques in preference to open bile duct exploration although this has never been formally compared. In the present era of evolving laparoscopic techniques, endoscopic methods are likely to be favored all the more as a minimally invasive approach (figs. 4 and 6). The successes, failures and complications of secondary bile duct operations are such that if endoscopic therapy can achieve the high success rates published by most established centers (155), this should be the treatment of first choice.

Biliary Strictures

The surgical management of post-operative biliary strictures is associated with a significant mortality and a requirement for repeated surgery in up to 35% of cases. A recent study (156) of attempted endoscopic stenting in 80 patients presenting with post-operative symptomatic biliary strictures (fig. 9), 46 patients had endoprostheses remaining after one year which were subsequently removed and further follow up obtained. Recurrent stricture was seen in eight patients requiring surgery in five and repeat endoscopic stenting in three. Two patients had extraction of recurrent gallstones. 13% of those 46 patients died of non-biliary related illness. The authors concluded that endoscopic stenting appears to be a viable alternative to a surgical approach in patients with post-operative benign biliary strictures but the surgical literature has taught us that very long term follow-up is needed before success can be claimed.

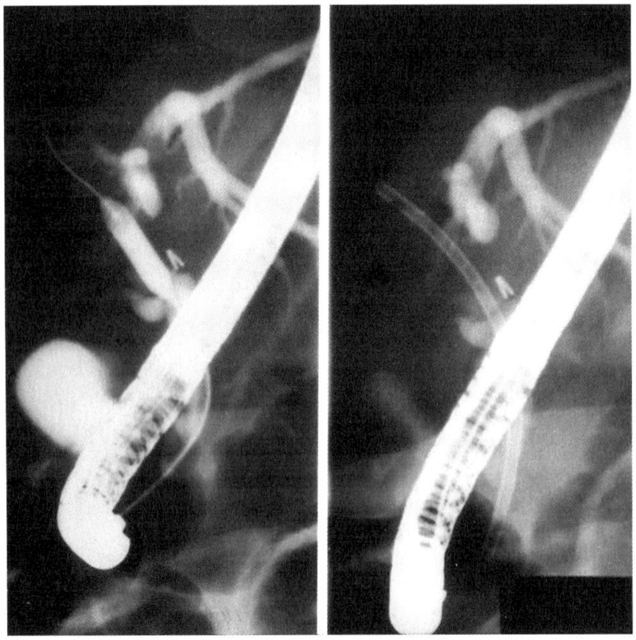

Fig. 9. Placement of a biliary endoprosthesis in a patient with a biliary stricture.

Bile Leak

Post-operative biliary leaks may occur by a variety of mechanisms including direct injury to bile duct system, dehiscence or «blowout» of the cystic stump, or disruption of a ductal anastomosis. Traditional treatment for persistent bile leaks has been reoperation. In the mid and late 1980s, reports on successful endoscopic treatment (fig. 10) of post-operative bile leaks appeared with decompression reported via endoscopic sphincterotomy alone, naso-biliary drainage or stent placement (157-164).

BENIGN BILIARY STRICTURE

The application of endoprostheses in benign strictures and sclerosing cholangitis has been limited to the short term and has often been combined with other endoscopic techniques such as sphincterotomy or balloon bilioplasty.

Post-Operative Biliary Strictures

See above.

Biliary Strictures and Chronic Pancreatitis

Common bile duct strictures may be seen in up to 27% of patients with chronic pancreatitis. Surgical decompression of symptomatic strictures is associated with a morbidity of approximately 25%. Deviere et al (165) recently reported endoscopic biliary stenting in 25 patients who presented with chronic pancreatitis and biliary stenosis with associated cholestasis. Whenever possible two stents were inserted. Patency of the prosthesis was evaluated by ultrasonography every three months, and blocked

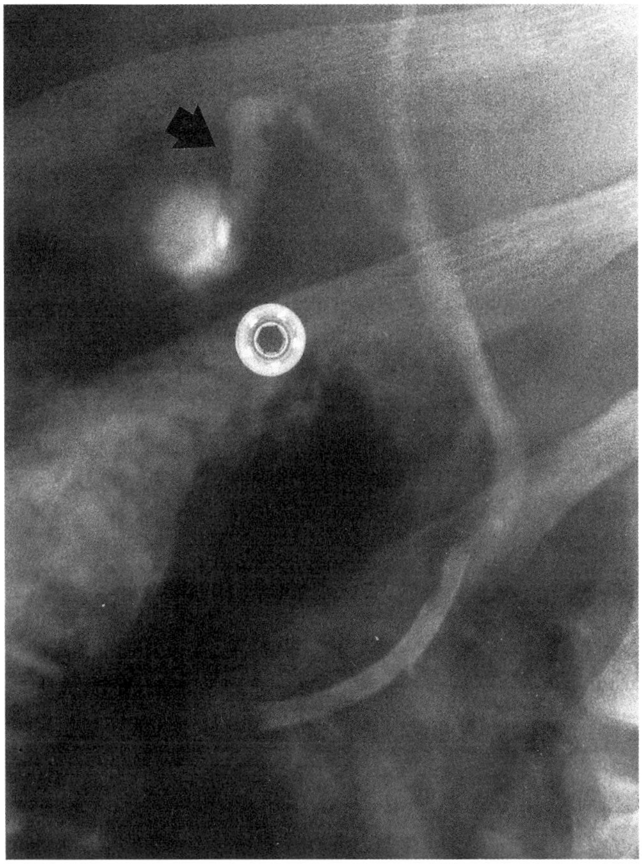

Fig. 10. Biliary endoprosthesis for the treatment of a bile leak (arrow).

stents were replaced endoscopically. There were no complications and cholestasis resolved in all cases. In follow up (mean 14 months), of the 25 patients that were initially treated, only three were able to have stents removed and remain asymptomatic, seven patients required surgery, ten patients had stents in place, two patients died and three were lost to follow up. Endoscopic stenting of common bile duct strictures in this patient population was very successful at treating the sequelae of cholangitis acutely, however, the long term follow up in this group was disappointing and the authors suggest reservation of this technique in this clinical scenario for temporizing measures only in patients who are not candidates for definitive surgical decompression. One potential role for endoscopic stenting in these patients is as a diagnostic test to determine whether or not chronic pain is originating from chronic pancreatitis or chronic biliary obstruction (166).

Sclerosing Cholangitis

Endoscopic intervention in sclerosing cholangitis, including endoscopic sphincterotomy, nasobiliary drainage, nasobiliary perfusion with antibiotics, saline and/or steroids, balloon dilatation of strictures and endoprosthesis placement, has been reported since 1983 (167-171). Johnson et al. (171) retrospectively evaluated 35 patients with primary sclerosing cholangitis and symptomatic dominant bile duct strictures that were treated endoscopically. Three patients died during the follow-up period, one of cholangiocarcinoma, one from ileal varices, and one of pneumonia and renal failure. One patient underwent successful liver transplantation. These authors demonstrate that endoscopic dilatation of dominant strictures in patients with primary sclerosing cholangitis results in clinical improvement as evaluated in this retrospective study, and argue that this form of therapy should precede a consideration for liver transplantation. They argue that stents are best avoided in this patient population as evidenced by a high incidence of procedure-related cholangitis. The impact of such interventions on overall prognosis is not clear but there does not seem to be any evidence that future considerations for liver transplantation are jeopardized. Given the low morbidity associated with endoscopic treatment of biliary strictures, it is a modality which should be considered as first line management and may, in some patients, be definitive (170-173).

MALIGNANT BILE DUCT STRICTURE

Once a decision has been made to provide palliation for malignant biliary obstruction, in the 80% or so of cases in whom this is possible without recourse to surgery, this should be achieved with minimum disturbance to the patient and with as good a quality of life as possible for the remaining weeks or months. The morbidity associated with endoscopic stent insertion varies from 0 to 36% (174-186) but major morbidity is probably well under 10%. Mortality within one month of the procedure is 10-18% and median survival is about six months (174-176). An endoscopic approach has been shown to be superior to surgical bypass (table 4)

Table 4. Randomized controlled trial of endoscopic *versus* surgical palliation in malignant biliary obstruction

	Endoscopy	Surgery
N	101	103
Success (%)	94	91
Complications (%)	10*	28
Procedure mortality (%)	4*	14
30 day mortality (%)	7*	17
Late jaundice (%)	18*	3
Duodenal obstruction (%)	6*	1
Hospital stay days	9*	13
Survival weeks	22*	26

* Statistically significant differences $p < 0.05$.
Data from reference 181 and P. B. Cotton (personal communication, 1992).

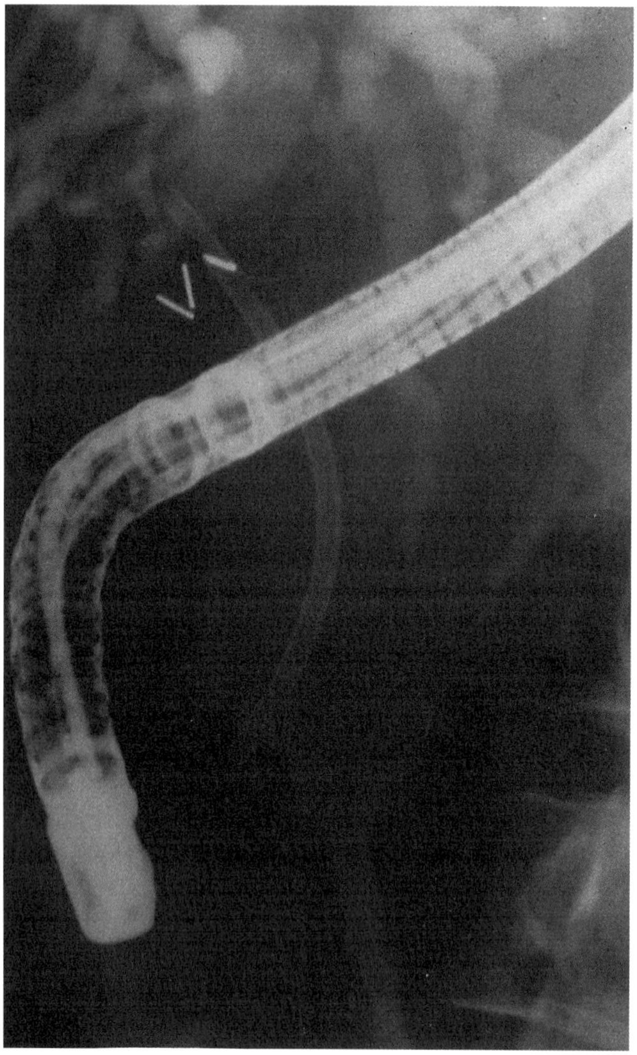

Fig. 11. Biliary endoprosthesis for the treatment of a malignant bile duct obstruction. Note the dilatation of intrahepatic bile ducts.

and percutaneous placement of endoprostheses (177, 178, 180, 181, 187).

Plastic Endoprostheses

The methodology and range of plastic endoprosthesis equipment currently available has been well standardized (174-182, 188). Experience with endoprosthesis insertion (fig. 11) suggests that, in centers performing it regularly, a technical success rate of at least 95% should be expected with relief of jaundice and pruritus in 80% or more (174-184) (table 5). Hydrophilic guidewires may speed the process and often permit access across strictures resistant to standard wires. Steerable and torque stable wires have made some difference to selective intrahepatic cannulation. A sphincterotome can also be used as a deflecting device. Two wires can be placed through the channel of a stenting endoscope into both hepatic ducts in hilar lesions. Many experts do not use sphincterotomy for stent insertion unless insertion of two stents is planned.

Stent occlusion may occur from one week to over 15 months after placement, with a mean of about five months (189-199) and patients can present with malaise, low-grade fever or mild disturbance of liver enzymes. Several variables may be involved: bile flow, bile composition, bacterial contamination and endoprosthesis characteristics such as length, shape, design, position, size, number and material (polyethylene and other similar polymers). Attempts at manipulating all of these have been made in vitro (189-195) with little impact on clinical practice although a newly developed Teflon stent

Table 5. Results of endoscopic palliation in malignant biliary obstruction

Tumor position	Ampullary	Low CBD	GB	Hilar
N	112	679	71	640
Success (%)	96	84-90	86	91-96
Complications (%)	8-32	10-19	14	8-60
30 day mortality (%)	1-3	10-17	13	10-33
Late jaundice (%)	36	37	25	40-68
Duodenal obstruction (%)	23	5-7.5	5	-
Survival months	9-14	4.5-6	5	2-6

Data from references 176, 179, 181, 184, 192.

shows promise (196). The maximum outside diameter of such stents is limited by the diameter of the instrument channel in the duodenoscope and 10 to 11.5 French stents are now standard and perform better than smaller diameter endoprostheses (192). Endoscopic replacement of a clogged stent is usually technically simple and is associated with resolution of symptoms. Macroscopically, the material in a blocked stent resembles biliary sludge or brown pigment stones consisting mainly of calcium bilirubinate with some calcium palmitate and unidentified organic material together with bacteria (189-192) (table 6). Bacteria form biofilms by polysaccharide production, which cements the bacterial cell to the surface and mediates adhesion to sister cells. The polysaccharide matrix protects the bacteria from the host defense mechanisms and from toxic substances such as antibiotics, biocides, and surfactants. It is most likely that this layer is the first step in the clogging process (189-191). Crystals of calcium bilirubinate, calcium palmitate and cholesterol are embedded within the matrix and the bacteria are attached to the stent surface by a fibrillar matrix. The use of antibiotics, antibiotic- or bacteriostatic-impregnated stents have not prevented this clogging phenomenon from occurring nor have the use of gallstone dissolution agents, mucolytic and choleretic (193-195).

The predictability of occlusion, with its serious complication of sepsis, militates in favor of planned removal and replacement at approximately four month intervals (174-177). The variability of stent survival, however, would support the conservative approach of close clinical follow-up to anticipate early symptoms of biliary obstruction or cholangitis (197-199).

Metallic Expandable Endoprostheses

In search of a solution to the problem of plastic stent occlusion, larger diameter expandable metallic stents have been developed. All types have been first deployed through the percutaneous transhepatic route (200-206) and some have not yet become available in an endoscopically usable form.

There is limited experience with the endoscopic Gianturco Z stent (Wilson-Cook) which is available as single 8 mm by 30 mm units when fully expanded (203, 207, 208) and which can be linked end to end to cover the necessary stricture length. The Strecker stent (Microvasive, Boston Scientific Corporation) has a single tantalum thread interlocking woven meshwork construction, attains a maximum diameter of 8 mm and is available in lengths of 4, 6 and 8 cm. It requires balloon expansion at the time of placement, there are technical failures in up to 18% and there is no subsequent self-expansion in its original form (199, 200, 209). One randomized trial (200) included these devices but used the endoscopic version in common bile duct lesions and the transhepatic version for hilar lesions compared with plastic stents inserted by the same routes. Unfortunately, all metallic stents (Strecker and Wallstent patients) were reported together suggesting an overall improvement in palliation with less time in hospital, a lower incidence of early cholangitis and a lower late occlusion rate.

Most experience has been gained with the self-expanding metallic Wallstent (Schneider Stent, Inc) which is delivered on an 8 French gauge system of 100 mm length but expands to 30 French gauge (fig. 12) in its fully expanded form of 42-68 mm length (199-216). Initial open studies were conducted in Europe (201, 209-211, 216) in a total of 293 patients with malignant biliary obstruction. Early morbidity was very low but late occlusion by tumor ingrowth or overgrowth appeared in 10% (figs. 13 and 14) but sludge occlusion was reported in only 2%. Three randomized controlled trials have now been reported (202, 213, 214) from the USA and Europe comparing Wallstents with plastic in 380 patients. Prolonged stent patency, lower

Table 6. Composition of stent occlusion material compared to bile (% dry weight) (191)

	Stent sludge	Bile
Bile acid	9 ± 4	56 ± 6
Cholesterol	5 ± 3	3
Lecithin	6 ± 3	20 ± 2
Bilirubin	12 ± 7	
Protein	25 ± 12	5 ± 1
Residue	20 ± 10	
Total	77 ± 20	84 ± 6

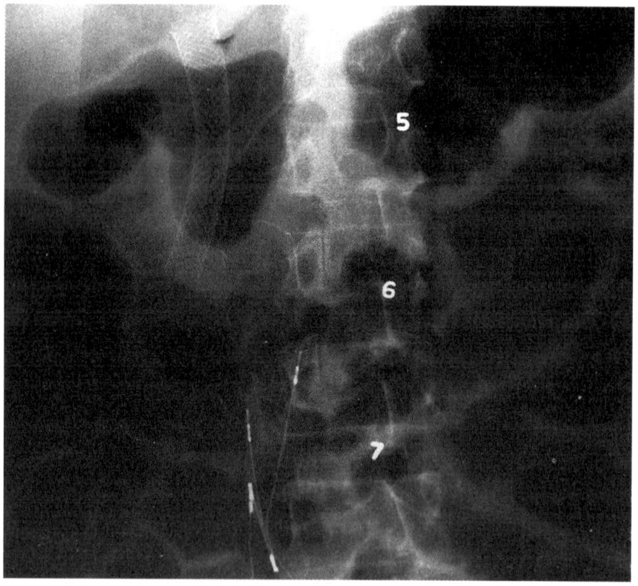

Fig. 12. Metallic expandable endoprosthesis (Wallstent).

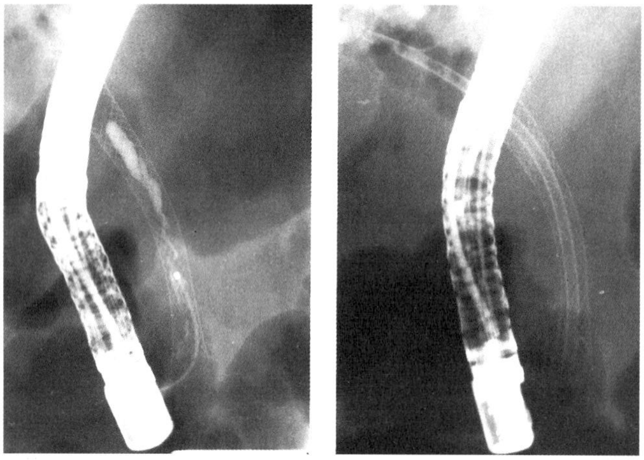

Fig. 13. Occlusion of a metallic Wallstent (left) and insertion of a new prosthesis inside the occluded one.

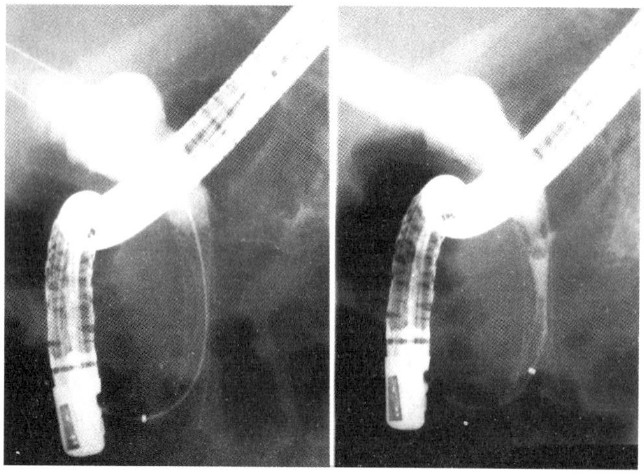

Fig. 14. Occlusion of a metallic Wallstent.

stent occlusions and other complications and a reduction in subsequent interventions for Wallstents were demonstrated with a significant impact on cost-effectiveness. The problem of tumor ingrowth through the meshwork may be overcome by the development of a silicone covering (217) or the emergence of newer metallic stents which do not have an open framework (218).

REFERENCES

1. Kawai K, Akasaka Y, Murakami K, Tada M, Kohle Y, Nakajima M. Endoscopic sphincterotomy of the ampulla of vater. Gastrointest Endosc 1974; 20:148-151.
2. Classen M, Demling L. Endokopische sphinkterotomie der papilla bateri und steinextraktion aus dem ductus choledochus. Dtsch Med Wochenschr 1974; 99:496-497.
3. Kullman E, Borch K, Lindstrom E, Ansehn S, Ihse I, Anderberg B. Bacteremia following diagnostic and therapeutic ERCP. Gastrointest Endosc 1992; 38:444-449.
4. Rossos PG, Kortan P, Haber G. Selective common bile duct cannulation can be simplified by the use of a standard papillotome. Gastrointest Endosc 1993; 39:67-69.
5. Siegel JH, Pullano W. Two new methods for selective bile duct cannulation and sphincterotomy. Gastrointest Endosc 1987; 33:438-440.
6. Shakoor T, Geenen JE. Pre-cut papillotomy. Gastrointest Endosc 1992; 38:623-627.
7. Dowsett JF, Vaira D, Hatfield RW, Cairns SR, Polydorou A, Frost R, Croker J, Cotton PB, Russell RCG, Mason RR. Endoscopic biliary therapy using the combined percutaneous and endoscopic technique. Gastroenterology 1989; 96:1180-1186.
8. Tweedle DEF, Martin KF. Needle knife papillotomy for endoscopic sphincterotomy and cholangiography. Gastrointest Endosc 1991; 37:518-521.
9. Siegel JH, Ben-Zvi JS, Pullano W. The needle knife: a valuable tool in diagnostic and therapeutic ERCP. Gastrointest Endosc 1989; 35:499-503.
10. Leung JWC, Banez VP, Chung SCS. Precut (needle knife) papillotomy for impacted common bile duct stone at the ampulla. Am J Gastroenterol 1990; 85:991-993.
11. Leese T, Neoptolemos JP, Carr-Locke DL. Successes, failures, early complications and their management following endoscopic sphincterotomy:results in 394 consecutive patients from a single center. Br J Surg 1985; 72:215-219.
12. Nakajima M, Kizu M, Akasaka Y, Kawai K. Five year experience of endoscopic sphincterotomy in Japan. Endoscopy 1979; 2:138-141.
13. Reiter JJ, Bayer HB, Mennicken C, Manegold PC. Results of endoscopic papillotomy: a collective ex-

perience from 9 endoscopic centers in West Germany. World J Surg 1978; 2:505-507.
14. Safrany L. Endoscopic treatment of biliary tract diseases. Lancet 1978; ii:983-985.
15. Siegel JH. Endoscopic papillotomy in the treatment of biliary tract disease: 258 procedures and results. Dig Dis Sci 1981; 26:1057-1064.
16. Cotton PB, Vallon AG. British experience with duodenoscopic sphincterotomy for removal of bile duct stones. Br J Surg 1981; 68:373-375.
17. Lambert ME, Betts CD, Hill J, Faragher EB, Martin DF, Tweedle DEF. Endoscopic sphincterotomy: the whole truth. Br J Surg 1991; 78:473-476.
18. Vaira D, Ainley C, Williams S, Cairns S, Salmon P, Russell C, D'Anna L, Dowsett J, Baillie J, Croker J, Cotton P, Hatfield A. Endoscopic sphincterotomy in 1,000 consecutive patients. Lancet 1989; ii:431-433.
19. Despland M, Clavien PA, Mentha G, Rohner A. Gallstone ileus and bowel perforation after endoscopic sphincterotomy. Am J Gastroenterol 1992; 87:886-887.
20. Lewis FW, Moloo N, Stiegmann GV, Goff JS. Splenic injury complicating therapeutic upper gastrointestinal endoscopy and ERCP. Gastrointest Endosc 1991; 37:632-633.
21. Tam F, Prindiville T, Wolfe B. Subcutaneous emphysema as a complication of endoscopic sphincterotomy of the ampulla of vater. Gastrointest Endosc 1989; 35:447-449.
22. Cotton PB, Lehman G, Vennes J, Geenen JE, Russell RCG, Meyers WC, Liguory C, Nickl N. Endoscopic sphincterotomy complications and their management: an attempt at consensus. Gastrointest Endosc 1991; 37:383-393.
23. Sherman S, Ruffolo TA, Hawes RH, Lehman GA. Complications of endoscopic sphincterotomy. A prospective series with emphasis on the increased risk associated with sphincter of oddi dysfunction and nondilated bile ducts. Gastroenterology 1991; 101:1068-1075.
24. Vaira D, Dowsett JF, Hatfield ARW, Cairns SR, Polydorou AA, Cotton PB, Salmon PR, Russell RCG. Is duodenal diverticulum a risk factor for sphincterotomy? Gut 1989; 30:939-942.
25. Shemesh E, Klein E, Czerniak A, Coret A, Bat L. Endoscopic sphincterotomy in patients with gallbladder in situ: The influence of periampullary duodenal diverticula. Surgery 1990; 107:163-166.
26. Spach DH, Silverstein FE, Stamm WE. Transmission of infection by gastrointestinal endoscopy and bronchoscopy. Ann Intern Med 1993; 118:117-128.
27. Moreira VF, Arribas R, Sanroman AL, Merono E, Larena C, García M, Torres G. Choledocholithiasis in cirrhotic patients: Is endoscopic sphincterotomy the safest choice? Am J Gastroenterol 1991; 86:1006-1009.
28. Sherman S, Hawes RH, Nisi R, Lehman GA. Endoscopic sphincterotomy-induced hemorrhage: treatment with multipolar electrocoagulation. Gastrointest Endosc 1992; 38:123-126.
29. Sherman S, Lehman GA. ERCP- and endoscopic sphincterotomy-induced pancreatitis. Pancreas 1991; 6:350-367.
30. Bedford RA, Johnson GK, Geenen JE, Lehman G, Frakes J, Ryan M, Silverman W, Cass O, Edmundowicz S, Payne M, Johanson J. Does the use of nonionic contrast prevent post-ERCP pancreatitis:Results of a prospective multicenter study. Gastrointest Endosc 1993; 39:315.
31. Barkin JS, Casal GL, Reiner DK, Goldberg RI, Phillips RS, Kaplan S. A comparative study of contrast agents for endoscopic retrograde pancreatography. Am J Gastroenterol 1991; 86:1437-1441.
32. Persson B, Slezak P, Efendic S, Haggmark A. Can somatostatin prevent injection pancreatitis after ERCP? Hepatogastroenterology 1992; 39:259-261.
33. Binmoeller KF, Harris AG, Dumas R, Grimaldi C, Delmont JP. Does the somatostatin analogue octreotide protect against ERCP induced pancreatitis? Gut 1992; 33:1129-1133.
34. Sternlieb JM, Aronchick CA, Retig JN, Dabezies M, Saunders F, Goosenberg E, Infantolino A, Ionna S, Maislin G, Wright S, Lipshutz WH. A multicenter, randomized, controlled trial to evaluate the effect of prophylactic octreotide on ERCP-induced pancreatitis. Am J Gastroenterol 1992; 87:1561-1566.
35. Lai ECS, Lo CM, Choi Tk, Cheng WK, Fan ST, Wong J. Urgent biliary decompression after endoscopic retrograde cholangiopancreatography. Am J Surg 1989; 157:121-125.
36. Hawes RH, Cotton PB, Vallon AG. Follow-up 6 to 11 years after duodenoscopic sphincterotomy for stones in patients with prior cholecystectomy. Gastroenterology 1990; 98:1008-1012.
37. Ikeda S, Tanaka M, Matsumoto S, Yoshimoto H, Itoh H. Endoscopic sphincterotomy: long-term results in 408 patients with complete follow-up. Endoscopy 1988; 20:13-17.
38. Lygidakis NJ. Surgical approaches to recurrent choledocholithiasis: choledochoduodenostomy versus T-tube drainage after choledochotomy . Am J Surg 1983; 145:636-639.
39. Baker AR, Neoptolemos JP, Leese T, James DC, Fossard DP. Long-term followup of patients with side to side choledochoduodenostomy and transduodenal sphincteroplasty. Ann R Coll Surg 1987; 69:253-257.
40. Ricci E, Bertoni G, Conigliaro R, Contini S, Mortilla MG, Bedogni G. Endoscopic sphincterotomy in billroth II patients: an improved method using a diathermic needle as sphincterotomy and a nosobiliary drain as guide. Gastrointest Endosc 1989; 35:47-50.
41. Shaw MJ, Dorsher PJ, Vennes JA. A new mechanical lithotripter for the treatment of large common duct stones. Am J Gastroenterol 1990; 85:796-798.
42. Siegel JH, Ben-Zvi JS, Pullano WE. Mechanical lithotripsy of common duct stones. Gastrointest Endosc 1990; 36:351-356.
43. Chung SCS, Leung JWC, Leong HT, Li AKC. Mechanical lithotripsy of large common bile duct stones using a basket. Br J Surg 1991; 78:1448-1450.

44. Van Dam J, Sivak MV. Mechanical lithotripsy of large common bile duct stones. Cleve Clin J Med 1993; 60:38-42.
45. Shaw MJ, Mackie RD, Moore JP, Dorsher PJ, Freeman ML, Meier PB, Potter T, Hutton SW, Vennes JA. Results of a multicenter trial using a mechanical lithotripter for the treatment of large bile duct stones. Am J Gastroenterol 1993; 88:730-733.
46. Birkett DH. Biliary laser lithotripsy. Surg Clin N Am 1992; 72:641-654.
47. Ell C, Lux G, Hochberger J, Muller D, Demling L. Laser lithotripsy of common bile duct stones. Gut 1988; 29:746-751.
48. Cotton P, Kozarek RA, Schapiro RH, Nishioka NS, Kelsey PB, Ball TJ, Putnam WS, Barkun A, Weinerth J. Endoscopic laser lithotripsy of large bile duct stones. Gastroenterology 1990; 99:1128-1133.
49. Ponchon T, Gagnon P, Valette PJ, Henry L, Chavaillon A, Thieulin F. Pulsed dye laser lithotripsy of bile duct stones. Gastroenterology 1991; 100:1730-1736.
50. Picus D. Intracorporeal biliary lithotripsy. Rad Clin N Am 1990; 28:1241-1249.
51. Siegel J, Ben-Zvi J, Pullano W. Endoscopic electrohydraulic lithotripsy. Gastrointest Endosc 1990; 36:134-136.
52. Hixson LJ, Fennerty MB, Jaffee PE, Pulju JH, Palley SL. Peroral cholangioscopy with intracorporeal electrohydraulic lithotripsy for choledocholithiasis. Am J Gastroenterol 1992; 87:296-299.
53. Leung JWC, Chung SSC. Electrohydraulic lithotripsy with peroral choledochoscopy. Br Med J 1989; 299:595-598.
54. Bonnel DH, Liguory CE, Cornud FE, Lefebvre JF. Common bile duct and intrahepatic stones: Results of transhepatic electrohydraulic lithotripsy in 50 patients. Radiology 1991; 180:345-348.
55. Gordon SJ, Stampfl DA, Grimm IS, Dahnert W, Goldberg BB, Taglienti G. Successful shock-wave lithotripsy of bile duct stones using ultrasound guidance. Dig Dis Sci 1991; 36:1102-1109.
56. Ponchon T, Martin X, Barkun A, Mestas JL, Chavaillon A, Boustiere C. Extracorporeal lithotripsy of bile duct stones using ultrasonography for stone localization. Gastroenterology 1990; 98:726-732.
57. Bland KI, Jones RS, Maher JW, Cotton PB, Pennell TC, Amerson R, Munson JL, Berci G, Fuchs GJ, Way LW, Graham JB, Lindenau BU, Moody FG. Extracorporeal shock-wave lithotripsy of bile duct calculi. Ann Surg 1989; 209:743-755.
58. Sauerbruch T, Stern M. Fragmentation of bile duct stones by extracorporeal shock waves. A new approach to biliary calculi after failure of routine endoscopic measures. Gastroenterology 1989; 96:146-152.
59. Weber J, Adamek HE, Riemann JF. Extracorporeal piezoelectric lithotripsy for retained bile duct stones. Endoscopy 1992; 24:239-243.
60. Palmer KR, Hofmann AF. Intraductal mono-octanoin for the direct dissolution of bile duct stones:experience in 343 patients. Gut 1986; 27:196-202.
61. Neoptolemos JP, Hall C, O'Connor, Murray WR, Carr-Locke DL. Methyl-tert-butyl-ether for treating bile duct stones: the British experience. Br J Surg 1990; 77:32-35.
62. Kaye GL, Summerfield JA, McIntyre N, Dooley JS. Methyl tert butyl ether dissolution therapy for common bile duct stones. J Hepatol 1990; 10:337-340.
63. Brandon JC, Teplick SK, Haskin PH, Sammon JK, Muhr WF, Hofmann AF, Gambescia RA, Zitomer N. Common bile duct calculi: Updated experience with dissolution with methyl tertiary butyl ether. Radiology 1988; 166:665-667.
64. Murray WR, Laferla G, Fullarton GM. Choledocholithiasis-in vivo stone dissolution using methyl tertiary butyl ether (MTBE). Gut 1988; 29:143-145.
65. Swobodnik W, Baumgaertel H, Janowitz P, Fuchs S, Ditschuneit H. Dissolution of calcified gallbladder stones by treatment with methyl-hexyl ether and urea-EDTA. Lancet 1988; ii:216.
66. Neoptolemos JP, Hofmann AF, Moossa AR. Chemical treatment of stones in the biliary tree. Br J Surg 1986; 73:515-524.
67. Leung JWC, Cotton PB. Endoscopic nasobiliary catheter drainage in biliary and pancreatic disease. Am J Gastroenterol 1991; 86:389-394.
68. Kiil J, Kruse A, Rokkjaer M. Large bile duct stones treated by endoscopic biliary drainage. Surgery 1989; 105:51-56.
69. Rustgi AK, Schapiro RH. Biliary stents for common bile duct stones. Gastrointest Endosc Clin North Am 1991; 1:79-91.
70. Nordback I. Management of unextractable bile duct stones by endoscopic stenting. Ann Chirurgiae Gynaecol 1989; 78:290-292.
71. Cotton PB, Forbes A, Leung JWC, Dineen L. Endoscopic stenting for long-term treatment of large bile duct stones: 2- to 5-year follow-up. Gastrointest Endosc 1987; 33:411-412.
72. Soomers AJ, Nagengast FM, Yap SH. Endoscopic placement of biliary endoprostheses in patients with endoscopically unextractable common bile duct stones. Endoscopy 1990; 22:24-26.
73. Foutch PG, Harlan J, Sanowski RA. Endoscopic placement of biliary stents for treatment of high risk geriatric patients with common duct stones. Am J Gastroenterol 1989; 84:527-529.
74. Johnson G, Geenen JE, Venu RP, Schmalz MJ, Hogan WJ. Treatment of non-extractable common bile duct stones with combination ursodeoxycholic acid (UDCA) plus endoprosthesis. Gastrointest Endosc 1991; 37:253.
75. Tritapepe R, di Padova C, di Padova F. Non-invasive treatment for retained common bile duct stones in patients with T tube in situ:saline washout after intravenous ceruletide. Br J Surg 1988; 75:144-146.
76. Josephs LF, Birkett DH. Laser lithotripsy for the management of retained stones. Arch Surg 1992; 127:603-605.
77. Burhenne JH. Percutaneous extraction of retained biliary tract stones. AJR 1980; 134:888-898.
78. Cotton PB. Retained bile duct stones: T-tube in pla-

ce, percutaneous or endoscopic management? Am J Gastroenterol 1990; 85:1075-1078.

79. Caprini JA. Biliary stone extraction. Am Surg 1988; 54:343-346.

80. Nussinson E, Cairns SR, Vaira D, Dowsett JF, Mason RR. A 10 year single centre experience of percutaneous and endoscopic extraction of bile duct stones with T tube in situ. Gut 1991; 32:1040-1043.

81. Tandon RK, Nijhawan S, Arora A. Management of retained common bile duct stones in patients with T-tube in situ: Role of endoscopic sphincterotomy. Am J Gastroenterol 1990; 85:1126-1131.

82. Bickerstaff KI, Berry AR, Chapman RW, Britton J. Early postoperative endoscopic sphincterotomy for retained biliary stones. Ann R Coll Surg Engl 1988; 70:350-351.

83. Soehendra N, Kempeneers I, Eichfuss HP, Reynders-Frederix V. Early postoperative endoscopy aafter biliary tract surgery. Endoscopy 1981; 13:113-117.

84. Simpson CJ, Gray GR, Gillespie G. Early endoscopic sphincterotomy for retained common bile duct stones. J R Coll Surg Edinburgh 1985; 30:288-289.

85. O'Doherty DP, Neoptolemos JP, Carr-Locke DL. Endoscopic sphincterotomy for retained common bile duct stones in patients with T-tube in situ in the early postoperative period. Br J Surg 1986; 73:454-456.

86. Danilewitz MD. Early postoperative endoscopic sphincterotomy for retained common bile duct stones. Gastrointest Endosc 1989; 35:298-299.

87. Lambert ME, Martin DF, Tweedle DEF. Endoscopic removal of retained stones after biliary surgery. Br J Surg 1988; 75:896-898.

88. Baillie J, Cairns S, Cotton P. Endoscopic management of choledocholithiasis during pregnancy. Surgery 1990; 171:1-4.

89. Binmoeller KF, Katon RM. Needle knife papillotomy for an impacted common bile duct stone during pregnancy. Gastrointest Endosc 1990; 36:607-609.

90. Beck G, Brodmekel G. Choledocholithiasis in pregnancy:Treatment by endoscopic sphincterotomy. Gastrointest Endosc 1991; 100:A252.

91. Brolin RE, Siemons GO, Fynan TM. Critical analysis of retained and residual common duct stones. Am Surg 1986; 52:588-593.

92. Danilewitz MD. Early postoperative endoscopic sphincterotomy for retained common bile duct stones. Gastrointest Endosc 1989; 35:298-299.

93. Cranley B, Logan H. Exploration of the common bile duct-the relevance of the clinical picture and the importance of preoperative cholnagiography. Br J Surg 1980; 67:869-872.

94. Sheridan WG, Williams HOL, Lewis MH. Morbidity and mortality of common bile duct exploration. Br J Surg 1987; 74:1095-1099.

95. Hill J, Martin F, Tweeddle DEF. Risks of leaving the gallbladder in situ after endoscopic sphincterotomy for bile duct stones. Br J Surg 1991; 78:554-557.

96. Siegel JH, Safrany L, Ben-Zvi JS, Pullano WE, Cooperman A, Stenzel M, Ramsey WH. Duodenoscopic sphincterotomy in patients with gallbladders in situ: Report of a series of 1272 patients. Am J Gastroenterol 1988; 83:1255-1258.

97. Escourrou J, Cordova JA, Lazorthes F, Frexinos J, Ribet A. Early and late complications after endoscopic sphincterotomy for biliary lithiasis with and without the gallbladder *in situ*. Gut 1984; 25:598-602.

98. Davidson BR, Neoptolemos JP, Carr-Locke DL. Endoscopic sphincterotomy for common bile duct calculi in patients with gallbladder in situ considered unfit for surgery. Gut 1988; 29:114-120.

99. Rosseland AR, Solhaug JH. Primary endoscopic papillotomy (EPT) in patients with stones in the common bile duct and the gallbladder in situ: A 5-8 year follow-up study. World J Surg 1988; 12:111-116.

100. Tanaka M, Ikeda S, Yoshimoto H, Matsumoto S. The long-term fate of the gallbladder after endoscopic sphincterotomy. Am J Surg 1987; 154:505-509.

101. Gracie W, Ransohoff D. The natural history of silent gallstones. N Engl J Med 1982; 307:798-800.

102. Worthley CS, Toouli J. Gallbladder non-filling: an indication for cholecystectomy after endoscopic sphincterotomy. Br J Surg 1988; 75:796-798.

103. Holbrook RF, Jacobson FL, Pezzuti RT, Howell DA. Biliary patency imaging after endoscopic retrograde sphincterotomy with gallbladder in situ: Clinical impact of nonvisualization. Arch Surg 1991; 126:738-742.

104. Neoptolemos JP, Carr-Locke DL, Fossard DP. Prospective randomized study of preoperative endoscopic sphincterotomy versus surgery alone for common bile duct stones. Br Med 1987; 294:470-474.

105. Stiegmann GV, Goff JS, Mansour A, Pearlman N, Reveille RM. Precholecystectomy endoscopic cholangiography and stone removal is not superior to cholecystectomy, cholangiography, and common duct exploration. Am J Surg 1992; 163:227-230.

106. The Southern Surgeons Club. A prospective analysis of 1518 laparoscopic cholecystectomies. N Engl J Med 1991; 324:1073-1078.

107. NIH Consensus Conference on Gallstones and Laparoscopic Cholecystectomy. Am J Surg 1993; 390-547.

108. Flowers JL, Zucker KA, Graham SM, Scovill WA, Imbembo AL, Bailey RW. Laparoscopic cholangiography:Results and indications. Ann Surg 1992; 215:209-216.

109. Sackier JM, Berci G, Phillips E, Carroll B, Shapiro S, Paz-Partlow M. The role of cholangiography in laparoscopic cholecystectomy. Arch Surg 1991; 126:1021-1026.

110. Hunter JG. Laparoscopic transcystic common bile duct exploration. Am J Surg 1992; 163:53-56.

111. Cotton PB, Baillie J, Pappas TN, Meyers WS. Laparoscopic cholectstectomy and the biliary endoscopist. Gastrointest Endosc 1991; 37:94-97.

112. Del Santo P, Kazarian KK, Rogers JF, Bevins PA, Hall JR. Prediction of operative cholangiography in patients undergoing elective cholecystectomy with

routine liver function chemistries. Surgery 1985; 98:7-11.
113. Hauer-Jensen M, Karesen R, Nygaard K, Solheim K, Amlie E, Havig O, Viddal KO. Predictive ability of choledocholithiasis indicators. Ann Surg 1985; 202:64-68.
114. Lacaine F, Corlette MB, Bismuth H. Preoperative evaluation of the risk of common bile duct stones. Arch Surg 1980; 115:1114-1116.
115. Neuhaus H, Feussner H, Ungeheuer A, Hoffmann W, Siewert JR, Classen M. Prospective evaluation of the use of endoscopic retrograde cholangiography prior to laparoscopic cholecystectomy. Endoscopy 1992; 24:745-749.
116. Aliperti G, Edmundowicz SA, Soper NJ, Ashley SW. Combined endoscopic sphincterotomy and laparoscopic cholecystectomy in patients with choledocholithiasis and cholecystolithiasis. Ann Intern Med 1991; 115:783-785.
117. Boulay J, Schellenberg R, Brady PG. Role of ERCP and therapeutic biliary endoscopy in association with laparoscopic cholecystectomy. Am J Gastroenterol 1992; 87:837-842.
118. Cotton PB. Removing duct stones without sphincterotomy. Gastrointest Endosc 1993; 39:312.
119. Ibuki Y, Kudo M, Todo A. Endoscopic retrograde extraction of common bile duct stones with drip infusion of isosorbide dinitrate. Gastrointest Endosc 1992; 38:178-180.
120. Staritz M, Poralla T, Dormeyer HH, Buschenfelde MZ. Endoscopic removal of common bile duct stones through the intact papilla after medical sphincter dilation. Gastroenterology 1985; 88:1807-1811.
121. Deslandres E, Gagner M, Pomp A, Rheault M, Leduc R, Clermont R, Gratton J, Bernard EJ. Intraoperative endoscopic sphincterotomy for common bile duct stones during laparosopic cholecystectomy. Gastrointest Endosc 1993; 39:54-58.
122. Opie EL. The etiology of acute hemorrhagic pancreatitis. Bull Johns Hopkins Hosp 1901; 12:182-188.
123. Moody FG, Senninger N, Runkel N. Another challenge to the Opie myth. Gastroenterology 1993; 104:927-931.
124. Acosta JM, Ledesma CL. Gallstone migration as a cause of acute pancreatitis. N Engl J Med 1974; 290:484-487.
125. Kelly TR. Gallstone pancreatitis: The timing of surgery. Surgery 1980; 88:34-350.
126. Stone HH, Fabian TC, Dunlop WE. Gallstone pancreatitis. Biliary tract pathology in relation to time of operation. Ann Surg 1981; 194:305-312.
127. Acosta JM, Rossi R, Galli OMR, Pellegrini CA, Skinner DB. Early surgery for acute gallstone pancreatitis: Evaluation of a systematic approach. Surgery 1978; 83:367-370.
128. Leese T, Shaw D. Comparison of three Glasgow multifactor prognostic scoring systems in acute pancreatitis. Br J Surg 1988; 75:460-462.
129. Osborne DH, Imrie CW, Carter DC. Biliary surgery in the same admission for gallstone-associated pancreatitis. Br J Surg 1981; 68:758-761.
130. Ranson JHC. The timing of biliary surgery in acute pancreatitis. Ann Surg 1979; 189:654-662.
131. Kim U, Bosner B. Timing of surgery for acute gallstone pancreatitis. Am J Surg 1988; 156:393-396.
132. Kelly TR, Wagner DS. Gallstone pancreatitis: A prospective randomized trial of the timing of surgery. Surgery 1988; 104:600-605.
133. Safrany L, Cotton PB. A preliminary report: Urgent duodenoscopic sphincterotomy for acute gallstone pancreatitis. Surgery 1981; 89:424-428.
134. Rosseland AR, Solhaug JH. Early or delayed endoscopic papillotomy (EPT) in gallstone pancreatitis. Ann Surg 1984; 199:165-167.
135. Shemesh E, Czerniak A, Schneabaum S, Nass S. Early endoscopic sphincterotomy in the management of acute gallstone pancreatitis in elderly patients. JAGS 1990; 38:893-896.
136. Neoptolemos JP, Carr-Locke DL, London NJ, Bailey IA, James D, Fossard DP. Controlled trial of urgent endoscopic retrograde chlangiopancreatography and endoscopic sphincterotomy versus conservative treatment for acute pancreatitis due to gallstones. Lancet 1988; ii:979-983.
137. Fan ST, Lai ECS, Mok FPT, Lo CM, Zheng SS, Wong J. Early treatment of acute biliary pancreatitis by endoscopic papillotomy. N Engl J Med 1993; 328:228-232.
138. Ros E, Navarro S, Bru C, Garcia-Puges A, Valderrama R. Occult microlithiasis in «idiopathic» acute pancreatitis: Prevention off relapses by cholecystectomy or ursodeoxycholic acid therapy. Gastroenterology 1991; 101:1701-1709.
139. Lee SP, Nicholls JF, Park HZ. Biliary sludge as a cause of acute pancreatitis. N Engl J Med 1992; 326:589-593.
140. May GR, Shaffer EH. Should elective endoscopic sphincterotomy replace cholecystectomy for the treatment of high-risk patients with gallstone pancreatitis? J Clin Gastroenterol 1991; 13:125-128.
141. Csendes A, Sepulveda A, Burdiles P, Braghetto I, Bastias J, Schutte H, Diaz JC, Yarmuch J, Maluenda F. Common bile duct pressure in patients with common bile duct stones with or without acute suppurative cholangitis. Arch Surg 1988; 123:697-699.
142. Reynold BM, Dargan EI. Acute obstructive cholangitis —A distinct clinical syndrome. Ann Surg 1959; 150:299-303.
143. Boey JH, Way LW. Acute cholangitis. Ann Surg 1980; 191:264-270.
144. Gould RJ, Vogelzang, Neimen HL, Pearl JG, Politcha SM. Percutaneous biliary drainage as an initial therapy of the biliary tract. Surg Gynecol Obstet 1985; 160:523-527.
145. Kadir S, Baassiri A, Barth KH, Kaufman SL, Cameron JL, White RT. Percutaneous transhepatic biliary drainage in the management of biliary sepsis. Am J Roentgenol 1982; 138:25-29.
146. Pessa ME, Hawkins IF, Vogel SB. The treatment of acute cholangitis. Percutaneous transhepatic bi-

liary drainage before definitive therapy. Ann Surg 1987; 205:389-392.
147. Ditzel H, Schaffalitzky de Muckadell OB. Endoscopic sphincterotomy in acute cholangitis due to choledocholithiasis. Hepatogastroenterology 1990; 37:204-207.
148. Leese T, Neoptolemos JP, Baker AR, Carr-Locke DL. Management of acute cholangitis and the impact of endoscopic sphincterotomy. Br J Surg 1986; 73:988-992.
149. Leung JW, Chung SCS, Sung JJY, Banez VP, Li AKC. Urgent endoscopic drainage for acute suppurative cholangitis. Lancet 1989; i:1307-1309.
150. Gogel HK, Runyon BA, Volpicelli NA, Palmer RC. Acute suppurative obstructive cholangitis due to stones:treatment by urgent endoscopic sphincterotomy. Gastrointest Endosc 1987; 33:210-213.
151. Nunez D, Guerra JJ, Al-Sheikh WA, Russell E, Mendez G Jr. Percutaneous biliary drainage in acute suppurative cholangitis. Gastrointest Radiol 1986; 11:85-89.
152. Ikeda S, Tanaka M, Itoh H, Kishikawa H, Nakayama F. Emergency decompression of bile duct in acute obstructive suppurative cholangitis by duodenoscopic cannulation: A lifesaving procedure. World J Surg 1981; 5:587-593.
153. Lai ECS, Mok FPT, Tan ESY, Lo CM, Fan ST, You KT, Wong J. Endoscopic biliary drainage for severe acute cholangitis. N Engl J Med 1992; 326:1582-1586.
154. NIH Consensus Development Conference on Laparoscopic Cholecystectomy, September 14-16, 1992. Am J Surg 1993; 165:390-398.
155. Carr-Locke DL. Endoscopic Approaches. In: Blumgart LH, Surgery of the Liver and Biliary Tract. London: Churchill Livingstone, 1987; chapter 47, 587-601.
156. Davids P et al. Benign postoperative biliary strictures: Endoscopic management and longterm follow-up. Gastrointest Endosc 1991; 37:A267.
157. Binmoeller K et al. Endoscopic management of postoperative biliary leaks: Review of 77 cases and report of two cases with biloma formation. Am J Gastroenterol 1991; 86:227-231.
158. Hoffman B, Cunningham J, Marsh W. Endoscopic management of biliary fistulas with small caliber stents. Am J Gastroenterol 1990; 85:705-707.
159. Golden E et al. Treatment of fistulas of the biliary tract by endoscopic insertion of endoprostheses. Surgery 1990; 170:418-423.
160. Feretis C et al. Postoperative external and internal biliary fistulas, unassociated with distal bile duct obstruction: Endoscopic treatment. Endoscopy 1990; 22:211-213.
161. Kozarek R, Traverso L. Endoscopic stent placement for cystic duct leak after laparoscopic cholecystectomy. Gastrointest Endosc 1991; 37:71-72.
162. Ward E et al. Persistent bile leak after liver transplantation: Biloma drainage and endoscopic retrograde cholangiopancreatographic sphincterotomy. Radiology 1991; 179:719-720.
163. Krige J et al. Endoscopic embolization of external biliary fistulae. Br J Surg 1990; 77:581-583.
164. Bjorkman DJ, Carr-Locke DL, Lichtenstein DR, Ferrari AP, Brooks, DC. Post-Laparoscopic Cholecystectomy Bile Leaks: A Short Stent is Enough. Am J Gastroenterol 1994 (in press).
165. Deviere J et al. Endoscopic biliary drainage in chronic pancreatitis. Gastrointest Endosc 1990; 36:96-100.
166. Meier P et al. Nonoperative biliary drainage differentiates chronic pancreatitis (CP) from biliary pain in CP patients with benign bile duct strictures. Gastrointest Endosc 1991; 37:A250.
167. Siegel JH, Guelrud M. Endoscopic cholangiopancreatoplasty: hydrostatic balloon dilation in the bile duct and pancreas. Gastrointest Endosc 1983; 29:99-103.
168. Grijm R, Huibregtse K, Bartelsman J et al. Therapeutic problems in primary sclerosing cholangitis. Dig Dis Sci 1986; 31:792-798.
169. Johnson GK, Geenen JE, Venu RP, Hogan WJ. Endoscopic treatment of biliary duct strictures in sclerosing cholangitis: follow-up assessment of a new therapeutic approach. Gastrointest Endosc 1987; 33:9-12.
170. Cotton PB, Nickl N. Endoscopic and radiologic approaches to therapy in primary sclerosing cholangitis. Semin Liver Dis 1991; 11:40-48.
171. Johnson GK, Geenen JE, Venu RP, Schmalz MJ, Hogan WJ. Endoscopic treatment of biliary duct strictures in sclerosing cholangitis: a larger series and recommendations. Gastrointest Endosc 1991; 37:38-43.
172. Craig P et al. Endoscopic therapy in the management of primary sclerosing cholangitis: Assessment of clinical response. Gastroenterology 1991; 100:A732.
173. Gaing AA, Geders JM, Cohen SA, Siegel JH. Endoscopic management of primary sclerosing cholangitis —Review and report of an open series. Am J Gastroenterol 1993; 88:2000-2008.
174. Cotton PB. Endoscopic methods for relief of malignant obstructive jaundice. World J Surg 1984; 8:854-861.
175. Huibregtse K, Katon RM, Coene PP, Tytgat GNJ. Endoscopic palliative treatment in pancreatic cancer. Gastrointest Endosc 1986; 32:334-338.
176. Siegel JH, Snady H. The significance of endoscopically placed prostheses in the management of biliary obstruction due to carcinoma of the pancreas: results of nonoperative decompression in 277 patients. Am J Gastroenterol 1986; 81:634-641.
177. Brandabur JJ, Kozarek RA, Ball TJ, Hofer BO, Ryan JA, Traverso LW, Freeny PC, Lewis GP. Nonoperative veruse operative treatment of obstructive jaundice in pancreatic cancer: Cost and survival analysis. Am J Gastroenterol. 1988; 83:1132-1139.
178. Sheperd HA, Royle G, Ross APR, Diba A, Arthur M, Colin-Jones D. Endoscopic biliary endoprosthesis in the palliation of malignant obstruction of the distal common bile duct —a randomised trial. Br J Surg 1988; 75:1166-1168.

179. Deviere J, Baize M, DeToeuf J, Cremer M. Long term follow-up of patients with hilar malignant stricture treated by endoscopic internal biliary drainage. Gastrointest Endosc 1988; 34:95-101.
180. Andersen JR, Sorensen SM, Kruse A, Rokkjaer M, Matzen P. Randomised trial of endoscopic endoprosthesis versus operative bypass in malignant obstructive jaundice. Gut 1989; 30:1132-1135.
181. Dowsett JF, Russell RCG, Hatfield ARW, Cotton PB, Speer AG, Houghton J, Lennon T, Stanesby L, Macrae K, Ahern R. Malignant obstructive jaundice: What is the best management? A prospective randomised trial of surgery vs. endoscopic stenting. Gut 1989; 30:128.
182. Cullingford GL, Srinivasan R, Carr-Locke DL. Endoscopic endoprosthesis for malignant biliary obstruction. Gut 1989; 30:A1458.
183. Mizuma Y, Ikeda E, Mukai H, Yasuda K, Nakajima M. ERBD vs PTBD in the managment of inoperable malignant obstructive jaundice. Gastroenteroly 1992; 102:A323.
184. Boender J, Nix GA, Schutte HE, Lameris JS, van Blankenstein M, Dees J. Malignant common bile duct obstruction: factors influencing the success rate of endoscopic drainage. Endoscopy 1992; 22:259-262.
185. Marsh WH, Cunningham JT. Endoscopic stent placement for obstructive jaundice secondary to metastatic malignancy. Am J Gastroenterol 1992; 87: 985-990.
186. Motte S, Deviere J, Dumonceau J-M, Serruys E, Thys J-P, Cremer M. Risk factors for septicemia following endoscopic biliary stenting. Gastroenterology 1991; 101:1374-1381.
187. Clarke BD, Lehman GA. «Cloggology» revisited: endoscopic or surgical decompression of malignant biliary obstruction. Am J Gastroenterolory 1990; 85:1533-1534.
188. Kadakia SC, Starnes E. Comparison of 10 Fr stent with 11.5 French gauge stent in patients with biliary tract diseases. Gastrointest Endosc 1992; 38:454-459.
189. Leung JWC, Ling TKW, Kung JLS, Vallance-Owen J. The role of bacteria in the blockage of biliary stents. Gastrointest Endosc 1988; 34:19-22.
190. Huibregtse K. Endoscopic Biliary and Pancreatic Drainage. Stuttgart: Georg Thieme, 1988.
191. Speer AG, Cotton PB, Rhode J, Seddon AM, Neal CR, Holton J, Costerton JW. Biliary stent blockage with bacterial biofilm. Ann Intern Med 1988; 108:546-553.
192. Speer AG, Cotton PB, MacRae KD. Endoscopic management of malignant biliary obstruction: stents of 10 French gauge are preferable to stents of 8 French gauge. Gastrointest Endosc 1988; 34:412-417.
193. Coene PPLO. Endoscopic Biliary Stenting: Mechanisms and possible solutions of the clogging phenomenon. MD Thesis. Den Haag: CIP-DATA Koninklijke Bibliotheek den Haag, 1990.
194. Sung JY, Shaffer EA, Lam K, Costerton JW. Inhibition of *E. coli* adhesion on biliary stents by bile salts with different hydrobicities. Gastrointest Endosc 1992; 38:263.
195. Hurwich DB, Poterucha JJ, Nixon DE, Cockerill FR, Moyer TP, Thistle JL. Preventing biliary stent occlusion. Gastrointest Endosc 1992; 38:263.
196. Seitz U, Vadeyar H, Soehendra N. Prolonged Patency with a New-Design Teflon Biliary Prosthesis. Endoscopy 1994; 26:478-482.
197. Johanson JF, Frakes JT. Optimal timing for stent replacement in malignant biliary strictures. Gastrointest Endosc 1992; 38:254.
198. Cessot F, Sauterau D, Le Sidaner A, Moesch C, Berry P, Florence J, Deviois B, Pillegand B. Obstruction delay of biliary endoprostheses. Gastroenteroly 1992; 102:A304.
199. Soehendra N. A new method for exchanging biliary stents. Endoscopy 1990; 22:271-272.
200. Yoshioka T, Sakaguchi H, Yoshimura H, Tamada T, Ohishi H, Uchida H, Wallace S. Expandable metallic biliary endoprostheses: preliminary clinical evaluation. Radiology 1990; 177:253-7.
201. Lammer J. Biliary endoprosthesis, plastic versus metal stents. Radiol Clin North Am 1990; 28:1211-1222.
202. Knyrim K, Wagner HJ, Starck E, Hertberg A, Pausch J, Vakil N. Metall oder Kunststoffendoprosthesen bei malignem Verschulssikterus. Ein randomisierter und prospektiver Vergleich. Dtsch Med Wochenschr 1992; 117:847-853.
203. Kozarek RA, Ball TJ, Patterson DJ. Metallic self-expanding stent application in the upper gastrointestinal tract: caveats and concerns. Gastrointest Endosc 1992; 38:1-6.
204. Salomonowitz EK, Antonucci F, Heer M, Stuckmann G, Egloff B, Zollikofer CL. Biliary obstruction: treatment with self-expanding metal prostheses. J Vasc Interv Radiol 1992; 3:365-370.
205. Jackson JE, Roddie ME, Chetty N, Benjamin IS, Adam A. The management of occluded metallic self-expandable biliary endoprostheses. Am J Roentgenol 1991; 157:291-292.
206. Nicholson DA, Chetty N, Jackson JE, Roddie ME, Adam A. Patency of side branches after peripheral placement of metallic biliary endoprostheses. J Vasc Interv Radiol 1992; 3:127-130.
207. Shim CS, Lee MS, Kim JH, Cho SW. Endoscopic application of Gianturco-Rosch biliary Z-stent. Endoscopy 1992; 24:436-439.
208. Kawase Y, Takemura T, Hashimoto T. Endoscopic implantation of expandable metal Z stents for malignant biliary strictures. Gastrointest Endosc 1993; 39:65-67.
209. Neuhaus H, Hagenmuller F, Classen M. Self-expanding biliary stents, preliminary clinical experience. Endoscopy 1989; 21:225-228.
210. Bethge N, Wagner HJ, Knyrim K, Zimmerman HB, Starck E, Pausch J, Vakil N. Technical Failure of Biliary Metal Stent Deployment in a Series of 116 Applications. Endoscopy 1992; 24:395-400.
211. Huibregtse K, Carr-Locke DL, Cremer M, et al. Bi-

liary Stent Occlusion —A Problem Solved with Self-Expanding Metal Stents? Endoscopy 1992; 24:391-394.
212. Cotton PB. Metallic Mesh Stents —Is the expanse worth the expense? Endoscopy 1992; 24:421-423.
213. Carr-Locke DL, Ball TJ, Connors PJ, Cotton PB, Geenen JE, Hawes RH, Jowell PS, Kozarek RA, Lehman GA, Meier PB, Ostroff JW, Shapiro HA, Silvis SE, Vennes JA. Multicenter randomized trial of Wallstent biliary endoprosthesis versus plastic stents. Gastrointest Endosc 1993; 39:310.
214. Davids PHP, Groen AK, Rauws EAJ, Tytgat GNJ, Huibregtse K. Randomized trial of self-expanding metal stents versus polyethylene stents for distal malignant biliary obstruction. Lancet 1992; 340:1488-1492.
215. Cremer M, Deviere J, Sugai B, Baize M. Expandable biliary metal stents for malignancies: endoscopic insertion and diathermic cleaning for tumor ingrowth. Gastrointest Endosc 1990; 36:451-457.
216. Dertinger S, Ell C, Fleig WE, Hochberger J, Karn M, Gurza L, Hahn EG. Long-term results using self-expanding metal stents for malignant biliary obstruction. Gastroenteroly 1992; 102:A310.
217. Sievert CE, Silvis SE, Vennes JA, Abeyta B, Brennecke LH. Comparison of covered vs uncovered wire stents in the canine biliary tract. Gastrointest Endosc 1992; 38:A262.
218. Goldin E, Wengrower D, Fich A, Safra T, Verstandig A, Globerman O, Beyar M. A new self-expandable and removable metal stent for biliary obstruction. Gastrointest Endosc 1992; 38:A251.

Surgical Treatment for Hepatocellular Carcinoma

M. Makuuchi

INTRODUCTION

During the last 30 years, great progress has been made in surgical resection of the liver. In the 1970s, four major hepatectomy procedures for patients without impaired liver function, but large tumors were established, namely right trisegmentectomy, right hepatectomy, left hepatectomy and left lateral segmentectomy (1). In the '80s, the following minor hepatectomies for small hepatocellular carcinoma with liver cirrhosis were developed: limited resection (2), subsegmentectomy (3), and segmentectomies (4, 5, 6). These small anatomical resections for liver cirrhosis involve a wider area of liver transection than major liver resections and they are more difficult to perform than the four conventional hepatectomy procedures described above. Small anatomical resections and limited resections without injuring major vessels, which should be preserved to maintain the function of the remaining liver, have become possible due to the introduction of intraoperative ultrasonography (7) and of vascular occlusion techniques for the cirrhotic liver. With the use of these procedures, systematic subsegmentectomy (3) and hepatectomies preserving the inferior right hepatic vein (8) were developed.

OUR EXPERIENCE OF HEPATECTOMY

During the last 14 years, we have laparotomized 1,301 patients for hepatectomy and hepatic resection was carried out in 1,188 of them. Therefore, the resectability was 91.4%. Hepatocellular carcinoma (HCC) was seen in 781 patients (60.0%) and the resectability of HCC was 93.3%. Of the patients with HCC, 556 (76.3%) had small HCCs less than 5 cm in diameter and 95.3% of them underwent hepatic resection.

SELECTION OF OPERATIVE PROCEDURES

Our criteria for hepatic resection are very simple (9): ascites, the serum total bilirubin level and the indocyanine green retention rate at 15 min (ICG 15 min, fig. 1). The indocyanine green plasma disappearance rate (K-ICG) is also calculated. The presence of ascites is a critical sign for hepatectomy and if it cannot be controlled easily with diuretics, hepatectomy is not indicated. The second parameter analyzed is serum bilirubin. Hepatic resection is not carried out when serum the total bilirubin persistently exceeds 2 mg/dl, with the single exception of patients with a tumor thrombus in the bile duct that causes obstructive jaundice. Limited resection and enucleation of the tumor can be performed in patients whose serum total bilirubin levels range from 1.1 to 1.4 mg/dl and from 1.5 to 1.9 mg/dl, respectively. When the total bilirubin value is normal, the ICG 15 min and K-ICG are used as parameters to select the type of hepatectomy. Right trisegmentectomy or right hepatectomy, which involve removing two thirds or more of the total non-cancerous liver, can be carried out if the ICG 15 min is less than 10% (K-ICG > 0.15 min). One third of the liver parenchyma can be resected in patients with an

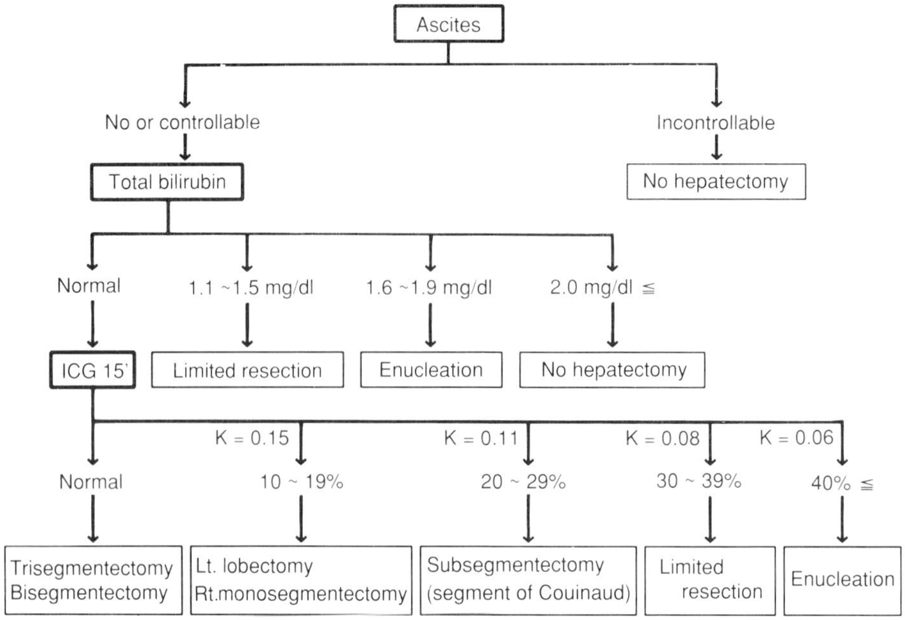

Fig. 1. Indications for hepatectomy and selection of operative procedures for patients with HCC and liver cirrhosis (9 with permission).

ICG 15 min value within the range 10 to 19% and the procedures used to do this are right posterior and anterior segmentectomies (right lateral and paramedian sectoriectomies) and left hepatectomy. For patients with an ICG 15 min value within the range of 20 to 29%, the segments of Couinaud are removed. Limited resection is indicated in patients whose ICG 15 min values are 30 to 39% and when the ICG 15 min value exceeds 40%, enucleation is performed.

PERIOPERATIVE CARE

The operation should not be carried out immediately after admission of patients with chronic hepatitis and liver cirrhosis. Two to three weeks of bed rest can improve the patient's general condition and decrease the serum transaminases value. If transaminases do not fall below 100 IU/l after bed rest, a central venous catheter is introduced and glucose solution together with glycyrrhizin are administered. Respiratory training and intestinal cleaning are carried out and a diuretic (potassium canrenonate, about 10 mg × ICG 15 min value) is administered.

Before starting liver transection, the level of anesthesia must be sufficient to decrease the thoracic and right atrial pressures. The respiratory tidal volume is kept at a minimal level by increasing the respiratory rate. This form of anesthetic management is most important to reduce backbleeding from the hepatic veins, which is the main cause of bleeding during inflow blood occlusion caused by the Pringle maneuver or selective vascular occlusion.

Intraoperative infusion of sodium should be restricted because considerable amounts of fresh frozen plasma (FFP), which has a high sodium content are used. The amount of blood and ascites lost is replaced by FFP, the amount of which transfused exceeds the amount of blood lost by 10 to 20%. When the hematocrit value is below 30%, whole blood is administered first. The total amount of fluid infused should be restricted to 4 ~ 4.5 ml/kg/h.

In patients who receive potassium canrenonate, the serum potassium levels should be checked carefully postoperatively. If potassium levels exceed 4.0 mEq/l just after hepatectomy, potassium-free solution is given. Acidosis due to transfusion is not corrected, because it converts to alkalosis spontaneously within 12 h after the operation and, moreover, the use of bicarbonate results in excessive sodium infusion. Bleeding from the drain and discharge of ascites are monitored. If blood loss exceeds 100 ml/h, excluding ascites, reoperation is indicated. About 15 ml/kg/day FFP is given until the total protein value reaches 6.5 g/dl. As an excess of FFP is given when a large volume of ascites is discharged, sodium-free electrolyte solution is infused at about 1 ml/kg/h. The total amount of water, including FFP, is restricted to 40 ~ 45 ml/kg/day. Adequate insulin should be administered to control the serum glucose level. Whole blood is not transfused postoperatively until the hematocrit value falls to 20%. Chloride-rich amino acid solution is administered to correct alkalosis and when the FFP transfusion is stopped this amino acid solution is switched to an acid-base-balanced one.

NEED FOR AND RESULTS WITH INTRAOPERATIVE ULTRASONOGRAPHY

Since the late 70s, patients with small HCC have been referred to hepatic surgeons. The first problem with resection of small HCC we encountered was that a considerable number of patients with cirrhosis had invisible and non-palpable HCCs (10). Of 781 patients with HCC, 368 (47.1%) had at least one invisible, non-palpable main HCC nodule. Four-hundred and one patients had a small HCC less than 5 cm in diameter and liver cirrhosis and 261 (65.1%) of them had at least one invisible, non-palpable HCC nodule. Intraoperative ultrasonography revealed these nodules with the surrounding vascular structures clearly. When a patient was referred to us by a hepatologist and the hepatic surgeon could not resect the tumor because of failure to identify its site, it was considered shameful. After returning the patient to the hepatologist, who then carried out further angiography, which often demonstrated a larger HCC, the hepatologist might never refer the patient to the surgeon again. Therefore, intraoperative ultrasonography became accepted and its use spread among Japanese and European surgeons in the early 80s.

Of 799 main small HCC nodules, preoperative ultrasonography, computed tomography and angiography detected 86.0, 86.5 and 73.0% respectively, whereas intraoperative ultrasonography revealed 97.9%. Hitherto, angiography was believed to be the most sensitive diagnostic modality because HCCs are hypervascular tumors. However, as small HCC nodules are often hypovascular and cirrhotic nodules are revealed as faintly stained areas, it is far more difficult to demonstrate small HCCs using arteriography than ultrasonography and computed tomography.

A tumor thrombus is one of the most common forms of tumor extension in patients with HCC. Among 781 patients with HCC who underwent surgery, 101 tumor thrombi were identified in 79 (10.1%) by perioperative examinations and found in the resected specimens. Preoperative ultrasonography demonstrated 28% of these thrombi and angiography, including arterial portography, disclosed 18%. Hepatic venography was performed in virtually no patients. Of the 101 tumor thrombi, 75 were located in the portal venous branches, 21 were budding into the hepatic veins, 4 were in the bile duct and one was located in the epiploic vein where the greater omentum adhered. Four of the 21 tumor thrombi in the hepatic veins were growing into the short hepatic veins. During pre- and intraoperative ultrasound examination, not only the portal venous branches in the liver but also the hepatic veins, including the short hepatic veins, and the bile duct should be scanned carefully.

Other uses of intraoperative ultrasound are demonstration of the transected plane of the liver (11) and intraoperative ultrasound-guided puncture techniques (7). As the transection line of the liver can be demonstrated clearly with ultrasound, we can assess the direction of liver transection and identify the vessels which appear on the divided surface of the liver and their positions accurately (fig. 2). The ultrasound-guided intraoperative puncture technique can facilitate puncture of the ductal structure of the liver and the tumor to enable biopsy specimens to be taken.

The findings described above show that intraoperative ultrasonography is indispensable as the final and definitive diagnostic procedure for patients with HCC undergoing hepatectomy and as a direct guide for hepatectomy procedu-

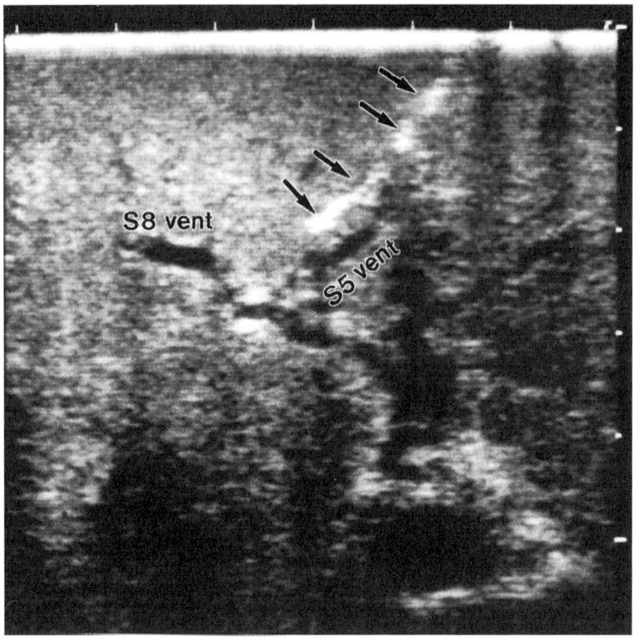

Fig. 2. Intraoperative ultrasonic demonstration of the transected surfaces of the liver. The divided surfaces of the liver appear as an echogenic line (arrows). The division of liver parenchyma will be reached to the bifurcation of the ventral branches of the S8 and S5 after it will be proceeded 1 cm more. S8 vent; Ventral branch of segment 8, S5 vent; ventral branch of segment 5. (Cited from Makuuchi M. Segmentectomy and Subsegmentectomy. In: Lygidakis NJ, Makuuchi M, eds. Pitfalls and Complications in the Diagnosis and Management of Hepatectomy and Pancreatic Diseases. Stuttgart: Thieme, 1993; 133-145, with permission.)

res. Now, performing hepatectomy without the assistance of intraoperative ultrasonography is unacceptable from both the medical and ethical points of view.

SYSTEMATIC SUBSEGMENTECTOMY

When HCC invades the portal venous branch, cancer cells become detached from the tumor, enter the blood stream and are carried to the distal branches. Then, some of them form daughter nodules or intrahepatic metastases (fig. 3). If an arterio-portal shunt and tumor thrombus are both present, tumor cells are regurgitated into the portal vein and spread over an even wider area (3). Therefore, the portal venous branch feeding the tumor should be ligated at some distance from the tumor. The ligation point should be as far from the tumor as the liver function permits and the liver parenchyma belonging to the ligated portal venous branch should be removed completely. Systematic subsegmentectomy was developed for this purpose.

When the systematic subsegmentectomy procedure is performed, the area containing the tumor is scanned by intraoperative ultrasound to evaluate the three-dimensional nature of the tumor and vessels. The feeding portal venous branch is punctured under ultrasound guidance at the point distal to where the portal venous branch is to be ligated (fig. 4) and blue dye is injected, which stains the surface of the hepatic portal unit containing the tumor, the stained area is marked with electrocautery and tattooing is carried out to identify the ligation point of the vessels. The liver is divided under hemihepatic vascular occlusion, and when the anterosuperior area has been totally resected, the whole lengths of the right and middle hepatic veins are exposed (fig. 5). The systematic sub-

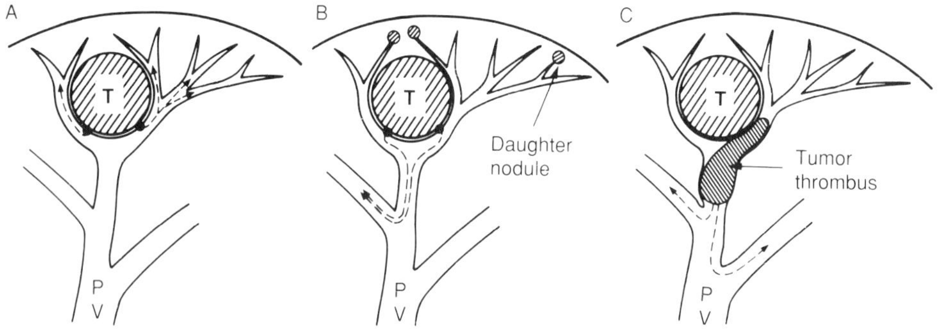

Fig. 3. Intrahepatic extension of HCC. A) A tumor invades the portal venous branches and tumor cells are carried to the periphery. B) These cells form microscopic tumor thrombi and then intrahepatic metastases. C) Tumor thrombi are also a source of wider tumor spread. T: tumor; PV: portal venous branch (3 with permission).

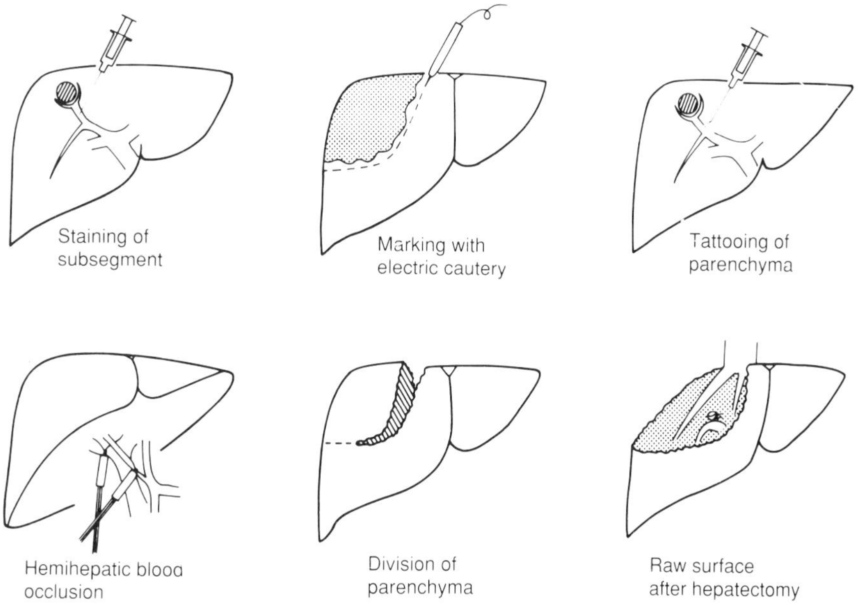

Fig. 4. Systematic subsegmentectomy opertive procedure (3 with permission).

segmentectomy procedure led to the introduction of the concept of anatomical resection involving hepatectomy smaller than Healey's segment in the right lobe.

The survival rates of patients who undergo systematic subsegmentectomy is significantly better than that after limited resection (fig. 6).

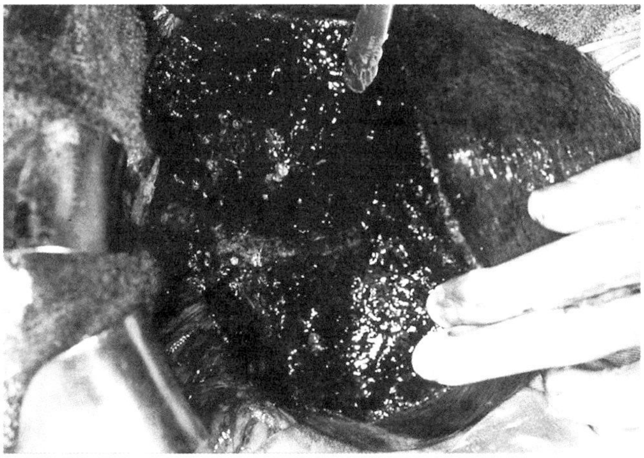

Fig. 5. The raw surface of the liver beyond segment 8 has been resected completely. (Cited from Makuuchi M. Segmentectomy and Subsegmentectomy. In: Lygidakis NJ, Makuuchi M, eds. Pitfalls and Complications in the Diagnosis and Management of Hepatobiliary and Pancreatic Diseases. Stuttgart: Thieme, 1993;133-145, with permission.)

HEPATECTOMIES PRESERVING THE INFERIOR RIGHT HEPATIC VEIN

Hepatectomies preserving the inferior right hepatic vein were also developed as a result of the introduction of intraoperative ultrasonography (8). In adition to the three principal (right, middle, and left) hepatic veins, there are several short hepatic veins. One of these the inferior right hepatic vein, which drains the dorsal part of segment 6, is thick in about 20 to 25% of patients. If the right hepatic vein is resected from its confluence to the inferior vena cava, segment 6 cannot be preserved in patients with the normal hepatic venous system pattern due to congestion. However, in patients with a thick inferior right hepatic vein, even if it is resected, segment 6 can be preserved.

Four types of operation preserving the inferior right hepatic vein, shown in figure 7, have been described. Type A involves resecting segments 7 and 8 together with the right hepatic vein. In the type B hepatectomy, the right anterior segment and segment 7 together with the right hepatic vein are removed. The type C resection involves taking out the left medial and right anterior segments, segment 7 and the middle and right hepatic veins. In the type D

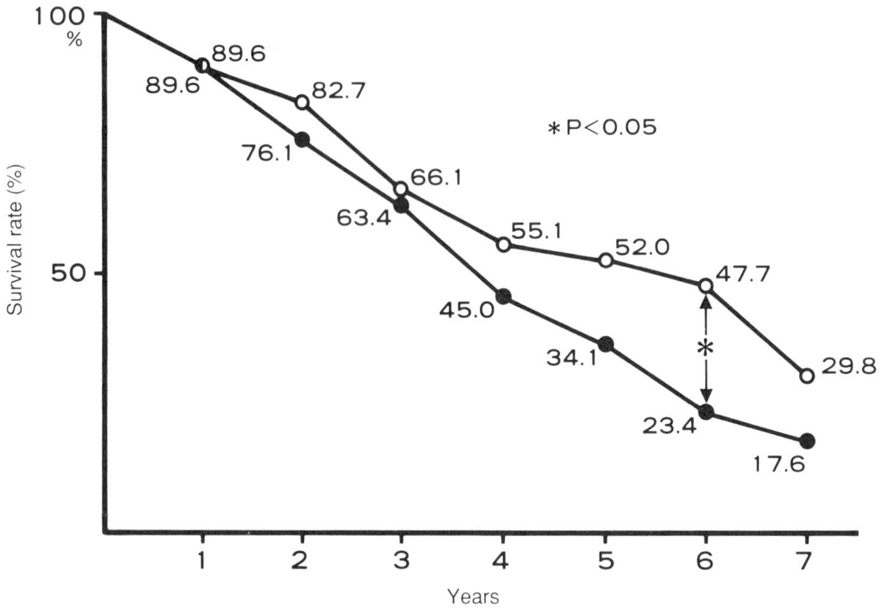

Fig. 6. Survival curves after systematic subsegmentectomy and limited resection. Survival is better after systematic subsegmentectomy (open circles) than limited resection (closed circles) and the difference is significant at 6 years postoperatively.

operation, the left trisegments and segment 7 with the right, middle, and left hepatic veins are removed *en bloc*. We carried out the A, B and C types of operation in the early 1980s, but have not tried yet the type D hepatectomy, which was first described by Baer et al. in 1991 (12). These

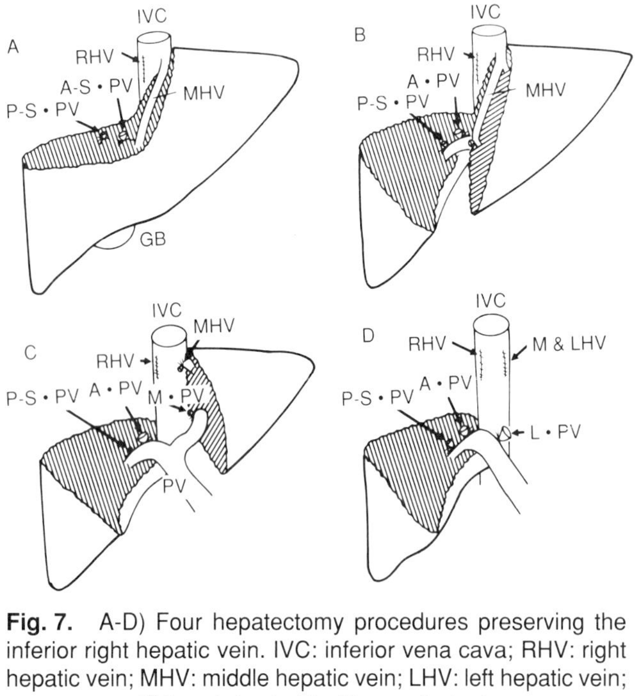

Fig. 7. A-D) Four hepatectomy procedures preserving the inferior right hepatic vein. IVC: inferior vena cava; RHV: right hepatic vein; MHV: middle hepatic vein; LHV: left hepatic vein; PV: portal vein (8 with permission).

somewhat complicated hepatectomy procedures became possible with the advent of intraoperative ultrasonography.

RESULTS WITH VASCULAR OCCLUSION TECHNIQUES

Until the 70s, it was believed that if vascular occlusion was used in patients with liver cirrhosis, post-operative liver dysfunction would follow. I thought that this was superstition and started to use hemihepatic (selective) vascular occlusion in 1980 (13). When the resection area extended to both sides of the liver, alternate hemihepatic vascular occlusion was undertaken. The aim of this procedure was to enable metabolism by one side of the liver to continue and minimize portal congestion. In patients who underwent hemihepatic vascular occlusion, the mean blood loss was lower (1,500 ml) as compared with hepatectomy without vascular occlusion (3,000 ml). Postoperative serum total bilirubin levels were also significantly lower and serum transaminase levels were unchanged or fell (14).

In the light of these data, it was speculated that if the volume of blood transfused was reduced, the increase in serum bilirubin levels could be suppressed. Therefore, the non-transfusion protocol was introduced (15, 16). With this protocol, whole blood is not transfused unless the hematocrit declines to 30% during the operation and 20% during the postoperative course. The blood lost is replaced by FFP. As a low hematocrit induces a hyperdynamic state, a volume of FFP 10 to 20% greater than the calculated amount of blood lost is transfused. The mean postoperative serum total bilirubin level after this protocol was significantly lower than that in patients who received blood transfusions. If severe pancreatitis develops after hepatectomy in cirrhotic patients, the prognosis is very poor. Therefore, we must select an operative procedure which does not result in increased postoperative serum amylase levels. The postoperative serum amylase level was compared with the preoperative level in patients with impaired liver function who underwent the Pringle maneuver or hemihepatic vascular occlusion. The mean postoperative amylase levels were significantly higher than the preoperative values in the former, but not in the latter. This may have been due to increased portal pressure during clamping of the hepatoduodenal ligament involved in the Pringle maneuver, which should be avoided, if possible, especially in patients with severe liver cirrhosis.

With the vascular occlusion techniques and non-transfusion protocol, 75~80% of hepatectomized patients do not receive blood transfusions and several do not even receive blood when extended right hepatectomy together with pancreatoduodenectomy is carried out. Since 1985, the operative mortality after hepatectomy in patients with cirrhosis has been less than 1%.

Fresh blood was used in such patients, because transfusion of blood stored for more than 3 days or packed red blood cells tended to increase serum bilirubin levels. The survival rate of patients who did not receive blood transfusions was found to be significantly better than that of those who did (17). When the blood loss was limited to 1,000 to 1,500 ml, the recurrence-free survival rate of the non-transfusion group was significantly better than that of the transfusion group (fig. 8). Some immunological factors may affect survival, which occurs with other types of cancer.

The use of vascular occlusion techniques and the non-transfusion protocol has decreased the operative mortality and improved long-term survival rates of patients with HCC.

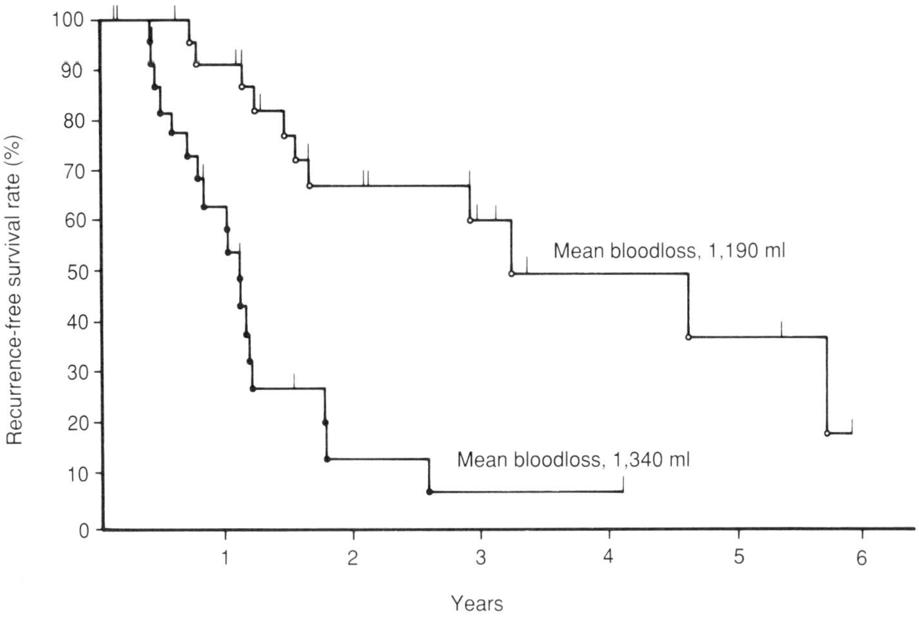

Fig. 8. Difference between recurrence-free survival after hepatic resection of patients who received blood transfusions (closed circles) and those who did not (open circles).

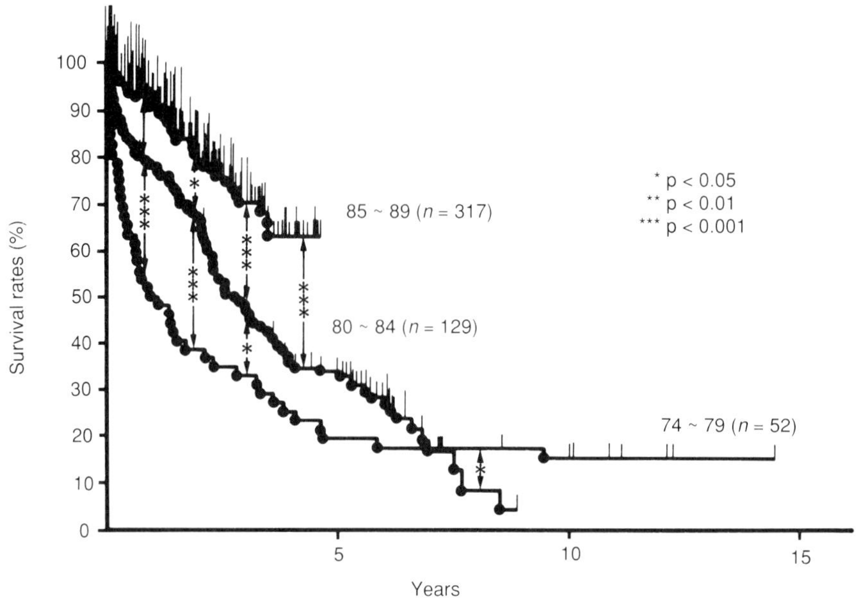

Fig. 9. Year trends of survival after hepatectomy.

SURVIVAL AFTER HEPATECTOMY

The survival rates of 498 patients with HCC who underwent hepatectomy in the National Cancer Center in Tokyo from 1974 to 1989 were 83.1, 57.2 and 40.6% after one, three and five years respectively. The survival decline slowed down slightly after four years, but did not stop until eight years. This may be due mainly to development of second and third primary lesions.

In our experience, after the late 80s, most of the resected HCCs were less than 5 cm in diameter. The survival rate five years after hepatectomy of patients with small HCC (≤ 5 cm) ranged from 35 to 50%. Reports from People's Republic of China quote a survial rate over 60% (9).

Prognostic factors associated with small HCC (≤ 5 cm) have been reported many authors. The tumor size, number of tumors, intrahepatic metastasis and vascular invasion have been generally accepted as significant prognostic factors. In our experience, liver cirrhosis, operative procedure and Edmondson-Steiner's grade are also significant (9). Other than these, year trends were one of the most important prognostic factors. Figure 9 shows survival curves for the '70s, '80 to '84, and '85 to '89. They clearly shift progressively to the right and differ significantly from each other. This was due to early detection, introduction of transcatheter arterial embolization (TAE) and improvements in surgical techniques, including intraoperative ultrasonography, vascular occlusion techniques and repeated resections.

EARLY HEPATOCELLULAR CARCINOMA

During laparotomy, intraoperative ultrasonography can demonstrate many new nodules not detected by preoperative examinations. However, ultrasound cannot define the histological nature of minute foci in the liver. In order to establish the histological nature of minute nodules, intraoperative thick needle (14G Trucut needle) biopsy has been carried out and large core specimens subjected to histological examinations. As a result of this thick needle biopsy and resection for minute nodules together with DNA analysis for the integration site of the HB virus, a new concept of early HCC has been established (18). The characteristics of early HCC are: *a*) lack of a fibrous capsule, *b*) contains Glissonean triads, and *c*) some part of the tumor consists of very well differentiated HCC (Edmondson-Steiner's grade I) and peripheral parts of the nodule are occupied by adenomatous hyperplasia. Most early HCCs were not enhanced by contrast media used for angiography and bolus injection computed tomographic

(CT) scaning (19) and differential diagnosis of borderline lesions and early HCC was found to be difficult using frozen and paraffin sections.

Large cirrhotic or hyperplastic nodules may undergo transformation to HCC. When the pathologist classified a nodule as atypical adenomatous hyperplasia or adenomatous hyperplasia with dysplastic changes, 10 of 24 such nodules transformed into HCC during the postoperative followup period. If the pathological diagnosis was a large regenerative nodule or adenomatous hyperplasia, 8 of 33 nodules transformed into HCC. Takayama et al found that the time for the nodule to become transformed to HCC became shorter as the cellularity and diameter of the nodule increased. The transformation index (the product of the diameter and cellularity of the nodule) and time required for transformation correlated significantly (20).

SELECTION OF TREATMENT MODALITY FOR MINUTE HCC

Recently, several authors claimed that percutaneous ethanol injection therapy (PEIT) could produce complete necrosis of small HCC and the prognosis associated with PEIT was equal to or better than that with surgical resection in patients with tumors no more than 3 cm in diameter and no more than 3 nodules (21, 22). During the last 5 years, data on more than 3,000 patients with HCC were collected by our study group which was sponsored by the Ministry of Health and Welfare of Japan and directed by Ryu. Figure 10 shows the survival curves of patients with tumors no more than 3 cm in diameter and no more than 3 nodules after undergoing hepatic resection, TAE and PEIT. During the first 3 years, PEIT yielded better survival rates than surgery, but after 3 years, the PEIT survival curve declined very rapidly and showed the same tendency as that of TAE. The mortality associated with PEIT was almost zero, whereas that with hepatectomy was 5%. As for background factors, the tumors treated by PEIT were smaller, there were fewer nodules and the PEIT group included patients with a higher rate of early HCC, and inevitably, this group included borderline lesions. The better or almost identical survival with PEIT compared with hepatic resection during the early phase is dependent on these factors, but the true efficacy of

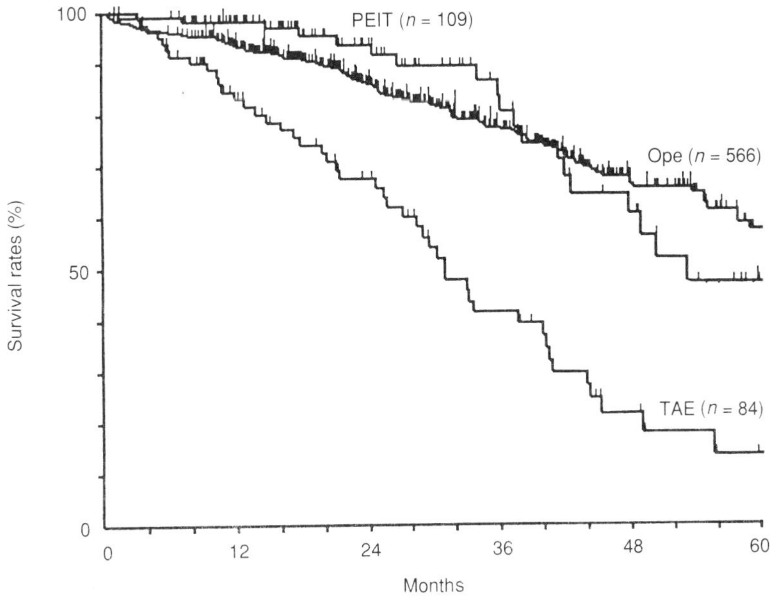

Fig. 10. Difference between survival rate of patients with tumors 1 to 3 cm in diameter and no more than 3 nodules treated by hepatic resection (Ope) trans-arterial embolization (TAE), and percutaneous ethanol injection therapy (PEIT). (Cited from the Reports on Projects of the Comprehensive Ten-year Strategy of Cancer Control sponsored by the Ministry of Health and Welfare of Japan, 1993; 176-181.)

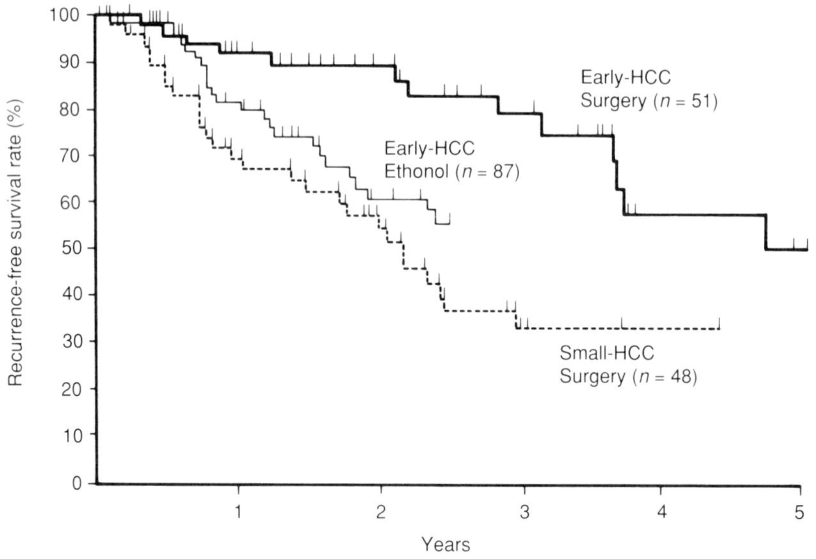

Fig. 10. Difference between recurrence-free survivals of patients with early HCC treated by surgery and PEIT. For reference, the recurrence-free survival curve after surgery in patients with conventional HCC (Edmondson-Steiner's grade II-IV) is shown. (These data originated from Dr. Michiie Sakamoto Department of Pathology, National Cancer Center Institute, Director of the Study Group on Minute Liver Cancer stonsored by the Ministory of Health and Welfare of Japan with permission.)

PEIT was apparent after three years when it was almost identical to that of TAE. Moreover, in our experience, the 5 year survival after surgical resection of early HCC is 100%. The relapse-free survival rate of patients with early HCC after hepatic resection was significantly better than that after PEIT in the study conducted by Sakamoto and his group (fig. 11).

Therefore, it can be concluded that surgery is the first-choice treatment, even for early HCCs, and the indications for PEIT are limited, especially in institutions where experienced hepatic surgeons are available.

CONCLUSIONS

In our experience of more than 1,000 hepatectomies, mortality after hepatectomy has declined markedly since 1980. Now, mortality, including hospital mortality, is less than 1%, even in patients with liver cirrhosis. This is due to the introduction of vascular occlusion techniques, the non-transfusion protocol and intraoperative ultrasonography and improved perioperative care. New operative procedures, such as systematic subsegmentectomy, hepatectomies preserving the inferior right hepatic vein, preoperative portal embolization and repeated hepatic resections have expanded the indications for hepatectomy and improved postoperative survival rates. Surgical resection is still the first-choice treatment for patients with minute and early HCCs. Liver transplantation can be considered as a surgical treatment for HCC, but due to the shortage of donors and the poorer prognosis of patients with HCC than benign hepatobiliary diseases, liver transplantation is unlikely to be carried out in such patients until the problem of organ procurement is solved.

REFERENCES

1. Fortner JG, Maclean BJ, Kim DK, Howland WS, Turnbull AD, Goldiner P, Carlon G, Beattie EJ Jr. The seventies evolution in liver surgery for cancer. Cancer 1981; 47:2162-2166.
2. Kanematsu T, Takenaka K, Matsumata T, Furuta T, Sugimachi K, Inokuchi K. Limited hepatic resection effective for selected cirrhotic patients with primary liver cancer. Ann Surg 1984; 199:51-56.
3. Makuuchi M, Hasegawa H, Yamazaki S. Ultrasonically guided subsegmentectomy. Surg Gynecol Obstet 1985; 161:346-350
4. Hasegawa H, Makuuchi M, Yamazaki S, Gunvén P. Central bisegmentectomy of the liver:Experience in 16 patients. World J Surg 1989; 13:786-790.
5. Kawasaki S, Makuuchi M, Harada H, Takayama T, Kosuge T. A new alternative hepatectomy method for resection of segment 3 and 4 of the liver. Surg Gynecol Obstet 1992; 175:267-269.

6. Makuuchi M, Hashikura Y, Kawasaki S, Tan D, Kosuge T, Takayama T. Personal experience of right anterior segmentectomy (Segments V and VIII) for hepatic malignancies. Surgery 1993; 114:52-58.
7. Makuuchi M. Abdominal intraoperative ultrasonography. Tokyo: Igaku-Shoin, 1987.
8. Makuuchi M, Hasegawa H, Yamazaki S, Takayasu K. Four new hepatectomy procedures for resection of the right hepatic vein and preservation of the inferior right hepatic vein. Surg Gynecol Obstet 1987; 164:68-72.
9. Makuuchi M, Kosuge T, Takayama T, Yamazaki S, Kakazu T, Miyagawa S, Kawasaki S. Surgery for small liver cancers. Semin Surg Oncol 1993; 9:298-304.
10. Makuuchi M, Hasegawa H, Yamazaki S. Intraoperative ultrasonic examination for hepatectomy. Jpn J Clin Oncol 1981; 11:367-390.
11. Makuuchi M, Hasegawa H, Yamazaki S, Takayasu K, Moriyama N. The use of operative ultrasound as an aid to liver resection in patients with hepatocellular carcinoma. World J Surg 1987; 11:615-621.
12. Baer HU, Dennison AR, Maddern GJ, Blumgart LH. Subtotal hepatectomy: a new procedure based on the inferior right hepatic vein. Br J Surg 1991; 78:1221-1222.
13. Yamazaki S, Makuuchi M, Abe I, Hasegawa H. Subsegmentectomy of the liver for small hepatocellular carcinoma. Operation 1981; 35:1199-1202 (in Japanese).
14. Makuuchi M, Mori T, Gunvén P, Yamazaki S, Hasegawa H. Safety of hemihepatic vascular occlusion during resection of the liver. Surg Gynecol Obstet 1987; 64:155-158.
15. Makuuchi M, Takayama T, Gunvén P, Kosuge T, Yamazaki S, Hasegawa H. Restrictive versus liberal blood transfusion policy for hepatectomies in cirrhotic patients. World J Surg 1989; 13:644-648.
16. Miyagawa S, Makuuchi M, Kawasaki S, Kakazu T. Changes in serum amylase level following hepatic resection in chronic liver disease. Arch Surg 1994; 129:634-638.
17. Yamamoto J, Kosuge T, Takayama T, Shimada K, Yamazaki S, Ozaki H, Yamaguchi N, Mizuno S, Makuuchi M. Perioperative blood transfusion promotes recurrence of hepatocellular carcinoma after hepatectomy. Surgery 1994; 115:303-309.
18. Kanai T, Hirohashi S, Upton MP, Noguchi M, Kishi K, Makuuchi M, Yamazaki S, Hasegawa H, Takayasu K, Moriyama N, Shimosato Y. Pathology of small hepatocellular carcinoma: A proposal for a new gross classification. Cancer 1987; 60:810-819.
19. Takayasu K, Wakao F. Moriyama N, Muramatsu Y, Sakamoto M, Hirohashi S, Makuuchi M, Kosuge T, Takayama T, Yamazaki S. Response of early-stage hepatocellular carcinoma and borderline lesions to therapeutic arterial embolization. AJR 1993; 160:301-306.
20. Takayama T, Makuuchi M, Hirohashi S, Sakamoto M, Okazaki N, Takayasu K, Kosuge T, Motoo Y, Yamazaki S, Hasegawa H. Malignant transformation of adenomatous hyperplasia to hepatocellular carcinoma. Lancet 1990; 336:1153-1155.
21. Livraghi T, Bolondi L, Lazzaroni S, Marin G, Morabito A, Papaccini GL, Salmi A, Torzilli G. Percutaneous ethanol injection in cirrhosis (a study on 207 patients). Cancer 1992; 69:925-929.
22. Shiina S, Tagawa K, Unume T, Fujino H, Uta Y, Niwa Y, Hata Y, Komatsu Y, Shiratori Y, Terano A, Sugimoto T. Percutaneous ethanol injection therapy of hepatocellular carcinoma:analysis of 77 patients. AJR 1990; 155:1221-1226.

Medical Treatment of Hepatocellular Carcinoma

J. Bruix, A. Castells, L. Boix, C. Brú

INTRODUCTION

For most groups the first therapeutic option for patients diagnosed with hepatocellular carcinoma (HCC) is surgical treatment, either resection or transplantation. If these options are considered contraindicated, patients are evaluated for medical treatment, there being several options that have been proposed to be effective. However, it should be stressed that most of these therapeutic alternatives have only been evaluated in uncontrolled studies. Thus, despite the fact that each therapy may bear significant antitumoral efficacy, there is no unequivocal evidence that medical treatment improves survival. In addition, when comparing results of different authors the reader should take into account the stage at which the patients have been diagnosed and treated. As known, most of the HCC arise on hepatic cirrhosis (1) and thus, to establish the baseline status and prognosis of patients we should consider not only the characteristics of the tumor, but also the functional status of the underlying liver (2, 3). In the present chapter we mainly review those medical options, which while having a potential antitumoral efficacy, do not require a sophisticated equipment to be applied, paying special attention not only to their usefulness, but also to their impact on survival.

PERCUTANEOUS ETHANOL INJECTION (PEI)

This therapeutic approach has been developed in the last decade and has achieved wide diffusion. In addition to being highly effective, it is easy to apply and has a reduced economic cost. Ethanol injection is done under continuous ultrasound guidance using thin needles (4-6). Some authors use special needles with several distal holes to facilitate ethanol injection within the tissue (7), but the injection of ethanol can be done using a common spinal needle. The amount of ethanol injected each session varies between 1 and several ml, depending on the size of the tumor and diffusion of the ethanol within the tissue (8). After injection, ethanol diffuses within the tumor and causes some degree of tissue necrosis. After repeated injections, the treated nodule is completely infiltrated and, at that time, it may become completely necrotic (figs. 1 and 2) (8-10). It should be noted that the number of sessions needed to achieve complete necrosis depends on the size of the nodule (5), and that some HCC may present septa, which may explain why some tumors are not completely necrosed despite numerous injections (10). In that regard, there are no widely accepted criteria to define the maximum number of sessions to be applied prior to classifying a patient as a treatment failure.

After successful tumor necrosis the nodule is smaller and the fine needle biopsy shows only necrotic material. However, the best method to assess the efficacy of the treatment is dynamic computed tomography (CT) (5, 10, 11). Thereby, if ethanol has prompted cell death and vascular obliteration, there will be no contrast uptake on dynamic CT, thus reflecting the absence of vascularization and the obtention of a complete response. Angiography would be

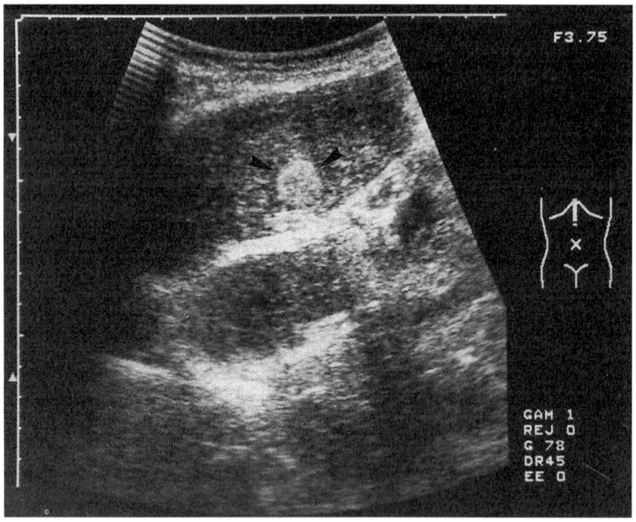

Fig. 1. Small hyperechoic hepatocellular carcinoma (arrowheads) of less than 3 cm in diameter located in the left lobe.

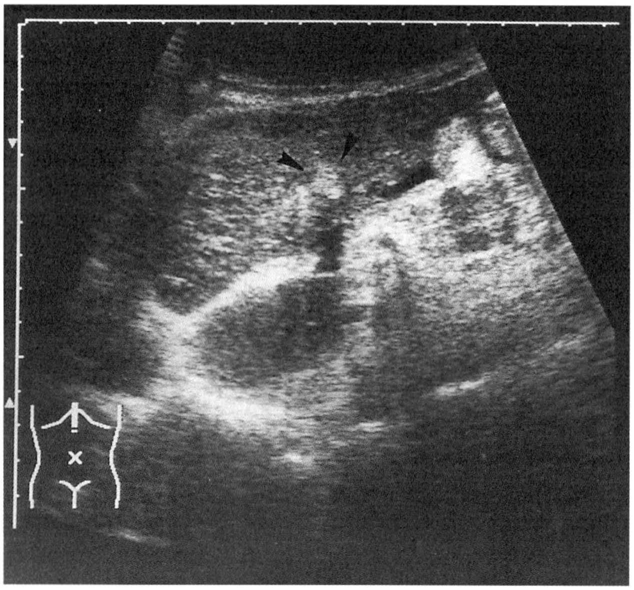

Fig. 2. After repeated injection of ethanol (6 injections) the nodule has been completely infiltrated and necrosed. The tumor has experienced a marked reduction in size (arrowheads); fine needle biopsy will obtain necrotic material and dynamic CT will show the absence of contrast uptake.

equally useful, but it is clearly more invasive (5). The usefulness of magnetic resonance (MRI) for this purpose is similar to that of dynamic CT (12).

The efficacy of PEI is mainly related to tumor size (10). While most tumors smaller than 3 cm are successfully necrosed, only a partial response can be achieved in tumors greater than 3 cm (10). Therefore it would seem appropriate to restrict PEI to those patients with solitary HCC smaller than 3 cm. However, despite this relationship between tumor size and treatment success, some groups still treat larger lesions and/or multinodular tumors (13). This requires the injection of large amounts of ethanol and/or an increase in the number of liver punctures to be done. Furthermore, injection of several ml of ethanol to treat large HCC during one session («one shot» PEI) should be done under general anesthesia (13). However, there is no evidence that treating these large/multinodular tumors with PEI really represents an advantage (both in efficacy and invasiveness) as compared to other options, such as arterial embolization, which also achieves extensive necrosis (14).

PEI is usually well tolerated (4, 5, 10). Tumor necrosis may induce non-septic fever mostly after the first ethanol injections. If patients are properly selected and have preserved clotting tests, the incidence of peritoneal bleeding is less than 10% and is usually self-limited. A third of the patients refer slight pain during ethanol injection, while severe pain due to ethanol leakage to the peritoneal cavity can be avoided by leaving the needle in place for 1-2 minutes after the injection. If the injection is not carefully monitored and/or the amount of ethanol is too high, the liquid may pass to vascular vessels inducing thrombosis. Bile duct injury is seldom encountered and finally, there are isolated reports of neoplastic seeding along the needle track (15).

After initial treatment success the patients should be carefully controlled to detect HCC recurrence, with the probability of presenting disease recurrence after 5 year follow-up exceeding 50% (16-18) and reaching 90% in some series (19). Recurrence may occur beside the treated nodule, probably reflecting the growth of unrecognized satellites, or in a different hepatic segment or lobe, reflecting either intrahepatic dissemination or the development of a second metachronic HCC. Tumoral portal thrombosis appearing after PEI may also be treated with ethanol injection (20). In some cases with successful treatment, the nodule may disappear as time goes by and to facilitate their follow-up some authors recommend the placement of a coil (7) or gelfoam (5) within the tumor in order to easily recognize the treated area after PEI.

There are no randomized studies comparing PEI against surgical resection or no treatment. Thus, most of the reports compare the outcome of PEI treated cases with that of contemporary or historical untreated subjects or patients submitted to surgical resection (16, 17, 21, 22). In most of the investigations the stage of the tumor at the time of treatment is the same, while the functional status of the liver is better preserved in surgically treated cases. However, despite this baseline difference, the survival of PEI treated cases is similar to that of operated patients, with survival reaching 50% after 5 year follow-up in some studies (16-19, 21, 22). Since the recurrence rate is also very similar after both treatments, it has been proposed that surgical resection should be substituted for PEI or, at least, restricted to those patients in whom perioperative morbidity and mortality are thought to be almost abolished.

Some authors have evaluated the usefulness of injecting agents other than ethanol. The use of boiling saline would have the advantage of its easier diffusion, the possibility of injecting a larger volume in each session without the risk of vascular damage and the absence of severe pain due to peritoneal leakage (23). Hot saline prompts heat-induced coagulation necrosis and it has been suggested to be as effective as ethanol injection (23). By contrast, the percutaneous injection of OK-432 (24), interleukin-2 and lymphokine activated killer cells (25) or chemotherapy (26) is of reduced efficacy. Finally, another approach to be evaluated is the percutaneous placement of an electrocautery with thermically induced tumor necrosis (27).

TRANSARTERIAL EMBOLIZATION

HCC receives its main blood supply through the hepatic artery and this was the rationale for the surgical ligation of this vessel as a treatment for this neoplasm. This surgical approach was abandoned because of its invasiveness, which prompted several complications. However, arterial obstruction can also be achieved during a catheterization of a peripheral artery (28). The catheter is advanced under fluoroscopic control up to the hepatic artery and after identifying the branch selectively feeding the tumor it is possible to obstruct the blood flow by injecting several agents. Most of the groups use gelatin particles (14, 28), but the usefulness of Ivalon (29), starch microspheres (30, 31), and autologous blood clots (32) have also been evaluated. The use of gelatin powder should be avoided since it may embolize very distal vessels and induce ischemic bile duct necrosis (33). Some authors combine distal embolization with gelatin with the proximal placement of a steel coil with the aim of intensifing the ischemic effect on the tumor (14, 34). There are no evidences, however, that this approach increases the efficacy (14). Hepatic artery obstruction with gelatin is frequently associated with the administration of chemotherapy mixed or not with lipiodol, aimed at combining the ischemic effect of the gelatin emboli with the toxic effect of the drugs injected, mostly adriamycin, mitomycin-C, SMANCS and cisplatin (2, 35-47). Theoretically, lipiodol would selectively place and retain the chemotherapy within the tumor, while the hepatic artery obstruction would prompt a slower elimination of the antineoplastic agents from the tumor, which results in an increased antitumoral action (46). However, there is no evidence that this so-called chemoembolization is really more effective than embolization alone (48).

TAE is usually well tolerated if patients are carefully selected. Patients submitted to TAE should have no contraindications for an arterial catheterization with administration of radiocontrast agents (severely impaired clotting tests, renal failure, advanced atheromatosis). A crucial point to be controlled prior to the procedure is the presence of a preserved portal blood flow. Accordingly, patients with portal thrombosis or hepatofugal portal blood flow or with portosystemic shunts should not be submitted to TAE, since they may develop severe hepatic failure due to acute liver ischemia. After TAE, most patients (80%) develop the so-called postembolization syndrome, which is characterised by fever, abdominal pain, nausea and, in some cases, ileus (14). This clinical picture resolves spontaneously in less than 72 hours and more severe complications such as abscess for-

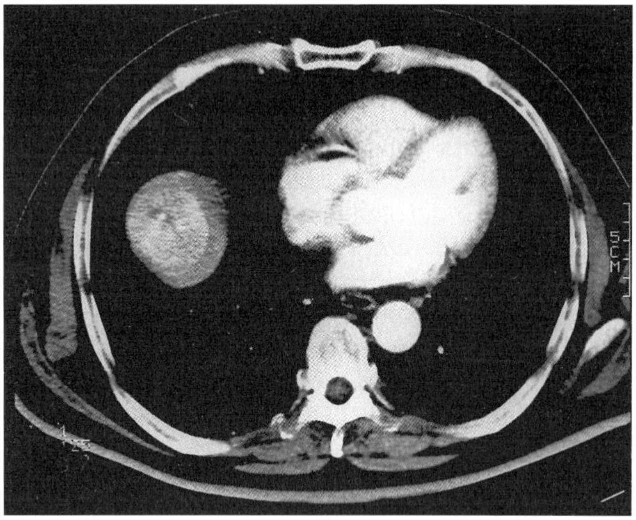

Fig. 3. Dynamic CT showing a hypervascular mass measuring 5 cm located in the dome of the right lobe.

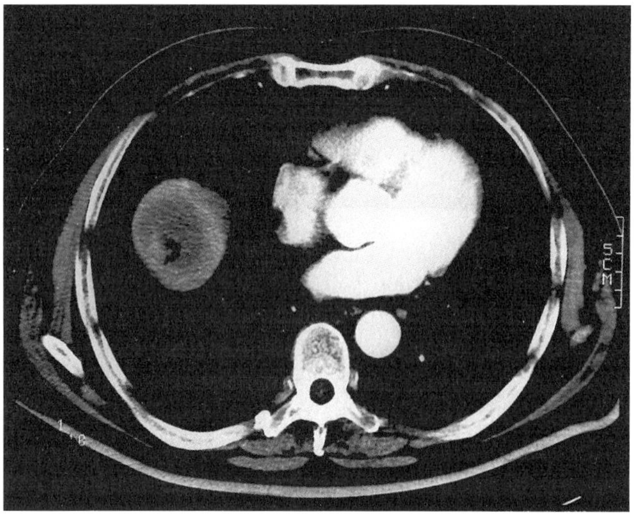

Fig. 4. After transarterial embolization the size of the tumor has been reduced and the absence of contrast enhancement on dynamic CT and the presence of bubbles reflect extensive tumor necrosis; some is recognized by the absence of contrast uptake within it.

mation, cholecystitis, liver failure or bleeding are rarely seen. Liver function is transiently impaired, but it recovers completely within one month (49). The development of fever reflects necrosis of the tumor and thus, rather than suggesting a potential infection, it constitutes a marker of treatment efficacy (50). Antibiotic prophylaxis is, therefore, not needed (50).

Whether associated to chemotherapy or not, TAE is highly effective, prompting extensive tumor necrosis with relevant tumor size reduction in 60-80% of patients (figs. 3 and 4) (14, 44, 51, 52). The highest effectiveness is achieved in nodular HCC showing the expansive pattern with capsule formation, while infiltrative or diffuse HCC are less likely to be necrosed (51-54). TAE prompts the necrosis of those parts of the tumor fed by the hepatic artery, while those nourished by the portal vein, such as the hepatic capsule and the satellites, remain alive. Furthermore, arterial collaterals develop early after hepatic artery obstruction and thus, undifferentiated clones tolerating low oxygen levels for some days may not experience necrosis. During follow-up these remnant tumor foci grow and are recognized as new tumor sites, that may merit further TAE treatment. Accordingly, repeated procedures may be performed in a given patient.

Unfortunately, there is no evidence that TAE, with or without chemotherapy, really improves survival in patients with HCC. Retrospective analyses comparing treated cases against historical untreated controls usually show increased survival (2, 14, 37), but the few available controlled studies comparing TAE or TAE plus chemotherapy against untreated controls have failed to demonstrate an improved survival (42, 55, 56). However, it should be noted that the procedure achieves partial response in most patients and this prompts slower tumor progression, which delays the appearance of tumor-related symptoms. Thus, despite the absence of a benefit in survival, TAE should be considered as an effective palliative treatment for HCC.

A clinical condition in which TAE has been shown to be highly effective is hemoperitoneum due to HCC rupture. In most patients with this severe complication, TAE is able to stop bleeding and some may thereafter benefit from elective surgical resection (57).

Some groups perform TAE prior to surgical treatment with the aim of preventing the growth of the tumor while patients are the waiting list for resection (58) or transplantation (59). However, there are no studies indicating the benefits of this policy and even some retrospective analyses have suggested that operated patients who had previously been treated with TAE have more complications during surgery and develop earlier recurrence during follow-up

(60, 61). Furthermore, chemoembolization has been associated with the appearance of sarcomatous change (62).

CHEMOTHERAPY

Several agents have been evaluated for the treatment of HCC (63-65). The results have not been encouraging with any of them. Only adriamycin and cisplatinum have been reported to induce significant and sustained positive responses, associated, however, to a high rate of side-effects (bone marrow suppression, cardiac toxicity, severe vomiting, mucositis, alopecia). To avoid them, the dosage of the drugs should be tailored to the patients liver function, with this dose reduction being associated to the loss of efficacy (66, 67). Thereby, while the rate of positive responses in patients receiving full dosage may reach 45%, the response rate in those with dose reduction is lower than 10%; the mean response rate being around 15% (63-67). The reason for the lack of antitumoral effect of chemotherapy is suggested to be due to the overexpression of the multidrug resistance gene (MDR), which prompts a rapid efflux of the anticancer agents out from the neoplastic cells (68), and it has recently been suggested that MDR gene overexpression might be mediated by p53 mutations (69).

To increase the amount of antineoplastic agent reaching the HCC and to reduce its systemic concentration and thus, side effects, some authors have administered the drugs selectively into the hepatic artery, with or without lipiodol (46, 70). This oily contrast is selectively retained within the HCC after its injection into the hepatic artery and thus, the antineoplastic agents mixed with it will also be stored within the neoplasm. However, it has been shown that adriamycin (the most frequently used agent) has a low extraction rate and therefore, after injection into the hepatic artery the first pass effect is minimal and accordingly, the systemic concentration of the drug is not diminished when compared to the intravenous route (71-74). Thereby, it has not been shown that the intra-arterial injection with or without lipiodol induces a higher response rate and/or a lower rate of side effects and/or improves survival (74, 75). Accordingly, future trials should be done to test new potentially effective drugs.

RADIOTHERAPY

The liver is sensitive to radiation and the risk of actinic toxicity precluded the use of high radiation doses above 3,000 rads, which would have achieved antitumoral effects (63, 76, 77). Using equipment that allows selective and fractionated exposure, the results are encouraging. Solitary HCC smaller than 5 cm may experience extensive necrosis and in 55% the size is reduced to less than half of its initial measurements (78). In larger HCC the antitumoral effect is almost the same, but the course of the disease is not modified. The side effects are minimal and consist in fever, anorexia and malaise (78). More severe findings are infrequent, but it must be kept in mind that the duodenum is fixed beneath the liver and depending on the location of the HCC, it is exposed to almost the same radiation as the neoplasm. Furthermore, despite being highly selective the radiation also affects the non-tumoral liver and until more data are available, this option should only be applied within research trials.

To achieve a highly selective irradiation of the tumor some authors have evaluated the efficacy of injecting yttrium-90 labeled microspheres into the hepatic artery (79) or ^{131}I-lipiodol (80). With this last option the results are promising since the rate of positive responses is high (more than half of the patients exhibit 50% tumor size reduction), whereas side-effects are minimal (80). However, it is necessary to wait for the results of controlled trials.

Another approach to achieve selective radiation is the administration of radio-labeled antibodies against components of the HCC (81, 82). The administration of ^{131}I-antialphafetoprotein or anti-ferritin antibodies has induced some positive responses and favored the use of this option in patients with advanced disease who may thereafter benefit from other treatment modalities. However, this therapy is still under debate. In addition, in repeated administrations the animal from which the antibodies are derived has to be changed, to avoid development of antibodies against the foreign proteins.

Finally, it is possible to place radioactive needles within the tumor (83). This is done under ultrasound guidance, but its efficacy is not well established and in addition, the needles to be used are thick and thus, the risk of bleeding is increased.

HORMONAL THERAPY

Sex hormone administration may favor the development of hepatic tumors and there are reports indicating the presence of sex hormone receptors in the HCC cells (84-86). However, while androgen receptors are detected in more than half of the cases, estrogen receptors are found at a significant concentration in a very low proportion of cases (84, 87). The role of these receptors in the natural history of the tumor is not known, but assuming that they may participate in the progression of the neoplasm, several authors have evaluated the potential usefulness of their blockade for the treatment of advanced HCC. Antiandrogenic therapy with several agents has never been shown to be effective, the highest reported rate of favorable responses being 20% (88-90). Moreover, the survival of HCC patients has not been shown to be improved (91). By contrast, the benefits of antiestrogenic treatment with tamoxifen, an estrogen receptor blocker, are more controversial. The drug is well tolerated and despite not inducing a noteworthy positive response (92-94), it has been suggested that chronic tamoxifen administration improves the survival of HCC patients (93, 94). Nevertheless, this has not been confirmed in a large double-blind controlled trial (95).

IMMUNOTHERAPY

Immunity is compromised in cirrhotic patients with HCC and this has prompted the evaluation of several immunomodulators such as BCG (96), interleukin and lymphokine-activated killer cells (97-103). Lymphokine-activated killer cells and recombinant interleukin-2 induce tumor size reduction in 10% of the HCC patients but this minimal benefit is associated with a high rate of side-effects (7-103). The usefulness of interferon is more controversial. Previous phase II trials failed to disclose a positive response to interferon administration (104, 105), but two recent controlled trials have reported that the survival of Interferon treated patients is significantly better as compared to patients treated with chemotherapy or to untreated controls (106, 107). Moreover, despite the usage of high doses of this agent the reported rate of side effects is negligible. Accordingly, the potential of this drug merits evaluation in large prospective trials.

REFERENCES

1. Johnson PJ, Williams R. Cirrhosis and the etiology of hepatocellular carcinoma. J Hepatol 1987; 4:140-147.
2. Okuda K, Ohtsuki T, Obata H, Tomimatsu, Okazaki N, Hasegawa H, Nakajima Y, Ohnishi K. Natural history of hepatocellular carcinoma and prognosis in relation to treatment. Study of 850 patients. Cancer 1985; 56:918-928.
3. Calvet X, Bruix J, Ginès P, Bru C, Solé M, Vilana R, Rodés J. Prognostic factors of hepatocellular carcinoma in the West. A multivariate analysis in 206 patients. Hepatology 1990; 12:753-760.
4. Livraghi T, Salmi A, Bolondi L, Marin G, Arienti V, Monti F, Vettori C. Small hepatocellular carcinoma: percutaneous alcohol injection results in 23 patients. Radiology 1988; 168:313-317.
5. Shiina S, Tagawa K, Unuma T, Terano A. Percutaneous ethanol injection therapy for the treatment of hepatocellular carcinoma. AJR 1990; 154:947-951.
6. Ohto M, Ebara M, Yoshikawa M, Okuda K. Radiation therapy and percutaneous ethanol injection for the treatment of hepatocellular carcinoma. In: Okuda K, Ishak KG, eds. Neoplasms of the Liver. Tokyo: Springer, 1987; 335-341.
7. Sheu JC, Huang GT, Chen DS, Sung JL, Yang PM, Wei TC, Lai MY, Su CT, Tsang YM, Hsu HC, Su IJ, Wu TT, Lin JT, Chung CN. Small hepatocellular carcinoma: Intratumor Ethanol Treatment using New Needle and Guidance Systems. Radiology 1987; 163:43-48.
8. Sheu JC, Sung JL, Huang GT, Chen DS, Yang PM, Lai MY, Wei TC, Su CT, Tsang YM, Lea CZ, Chen JC, Hsu HC. Intratumor injection of absolute ethanol under ultrasound guidance for the treatment of small hepatocellular carcinoma. Hepatogastroenterology 1987; 34:255-261.
9. Shiina S, Tagawa K, Niwa Y, Unuma T, Komatsu Y, Yoshiuro, Hamada H, Takahashi M, Shiratori Y, Terano A, Omata M, Kawauchi N, Inoue H. Percutaneous ethanol injection for hepatocellular carcinoma: results in 146 patients. AJR 1993; 160:1023-1028.
10. Vilana R, Bruix J, Bru C, Ayuso MC, Solé M, Rodés

J. Tumor size determines the efficacy of percutaneous ethanol injection for the treatment of small hepatocellular carcinoma. Hepatology 1992; 16:353-357.
11. Joseph FB, Baumgarten DA, Bernardino ME. Hepatocellular carcinoma: CT appearance after percutaneous ethanol ablation therapy. Radiology 1993; 186:553-556.
12. Sironi S, De Cobelli F, Livraghi T, Villa G, Zanello A, Taccagni G, DelMaschio A. Small hepatocellular carcinoma treated with percutaneous ethanol injection: unenhanced and gadolinium-enhanced MR imaging follow-up. Radiology 1994; 192:407-412.
13. Livraghi T, Lazzaroni S, Pellicano S, Rabassi S, Torzilli G, Vettori C. Percutaneous ethanol injection of hepatic tumors: single-session therapy with general anesthesia. AJR 1993; 161:1065-1069.
14. Bruix J, Castells A, Montanyà X, Calvet X, Bru C, Ayuso MC, Jover LL, García L, Vilana R, Boix L, Rodés J. Phase II study of transarterial embolization in European patients with hepatocellular carcinoma: need for controlled trials. Hepatology 1994; 20:643-650.
15. Cedrone A, Rapaccini GL, Pompili L, Grattagliano A, Aliotta A, Trombino C. Neoplastic seeding complicating percutaneous ethanol injection for treatment of hepatocellular carcinoma. Radiology 1992; 183:787-788.
16. Castells A, Bruix J, Bru C, Fuster J, Vilana R, Navasa M, Ayuso MC, Boix L, Visa J, Rodés J. Treatment of small hepatocellular carcinoma in cirrhotic patients: A cohort study comparing surgical resection and percutaneous ethanol injection. Hepatology 1993; 18:1121-1126.
17. Kotoh K, Sakai H, Sakamoto S, Nakayama S, Satoh M, Morotomi I, Nawata H. The effect of percutaneous ethanol injection therapy on small solitary hepatocellular carcinoma is comparable to that of hepatectomy. Am J Gastroenterol 1994; 89:194-198.
18. Ebara M, Ohto M, Sugiura N, Kita K, Yoshikawa M, Okuda K, Kondo F, Kondo Y. Percutaneous ethanol injection for the treatment of small hepatocellular carcinoma. Study of 95 patients. J Gastroenterol Hepatol 1990; 5:616-626.
19. Tanikawa K, Majima Y. Percutaneous ethanol injection therapy for recurrent hepatocellular carcinoma. Hepatogastroenterology 1993; 40:324-327.
20. Livraghi T, Grigioni W, Mazziotti A, Sangalli G, Vettori C. Percutaneous alcohol injection of portal thrombosis in hepatocellular carcinoma: a new possible treatment. Tumori 1990; 76:394-397.
21. Yamazaki S, Hasegawa H, Makuuchi M, Takayama T, Kosuge T, Shimada K. Choice of treatments for small hepatocellular carcinoma: hepatectomy, embolization or ethanol injection. J Gastroenterol Hepatol 1991; 6:408-413.
22. Livraghi T, Bolondi l, Lazzaroni S, Marin G, Morabito A, Rapaccini G, Salmi A, Torzilli G. Percutaneous ethanol injection in the treatment of hepatocellular carcinoma in cirrhosis. A study of 207 patients. Cancer 1992; 69:925-929.
23. Honda N, Guo Q, Uchida H, Ohishi H, Hiasa Y. Percutaneous hot saline injection therapy for hepatic tumors: an alternative to percutaneous ethanol injection therapy. Radiology 1994; 190:53.57.
24. Huang Gt, Yang Pm, Sheu JC, Hsu JL, Sung JL, Wang TH, Chen DC. Intratumor injection of OK-432 for the Treatment of small hepatocellular carcinoma. Hepatogastroenterology 1990; 37:439-532.
25. Gandolfi L, Salmi L, Pizza GC, Bertoni F, Miratori R, DeVinci C, Bachini, Morelli MC, Corrado G. Intratumoral echo- guided injection of interleukin-2 and lymphokine-activated killer cells in Hepatocellular Carcinoma. Hepatogastroenterology 1989; 36:352-356.
26. Livraghi T, Baietta E, Matricardi L, Villa E, Lovati R, Vettori C. Fine needle percutaneous intratumoral chemotherapy under ultrasound guidance: a feasibility study. Tumori 1986; 72:81-86.
27. Rossi S, Fornari F, Buscarini L. Percutaneous ultrasound-guided radiofrequency electrocautery for the treatment of small hepatocellular carcinoma. J Intervent Radiol 1993; 8:97-103.
28. Takayasu K, Suzuki M, Uesaka K, Muramatsu Y, Moriyama N, Yoshida T, Yoshino M, Okazaki N, Hasegawa H. Hepatic artery embolization for inoperable hepatocellular carcinoma; prognosis and risk factors. Cancer Chemother Pharmacol 1989; 23:S123-S125.
29. Chuang VP, Wallace S, Soo CS, Charnsangavej C, Bowers T. Therapeutic Ivalon embolization of hepatic tumors. AJR 1982; 138:289-294.
30. Taguchi T. Chemo-occlusion for the treatment of liver cancer. A new technique using degradable starch microspheres. Clin Pharmacokinet 1994; 26:275-291.
31. Andersson M, Aronsen KF, Balch C, Domellof, Eksborg S, Hafstrom LO, Howell SB, Karesen R, Midander, Teder H. Pharmacokinetics of intra-arterial mitomycin C with or without degradable starch microspheres (DSM) in the treatment of non-resectable liver cancer. Acta Oncol 1989; 28:219-222.
32. Gunji T, Kawauchi N, Ohnishi S, Ishikawa T, Nakagama H, Kaneko T, Moriyama T, Matsuhashi N, Yazaki Y, Imawari M. Treatment of hepatocellular carcinoma associated with advanced cirrhosis by transcatheter arterial chemoembolization using autologous blood clot: a preliminary report. Hepatology 1992; 15:252-257.
33. Makuuchi M, Sukigara M, Mori T, Kobayashi J, Yamazaki S, Hasegawa H, Moriyama N, Takayasu K, Hirohashi S. Bile duct necrosis: Complication of transcatheter arterial embolization. Radiology 1985; 156:331-334.
34. Charnsangavej C, Chuang VP, Wallace S, Soo CS, Bowers T. Transcatheter management of primary carcinoma of the liver. Radiology 1983; 147:51-55.
35. Stuart K, Stokes K, Jenkins R, Trey Ch, Clouse M. Treatement of hepatocellular carcinoma using doxorubicin ethiodized oil gelatin powder chemoembolization. Cancer 1993; 72:3202-3209.
36. Okuda K, Ohnishi K, Takayasu K. Arterial emboli-

zation in the treatment of hepatocellular carcinoma. In: Okuda K, Ishak KG, eds. Neoplasms of the Liver. Tokyo: Springer, Verlag 1987; 327-334.

37. Vetter D, Wenger JJ, Bergier JM, Doffoel M, Bockel R. Transcatheter oily chemoembolization in the management of advanced hepatocellular carcinoma in cirrhosis: results of a Western comparative study in 60 patients. Hepatology 1991; 13:427-433.

38. Kasugai H, Kojima J, Tatsuta M, Okuda S, Sasaki Y, Imaoka S, Fujita M, Ishiguro S. Treatment of hepatocellular carcinoma by transcatheter arterial embolization combined with intraarterial infusion of a mixture of cisplatin and ethiodized oil. Gastroenterology 1989; 97:965-971.

39. Lin DY, Liaw YF, Lee TY, Lai CM. Hepatic arterial embolization in patients with unresectable hepatocellular carcinoma —A randomized controlled trial. Gastroenterology 1988; 94:453-456.

40. Sato Y, Fujiwara K, Ogata I, Ohta Y, Hayashi S, Oka Y, Furui S, Oka H. Transcatheter arterial embolization for hepatocellular carcinoma. Benefits and limitations for unresectable cases with liver cirrhosis evaluated by comparison with other conservative treatments. Cancer 1985; 55:2822-2825.

41. Yamada R, Sato M, Kawabata M, Nakatsuka H, Nakamura K, Takashima S. Hepatic artery embolization in 120 patients with unresectable hepatoma. Radiology 1983; 148:397-401.

42. Pelletier G, Roche A, Ink O, Anciaux ML, Derhy S, Rougier P, Lenoir C, Attali P, Etienne JP. A randomized trial of hepatic arterial chemoembolization in patients with unresectable hepatocellular carcinoma. J Hepatol 1990; 11:181-184.

43. Ikeda K, Kumada H, Saitoh S, Arase Y, Chayama K. Effect of repeated transcatheter arterial embolization on the survival time in patients with hepatocellular carcinoma. Cancer 1991; 68:2150-2154.

44. Mondazzi L, Bottelli R, Brambilla G, Rampoldi A, Rezakovic I, Zavaglia C, Alberti A, Ideo G. Transarterial oily chemoembolization for the treatment of hepatocellular carcinoma: a multivariate analysis of prognostic factors. Hepatology 1994; 19:1115-1123.

45. Venook AP, Stagg RJ, Lewis BJ, Chase JL, Ring EJ, Maroney TP, Hohn DC. Chemoembolization of hepatocellular carcinoma. J Clin Oncol 1990; 8:1108-1114.

46. Takayasu K, Shima Y, Muramatsu Y, Moriyama N, Yamada T; Makuuchi M, Hasegawa H, Hirohashi S. Hepatocellular carcinoma: Treatment with intraarterial iodized oil with and without chemotherapeutic agents. Radiology 1987; 162:345-351.

47. Jinno K, Moriwaki S, Tanada M, Wada T, Mandai K, Okada Y. Clinicopathological study on combination therapy consisting of arterial infusion of lipiodol-disolved SMANCS and transcatheter arterial embolization for hepatocellular carcinoma. Cancer Chemother Pharmacol 1992; 31:S7-S12.

48. The Cooperative Study Group for Liver Cancer Treatment of Japan. Prospective and randomized clinical trial for the treatment of hepatocellular carcinoma —a comparison lipiodol-transcatheter arterial embolization with and without adriamycin. Cancer Chemother Pharmacol 1992; 31:S1-S6.

49. Miyoshi S, Minami Y, Kawata S, Imai Y, Sitoh S, Noda S, Tamura S, et al. Changes in hepatic functional reserve after transcatheter embolization of hepatocellular carcinoma. Assessment by maximal removal of indocyanine green. J Hepatol 1988; 6:332-336.

50. Castells A, Bruix J, Ayuso Mc, Brú C, Montanyà X, Boix L, Rodés J. Transarterial embolization for hepatocellular carcinoma. Antibiotic prophylaxis and clinical meaning of postembolization fever. J Hepatol (in press)

51. Nakamura H, Tanaka T, Hori S, Yoshioka H, Kuroda C, Okamura J, Sakurai M. Transcatheter embolization of hepatocellular carcinoma: Assessment of efficacy in cases of resection following embolization. Radiology 1983; 147:401-405.

52. Hsu HC, Wei TC, Tsang YM, Wu MZ, Lin YH, Chuang SM. Histologic assessment of resected hepatocellular carcinoma after transcatheter hepatic arterial embolization. Cancer 1986; 57:1184-1191.

53. Kuroda C, Sakurai M, Monden M, Marukawa T, Hosoki T, Tokunaga K, Wakasa K, Okamura J, Kozuka T. Limitation of transarterial chemoembolization using iodized oil for small hepatocellular carcinoma. Cancer 1991; 67:81-86.

54. Wakasa K, Sakurai M, Kuroda C, Marukawa T, Monden M, Okamura J, Kurata A. Effect of transcatheter arterial embolization on the boundary architecture of hepatocellular carcinoma. Cancer 1990; 65:913-919.

55. Groupe Francophone d'Etude et de Traitement du Carcinome Hepatocellulaire. Treatment of unresectable hepatocellular carcinoma by lipiodol-targeted transcatheter arterial chemoembolization. A multicenter randomized trial. Hepatology 1993; 18:58A.

56. Castells A, Bruix J, Montanyà X, Brú C, Ayuso MC, Boix L, Rodés J. Transarterial embolization in patients with advanced hepatocelllar carcinoma. Preliminary analysis of a randomized controlled trial. J Hepatol 1994; 21:S22.

57. Sato Y, Fujiwara K, Furui S, Ogata I, Oa Y, Hayashi S, Ohta Y, Iio M, Oka H. Benefit of transcatheter arterial embolization for ruptured hepatocellular carcinoma complicating liver cirrhosis. Gastroenterology 1985; 89:157-159.

58. Bismuth H, Morino M, Sherlock D, Castaing D, Miglietta C, Cauquil P, Roche A. Primary treatment of hepatocellular carcinoma by arterial chemoembolization. Am J Surg 1992; 163:387-394.

59. Stone MJ, Klintmalm GBG, Polter D, Husberg BS, Mennel RG, Ramsay MAE, Flemens EE, Goldstein RM. Neoadjuvant chemotherapy and liver transplantation for hepatocellular carcinoma. Results in 20 patients. Gastroenterology 1992; 103:196-202.

60. Nagasue N, Galizia G, Kohno H, Chang YC, Hayashi T, Yamanoi A, Nakamura T, Yuaya H. Adverse effects of preoperative hepatic artery chemoembolization for resectable hepatocellular carcinoma: a

retrospective comparison of 138 liver resections. Surgery 1989; 106:81-86.
61. Adachi E, Matsumata T, Nishizaki T, Hashimoto H, Tsuneyoshi M, Sugimachi K. Effects of preoperative transcatheter hepatic arterial chemoembolization for hepatocellular carcinoma. Cancer 1993; 72:3593-3598.
62. Kojiro M, Sugihara S, Kakizoe S, Nakashima O, Kiyomatsu K. Hepatocellular carcinoma with sarcomatous change: a special reference to the relationship with anticancer therapy. Cancer Chemother Pharmacol 1989; 23:S4-S8.
63. Nerenstone SR, Ihde DC, Friedman MA. Clinical trials in primary hepatocellular carcinoma: current status and future directions. Cancer Treat Rev 1988; 1-31.
64. Friedman MA. Primary hepatocellular cancer. Present results and future prospects. Int J Radiat Oncol Biol Phys 1983; 9:1841-1850.
65. Okazaki N, Okada S, Nose H, Aoki K. Systemic chemotherapy for hepatocellular carcinoma. In: Tobe T, Kameda H, Okudaira M, Ohto H, Endo Y, Mito M, Okamoto E, Tanikawa K, Kojiro M, eds. Primary Liver Cancer in Japan. Tokyo: Springer, 1992; 301-306.
66. Johnson PJ, Alexopoulos A, Johnson RD, Williams R. Significance of serum bilirrubin level in response of hepatocellular carcinoma to doxorubicin. J Hepatol 1986; 3:149-153.
67. Sciarrino E, Simonetti R, LeMoli S, Pagliaro L. Adriamycin treatment for hepatocellular carcinoma —experience with 109 patients. Cancer 1984; 56:2751-2755.
68. Abraham EH, Prat AG, Gerweck L, Seneveratne T, Arceci RJ, Kramer R, Guidotti G, Cantiello HF. The multidrug resistance gene product functions as an ATP channel. Proc Natl Acad Sci USA 1993; 90:312-316.
69. Harris CC, Hollstein M. Clinical implication of the p53 tumor-suppressor gene. N Engl J Med 1993; 329:1318-1327.
70. Kanematsu T, Furuta T, Takenaka K, Matsumata T, Yoshida Y, Nishizaki T, Hasuo K, Sugimachi K. A 5-year experience of lipiodolization:selective regional chemotherapy for 200 patients with hepatocellular carcinoma. Hepatology 1989; 10:98-102.
71. Ensminger Wd, Gyves JW. Clinical pharmacology of hepatic arterial chemotherapy. Semin Oncol 1983; 10:176-182.
72. Ballet F, Barbare JC, Poupon R. Hepatic extraction of adriamycin in patients with hepatocellular carcinoma. Eur J Cancer Clin Oncol 1984; 20:761-764.
73. Lee YTN, Chan KK, Harris PA, Cohen JL. Distribution of adriamycin in cancer patients. Tissue uptakes, plasma concentration after IV and hepatic IA administration. Cancer 1980; 45:2231-2239.
74. Johnson PJ, Kalayci C, Dobbs N, Raby N, Metivier EM, Summers L, Harper P, Williams R. Pharmacokinetics and toxicity of intrarterial adriamycin for hepatocellular carcinoma. Effect of coadministration of lipiodol. J Hepatol 1991; 13:120-127.
75. Kalayci C, Johnson PJ, Raby N, Metivier EM, Williams R. Intraarterial adriamycin and lipiodol for inoperable hepatocellular carcinoma: a comparison with intravenous adriamycin. J Hepatol 1990; 11:349-353.
76. Murray-Lyon IM. Primary and secondary cancer of the liver. In: Gazet JC, ed. Carcinoma of the Liver, Biliary Tract and Pancreas. London: Edward Arnold, 1983; 1-81.
77. El-Domeiri, Huvos A, Goldsmith H, Foote F. Primary malignant tumors of the liver. Cancer 1971; 27:7-11.
78. Takara K, Ohto M, Yoshikawa M, Ebara M, Okuda K, Itami J, Arimizu N. Clinical and pathological study of irradiation therapy in 24 patients with hepatocellular carcinoma. Jpn J Gastroenterol 1986; 83:1473-1482.
79. Houle SH, Yip TCK, Shepherd FA. Hepatocellular carcinoma: Pilot trial of treatment with Y-90 microspheres. Radiology 1989; 172:857-860.
80. Raoul JI, Bretagne JF, Caucanas JP et al. Internal radiation therapy for hepatocellular carcinoma. Results of a French multicenter phase II trial of transarterial injection of Iodine 131 labeled lipiodol. Cancer 1992; 69:346-352.
81. Order SE, Stillwagon GB, Klein JL, Leichner PK, Siegelman SS, Fishman EK, Ettinger DS, HaulkT, Kapher K, Finney K, Surdyke M, Self S, Leibel S. Iodine 131 antiferritin. A new treatment modality in hepatoma: a Radiation Therapy Oncology Group Study. J Clin Oncol 1985; 3:1573-1582.
82. Sitzmann JV, Order SE, Klein JL, Leichner PK, Fishman EK, Smith GW. Conversion by new treatment modalities of nonresectable to resectable hepatocellular cancer. J Clin Oncol 1987; 1566-1573.
83. Burton MA, Gray BN, Klemp PF, Kelleher DK, Hardy N. Selective internal radiation therapy: distribution of radiation in the liver. Eur J Cancer Clin Oncol 1989; 25:1487-1491.
83. Dritschilo A, Grant EG, Harter KH, Holt RW, Rustgi SN, Rodgers JE. Interstitial radiation therapy for hepatic metastases: sonographic guidance for applicator placement. AJR 1986; 146:275-278.
84. Nagasue N, Ito A, Yukaya H, Ogawa Y. Estrogen receptors in hepatocellular carcinoma. Cancer 1986; 57:87-91.
85. Nagasue N, Ito A, Yukaya A, Ogawa Y. Androgen receptors in hepatocellular carcinoma and surrounding parenchyma. Gastroenterology 1985; 89:643-647.
86. Ohnishi S, Murakami T, Moriyama T, Mitamura K, Imawari M. Androgen and estrogen receptors in hepatocellular carcinoma and in the surrounding noncancerous liver tissue. Hepatology 1986; 6:440-443.
87. Boix L, Bruix J, Castells A, Fuster J, Bru C, Visa J, Rivera F, Rodés J. Sex hormone receptors in hepatocellular carcinoma. Is there a rationale for hormonal treatment? J Hepatol 1993; 17:187-191.
88. Guechot J, Peigney N, Ballet F, Vaubordulle M, Giboudeau J, Poupon R. Effect of D-tryptophan-6-lu-

teinizing hormone-releasing hormone on the tumoral growth and plasma sex steroids levels in cirrhotic patients with hepatocellular carcinoma. Hepatology 1989; 10:346-348.

89. Gupta S, Korula J. Failure of ketoconazole as antiandrogen therapy in nonresectable primary hepatocellular carcinoma. J Clin Gastroenterol 1988; 10:651-654.

90. Forbes A, Williams ML, Iqbal MJ, Johnson PJ, Williams R. Response to cyproterone acetate treatment in primary hepatocellular carcinoma is related to fall in free 5 alpha-dihydrotestosterone. Eur J Cancer Clin Oncol 1987; 23:1659-1664.

91. Bleiberg H, Grimaldi C, Gay F, Messner M, Rougier P, Kok TC, Cirera L, Cervantes F, DeGreve J, Paillot B, Sahmoud T, Selleslags J. Double blind clinical trial of antiandrogen therapy vs. placebo in unresectbale hepatocellular carcinoma (Abstr). Proceedings of 29th Annual Meeting of Am Soc Clin Oncol, 1993; 12:193.

92. Engstrom PF, Levin B, Moertel CG, Schutt A. A phase II trial of tamoxifen in HCC. Cancer 1990; 65:2641-2643.

93. Farinati F, Salvagnini M, de Maria N, Fornasiero A, Chiaramonte M, Rossaro L, Naccarato R. Unresectable hepatocellular carcinoma: a prospective controlled trial with tamoxifen. J Hepatol 1990; 12:297-301.

94. Martínez-Cerezo F, Tomás A, Donoso L, Enríquez J, Guarner C, Balanzó J, Martínez A, Vilardell F. Controlled trial of tamoxifen in patients with advanced hepatocellular carcinoma. J Hepatol 1994; 20:702-706.

95. Bruix J, Castells A, Bru C, Ayuso MC, Boix L, Roca M, Rodés J. Treatment of advanced hepatocellular carcinoma with tamoxifen. Results of a randomized double-blind placebo controlled trial in 120 patients. Hepatology 1994; 20:279A.

96. Lin ZY, Tang ZY. Immunity to subclinical hepatocellular carcinoma. In: Tang ZY, ed. Subclinical hepatocellular carcinoma. Beijing: Springer, 1985; 124-161.

97. Lotze MT, Mule JJ. In: Rosenberg SA, moderator. New approaches to the immunotherapy of cancer using interleukin-2. Ann Intern Med 1988; 108:853-864.

98. Van Haelst-Pisani CM, Pisani RJ, Kovach JS. Cancer Immunotherapy: Current status of treatment with interleukin-2 and lymphokine-activated killer cells. Mayo Clin Proc 1989; 64:451-465.

99. Okuno N, Takagi H, Nakamura T, Nakamura Y, Iwasa Z, Yasutomi M. Treatment for unresectable hepatoma via selective hepatic arterial infusion of lymphokine-activated killer cells generated from autologous spleen. Cancer 1986; 58:1001-1006.

100. Hsieh KH, Shu S, Lee CS, Chu CT, Yang CS, Chang KJ. Lysis of primary hepatic tumours by lymphokine activated killer cells. Gut 1987; 28:117-124.

101. Fagan EA, Pulley M, Limb A, Wolstencroft R, Cranenburgh C, DeVinci C, Karani J, Michell M, Nunnerley H, Zaman S, Williams R. Adoptive immunotherapy administered via the hepatic artery and intralesional interleukin-2 in hepatocellular carcinoma. Cancer Treat Rev 1989; 16:151-160.

102. Ichida T, Higuchi K, Arakawa K, Ohta H, Sugiyama K, Miyagiwa M, Nohzawa A, Satoh T, Sasaki H, Ichida F. Treatment of hepatocellular utilizing lymphokine-activated killer cells and interleukin-2. Cancer Chemother Pharmacol 1989; 23:S45-48.

103. Onishi S, Saibara T, Fujikawa M, Sakaeda H, Matsuura Y, Matsunaga Y, Yamammoto Y. Adoptive immunotherapy with lymphokine-activated killer cells plus recombinant interleukin-2 in patients with unresectable hepatocellular carcinoma. Hepatology 1989; 10:349-353.

104. Sachs E, Di Biscleglie AM, Dusheiko GM et al. Treatment of hepatocellular carcinoma with recombinant leucocyte interferon. Br J Cancer 1985; 52:111-116.

105. Nair PV, Tong MJ, Kempf R, Co R, Lee SD, Venturi CL. Clinical, serological and immunologic effects of human leukocyte interferon in HBsAg-positive primary hepatocellular carcinoma. Cancer 1985; 56:1018-1022.

106. Lai CL, Wu PC, Lok ASF et al. Recombinant alpha-interferon is superior to doxorubicin for inoperable hepatocellular carcinoma: a prospective randomised trial. Br J Cancer 1989; 60:928-933.

107. Lai ChL, Lau JYN, P-Ch Wu et al. Recombinant Interferon-alfa in inoperable hepatocellular carcinoma: a randomized controlled trial. Hepatology 1993; 17:389-394.

Section 9

Other Treatments in Liver Diseases

Treatment of Acute Liver Failure

R. Williams

Since 1973, we have had at King's College Hospital a specifically-designed unit for the treatment of acute liver failure (ALF), initially with two beds and extended in 1992 to a 5-bedded unit, the treatment of ALF in the UK having been recognised as a supraregional (national) specialty in 1986. The value of such a unit comes not only from the availability of all the specialised monitoring and treatment facilities that these very sick patients require, but also on the expertise of the medical and nursing staff that comes from the referral of a sufficient number of patients.

Some evidence to justify the effort and expense of such a Unit is shown in figure 1, which gives overall survival figures since it was first opened. Only those patients who developed grade III-IV encephalopathy are included —the most severely affected cases of acute liver failure and for which most current text books and review articles still quote an 80-90% mortality. These survival figures are for all aetiologies, and for some the outcome is even better, for instance paracetamol overdose cases with grade III-IV encephalopathy in the most recent 2-year period had a survival of 64%.

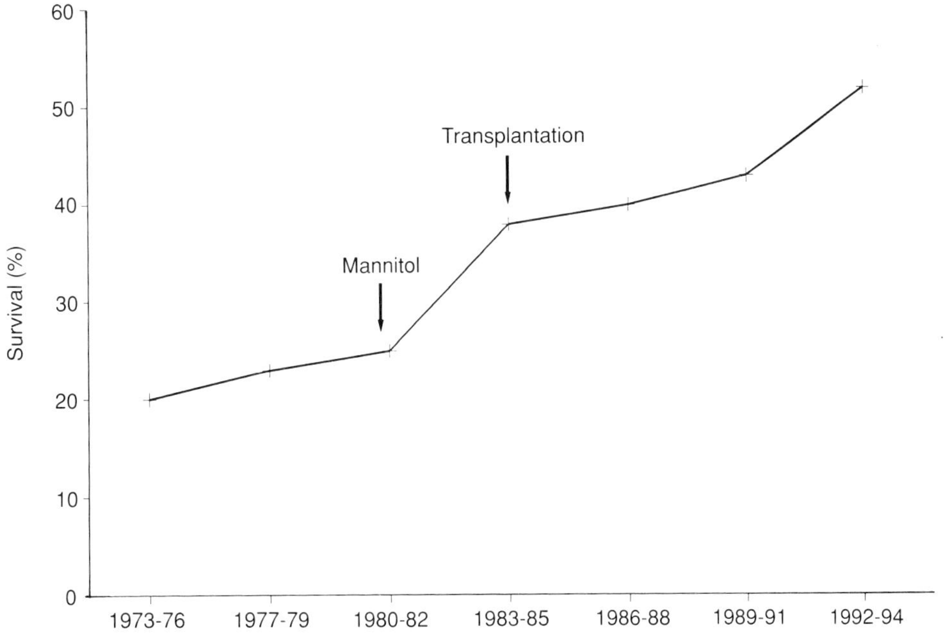

Fig. 1. Survival percentages for all aetiologies of fulminant hepatic failure in patients with grades III-IV encephalopathy only, since Liver Failure Unit opened in 1973. Total of 1,231 patients shown.

CLASSIFICATION AND AETIOLOGICAL CONSIDERATIONS

In addition to the encephalopathy, the clinical syndrome of fulminant hepatic failure (FHF) —first described by Trey and Davidson in 1970 (1)— is marked by severe coagulation and metabolic disturbance, together with cardiorespiratory and renal failure. A group of patients, in whom the appearance of encephalopathy is more delayed, was termed by us in 1986 «late-onset hepatic failure» (LOHF) to emphasize the similarities with FHF (2). In recent years we have learned that the cases of FHF with the most rapid loss of consciousness, paradoxically, have a somewhat better chance of survival (3), and this, together with the results of a statistical analysis of data from some 600 patients with FHF and LOHF, led us to propose last year with Schalm from Holland a new classification to encompass both conditions (4). Acute liver failure is the core term and is prefixed by hyper- and sub- to describe two cohorts at the opposite ends of the clinical spectrum that exhibit significant deviations from the trends seen overall (table 1). There is some correlation between the clinical category and the underlying aetiology. Thus 56% of the hepatitis A cases have a hyperacute course and only 14% the subacute one, whereas the reverse applies to non-A non-B fulminant hepatitis where the greatest percentage follows a subacute course.

As shown by a breakdown of the 342 admissions to the Liver Failure Unit during the period 1992-1994 (table 2), paracetamol overdose is the most common cause of FHF in the UK, although no longer can this be described as the English disease as cases are being reported from all over the world. In the majority of cases in the fulminant viral hepatitis group the cause was not identified, i.e. they are not hepatitis A, B, C, D, E, or F (5). This applies also to series reported from the USA and continental Europe, although in Japan most of these cases appear to have hepatitis C infection, as shown by PCR testing. Dual infection with hepatitis B and C has been described in fulminant viral hepatitis by Benhamou's group at Clichy (6). Recognition of the variety of aetiologies in the «others» category may allow specific therapy to be directed, as for instance in lymphoma, which could be life-saving for the individual patient. Aetiology has a considerable influence on the outcome; indeed, in a multivariate analysis of 588 patients with FHF from this Unit, aetiology was identified as the single most important independent predictor of outcome. The best prognosis is seen in acute fatty liver of pregnancy, whilst amongst the viral causes hepatitis A has the best outcome, hepatitis B intermediate and non-A, non-B the worst. The prognosis for drug induced FHF including that of halothane is the worst of all the aetiological groups. Fulminant Wilson's disease is almost always fatal and the

Table 1. New classification of acute liver failure, based on time from first sign of jaundice to appearance of encephalopathy, with frequency of main aetiological group (4)

	Hyperacute 0-7 days (%)	Acute 7-28 days (%)	Subacute 5-26 weeks (%)
Hepatitis A	55.2	31	13.8
Hepatitis B	62.5	29.9	8.3
NANB Hepatitis	13.6	38.8	47.6
Idiosyncratic drug reactions	35.2	52.9	11.7

Table 2. Aetiology of 342 cases of acute liver failure admitted to the Liver Failure Unit, King's College Hospital, 1993-1994

Overdose	
Paracetamol	250
Ecstasy	2
Viral hepatitis	
A	8
B	8
Non-A, B, C, D, E	28
Other causes	
Wilson's	3
Fatty liver of pregnancy	7
Lymphoma/malignant infiltration	7
Sepsis	2
Budd-Chiari Syndrome	5
Ischaemic hepatitis	9
Miscellaneous	6
Idiosincratic drug reactions	
Lamotrigine, cyproterone, NSAI, cloroquine, rifampicin/isoniacid, halothane, flucloxacillin	7

rapid detection of signs pointing to this aetiology (ie haemolysis, splenomegaly and Kaiser Fleischer rings) is vital so that patients can be listed for transplantation.

ASSESSMENT OF PROGNOSIS AND CRITERIA FOR EMERGENCY TRANSPLANTATION

Apart from taking account of aetiology and rapidity of onset, how in individual cases of ALF can the likely prognosis be assessed, and with this the need for an emergency liver transplant? The decision needs to be taken as early as possible, thereby giving the best possible chance for obtaining a donor organ. The degree of prolongation of prothrombin time has been recognised for many years as a good indicator of prognosis, and this came out strongly in a multivariate statistical analysis of possible prognostic criteria carried out by O'Grady and others (7), which formed the basis for the King's criteria for transplantation in ALF. In that analysis the prolongation of prothrombin time and the more recently introduced international normalised ratio (INR), were shown to be an independent predictor of outcome in all aetiological groups. Although in the paracetamol overdose group no particular cut off level of INR could be determined, a rise in INR at day 3 to 4 following overdose was associated with a 7% survival rate compared to one of 79% in those whose INR fell at that time (8). In a detailed study of 22 patients with paracetamol-induced FHF carried out in this Unit, factor V levels were lower in the patients who died but there was considerable overlap with the survivors (9). Factor VIII/V ratio was a better predictor of outcome, in contrast with either level alone. The height of serum bilirubin was as powerful as the INR in patients with a drug induced or viral aetiology. Some patients, however, succumb before the serum bilirubin has risen significantly and this is more frequently seen in paracetamol-induced hepatic damage of the hyperacute liver failure type (4).

The King's criteria for transplantation have now been validated prospectively in a number of centres worldwide (10). In the non-paracetamol overdose category, whether on the height of the prothrombin time alone or on the basis of age, aetiology, jaundice to encephalopathy time, prothrombin prolongation and height of serum bilirubin (3 out of these 5) a fatal outcome can be predicted with a high degree of certainty. With the paracetamol overdose cases it is more difficult, apart from in the small group with an uncontrollable acidosis at the time of presentation indicative of virtually complete hepatic necrosis. For the others, even with a prolonged prothrombin time, renal failure and grade III-IV encephalopathy, the positive predictive value is only 67%.

The Clichy group has found (11) that along with encephalopathy, measurement of Factor V, with its short half life, is the most certain indicant. The cut-off level taken —below 20% or less than 30%— is dependent on the age of the patient (< 30 and > 30 years, respectively). At Pittsburgh, the decision to transplant is based on the extent of reduction in the size of the liver as determined by CT scanning at the time an organ becomes available (12). Patients with a liver volume of less than 700 cc should be listed for transplantation whilst those with volumes between 700-900 cc can be observed although are likely to require transplantation. However, a Japanese group (13) found that use of computed tomography in assessing both liver size and functional volume was insufficiently precise to discriminate survivors from non-survivors. Moving a patient with developing cerebral oedema can be dangerous, and there are also risks in determining the extent of cell necrosis by liver biopsy —50% or more of the hepatic lobules indicating the need for transplantation.

DETAILED MANAGEMENT INCLUDING MULTI-ORGAN INVOLVEMENT

Infection

As an immediate consequence of the acute liver injury, host defences against infection are severely compromised and with secondary bacterial infection there is endotoxaemia, activation of macrophages, release of cytokines and tumour necrosis factor. The resulting clinical picture is similar to that of septic shock with hypotension and other circulatory changes leading to tissue hypoxia and damage to a number of organs as well as the gut, and with further ischaemic injury of the liver —a vicious cycle indeed.

With sepsis so important in pathogenesis and with recurrent pulmonary infections and septicaemic episodes the major cause of morbidity and death in ALF, effective management or, better, prevention of infection is essential to improving survival figures. In the most recent trial (manuscript in preparation) carried out in the Liver Failure Unit at King's, prophylaxis with the full SDD (selective decontamination of digestive tract) regime was compared with amphotericin B alone, both groups of patients also getting i.v. antibiotics at the first signs of an infection. A worrying development is the emergence of a significant number of infections from multiple resistant strains, especially *Enterococcus faecium* and *Klebsiella*, which may hamper further improvements to antibiotic regimes.

Hypotension and other circulatory changes

The severity of the vasodilatation and associated circulatory disturbances are closely related to the extent of underlying hepatic damage. Along with this oxygen consumption and oxygen extraction is decreased —similar to that found in other critically ill patients. As a consequence of the tissue hypoxia, there is a switch to anaerobic metabolism and a build up of lactate. Bihari was the first to draw attention to the importance of microcirculatory disturbance in ALF, showing also that an infusion of prostacyclin (a microcirculatory vasodilator) resulted in significant increases in oxygen consumption consequent on the increase in oxygen delivery (14). More recently Wendon has shown (manuscript in preparation) that both adrenaline and noradrenaline are effective in maintaining systemic blood pressure. Their use is accompanied by a fall in oxygen consumption presumably as a result of an effect on tissue perfusion and this can be prevented by giving prostacyclin at the same time.

In septic shock there is a massive release of nitric oxide from endotoxin-induced expression of the inducible nitric oxide synthase in vascular endothelial cells and smooth muscle cells. Infusion of low doses of LNMMA —a competitive antagonist— have been shown to restore the blood pressure and responsiveness to pressor agents and it has been suggested that the same mechanisms pertain in the circulatory disturbance of ALF. Recent data from Wendon (manuscript in preparation) shows that LNMMA does have a pressor effect although much larger doses are required and there is also a detrimental effect on oxygen consumption.

Of considerable importance was the demonstration by Harrison and Wendon that infusion of N-acetylcysteine improves blood flow as well as oxygen delivery and extraction by the tissues in both the systemic and cerebral circulations (15). The clinical benefits that result were shown in a controlled clinical trial carried out in ALF due to paracetamol overdose. The decreased frequency of multi-organ failure, particularly cerebral oedema, hypotension and renal failure, and the improved survival in the treated group was statistically highly significant (16). These important effects are quite separate from the better known antidote action of N-acetylcysteine when given within 12-15 hours of the overdose. Similar beneficial effects have been demonstrated in cases of ALF from fulminant viral hepatitis and the mechanism, we have postulated, is an enhancement of endothelial-derived relaxant factor (nitric oxide) at tissue level.

Cerebral Oedema and Ischaemia

The occurrence of cerebral oedema is an almost inevitable part of the progressive encephalopathy of ALF and if the accompanying elevation in intracranial pressure (ICP) cannot be controlled, brain stem coning is likely. Patients showing signs of grade III or IV coma should be ventilated both to protect their airway and also to allow optimal management of cerebral oedema and the raised intra-cranial pressure. Nursing should be at an angle of 20°, in order to maximise cerebral perfusion pressure (CPP), and patients should be subjected to the minimum of tactile stimuli (17). Once ventilated, an extradural catheter should be inserted, this will allow rapid treatment of rises in ICP before the onset of pupillary abnormalities and maintenance of cerebral perfusion pressure at greater than 50 mmHg. The monitoring of ICP is much safer now using the Camino technique, in which a 2 mm catheter is introduced into the subdural space by a small drill.

Although it has been reported that patients in grade IV encephalopathy have an elevated cerebral blood flow, thereby contributing to the rise in intracranial pressure, the most recent studies carried out by us have shown that cerebral blood flow is almost invariably reduced (18).

Monitoring of the cerebral state requires an appreciation also of the dangers of ischaemia, particularly epileptiform activity. This is difficult to detect clinically in the paralysed, ventilated patient, and an EEG monitor is of considerable value. The early recognition of this complication and its control by diazemols and/or phenytoin is of vital importance in minimising the likelihood of secondary cerebral oedema. With fitting, the jugular bulb oxygen saturation is decreased as a result of an increase in blood flow and oxygen consumption in the brain. First line management of a raised ICP is the infusion of mannitol, 0.5 g/kg as a bolus over 10 minutes. Plasma osmolarity should be checked and the patient can be given further doses until a plasma osmolarity of 320 mOsm is reached. In patients who are not diuresing or in those with incipient renal failure, ultrafiltration or arterio-venous haemodiafiltration is commenced to allow for the removal of 2-3 × the volume of mannitol infused. Thiopentone may be useful in patients who are resistant to therapy with mannitol (19). The prophylactic use of dexamethasone is of no benefit and hyperventilation should be avoided as it lowers CBF further. N-acetylcysteine has no effect on intracranial pressure but the increase in cerebral blood flow produced may prevent or delay the development of cerebral oedema.

RENAL FAILURE, AND METABOLIC AND RESPIRATORY COMPLICATIONS

A urine output of less than 300 ml/24 hours and serum creatinine of greater than 300 mmol/l, in the presence of adequate intravascular filling pressures occurs in about 70% of patients with paracetamol overdose and in about 30% of other cases of FHF (20). In such cases machine-driven haemodialysis should be avoided, since hypotension is a frequent complication, and in association with surges in intra-cranial pressure that can also be seen with machine-driven replacement therapy (21) may result in significant falls in cerebral perfusion pressure. Anticoagulation is normally achieved with heparin, but in patients with a severe coagulopathy, the use of prostacyclin and low dose heparin may be preferable.

Hypoglycaemia is a consequence of increasing circulating insulin, impaired gluconeogenesis and an inability to mobilise glycogen stores. Blood glucose should be monitored hourly and 50 ml of 50% dextrose administered if the blood glucose falls below 3.5 mmol/l. Normoglycaemia is often best achieved by use of a continuous infusion of either 10 or 20% glucose. A common occurrence is hypophosphataemia, especially in those patients who are still passing urine; intravenous supplementation is required.

A metabolic acidosis is a relatively frequent finding which until recently was attributed to impaired lactate metabolism consequent on liver dysfunction. Recent work has demonstrated that much of the acidosis is related to the presence of tissue hypoxia and increased peripheral lactate production (22).

Arterial hypoxaemia is frequently present and is multifactorial in origin. Aspiration of gastric contents, bacterial infection, intrapulmonary haemorrhage, atelectasis, V/Q mismatch and more rarely the development of adult respiratory distress syndrome are all contributory factors.

Coagulopathy

The risk of bleeding appears to correlate not so much with prothrombin time but with thrombocytopenia and the presence of overt disseminated intravascular coagulation. The prophylactic use of fresh frozen plasma in the absence of bleeding is not associated with a reduction in either morbidity nor mortality (23). Platelet infusions are indicated in severe thrombocytopenia and are supplemented if there is evidence of bleeding or if the count is below 50 per mm^3 prior to an invasive procedure being undertaken. Gastro-intestinal haemorrhage is usually related to the development of gastric erosions, although the frequency with which this occurs has been much decreased since the prophylactic use of H2 antagonists and agents such as sucralfate.

OVERALL OUTCOME AND RESULTS OF TRANSPLANTATION

The outcome in 342 cases of ALF admitted over the last two years is shown in table 3. Forty-four of the 252 cases of the paracetamol overdose cases fulfilled transplant criteria, the percentage being higher in fulminant viral hepatitis (27/46) and lower in the idiosyncratic drug reaction and others category (6/46). Of the 77 cases fulfilling transplant criteria, 53 were listed on the super urgent priority list to await an organ donation. Apart from the small number of paracetamol overdose cases in whom transplantation was contraindicated on psychiatric grounds, the main reason for not listing was the finding of other serious medical problems, for instance heart disease, or the occurrence as part of the ALF of uncontrollable sepsis, refractory hypotension or an apparently irretrievable cerebral state. The latter reasons also explain why not all those listed were finally transplanted (39/53).

The 79% survival of those who were transplanted is an excellent figure considering how ill they were at the time of operation, and is only some 10% lower than for an elective transplant in our programme. Four of the 24 cases fulfilling criteria but not listed, and one of the 12 listed but not transplanted survived (5/38; 13%). The latter figure is further evidence of the accuracy of the King's criteria in determining a poor prognosis. That some cases still survived from those two groups emphasises the need to continue treatment. The 61% survival for those not reaching transplant criteria would suggest that if less severe criteria with good predictive value could be identified, allowing more of those cases to be transplanted, the overall survival would be further increased.

Table 3. Outcome of 344 admissions with acute liver failure during 1992-1994

	N	Fulfilled Criteria	Listed	Transplanted
Paracetamol/ drug overdose	252	44	29	21
Viral hepatitis	46	27	18	13
Idiosyncratic reactions/others	46	6	6	5

To investigate the influence of pretransplant clinical status on the post-operative course, we have analysed the outcome of our first 100 consecutive adult patients who underwent emergency transplantation for acute liver failure in relation to aetiology, severity of liver failure and associated systemic critical illness (Devlin et al, manuscript submitted to publication). The results showed that in patients transplanted for non-paracetamol liver failure, no *static* variable determinable on admission to hospital (including age, sex, year of transplant, time from hospital admission to transplant, fulminant or late-onset presentation) other than aetiology correlated with two-month patient survival. Fulminant Wilson's disease had a high survival rate (100%) and idiosyncratic drug reactions a lower one (12.5%). At the time of transplantation, of the 4 *dynamic* variables significant in a univariate analysis only the creatinine level was an independent variable in a stepwise logistic regression. In patients transplanted for paracetamol overdose, «overdose to hepatectomy period» was the only significant static variable and of the dynamic variables at the time of transplantation, only the Apache 111 score ($p < 0.05$) was an independent variable in the regression model.

Other recent data relates to the efficacy and safety of an FK506 based immunosuppression regimen in transplanted acute liver failure patients compared to one based on cyclosporin A. In the European study a consistent trend towards improved patient and graft survival noted in the FK506 treated group was apparent from the first post-operative week (e.g., patient survival: at day 7 95.5% vs. 82.1% and at month 6 72.7% vs. 60.7%). Acute rejection was less frequent in the FK506 group with a cumulative intractable rejection rate at 6 months of 6.2% vs. 22.6%. The FK506 treatment group had improved graft function, lower steroid requirements and fewer infection episodes.

One approach that can be utilised for patients whose condition becomes too unstable for transplantation is the removal of the necrotic liver by surgical hepatectomy and a portacaval anastomosis. The patients can improve to a remarkable extent, presumably because toxic substances are no longer being released from the liver into the circulation. Values for mean arterial pressure, oxygen extraction and systemic vascular resistance are increased (Wendon et al, manuscript submitted to publication), and cerebral oedema usually becomes more easily controllable. The window of opportunity thereby obtained for transplantation is limited to 24-36 hours.

The most frequent contra-indication to proceeding with liver transplantation is active ongoing infection. If the patient has received 24 hours of antibiotics and their clinical course is stable it may be reasonable to proceed. Although haemodynamic indices nearly always improve following removal of the necrotic liver at transplantation but rapidly increasing requirements for vasopressor support in the form of adrenaline or noradrenaline should be considered a relative contra-indication. Progressive deterioration in respiratory function with increasing oxygen requirements and particularly the finding of an ARDS picture and an inspired oxygen of greater than 0.6 is an absolute contra-indication to transplantation. On the cerebral side, the development of fixed pupils for prolonged periods of time (one hour or more) is a contra-indication, as are prolonged elevations of ICP to levels greater than 35 mmHg. A CPP of less than 40 mmHg for longer than one hour makes full neurological recovery unlikely.

USE OF BIOARTIFICIAL LIVER

Two devices are currently undergoing clinical trial. One pioneered by Demetriou in the USA is based on culture of porcine hepatocytes. Separated plasma is passed first through a adsorbent charcoal column to remove toxic substances that might otherwise damage the cultured hepatocytes and then through the hollow fibres in the device containing the cultured hepatocytes. Patients treated in this way were successfully maintained until a transplant could be carried out and an improvement in encephalopathy grade along with the normalisation of intracranial pressure were among the striking benefits claimed by the investigators (24). The other device, known as ELAD (Extracorporeal Liver Assist Device), is the one that we are now evaluating in a controlled clinical trial is based on cultured human hepatoblastoma cells. It was developed by Sussman and colleagues in

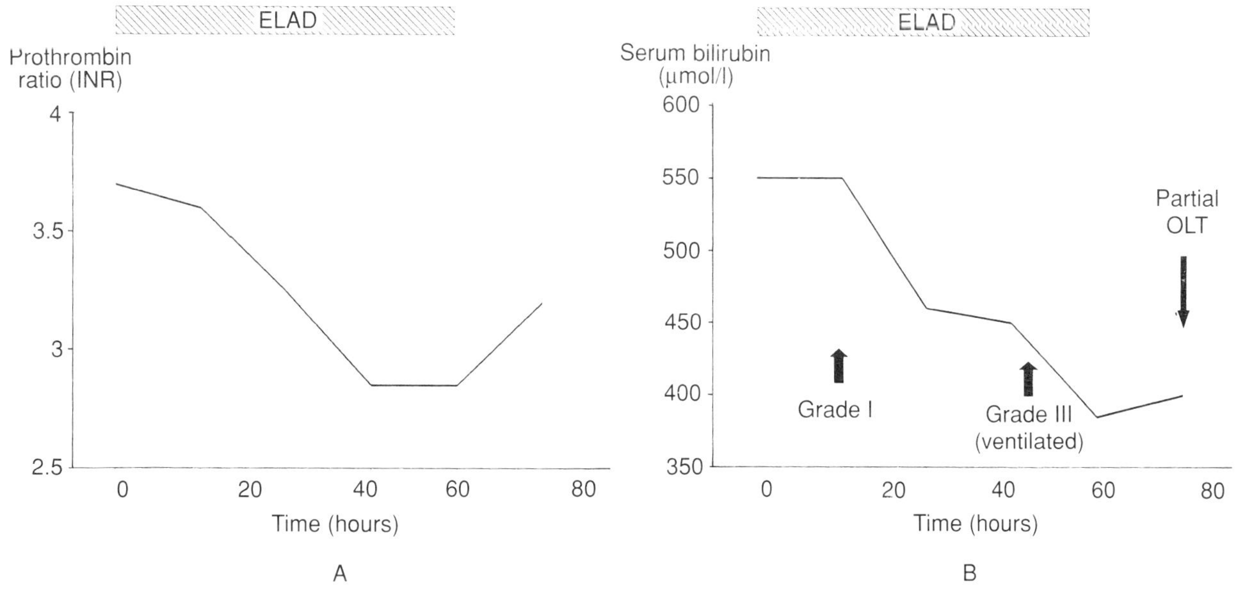

Fig. 2. Improvement in prothrombin ratio (A) and serum bilirubin (B) in a 14 year old boy with non-A non-B acute liver failure while the Extracorporeal Liver Assist Device (ELAD). OLT: orthotopic liver transplantation.

Houston (25). Each column contains 200 g of cells so that a circuit based on a perfusion of two columns should give approximately 20-30% of normal liver function. Ultrafiltrate is drawn into extracapillary space containing the hepatocytes at about 20 ml/min and reinfused into the return blood line after passing through a filter system to prevent any passage of the hepatoblastoma cells into the patient.

Figure 2 gives one illustration of its use was in a 14 year old UK-born Indian boy with acute liver failure from a non-A non-B fulminant hepatitis. Both the INR and serum bilirubin level fell whilst on the device which he stayed on for some 66 hours. His encephalopathy grade nevertheless showed some deterioration, but as he still did not completely fulfil transplant criteria it was decided to proceed with a partial rather than a complete orthotopic liver transplantation. In this procedure the left lobe of the patient's own liver is removed and the comparable part of the donor organ is placed in the same situation. The potential for complete recovery of the patient's own liver remains and if and when this occurs, the graft can be allowed to atrophy by withdrawing immunosuppression or it can be removed surgically. Worldwide at least 10 cases have now been treated by auxiliary liver transplantation, with recovery of the patient's own liver in a number (26, 27).

In conclusion, the research carried out to date has led to many improvements in patient care and the outlook for persons who develop this most devastating of illnesses is now very much better. Nevertheless, ALF will always remain a condition that places a great demand on resources, and on the expertise and dedication of those involved in the care of the patients.

REFERENCES

1. Trey C, Davidson C. The management of fulminant hepatic failure. In: Popper H, Schaffner F, eds. Progress in Liver Disease. New York: Grune and Stratton, 1970, 282-298.
2. Gimson AES, O'Grady JG, Ede RJ, Portmann B, Williams R. Late-onset hepatic failure: Clinical, serological and histological features. Hepatology 1986; 6:288-294.
3. Takahashi Y, Shimizi M. Aetiology and prognosis of fulminant hepatic viral hepatitis in Japan: a multicentre study. J Gastroenterol Hepatol 1991; 6:159-164.
4. O'Grady JG, Schalm S, Williams R. Acute liver failure: Redefining the syndromes. Lancet 1993; 342: 273-275.
5. Fagan EA. Acute liver failure of unknown pathogenesis: The hidden agenda. Hepatology 1994; 19: 1307-1312.
6. Feray C, Gigou M, Samuel D, et al. Hepatitis C virus RNA and hepatitis B virus DNA in serum and liver of patients with fulminant hepatitis. Gastroenterology 1993; 104:549-55.
7. O'Grady JG, Alexander GJ, Hayllar KM, Williams R. Early indicators of prognosis in fulminant hepatic faiure. Gastroenterology 1989; 97:439-445.
8. Harrison P, O'Grady J, Alexander G, Williams R. Serial prothrombin times: a prognostic indicator in paracetamol-induced fulminant hepatic failure. Br Med J 1990; 301:964-966.
9. Pereira L, Langley P, Hayllar K, Tredger J M, Williams R. Coagulation factors V and VIII/V ratio as predictors of outcome in paracetamol-induced fulminant hepatic failure: relationship to other prognostic indicators. Gut 1992; 33:98-102.
10. Pauwels A, Mostefa-Karan, Florent C, Levy VG. Emergency liver transplantation for acute liver failure: evaluation of London and Clichy criteria. J Hepatol 1993; 17:124-127.
11. Bernuau J, Samuel D, Durand R, Saliba F, Bourliere M, Adam R, Gugenheim J, Castaing D, Bismuth H, Rueff B, Erlinger S, Benhamou JP. Criteria for emergency liver transplantation in patients with acute viral hepatitis and factor V below 50% of normal: A prospective study. Hepatology 1991; 14:49.
12. Van Thiel DH. When should a decision to proceed with transplantation actually be made in cases of fulminant or subfulminant hepatic failure; at admission to hospital or when a donor organ is made available? J Hepatol 1993; 17:1-2.
13. Kumahara T, Muto Y, Moriwaki H, Yoshida T, Tomita E. Determination of an integrated CT number of the whole liver in patients with severe hepatitis: an indicator of the functional reserve of the liver. Gastroenterol Jpn 1989; 24:290-297.
14. Bihari D, Smithies M, Gimson A, Tinker J. The effects of vasodilation with prostacyclin on oxygen delivery and uptake in critically ill patients. N England J Med 1987; 317: 397-403.
15. Harrison PM, Wendon JA, Gimson AES, Alexander GJM, Williams R. Improvement by acetylcysteine of haemodynamics and oxygen transport in fulminant hepatic failure. N Engl J Med 1991; 324:1852-1858.
16. Keays R, Harrison PM, Wendon JA, Gimson AES, Alexander GJM, Williams R. Intravenous acetylcysteine in paracetamol induced fulminant hepatic failure: a prospective controlled trial. Br Med J 1991; 303:1026-1029.
17. Davenport A, Will EJ, Davison AM. Effect of posture on intracranial pressure and cerebral perfusion pressure in patients with fulminant hepatic and renal failure after acetaminophen self-poisoning. Crit Care Med 1990; 18:286-289.
18. Wendon JA, Keays R, Harrison PM, Gimson AE, Wi-

lliams R. Cerebral blood flow and cerebral metabolism in fulminant hepatic failure. Hepatology 1994; 19:1407-1413.
19. Forbes A, Alexander GJ, O'Grady JG, Keays R, Gullan R, Dawling S, Williams R. Thiopental infusion in the treatment of intracranial hypertension complicating fulminant hepatic failure. Hepatology 1989; 10:306-310.
20. O'Grady JG, Williams R. Management of acute liver failure. Schweiz Med Wochenschr 1986; 116: 541-544.
21. Davenport A, Will E, Davidson A et al. Changes in intracranial pressure during machine and continuous haemofiltration. Crit Care Med 1989; 12:439-444.
22. Bihari D, Gimson AE, Lindridge J, Williams R. Lactic acidosis in fulminant hepatic failure. Some aspects of pathogenesis and prognosis. J Hepatol 1985; 1:405-416.
23. Gazzard B, Henderson J, Williams R. Early changes in coagulation following paracetamol overdose and a controlled trial of fresh frozen plasma therapy. Gut 1975; 16:617-620.
24. Rozga J, Podesta L, LePage E, Morsiani E, Moscioni AD, Hoffman A et al. A bioartificial liver to treat severe acute liver failure. Ann Surg 1994; 219:538-546.
25. Sussman NL, Gislason GT, Conlin CA, Kelly JH. The Hepatix extracorporeal liver assist device: Initial clinical experience. Artificial Organs 1994; 18:390-396.
26. Terpstra OT. Auxiliary liver grafting: a new concept in liver transplantation. Lancet 1994; 342:758.
27. Boudjema K, Jaeck D, Simeoni U et al. Temporary auxiliary liver transplantation for subacute liver failure in a child. Lancet 1993:342; 778-779.

Treatment of Autoimmune Hepatitis

A. Schüler, M. P. Manns

INTRODUCTION

Autoimmune hepatitis (AIH) is a chronic necro-inflammatory disorder of unknown etiology. The disease is characterized by autoimmunologic features including the presence of circulating autoantibodies, high serum immunoglobulins, and, in about 40%, autoimmune diseases of other organs. In general there is a therapeutic response to immunosuppressive therapy. Overlap with other autoimmune liver diseases like primary biliary cirrhosis and primary sclerosing cholangitis may occur, obscuring the classic boundaries among these clinical entities.

CLINICAL SIGNIFICANCE OF DISEASE-ASSOCIATED MHC-HAPLOTYPES IN AUTOIMMUNE HEPATITIS

Autoimmune hepatitis is associated with alleles of the major histocompatibility complex (MHC) (1) that influence disease susceptibility (2, 3), clinical manifestations (4, 5) and prognosis (6, 7).

HLA A1, B8 and DR3 are recognized more often in young patients who have severe inflammatory activity at presentation (4), relapse after withdrawal of immunosupressive therapy (4) and require liver transplantation more often than patients with other HLA haplotypes (6, 7).

Patients with the haplotype DR4, which is the predominant allele in Japanese patients, are older and more commonly women. These patients exhibit higher serum immunoglobulin G levels and a greater frecuency of concurrent immunologic diseases (8). Disease remission during corticosteroid treatment seems to occur more often in HLA DR4 than in other phenotypes. On the other hand, treatment failure is less common.

Patients with HLA B8 phenotype have more active biochemical and histological features at diagnosis but there is no close relation with treatment outcome (9). Recent studies suggest HLA A11 to be associated with extrahepatic autoimmunologic manifestations and HLA DR4 showed a strong synergistic effect when present with HLA A11. These findings implicate a separate clinical entity for extrahepatic manifestations (10, 11).

CLASSIFICATION OF AUTOIMMUNE HEPATITIS

Autoimmune hepatitis is classificated by the occurrence of characterizing autoantibodies. It may be divided into several subgroups due to serological markers. Until now it is unknown, whether that has any therapeutic, aetiological or pathological relevance.

Type 1 autoimmune hepatitis corresponds most closely with the early definition of classic «lupoid» hepatitis. Antinuclear antibodies (ANA) are the major serological marker for this subgroup, many of whom exhibit in addition smooth muscle autoantibodies (SMA) (12, 13). The typical patient is a young woman presenting with an either acute or chronic hepatitis, accompanied by fluctuating jaundice, cushingoid appearance, lethargy, arthralgia, striae, hirsutism and acne. In addition some patients present with concomitant autoimmune thyroid disease and hemolytic anemia. Serum transaminases and polyclonal hypergammaglobulinemia are grossly raised. This disease subtype commonly shows a rapid response to immunosupresive therapy but 50% of the patients experience early relapse after treatment withdrawal.

Type 2 autoimmune hepatitis is characterized by liver-kidney microsomal autoantibodies type 1 (anti-LKM-1). Anti-LKM-1 reacts with cytochrome P450 IID6 (14) affecting mostly young women. In up to 7% of cases, chronic hepatitis C may be associated with LKM-1 antibodies, as detected by immunofluorescence (15). The fine specificity of antigen binding of these LKM-1 antibodies, associated with hepatitis C, revealed, that only a minority of sera binds to cytochrome 450 II D6 while other sera react with so far unidentified antigens at 59 and 70 kD (16). However, 50% of LKM-1 positive sera do not react in western blot and recognize conformational epitopes (16). These patients with chronic hepatitis C may be treated with interferon although the risk for increased side effects, such as increase in transaminases may be enhanced (Bianchi et al.; personal communication). These patients should not be termed chronic autoimmune hepatitis type 2b anymore (17, 18) (table 1). Anti-LKM-3 antibodies were found to be associated with delta hepatitis, requiring high dose interferon as the first line therapy. LKM-3 antibodies recognize UDP glucoronosyl transferases (19). Type 2 autoimmune hepatitis appears to be much less frequent than type 1 and has been described predominantly in continental Europe. Clinically, this variant shows distincitive features. It tends to predominate in the pediatric age group (20) and is more often associated with extrahepatic autoimmune disease like autoimmune thyroid disease, vitiligo and diabetes (table 2). The disease course is often acute, with severe histologic changes and a marked tendency to progress rapidly to cirrhosis. Patients usually respond well to immunosuppression.

Table 1. Hepatitis C virus in autoimmune hepatitis

	HCV negative	HCV positive
Age	Young	Older
Sex	Female	No predominance
ALT	↑↑↑	↑
LKM-1 titer	+++	+
Immunosupression	+	?
Interferon	ø	(+)
HLA DR3	++	+
C4A-Q0	+	+

Table 2. Extrahepatic symptoms in autoimmune hepatitis

Frequent symptoms	Rare symptoms
Fatigue	Pericarditis
Anorexia	Myocarditis
Abdominal pain	Leg ulcers
Acne	Pulmonary complications
Fever	Uveitis
Arthralgia	Mixed connective tissue disease
Vitiligo	
Autoimmune thyroid disease	Macroglobulinemia
Skin rashes	Lichen planus
Diabetes	Febrile panniculitis
Hirsutism, cushingoid features	

Type 3 autoimmune hepatitis is characterized by autoantibodies against a soluble liver antigen (SLA) (21) or liver-pancreas antigen (22). Other autoantibodies like ANA, SMA or AMA may be found in this group. There is no evidence that these patients differ in the clinical course or treatment response from those with type I autoimmune hepatitis. There is increasing evidence that some patients with cryptogenic cirrhosis exhibit clinical and laboratory features resembling those of autoimmune hepatitis including steroid treatment sensivity (23, 24).

DIAGNOSTIC CRITERIA FOR AUTOIMMUNE HEPATITIS

Before treatment of autoimmune hepatitis is started, other pathogenetic factors of chronic hepatitis have to be excluded, as defined by the International Autoimmune Hepatitis Group (25) (table 3). Liver biopsy reveals the extent of tissue inflammation and preexisting fibrosis and cirrhosis, which has been shown to be a major determinant of prognosis. Confidence in the diagnosis «autoimmune hepatitis» is increa-

Table 3. Diagnostic criteria for autoimmune hepatitis

Parameters	Definite	Probable
Liver histology	CAH (as defined previously) of moderate or severe activity with piecemeal necrosis, with or without lobular hepatitis or central-portal bridging necrosis, but without biliary lesions, granulomas, siderosis, copper deposits or any other change suggestive of a different etiology	Same as for «definite»
Serum biochemistry	Any abnormality in serum aminotransferases, especially (but not exclusively) if the serum alkaline phosphatase activity is not markedly elevated. Normal serum concentrations of α_1-antitrypsin, copper and ceruloplasmin	Same as for «definite», but patients with abnormal serum concentrations of copper and ceruloplasmin may be included, *provided thath Wilson's disease has been excluded by the absence of Kayser-Fleischer ring and no markedly increased urinary copper excretion after challenge with* D-*penicillamine*
Serum immunoglobulins	Total globulin or γ-blobulin or IgG concentrations greater than 1.5 times the upper normal limit	Any elevation of serum globullin or γ-globulin or IgG concentrations above the upper normal limit
Serum autoantibodies	Seropositivity for ANA, SMA or LKM-1 antibodies at titers greater thgan 1:80 in adults or greater than 1:20 in children, as determined by indirect immunofluorescence on rodent tissue sections	Seropositivity for ANA, SMA or LKM -1 antibodies at titers of 1:40 or greater in adults, or in children, ANA or LKM-1 at 1:10 or greater, SMA at 1:20 or greater or both. Patients who are seronegative for ANA, and LKM-1, SMA but who are seropositive for any other defined «liver autoantibody» may be included
Viral markers	Seronegativity for IgM hepatitis A virus antibody, HBsAg, IgM HBc antibody and HCV antibody (by at least second-generation assays), as well as for markers or current infections with other hepatotropic viruses (e.g., cytomegalovirus and Epstein-Barr virus). No history of parenteral exposure to blood or blood products	Same as for «definite», but patients who are seropositive for HCV antibody may be, included *until it is confirmed that this positivity reflects existing HCV infection*
Other etiological factors	Average alcohol consumption less than 35 g/day in male and 25 g/day in female patients. No history of recent use of known hepatotoxic drugs	Alcohol consumption less than 50 g/day in male and 40 g/day in female patients and no recent use of known hepatotoxic drugs. Patients who have recently taken potentially hepatotoxic drugs may be included, *if clear evidence exists of continuing liver damage after abstinence from alcohol or withdrawal of the drug*

From Johnson PJ, McFarlane IG. Meeting report: International Autoimmune Hepatitis Group. Hepatology 1993; 18:998-1005.

sed, if the patient has autoantibodies, hypergammaglobulinemia or concomitant autoimmune disorders. The spectrum of patients comprises young women with acute hepatitis, older women in the postmenopausal phase, who perhaps are more likely to develop treatment-related complications (26) and the patient with end-stage liver disease, suffering from ascites, hepatic encefalopathy, muscle dystrophia and gastrointestinal hemorrhage. Diagnosis sometimes is also made in later stages of the disease.

UNTREATED AUTOIMMUNE HEPATITIS

The severity and poor prognosis of autoimmune hepatitis was demonstrated in early studies with a minority of patients reaching ten year survival (27, 28). A poor prognosis was also seen in the untreated arm of controlled clinical studies performed in the 1970s (29, 30). In the Royal Free trial, 15 of 24 patients died within 4 years and in the Mayo Clinic trial survival in the untreated group was 50% at two years.

The fact, that in the 1990s survival in patients without cirrhosis was estimated more than 95% in 5 years (31) may reflect earlier and safer diagnosis of autoimmune hepatitis and detection of more patients with mild disease lacking from early progression to cirrhosis. In addition other causative factors like hepatitis virus B and C infection can be excluded more safely nowadays.

TREATED AUTOIMMUNE HEPATITIS

Keating et al. found an 87% 5-year survival in autoimmune hepatitis and 65% in cryptogenic cirrhosis (24). Anti-LKM positive autoimmune hepatitis is associated with a worse survival of about 75% after 10 years. Reduced survival in the last two disease groups seems to be the result of a higher frequency and earlier development of cirrhosis.

In general there is no convincing reason to establish special treatment regimen for different subgroups of autoimmune hepatitis, once replicating hepatotropic virus infection are excluded by all means. Immunogenetic factors may be helpful in regard to final approve of diagnosis, prognosis and treatment.

Immunosuppressive therapy is required for all immunoserologic groups, whereas spontaneous remission is rare. The large treatment trials gave evidence that immunosuppressive therapy prolongs survival, diminishes the extent of hepatic inflammation and fibrosis and decelerates progression to cirrhosis. Furthermore spontaneous exacerbations of untreated autoimmune hepatitis may be prevented. Remission rates after by initial therapy (prednisone or a combination of prednisone and azathioprine) range between 60-80% (7).

TREATMENT WITH CORTICOSTEROIDS AND/OR AZATHIOPRINE

The beneficial effect of corticosteroid treatment on AIH has been established in the large treatment trials. In the Mayo Clinic trials inclusion criteria focused on patients with rather severe disease and histologically-proven chronic active hepatitis. Patients with end-stage disease were excluded. One dilemma is how and when to establish corticosteroid therapy in the dominating group of patients with mild disease, mild histologic activity (absence of piecemeal necrosis and bridging necrosis) and few, if any, symptoms due to the lack of treatment studies in this group (32). The boundaries between disease activity, benign nonprogressive histological findings and progressive chronic hepatitis are not clearly defined (33, 34). It is unknown, whether patients with chronic persistent hepatitis (no piecemeal necrosis, intact limiting plate of liver cells between portal zones and liver cell columns, expansion of the portal zone by mononuclear cells and some fibrosis) or minimal chronic active hepatitis will develop cirrhosis and therefore should be candidates for corticosteroid treatment. The decision to treat these cases is often guided by symptoms. Asymptomatic patients may be observed without treatment but require careful monitoring for any sign of disease progression. On the other hand, patients with cirrhosis or chronic active hepatitis clearly have a poorer prognosis at the onset of treatment.

Initiation of corticosteroid therapy commonly improves the symptoms and causes decreasing transaminase activities. Hypergammaglobulinemia falls more slowly. In general remission occurs within 1-3 months of initiation of therapy. In a small group remission has been reported only after 2-4 years (7). Patients who do not achieve remission within 4 years are less likely to respond completely later and have to be regarded as treatment failures (7). As a matter of fact there is no evidence that progression to cirrhosis will finally be avoided (35), even in patients with biochemical and clinical remission.

Corticosteroids are generally considered as the first line therapy but there are no universal guidelines as to the initial dose or whether azathioprine should be added from the beginning. Azathioprine alone is not capable to induce a remission. In the Mayo trial there was even no better effect compared to placebo. Azathioprine alone may be used to maintain remission once it has been induced by corticosteroids (36). In the Mayo Clinic trial treatment was started with 60 mg prednisone daily for the first week, followed by 40 mg/day for the second week and 30 mg/

day for the next two weeks. The maintenance dose was 20 mg. In the prednisone/azathioprine group prednisone was started with 30 mg/day for the first week, followed by 20 mg/day for the next week and 15 mg/day for week 3 and 4. The maintenance dose was 15 mg/day. Azathioprine was added with 50 mg/day from the beginning. In the Royal Free Hospital trial lower initial doses with 15 mg prednisolone led to comparable results (29).

Both prednisone and prednisolone have been used in the treatment trials and no significant therapeutic differences were observed. Alternate day therapy regimen have been used in order to minimize steroid side effects but convincing studies are still lacking. There is no convincing evidence that prednisolone is more beneficial even in advanced disease states, compared to prednisone, which, as a prodrug, has to be converted into the biochemically active metabolite prednisolone.

DURATION OF THERAPY

It is estimated, that about 70% of patients with autoimmune hepatitis require lifelong immunosupressive therapy. A most important therapeutic concept in autoimmune hepatitis is to treat with sufficient doses for enough time. The most reliable determinant of sufficient therapy is to keep ALT activity below two times the upper normal limit (37). Patients with cirrhosis at the onset of therapy rarely stay in remission after treatment withdrawal and almost always require maintenance therapy.

Premature discontinuation of immunosupressive therapy endangers remission due to the frequent occurrence of inflammatory relapse in up to 87%, even after several years of treatment (38-40). In a smaller group of patients remission persists after treatment withdrawal.

Therefore, in general, treatment should last for a minimum of two years before treatment withdrawal by tapering the steroid dose may be attempted. Frequent monitoring of liver enzyme activities is strictly required during this phase in order to recognize disease relapse. Once relapse has occured and successfully been brought back into remission, no further attempt for another withdrawal should be tried.

Adjustment of the maintenance dose should primarily be based on the ALT-level. In many cases very low stroid doses (2.5-10 mg prednisolone) are sufficient to maintain remission and to prevent disease relapse. When using a combination therapy, corticosteroid dose should be reduced and azathioprine should be kept at a constant level.

REMISSION

Guidelines for definition of complete, partial and no response have been published by the International Autoimmune Hepatitis Group and are given in table 4 (25).

THERAPY COMPLICATIONS

Corticosteroid therapy is associated with a variety of dose-related side effects like hypertension, diabetes mellitus, cataract, acne, striae, weight gain, predisposition to infections and osteoporosis as a major limiting factor (41, 42). Azathioprine may induce bone marrow suppression, especially thrombocytopenia and severe toxic cholestatic liver disease. The risk of development of malignancies does not seem to be increased in long term low dose treatment, but may not be excluded in general.

ALTERNATIVE THERAPEUTIC REGIMEN

Cyclosporine may induce remission in a few corticosteroid-insensitive patients but is associated with a variety of severe side effects like hypertension, hypercholesterolemia and the danger for developing malignancy, which seems to render this treatment modality difficult for long term use (43).

Treatment with thymic extract, d-penicillamine and flavinoids as free radical scavenger failed to prove efficacy (44-46).

BUDESONIDE

Budesonide is a 16-alpha-hydroxyprednisolone derivate with strong topical activity. The marked 90% first pass hepatic metabolisation causes a short half life, combined with lower

Table 4. Definitions of response to therapy in autoinmune hepatitis

Complete	Either or both of the following: marked improvement of symptoms and return of all liver test values completely to normal within 1 yr and sustained for at least a further 6 mo on maintenance therapy, or a liver biopsy specimen at some time during this period showing at most minimal activity	*or*	Either or both of the following: marked improvement of symptoms together with at least 50% improvement of all liver test results during the first month of treatment, with AST and ALT levels continuing to fall to less than twice the upper normal limit within 6 mo during any reductions toward maintenance therapy or a liver biopsy showing only minimal activity within 1 yr
Partial	Improvement of symptoms together with at least 50% improvement of all liver test results during the first 2 mo of treatment with continuing decreases thereafter, but with AST and ALT levels still not completely normal by 1 yr	*or*	Improvement of symptoms and return of all liver test values to normal within 6 mo, but with a liver biopsy specimen still showing continuing activity
No	Either or both of the following: liver test values still greater than 30% of presenting value after 1 mo of treatmen regardless of symptomatic improvement or a liver biopsy showing no significant change in activity after 6 mo of standard therapy regardless of liver test values	*or*	Greater than 50% improvement in liver test values during the first 1 or 2 mo but not becoming completely normal and with no further improvement by 6 mo, whether steroid dosage is increased and whether symptoms have resolved
Treatment failure	Deterioration of patient's condition despite improvement in some parameters of disease activity		
Relapse	Either or both of the following: an increase in serum AST and ALT levels of greater than twice the upper normal limit or a liver biopsy specimen showing active disease, with or without reappearance of symptoms, after a «complete» response as defined above	*or*	Reappearance of symptoms of sufficient severity to require increased (or reintroduction of) immunosupression, accompanied by any increase in serum AST and ALT levels, after a «complete» response as defined above

From Johnson PJ, McFarlane IG. Meeting report: International Autoimmune Hepatitis Group. Hepatology 1993; 18:998-1005.

systemic side effects. First unpublished results from our department reveal the effectivity of budesonide to reach remission in autoimmune hepatitis and to reduce cushingoid side effects, especially in patients without cirrhosis.

A short case report of two of our Budesonide-treated patients with acute autoimmune hepatitis is presented in order to demonstrate the efficacy of short half life corticosteroids in the treatment of autoimmune hepatitis.

The first patient was a 65-year old woman in whom the first diagnosis of acute hepatitis was made in 1990, initially termed non-A non-B non-C hepatitis (chronic active hepatitis, AST 213 U/I, ALT 423 U/I, gamma globulin 24%). High titers of smooth muscle antibodies and not significantly demonstrable titers of antinuclear antibodies gave first hints for autoimmune hepatitis. Serum transaminase activities slowly returned to normal range within 2 years without immunosuppressive treatment. At the end of 1992 ALT rose to 717 U/I, AST to 343 U/I and gamma globulins were significantly elevated (29%). Another clinical evaluation led to the diagnosis of autoimmune hepatitis type 1 (ANA 1:160; differentiation on Hep2 cells: 1:80; homogenous pattern; SMA 1:80). Treatment with 9 mg Budesonide in three doses per day led to rapid normalization of liver transaminases within 4 weeks. Remission could be maintained with reduced doses of 3 mg per day. Initial development of cushingoid side effects was diminished by dose reduction and recovering liver function.

The second patient was a 21-year old women with acute autoimmune hepatitis type 3, firstly diagnosed in September 1993: ANA 1:160; differentiation on Hep2 cells > 1:160; SLA (ELISA) positive (86%). Initially she presented with acute hepatitis, jaundice, malaise and nausea. HLA-typing revealed haplotype HLA-A1, B8, DR3. Liver transaminases were strongly elevated (ALT 700 U/I, AST 362 U/I, bilirubin 51 umol/l and gamma globulin 32%).

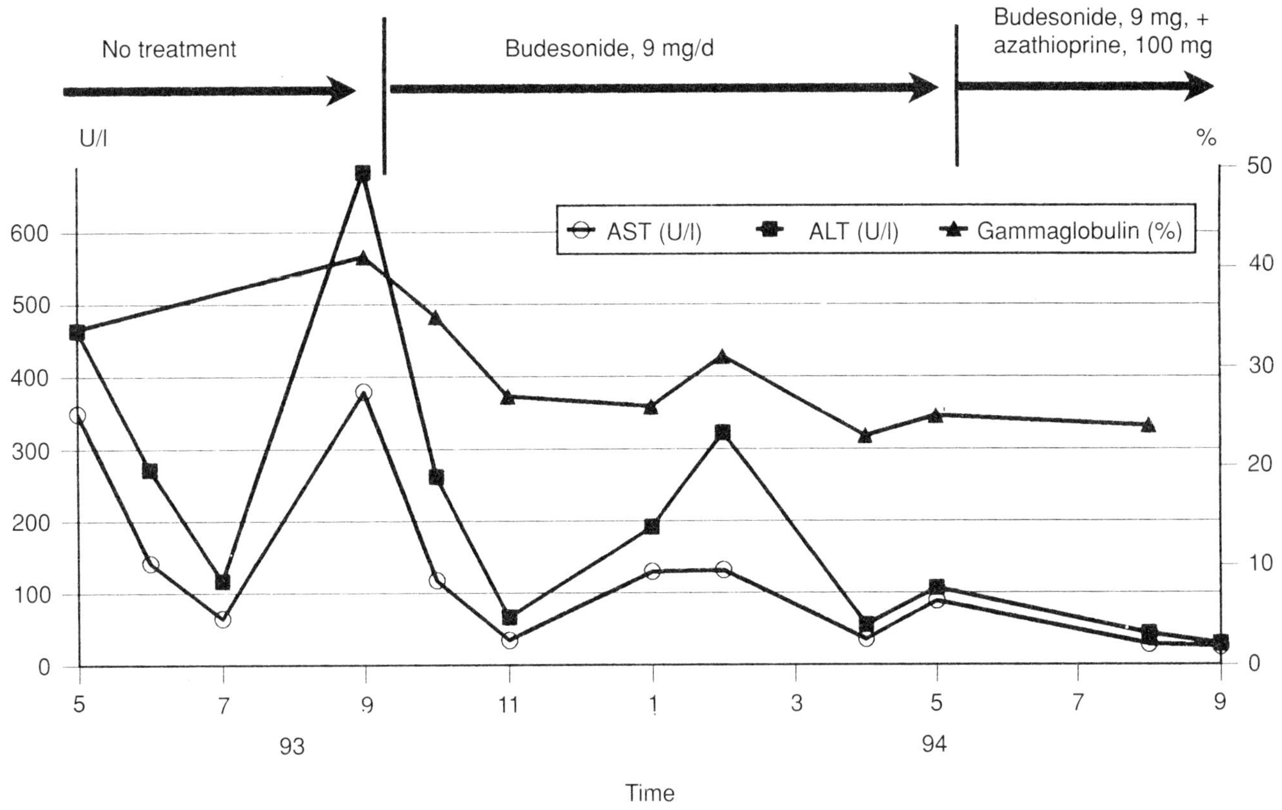

Fig. 1. Course of serum transaminases and gammaglobulin concentration in a patient with autoimmune hepatitis treated with budesonide.

Treatment with 9 mg Budesonide was started and liver enzyme activities fell during the following 2 months (ALT 66 U/I, AST 34 U/I, gamma globulin 27%) (fig. 1). During the next 2 months she experienced a relapse under corticosteroid therapy (ALT 191 U/I, AST 129 U/I, gamma globulin 26%). Liver enzymes fell during the next 2 months at the same dose but rose again in May 1994. At this time 100 mg azathioprine was added and liver transaminases decreased to a slightly elevated level which persisted until now (ALT 29 U/I, AST 29 U/I, gamma-globulin 22%). This case clearly may be attributed to the kind to autoimmune hepatitis, in which only a high dose combination immunosuppressive therapy may enforce remission. After start of Budesonide, disease symptoms quickly resolved and the patient felt well all the time and did not develop cushingoid habitus or weight gain.

These preliminary results demonstrate that treatment with Budesonide can induce remission in acute autoimmune hepatitis. Corticosteroide side effects are low or seem to be tolerable and may depend on the metabolizing capacity of the liver, which might be influenced by the degree of inflammation or preexisting fibrosis or cirrhosis.

TREATMENT WITH ANTI-CD4-ANTIBODIES

Individual cases have been treated with anti-CD4 monoclonal antibodies. Treatment success, however, was not convincing (47).

LIVER TRANSPLANTATION FOR AUTOIMMUNE HEPATITIS

Orthotopic liver transplantation (OLT) is now an established treatment for patients with end-stage disease when immunosuppresive therapy has failed to prevent cirrhosis. A higher frequency of the HLA phenotype A1 B8 DR3 in the transplantation group may reflect a more aggressive course of the disease in these patients (48). In contrast to other liver diseases there have been no valuable prognostic indices for liver transplantation in autoimmune hepatitis for a long time, and the results of the procedure in these patients are uncertain. First hints for possible recurrence in the liver graft have been reported (49).

Sánchez-Urdazpal et al. (7) consider patients, who do not achieve disease remission within 4 years unklikely for ultimate remission. These patients should be candidates for OLT in case of liver decompensation. In this study patients undergoing OLT had a lower mortality rate compared to patients with similar disease stage undergoing protracted immunosuppressive therapy. The five-year survival rate was 92% and was comparable to patients who achieved remission under immunosuppressive therapy. These results suggest that OLT is an appropriate procedure for patients with advanced autoimmune hepatitis. It is possible that combined immunosuppressive therapy for the prevention of graft rejection completely suppresses the perhaps still existing pathogenetic mechanisms of autoimmune hepatitis and that lower doses of these drugs may lead to recurrence of the disease (7), but those implications should not influence the transplant decision. End-stage autoimmune hepatitis is almost an ideal indication for liver transplantation.

REFERENCES

1. Manns MP, Krüger M. Immunogenetics of chronic liver disease. Gastroenterology 1994; 106:1676-1697.
2. Mackay IR, Morris PJ. Association of autoimmune active chronic hepatitis with HL-A 1,8. Lancet 1972; ii:793-795.
3. Seki T, Kiyosawa K, Inoko H, Ota M. Association of autoimmune hepatitis with HLA-Bw54 and DR4 in Japanese patients. Hepatology 1990; 12:1300-1304.
4. Czaja AJ, Rakela J, Hay JE, Moore SB. Clinical and prognostic implications of HLA B8 in corticosteroid-treated severe autoimmune chronic active hepatitis. Gastroenterology 1990; 98:1587-1593.
5. Czaja AJ, Carpenter HA, Santrach PJ, Moore SB, Taswell HF, Homburger HA. Evidence against hepatitis viruses as important causes of autoimmune hepatitis in the United States. J Hepatol (in press).
6. Donaldson PT, Doherty DG, Hayllar KM, McFarlane IG, Johnson PJ, Williams R. Susceptibility to autoimmune chronic active hepatitis: human leukocyte antigens DR4 and AI-B8-DR3 are independent risk factors. Hepatology 1991; 13:701-706.
7. Sánchez-Urdazpal L, Czaja AJ, van Hoek B, Krom RAF, Wiesner RH. Prognostic features and role of liver transplantation in severe corticosteroid-treated autoimmune chronic active hepatitis. Hepatology 1991; 15:215-221.
8. Czaja AJ, Carpenter HA, Santrach PJ, Moore SB. Significance of HLA DR4 in type I autoimmune hepatitis. Gastroenterology 1993; 105:1502-1507.
9. Czaja AJ, Rakela J, Hay JE, Moore SB. Clinical and prognostic implications of HLA B8 in corticosteroid treated severe autoimmune chronic active hepatitis. Gastroenterology 1990; 98:1587-1593.
10. Marcos Y, Fainboim HA, Capuccio M, Findor J, Daruich J, Reyes B, Paudo M, Theiler GC, Méndez M. Two-locus involvement in the association of human leukocyte antigen with the extrahepatic manifestations of autoimmune chronic active hepatitis. Hepatology 1994; 19:1371-1374.
11. Czaja AJ, Carpenter HA, Santrach PJ, Moore SB. Extrahepatic immunological features of chronic active hepatitis: genetic predispositions and prognostic implications. Hepatology 1992; 16:190A (Abstr).
12. Whittingham SF, Irwin J, Mackay IR, Smalley M. Smooth muscle autoantibody in «auto-immune» hepatitis. Gastroenterology 1966; 51:499-505.
13. Gabbiani G, Ryan GB, Lamelin JP, Vassalli P, Majno G, Bouvier CA, Cruchaud A, Luscher EF. Human smooth muscle autoantibody. Its identification as anti-actin antibody and a study of ist binding to «non-muscular» cells. Am J Pathol 1973; 72:473-488.
14. Manns MP, Johnson EF, Griffen KJ, Tan EM, Sullivan KF. Major antigen of liver kidney microsomal antibody in idiopatic autoimmune hepatitis is citochrome P450db1. J Clin Invest 1989; 83:1066-1072.
15. Manns MP. Autoantibodies in chronic hepatitis: diagnostic reagents and scientific tools to study etiology, pathogenesis and cell biology. Prog Liver Dis (in press).
16. Durazzo M, Philipp T, van Pelt FNAM, Lüttig B, Borghieso E, Michel G, Schmidt E, Loges S, Rizzetto M, Manns MP. Heterogeneity of microsomal autoantibodies (LKM) in chronic hepatitis C and D virus infection. Gastroenterology (in press).
17. Michel G, Ritter A, Gerken G, Meyer zum Büschenfelde K-H, Decker R, Manns M. Anti-GOR and hepatitis C virus in autoimmune liver diseases. Lancet 1992; 339:267-269.
18. Desmet V, Gerber MA, Hoofnagle JH, Manns M, Scheuer P. Classification of chronic hepatitis: Diagnosis, grading and staging. Hepatology 1994; 19:1513-1520.
19. Phillip T, Durazzo M, Trautwein C, Alex B, Straub P, Lamb JG, Johnson EF, Tukey RH, Manns MP. Recognition of uridine diphosphate glucuronosyl transferases by LKM-3 antibodies in chronic hepatitis D. Lancet 1994; 334:578-581.
20. Odievre AM, Maggiore G, Homberg JC, Saadoun F, Courouce AM, Yvart J, Hadchouvel M, Allagille D.

Seroimmunologic classification of chronic hepatitis in 57 children. Hepatology 1983; 3:407-411.
21. Manns M, Gerken G, Kyriatsoulis A. Characterization of a new subgroup of autoimmune chronic active hepatitis by autoantibodies against a soluble liver antigen. Lancet 1987; i:292-294.
22. Stechemesser E, Klein R, Berg PA. Characterization and clinical relevance of liver-pancreas antibodies in autoimmune hepatitis. Hepatology 1993; 18:1-9.
23. Johnson PJ, McFarlane IG, McFarlane BM, Williams R. Autoimmune features in patients with idiopathic chronic active hepatitis who are seronegative for conventional autoantibodies. J Gastroenterol Hepatol 1990; 5:244-251.
24. Keating JJ, O'Brien CJ, Stellon AJ, Portmann BC, Johnson RD, Johnson PJ, Williams R. Influence of aetiology, clinical and histological features on survival in chronic active hepatitis: An analysis of 204 patients. Q J Med 1987; 62:59-66.
25. Johnson PJ, McFarlane IG. Meeting report: International Autoimmune Hepatitis Group. Hepatology 1993; 18:998-1005.
26. Wang K, Czaja AJ. Prognosis of corticosteroid-treated hepatitis B surface antigen-negative chronic active hepatitis in postmenopausal women: A retrospective analysis. Gastroenterology 1989; 97:1288-1293.
27. Read AE, Sherlock S, Harrison CV. Active «juvenile» cirrhosis considered as part of a systemic disease and the effect of corticosteroid therapy. Gut 1963; 378-393.
28. Mistilis SP, Blackburn CRB. The treatment of active chronic hepatitis with 6-mercaptopurine and azathioprine. Austral Ann Med 1967; 16:305-311.
29. Cook GC, Mulligan R, Sherlock S. Controlled prospective trial of corticosteroid therapy in active chronic hepatitis. Q J Med 1971; 40:159-185.
30. Soloway RD, Summerskill WHJ, Baggenstoss AH, Geall MG, Gitnick GL, Elveback LR, Schoenfield LJ. Clinical, biochemical and histological remission of severe chronic active liver disease: A controlled trial of treatments and early prognosis. Gastroenterology 1972; 63:820-833.
31. Czaja AJ. Auto-immune chronic active hepatitis: A specific entity? The negative argument. J Gastroenterol Hepatol 1990; 5:342-351.
32. Koretz RL, Lewin KJ, Higgins J, Fagen ND,Gitnick GL. Chronic active hepatitis. Who meets treatment criteria? Dig Dis Sci 1980; 25:695-699.
33. Cooksley WGE, Breadbear RA, Robinson W, Harrison M, Halliday JW, Powell LW, Ng HS. The prognosis of chronic active hepatitis without cirrhosis in relation to bridging necrosis. Hepatology 1986; 6:345-348.
34. Combes B. The initial morphologic lesion in chronic hepatitis. Important or unimportant? Hepatology 1986; 6:518-522.
35. Davis GL, Czaja AJ. Immediate and long-term results of corticosteroid therapy for severe idiopathic chronic active hepatitis. In: Czaja AJ, Dickson ER eds. Chronic active hepatitis: The Mayo Experience. New York: Marcel Dekker, 1986; 269-283.
36. Stellon AJ, Keating JJ, Johnson PJ, McFarlane IG, Williams R. Maintenance of remission in autoimmune chronic active hepatitis with azathioprine after corticosteroid withdrawal. Hepatology 1988; 8:781-784.
37. Czaja AJ, Wolf AM, Baggenstoss AH. Laboratory assessment of severe chronic active liver disease during and after corticosteroid therapy: Correlation of serum transaminase and gamma globulin level with histologic features. Gastroenterology 1981; 80:678-692.
38. Hegarty JE, Nouri-Aria KT, Portmann B, Eddleston ALWF, Williams R. Relapse following treatment withdrawal in patients with autoimmune chronic active hepatitis. Hepatology 1983; 3:685-689.
39. McCullough AJ, Czaja AJ. Relapse following treatment withdrawal in autoimmune chronic active hepatitis. Hepatology 1984; 4:747-748.
40. Czaja AJ, Beaver SJ, Shiels MT. Sustained remission after corticosteroid therapy of severe hepatitis B surface antigen-negative chronic active hepatitis. Gastroenterology 1987; 92:215-219.
41. Uribe M, Go VLW, Kulge D. Prednisone for chronic active hepatitis: Pharmacokinetics and serum binding in patients with chronic active hepatitis and steroid major side effects. J Clin Gastroenterol 1984; 6:331-335.
42. Stellon AJ, Davies A, Compston J, Williams R. Bone loss in autoimmune chronic hepatitis on a maintenance corticosteroid therapy. Gastroenterology 1985; 89:1078-1083.
43. Hyams JS, Ballow M, Leichtner AM. Cyclosporine treatment of autoimmune chronic active hepatitis. Gastroenterology 1987; 93:809-893.
44. Hegarty JE, Nouri-Aria KT, Eddleston ALWF, Williams R. Controlled trial of a thymic hormone extract (Thymostimulin) in «autoimmune» chronic active hepatitis. Gut 1977; 25:279-283.
45. Stern RB, Wilkinson SP, Howorth PJN, Williams R. Controlled trial of synthetic D-penicilamine and prednisone in maintenance therapy for active chronic hepatitis. Gut 1977; 18:19-22.
46. Bar-Meir S, Halpern Z, Gutman M, Shpirer Z, Baratz M, Bass D. Effect of (+)-cyanidanol-3 on chronic active hepatitis: A double blind controlled trial. Gut 1985; 26:975-979.
47. Kakavand B, Reiter C, Riber EP, Riethmüller G, Sanders M, Eisenburg J. Therapeutic CD4 T-cell depletion with chimeric monoclonal CD4 antibodies for therapy of autoimmune chronic hepatitis (Abstr). 8th Spring Meeting of the Gesellschaft für Immunologie. München, 1992.
48. Donaldson PT, Doherty DG, Hayllar KM, McFarlane IG, Johnson PJ, Williams R. Susceptibility to autoimmune chronic active hepatitis: human leukocyte antigens DR4 and A1-B8-DR3 are independent risk factors. Hepatology 1991; 13:701-706.
49. Neuberger J, Portmann B, Calne R, Williams R. Recurrence of autoimmune chronic active hepatitis following orthotopic liver grafting. Transplantation 1984; 37:363-365.

Ursodeoxycholic Acid in the Treatment of Chronic Cholestasis and other Chronic Liver Diseases

R. Poupon, R. E. Poupon

INTRODUCTION

Cholestasis can be defined as the clinical, biochemical and histological manifestations of defective bile acid transport from the liver to the intestine. Chronic cholestatic conditions of the liver form a homogeneous group of diseases with several points in common. Most result from the destruction of intrahepatic or extrahepatic bile ducts, or a developmental defect. Most chronic cholestatic conditions can progress towards cirrhosis (biliary cirrhosis) and hepatocellular insufficiency.

Table 1 lists the chronic cholestatic conditions of adults that can progress towards biliary cirrhosis and liver failure. In the case of primary biliary cirrhosis (PBC), graft rejection, graft-versus-host disease (GVDH), most types of drug-induced cholestasis and liver involvement by sarcoidosis, the initial abnormality is inflammation and destruction of the interlobular bile ducts. In primary sclerosing cholangitis, the initial abnormality is sclerosis of the extrahepatic or intrahepatic bile ducts. Long-term parenteral feeding can lead to chronic cholestasis. Cholestasis of pregnancy, some cases of drug-induced cholestasis (especially those due to combined oral contraceptives) and recurrent benign cholestasis are clinical situations associated with "pure" cholestasis, with no bile duct lesions. These forms do not progress towards cirrhosis or hepatocellular failure. The main causes of chronic cholestatic conditions in children are congenital or acquired lack of bile ducts, the latter sometimes resulting from metabolic or infectious insult. As in adults, most of these pathological conditions can progress towards biliary cirrhosis.

The rate of progression towards the terminal stage varies from patient to patient and depends on the nature of each disease and probably on the degree of bile duct destruction. For example, in PBC, follow-up studies of patients in controlled trials have shown that within about 4 years approximately 40% develop cirrhosis and 20% reach the terminal stage requiring transplantation (1). Very similar results have been reported in sclerosing cholangitis (2-4). Most children with bile duct atresia develop liver failure before the age of 3 years if transplantation is not performed.

Table 1. Causes of chronic cholestasis

In adulthood	In infancy and childhood
Primary biliary cirrhosis	Bile duct atresia
Allograft rejection	Syndromic bile duct paucity
Graft-versus-host disease	Non-syndromic bile duct paucity
Drug-induced cholestasis	Metabolic
Idiopathic ductopenia	Infection
Primary sclerosing cholangitis	Familial intrahepatic
Drug-induced cholestasis	Cystic fibrosis
Stenosis, strictures	
Parenteral nutrition	

Terminal-stage chronic cholestatic conditions are an ideal indication for liver transplantation. This transforms the prognosis, increasing the 5-year survival rate to 70-80% if transplantation is done in good conditions.

RATIONALE FOR THE USE OF UDCA IN CHOLESTATIC DISORDERS

UDCA (3α,7β-dihydroxy-5β-cholanic acid) is a natural bile acid in many mammals, but is only present in very small quantities in humans. UDCA is formed by 7β-epimerisation of chenodeoxycholic acid, one of the two principal human bile acids, by certain intestinal organisms. Given its structural similarities with chenodeoxycholic acid, it was postulated that it might also dissolve cholesterol gallstones, and this was confirmed in therapeutic trials. Two lessons were learned from these trials: first, UDCA was capable of modifying the composition of circulating bile acids in humans, becoming the predominant bile acid species; and second, it was found to have no toxicity whatsoever, in contrast to chenodeoxycholic acid (5-7).

There are several lines of evidence indicating that the defective bile acid elimination in cholestatic conditions could be responsible for a major part of the clinical, biochemical and histopathological manifestations, as well as their progression towards cirrhosis and hepatocellular failure. During the course of chronic cholestatic conditions, bile acids accumulate in the liver, the systemic circulation and peripheral tissues (8-11). In the liver, concentrations close to 500 to 600 nmol/g are sometimes observed. Since the pioneering work by Holsti (12), it has been shown repeatedly that bile acids administered to animals, the isolated perfused liver or hepatocyte cultures are hepatotoxic. When given chronically to certain animal species, they induce ductular lesions, fibrosis, and even cirrhosis (13). In humans, the administration of chenodeoxycholic and deoxycholic acids can increase transaminase activity and lead to histological changes in the liver (14, 15). The toxic effects of bile acids include a series of phenomena observed during cholestasis and *in vitro*: increased membrane fluidity, increased membrane permeability (especially to calcium), impaired oxidative phosphorylation, decreased mono-oxygenase activities, inhibition of γ-glutamyl transpeptidase and glutathione transferase activities, changes in cytoskeleton organization, induction of free radical injury, changes in DNA superstructure and, finally, cell apoptosis and necrosis. These deleterious effects are apparently influenced by three main factors: *a*) the chemical structure and the degree of hydrophobicity of the bile acid; *b*) the nature of the cells or tissue exposed to bile acids, and *c*) the concentration-time product in or around the cells.

Contrary to endogenous human bile acids, and particularly, chenodeoxycholic acid, UDCA is strongly hydrophilic and is not toxic *in vitro* or in humans. In particular, UDCA has no toxicity up to concentrations of 500 μmol/l in several *in vitro* models. In humans, UDCA is at least partly transformed into lithocholic acid. However, humans rapidly detoxify and excrete lithocholate, which therefore does not accumulate in the enterohepatic circulation (16).

Although we do not know precisely how bile acid acid accumulation damages the liver, it is now possible to sketch a simplified mechanism of action of UDCA in cholestasis. UDCA inhibits the intestinal absorption and increases the canalicular excretion of cholic and chenodeoxycholic acids. Inhibition of bile acid intestinal absorption is well documented. During UDCA therapy, the fractional turn over rate and ileal excretion of cholic and chenodeoxycholic acids increase. However, several evidence suggest that the decreased intestinal absorption is not the only explanation for the hepatoprotective effect of UDCA in cholestasis. For example, cholestyramine which also reduces bile acid concentrations does not have frank beneficial effects in chronic cholestatic conditions. Indeed, several lines of evidence suggest that UDCA protects the liver through an increase in the intrinsic ability to secrete bile acids and other organic anions into bile. The mechanisms of this peculiar property is dicussed elsewere in detail. Other possible mechanisms involve immune modulation —UDCA reduces both cholestasis and abnormal expression of HLA class I molecules on hepatocytes (17, 18), and also possibly on biliary cells— and stabilization of hepatocellular membranes (19, 20).

TREATMENT OF ADULT CHOLESTATIC DISORDERS

Primary Biliary Cirrhosis

Immunosuppressive treatments have been used in controlled trials for the treatment of PBC. Colchicine has been used for its antifibrotic and anti-inflammatory properties. Most of these drugs, especially cyclosporin, had a certain effect on laboratory parameters, but not on the prognosis of the disease.

In 1987, we postulated that long-term treatment with UDCA might displace endogenous bile acids and thus, reverse their suspected cytotoxicity. In a pilot study of patients with PBC, UDCA indeed led to major sustained improvements in liver function tests (21). To determine whether UDCA would slow the progression of PBC towards the terminal phase, we conducted a 2-year multicenter, double-blind, controlled trial in which patients with PBC were randomized to receive either UDCA or a placebo (22). Patients were admitted to the trial regardless of the duration of symptoms and histological severity. The end-point chosen to define failure of UDCA treatment was one of the following criteria: hyperbilirubinemia, clinical complication (variceal bleeding, ascites, encephalopathy) or a major adverse effect. Following randomization, 73 patients with PBC received UDCA (13-15 mg/kg/d) and 73 placebo. At entry, the two groups were well matched for age, sex, time since initial diagnosis and histological severity: in the UDCA group 50% of the patients had Stage I-II disease, compared with 56% in the placebo group. At the end of the trial, the risk of failure was significantly (about 3-fold) higher in the placebo group than in the UDCA group. One patient in each group withdrew because of adverse effects. After 2 years of treatment, the proportion of treated patients with clinically overt disease had fallen significantly; in particular, there was a clear improvement in terms of the severity of pruritus. Patients receiving UDCA showed significant improvements in serum bilirubin level, alkaline phosphatase, transaminases, γ-glutamyl transpeptidase activity, cholesterol and immunoglobulin M levels, the anti-mitochondrial antibody titer and the Mayo risk score. There was a significant improvement in the mean histologic score and in all the histological features, except fibrosis, in the group given UDCA.

Because of patient selection and short duration of follow-up, there were few liver transplantations, preventing any comparison of the two groups of treatment on the basis of this criterion (22). Given the benefit of UDCA, patients completing the study received UDCA in an open fashion and were monitored for a further 2 years. At 4 years, there had been 4 liver transplantations in the original UDCA group, compared with 13 in the original placebo group. The incidence of liver transplantation was significantly lower in the patients who received UDCA for 4 years than in those initially receiving the placebo ($p = 0.003$, relative risk 0.21 [CI, 0.09-0.76]). Thus, long-term UDCA therapy slows the progression of the disease (23).

During the study period, other trials of UDCA in PBC were set up (24-27). The data so far available consistently show an improvement in biochemical parameters. By contrast, improvements in clinical and histologic parameters are inconsistently found (28) ; however, it must be emphasized that these trials lack the power required to conclude that UDCA has no effect on these parameters. The recent results of two large North-American trials (29, 30) indicate that UDCA delayed the progression of the disease but without reducing the need for liver transplantation. The apparent discrepancies with our results could be related to the duration of the treatment and/or selection of patients: a long-term follow-up is needed to show a potential effect on liver transplantation occurrence and UDCA is not expected to reverse the terminal phase of PBC. Further studies are required to better define the patients who are relevant of medical or surgical treatments and to assess the additional benefit of combined medical treatments.

Primary Sclerosing Cholangitis

Since sclerosing cholangitis and PBC share certain features, we studied the clinical and biochemical effects of UDCA administration in patients with sclerosing cholangitis (31). In an uncontrolled study (15 patients given 8-16 mg/kg/day UDCA), the proportion of patients suffering from fatigue or pruritus after 6 months of treatment fell from 60 to 20% and from 33 to 20%, respectively. Serum levels of alkaline phosphatases, γ-glutamyl transpeptidase (GGT) and transaminases also fell significantly. No exacerbation of associated disorders or side effects of UDCA were observed. The efficacy of UDCA was suggested by *a*) the clear improvement in patients in whom the cholestasis had been stable for at least 6 months, *b*) the absence of similar spontaneous improvements during the natural history of the disease and *c*) aggravation of liver test results following the discontinuation of UDCA in three patients.

Two other pilot studies have confirmed these results. One (32) in which 12 patients were treated for a mean period of 30 months with 10 mg/kg/day UDCA, confirmed the improvement of biochemical test results after six months of treatment, and the further improvement with long-term treatment. The other (33), in which 22 patients received UDCA for one year and were then randomized to receive either UDCA or a placebo for a further year, was interrupted for ethical reasons, i.e. the aggravation of the disease in patients receiving the placebo. A placebo-controlled study led to the conclusion that UDCA reduces disease activity in patients with sclerosing cholangitis (18). After one year of treatment, the patients in the UDCA group showed improvements relative to the placebo group with respect to serum levels of bilirubin, alkaline phosphatase, GGT and transaminases. Histological features, evaluated with a multiparametric score, also improved.

Although the effectiveness of UDCA in sclerosing cholangitis has been demonstrated, it is less valuable in this condition than in PBC. Indeed, patients with sclerosing cholangitis frequently develop a cholangiocarcinoma and liver transplantation is more widely indicated than in PBC; thus, UDCA therapy is aimed mainly at obtaining an improvement in the quality of life and in the patient's condition, with a view to transplantation.

Intrahepatic Cholestasis of Pregnancy

Intrahepatic cholestasis of pregnancy is a condition of unknown origin, characterized by pruritus and abnormal liver test results, with a predominantly cholestatic pattern. It appears during the second half of pregnancy in previously healthy women. After delivery, the pruritus resolves rapidly, and biochemical parameters return to normal. Besides the discomfort for the mothers, this disease causes an increased rate of fetal distress, premature delivery and perinatal mortality; there is no effective treatment.

In an open study, UDCA administration to eight patients with intrahepatic cholestasis of pregnancy led to an improvement in pruritus and laboratory test results. UDCA was well tolerated, and had no apparent toxicity for either the mother or the child (34). Unfortunately, data concerning bile acid composition before and during UDCA therapy were lacking.

In a case of triple pregnancy complicated by early cholestasis, UDCA administration normalized maternal liver function (35). The marked improvement in clinical and biochemical parameters, including serum bile acid levels, suggests a role of endogenous bile acids in the onset of this form of cholestasis.

Chronic Hepatitis

In this setting, there is no clear rationale for the use of UDCA. A large number of studies have reported a reduction of ALT and GGT activities in patients with chronic active hepatitis during UDCA administration (36-44). No firm conclusions have been drawn from these studies for the following reasons: low and variable doses of UDCA, short follow-up, small number of subjects, absence of histological evaluation and absence of bile acid assays. Two recent double-blind studies (45, 46), carried out over a one year period, confirmed that UDCA administration reduces ALT and GGT activities. There was, however, no improvement in liver histology, in particular Knodell' score. UDCA therapy is unlikely to affect the course of this disease.

Other settings

Liver graft rejection. Acute and chronic liver graft rejection is a frequent complication of liver transplantation, affecting 50-75% of patients and justifying aggressive treatment. UDCA could be effective in this setting for the following reasons: *a*) there is a striking similarity between the characteristic lesions of PBC and those of liver rejection, *b*) in both cases, there is abnormal expression of Class I and II HLA molecules in the liver, and *c*) both conditions are associated with cholestasis and the destruction of interlobular bile ducts. In PBC, UDCA reduces HLA Class I expression in the liver (17), prevents duct destruction and improves the cholestasis.

The results of a pilot study (47) are in favour of such an action. During the first month after liver transplantation, 2 episodes of rejection were observed in 18 consecutive patients who received UDCA, compared with 6 out of 8 previous patients who had received the usual immunosuppressive treatments. However, these results were not confirmed in a subsequent study (48). During the 6 months after liver transplantation, 12 rejection episodes were observed among eight of 15 patients treated with UDCA, while 10 episodes occurred in seven of 14 untreated patients. Unfortunately, the interpretation of these results is limited by the absence of randomization and the lack of data concerning the bioavailability of UDCA during the post-operative period.

Chronic graft-versus-host disease of the liver. The natural history of GVHD of the liver suggests that biliary cirrhosis may be the end-stage. On the basis of biochemical, clinical and histological similarities between GVHD and PBC, the efficacy of UDCA was tested in the therapy of GVHD of the liver (49). UDCA (10-15 mg/kg/day) was given for 6 weeks to 12 patients who had failed to respond to immunosuppressive therapy. Biochemical parameters improved during UDCA and returned to pre-treatment values after discontinuation of the treatment. This preliminary study requires confirmation in longer-term controlled trials.

Cyclosporin-induced cholestasis. Cholestasis induced by cyclosporin A following liver transplantation may be improved by the administration of UDCA (50). The study concerned 13 heart-transplant recipients, 5 of whom developed cholestasis during immuno-suppressive therapy including cyclosporin A. All 5 patients received UDCA; although no change in blood cyclosporin levels was observed, alkaline phosphatase, GGT and transaminase activities, as well as bilirubinemia, were markedly reduced. When UDCA was discontinued, all five patients redeveloped cholestasis, which again resolved when on UDCA.

Parenteral nutrition-associated cholestasis. Cholestasis can occur during long-term parenteral nutrition, and no treatment is known to be effective. A case report and, very recently, a cross-over study, suggest that UDCA could prevent or improve abnormalities in liver tests in this setting (51, 52).

Benign recurrent intrahepatic cholestasis. Benign recurrent intrahepatic cholestasis is characterized by the abrupt onset of severe cholestasis, which spontaneously subsides after several weeks, in otherwise healthy subjects. These acute attacks have been attributed to unknown factors impairing bile acid transport at the canalicular level in genetically susceptible subjects. All treatments so far evaluated have proven unsatisfactory. Recently, a contracted bile acid pool size was reported in these patients (53) and thus the use of UDCA was suggested. On the basis of a detailed clinical report, it appears that UDCA is unable to prevent acute cholestatic episodes (54). In contrast, in a case report, UDCA was found to have a beneficial effect over 4 years (55). However, because the course of this disease is highly variable, it is difficult to prove or disprove the efficacy of UDCA.

Alcoholic cirrhosis. A placebo-controlled, cross-over study (56) showed that the administration of UDCA for four weeks led to a reduction in serum bilirubin concentrations, as well as ALT, GGT and alkaline phosphatase activities in patients with alcoholic cirrhosis and who continue to drink excessively.

TREATMENT OF CHILDHOOD CHOLESTATIC DISEASES

Cystic Fibrosis

With the improved efficacy of treatments for pulmonary conditions, the survival of patients with cystic fibrosis has increased considerably. In contrast, hepatobiliary complications are more and more frequent: about 25% of adult patients have biliary abnormalities which, in 5-10% of the cases, progresses to cirrhosis.

In young patients with cystic fibrosis and severe cholestasis, UDCA not only improved conventional liver tests, but also improved nutritional parameters (57, 58). As in other cholestatic diseases, it seems likely that the beneficial effect of UDCA on cholestasis involves similar mechanisms, including an improvement in hepatic excretory function (58, 59) and, as a possible consequence, an improvement in biliary drainage. In contrast, why UDCA should act on nutritional status is less clear. An improvement in intestinal fat absorption can be ruled out because of the lack of change in fecal fat excretion (60), and the fact that UDCA inhibits intestinal cholesterol absorption. The most reasonable hypothesis is that nutritional status improves following improvement in liver function.

Other Childhood Cholestatic Diseases

Controlled studies are currently underway to evaluate the effects of UDCA in intrahepatic bile-duct paucity syndromes, including Alagille's syndrome and Byler's disease (61). Preliminary results show that UDCA has a spectacular effect on pruritus, laboratory test results, jaundice and nutritional status. Similar effects have been reported in patients with extrahepatic bile duct atresia (62, 63), in whom treatment with UDCA enabled Kasai's operation to be performed in excellent conditions.

Inborn Errors of Bile Acid Metabolism

Childhood cholestatic diseases characterized by errors of bile acid synthesis (3β-hydroxysteroid dehydrogenase and Δ^4-3-oxosteroid-5-α-reductase deficits, Zellweger's syndrome) manifest clinically as neonatal cholestasis, which can progress towards cirrhosis and death, and biologically as a predominance of atypical bile acids (64). Cholestasis could result from either the inability of the liver to synthesize primary bile acids (essential for bile secretion) or from the toxicity of the atypical bile acids. Treatment with UDCA together with cholate and/or chenodeoxycholate could be effective (65).

CONCLUSION AND PERSPECTIVES

Until the 1980s, the role of bile acids in the initiation of liver injury in humans was only suspected on the basis of the toxicity of whole bile and bile salts and studies showing elevations in serum and tissue levels of bile salts in liver diseases. The beneficial effects of UDCA in PBC have provided the first firm evidence that in some way, bile acids may be related to liver injury in humans.

These observations raise a series of questions and challenges in clinical, cellular and molecular research. For example, is UDCA capable of modifying the progression and prognosis of other cholestatic conditions of children and adults and, more generally, liver diseases in which the enterohepatic bile acid circulation is disturbed? Is it possible and warranted to design UDCA analogs with stronger activities and more specific targets? And how might UDCA and these analogs modulate fundamental cell or organelle functions and cell-to-cell relationships in the normal and cholestatic liver?

REFERENCES

1. Christensen E, Crowe J, Doniach D, Popper H, Ranek L, Rodés J, Tygstrup N, Williams R. Clinical pattern and course of disease in primary biliary cirrhosis based on an analysis of 236 patients. Gastroenterology 1980; 78:236-246.
2. Dickson ER, Murtaugh PA, Wiesner RH, Grambsch PM, Fleming T, Ludwig J, LaRusso NF, Malinchoc M, Chapman RW, Kaplan MM, Maddrey WC, Williams R, Farrant M, Langworthy A. Primary sclerosing cholangitis: refinement and validation of survival models. Gastroenterology 1992; 103:1893-1901.
3. LaRusso NF, Weisner RH, Ludwig J, MacCarty RL, Beaver SJ, Zinsmeister AR. Prospective trial of penicillamine in primary sclerosing cholangitis. Gastroenterology 1988; 95:1036-1042.
4. Wiesner RH, Grambsch PM, Dickson ER, Ludwig J, MacCarty RL, Hunter EB, Fleming TR, Fisher LD, Beaver SJ, LaRusso NF. Primary sclerosing cholangitis: natural history, prognostic factors and survival analysis. Hepatology 1989; 10:430-436.
5. Bachrach WH, Hofmann AF. Ursodeoxycholic acid in the treatment of cholesterol cholelithiasis. Part I. Dig Dis Sci 1982; 24:737-761.

6. Bachrach WH, Hofmann AF. Ursodeoxycholic acid in the treatment of cholesterol cholelithiasis. Part II. Dig Dis Sci 1982; 24:833-856.
7. Poupon RE, Poupon R. Ursodeoxycholic acid for treatment of cholestatic diseases. In: Boyer JL, Ockner RK, eds. Progress in Liver Diseases. Philadelphia: WB Saunders, 1992; 219-117.
8. Greim H, Czygan P, Schaffner F, Popper H. Determination of bile acids in needle biopsies of human liver. Biochem Med 1973; 8:280-286.
9. Akashi Y, Miyazaki H, Yanagisawa J, Nakayama F. Bile acid metabolism in cirrhotic liver tissue-altered synthesis and impaired hepatic secretion. Clin Chim Acta 1987; 168:199-206.
10. Hendenborg G, Norlander A, Norman A. Bile acid conjugates present in tissues during extrahepatic cholestasis. Scand J Clin Lab Invest 1986; 46:539-544.
11. Dupont J, Garcia PA, Hennig B, Dood NK, Yon Oh S, Sizer CE, Goswami SK, Hyde WG. Bile acids in extrahepatic tissues. In: Setchell KDR, Kritchevsky D, Nair PP, eds. The Bile Acids: Chemistry, Physiology, and Metabolism. New York: Plenum Press, 1987; 341-369.
12. Holsti P. Experimental cirrhosis of the liver in rabbits induced by gastric instillation of dessicated whole bile. Acta Path Microbiol Scand 1956; 112:1-67.
13. Palmer RH. Bile acids, liver injury, and liver disease. Arch Intern Med 1972; 130:606-617.
14. LaRusso NF, Szczepanik PA, Hofmann AF. Effect of deoxycholic acid ingestion on bile acid metabolism and biliary lipid secretion in normal subjects. Gastroenterology 1977; 72:132-140.
15. Schoenfield LJ, Lachin JM. Chenodiol (chenodeoxycholic acid) for dissolution of gallstones: the National Cooperative Gallstone Study: a controlled trial of efficacy and safety. Ann Intern Med 1981; 95:257-282.
16. Cowen AC, Korman MG, Hofmann AF, Cass OW, Coffin SB. Metabolism of lithocholate in healthy man. Gastroenterology 1975; 69:62-76.
17. Calmus Y, Gane P, Rouger P, Poupon R. Hepatic expression of class I and class II major histocompatibility complex molecules in primary biliary cirrhosis: effect of ursodeoxycholic acid. Hepatology 1990; 11:12-15.
18. Beuers U, Spengler U, Kruis W, Aydemir Ü, Wiebecke B, Heldwein W, Weinzeirl M, Pape GR, Sauerbruch T, Paumgartner G. Ursodeoxycholic acid for treatment of primary sclerosing cholangitis: a placebo-controlled trial. Hepatology 1992; 16:707-714.
19. Güldütuna S, Immer G, Imohof B S, You T, Leuschner U. Molecular aspects of membrane stabilization by ursodeoxycholate. Gastroenterology 1993; 104:1736-1744.
20. Heuman DM. Hepatoprotective properties of ursodeoxycholic acid. Gastroenterology 1993; 104: 1865-1870.
21. Poupon R, Chrétien Y, Poupon RE, Ballet F, Calmus Y, Darnis F. Is ursodeoxycholic acid an effective treatment for primary biliary cirrhosis? Lancet 1987; i:834-836.
22. Poupon RE, Balkau B, Eschwège E, Poupon R and the UDCA-PBC Study Group. A multicenter, controlled trial of ursodiol for the treatment of primary biliary cirrhosis. N Engl J Med 1991; 324:1548-1554.
23. Poupon RE, Poupon R, Balkau B and the UDCA-PBC Study Group. Ursodiol for the long-term treatment of primary biliary cirrhosis. N Engl J Med 1994; 330:1342-1347.
24. Leuschner U, Fischer H, Kurtz W, Güldütuna S, Hübner K, Hellstern A, Gatzen M, Leuschner M. Ursodeoxycholic acid in primary biliary cirrhosis - Results of a controlled double-blind trial. Gastroenterology 1989; 97:1268-1274.
25. Oka H, Toda G, Ikeda Y, Hashimoto N, Hasumura Y, Kamimura T, Ohta Y, Tsuji T, Hattori N, Nashima T, Nishioka M, Ito K, Sasaki H, Kakumu S, Kuroki T, Fujisawa K, Nakanuma Y. A multicenter double-blind controlled trial of ursodeoxycholic acid for primary biliary cirrhosis. Gastroenterol Jpn 1990; 25:774-780.
26. Combes B, Carithers RL, McDonald MF, Maddrey WC, Munoz SJ, Boyer J, Peters MG, Luketic V. Ursodeoxycholic acid in patients with primary biliary cirrhosis. Hepatology 1991; 14:91A (Abstr).
27. Battezzati P, Podda M, Bianchi F, Naccarato R, Orlandi F, Surrenti C, Pagliaro L, Manenti F, and the Italian Multicenter Group for the Study of UDCA in PBC. Ursodeoxycholic acid for symptomatic primary biliary cirrhosis - Preliminary analysis of a double-blind multicenter trial. J Hepatol 1993; 17:332-338.
28. Turner IB, Myzsor M, Mitchison HC, Bennett MK, Burt AD, James OFW. A two year controlled trial examining the effectiveness of ursodeoxycholic acid in primary biliary cirrhosis. J Gastroenterol Hepatol 1994; 9:162-168.
29. Heathcote EJ, Cauch-Dubek K, Walker V, Bailey RJ, Blendis LM, Ghent CN, Michielletti P, Minuk GY, Pappas SC, Scully LJ, Steinbrecher UP, Sutherland LR, Williams CN, Witt-Sullivan H, Worobetz LJ, Milner RA, Wanless IR. The Canadian multicenter double-blind randomized controlled trial of ursodeoxycholic acid in primary biliary cirrhosis. Hepatology 1994; 19:1149-1156.
30. Lindor KD, Dickson ER, Baldus WP, Jorgensen RA, Ludwig J, Murtaugh PA, Harrisson JM, Wiesner RH, Anderson ML, Lange SM, LeSage G, Rossi SS, Hofmann AF. Ursodeoxycholic acid in the treatment of primary biliary cirrhosis. Gastroenterology 1994; 106:1284-1290.
31. Chazouillères O, Poupon R, Capron JP, Metman EH, Dhumeaux D, Amouretti M, Couzigou P, Labayle D, Trinchet JC. Ursodeoxycholic acid for primary sclerosing cholangitis. J Hepatol 1990; 11:120-123.
32. O'Brien CB, Senior JR, Arora-Mirchandani R, Batta AK, Salen G. Ursodeoxycholic acid for the treatment of primary sclerosing cholangitis: a 30-month pilot study. Hepatology 1991; 14:838-847.
33. Stiehl A, Walker S, Stiehl L, Rudolph G, Hofmann W, Theilmann L. Effect of ursodeoxycholic acid on liver and bile duct disease in primary sclerosing cho-

langitis. A 3-year pilot study with a placebo-controlled study period. J Hepatol 1994; 20:57-64.
34. Palma J, Reyes JH, Ribalta J, Iglesias J, Gonzales MC, Hernandez I, Alvarez C, Molina C, Danitz AM. Effects of ursodeoxycholic acid in patients with intrahepatic cholestasis of pregnancy. Hepatology 1992; 15:1043-1047.
35. Marpeau L, Chazouillères O, Rhimi Z, Poupon R, Pigne A, Barrat J. Pregnancy-associated idiopathic intrahepatic cholestasis. Hypotheses of physiopathology: a therapeutic case report. Fetal Diagn Ther 1991; 6:120-125.
36. Bellentani S, Tabarroni G, Barchi T, Ferretti I, Fratti N, Villa E, Manenti F. Effect of ursodeoxycholic acid treatment on alanine aminotransferase and γ-glutamyltranspeptidase serum levels in patients with hypertransamisemia. J Hepatol 1989; 8:7-12.
37. Podda M, Ghezzi C, Battezzati PM, Crosignani A, Zuin M, Roda A. Effects of ursodeoxycholic acid on serum liver enzymes and bile acids in chronic hepatitis. Gastroenterology 1990; 98:1044-1050.
38. Idéo G, Bellati G, Pedraglio E, Botelli R, Maggi G. Efficacy of ursodeoxycholic acid in lowering alanine aminotransferase and gamma-glutamyl transpeptidase serum levels in patients with chronic active hepatitis and primary biliary cirrhosis. Curr Ther Res 1990; 47:62-66.
39. Buzzelli G, Moscarella S, Focardi G, Dattolo P, Giusti A, Relli P, Rusticali AG, Gentilini P. Long-term treatment with ursodeoxycholic acid in patients with chronic active hepatitis. Curr Ther Res 1991; 50:635-642.
40. Floreani A, Chiaramonte M, Fabris P, Ngatchu T, Naccarato R. Poor effect of ursodeoxycholic acid in anti-hepatitis C virus-positive chronic liver disease. Curr Ther Res 1991; 50:579-585.
41. Attili AF, Carli L, Recipe AM, Varriale M, Callea F. Effect of ursodeoxycholic acid (UDCA) on serum enzymes and liver histology in patients with chronic active hepatitis (CAH). J Hepatol 1991; 13 (Suppl 2):92 (Abstr).
42. Portincasa P, Palmieri V, Doronzo F, Vendemiale G, Altomare E, Sabba C, Palasciano G, Albano O. Effect of tauroursodeoxycholic acid on serum liver enzymes and dyspeptic symptoms in patients with chronic active hepatitis. Curr Ther Res 1993; 53:521-531.
43. Takikawa H, Yamanaka M, Miyake K, Kako M, Ohki H, Narita, Sugata F, Yoshiba M, Sekiyama K, Aoyagi T, Nakajima H, Kamii K, Matsumoto K. Ursodeoxycholic therapy for chronic type C hepatitis: a multicenter, dose-finding trial. Curr Ther Res 1994; 55:16-21.
44. Takano S, Ito Y, Yokosuka O, Ohto M, Uchiumi K, Hirota K, Omata M. A multicenter randomized controlled dose study of ursodeoxycholic for chronic hepatitis C. Hepatology 1994; 20:558-564.
45. Bellentani S, Podda M, Tiribelli C et al. Ursodiol in the long-term treatment of chronic hepatitis: a double-blind multicenter clinical trial. J Hepatol 1993; 19:459-464.
46. Attili AF, Rusticali A, Varriale M, Carli L, Repice AM, Callea F. The effect of ursodeoxycholic on serum enzymes and liver histology in patients with chronic active hepatitis. A 12-month double-blind, placebo-controlled trial. J Hepatol 1994; 20:315-320.
47. Svanvik J, Frimman S, Persson H, Schertén T, Karlberg I. Does adjuvant ursodeoxycholic acid prevent acute rejection in liver transplant recipients? In: Paumgartner G, Stiehl A, Gerok W, eds. Bile Acids as Therapeutic Agents: From Basic Science to Clinical Practice. Dordrecht: Kluwer Ac. 1990; 357-360.
48. Sama C, Mazzioti A, Grigioni W, Morselli Labate AM, Chianura A, Stefanini GF, Barbara L, Gozzetti G. Ursodeoxycholic acid administration does not prevent rejection after OLT. J Hepatol 1991; 13 (Suppl 2):68 (Abstr).
49. Fried RH, Murakami CS, Fisher LD, Willson RA, Sullivan KM, McDonald GB. Ursodeoxycholic acid treatment of refractory chronic graft-versus-host disease of the liver. Ann Intern Med 1992; 116:624-629.
50. Kallinowski B, Theilmann L, Zimmermann R, Gams E, Kommerell B, Stiehl A. Effective treatment of cyclosporine-induced cholestasis in heart-transplanted patients treated with ursodeoxycholic acid. Transplantation 1991; 51:1128-1129.
51. Lindor KD, Burnes J. Ursodeoxycholic acid for the treatment of home parenteral nutrition associated cholestasis - A case report. Gastroenterology 1991; 101:250-253.
52. Beau P, Labat-Labourdette J, Ingrand P, Beauchant M. Is ursodeoxycholic acid an effective therapy for total parenteral nutrition-related liver disease? J Hepatol 1994; 20:240-244.
53. Bijleveld C, Vonk R, Kuipers F, Havinga R, Boverhof R, Koopman B, Wolthers B, Fernades J. Benign recurrent intrahepatic cholestasis: altered bile acid metabolism. Gastroenterology 1989; 97:427-432.
54. Crosignani A, Podda M, Bertoloni E, Battezzati PM, Zuin M, Setchell KDR. Failure of ursodeoxycholic acid to prevent a cholestatic episode in a patient with benign recurrent intrahepatic cholestasis: a study of bile acid metabolism. Hepatology 1991; 13:1076-1083.
55. Maggiore G, De Giacomo C. Efficacy of ursodeoxycholic acid in preventing cholestatic episodes in a patient with benign recurrent intrahepatic cholestasis. Hepatology 1992; 16:504(Letter).
56. Plevris JN, Hayes PC, Bouchier IAD. Ursodeoxycholic acid in the treatment of alcoholic liver disease. Eur J Gastroenterol Hepatol 1991; 3:653-656.
57. Colombo C, Setchell K, Podda M, Crosignani A, Roda A, Curcio L, Ronchi M, Giunta A. Effects of ursodeoxycholic acid therapy for liver disease associated with cystic fibrosis. J Pediatr 1990; 117:482-489.
58. Cotting J, Dufour J, Lentze M, Paumgartner G, Reichen J. Ursodeoxycholate in the treatment of cholestatis in cystic fibrosis. A two-year experience and review of the literature. In: Lentze M, Reichen J, eds. Paediatric Cholestasis. Novel Approaches to Treatment. Dordecht: Kluwer Ac. 1992; 345-353.
59. Colombo C, Crosignani A, Assaisso M, Battezzati PM, Podda M, Giunta A, Zimmernechemias L, Setchell KDR. Ursodeoxycholic acid therapy in cystic fi-

brosis associated liver disease —A dose-response study. Hepatology 1992; 16:924-930.
60. Bittner P, Posselt HG, Sailer T, Ott H, Magdorf K, Wahn U, Arleth S, Bertele-Harms RM, Wolf A, Krawinkel M, Linderman H. The effect of ursodeoxycholic acid in cystic fibrosis and hepatopathy: results of a placebo-controlled study. In: Paumgartner G, Stiehl A, Gerok W, eds. Bile Acids as Therapeutic Agents: From Basic Science to Clinical Practice. Dordrecht: Kluwer Ac. 1990; 345-356.
61. Balistreri WF, A-Kader HH, Ryckman FC, Whitington PF, Heubi JE, Setchell KDR. Biochemical and clinical response to ursodeoxycholic acid administration in paediatric patients with chronic cholestasis. In: Paumgartner G, Stiehl A, Gerok W, eds. Bile acids as Therapeutic Agents: From Basic Science to Clinical Practice. Dordrecht: Kluwer Ac. 1990; 323-333.
62. Nittono H, Tokita A, Hayashi M, Nakatsu N, Obinata K, Watanabe T, Yamashiro Y, Yabuta K, Miyano T. Ursodeoxycholic acid in biliary atresia. Lancet 1988; i:528(Letter).
63. Ullrich D, Rating D, Schröter W, Hanefeld F, Bircher J. Treatment with ursodeoxycholic acid renders children with biliary atresia suitable for liver transplantation. Lancet 1987; ii:1324(Letter).
64. Setchell KDR, Bragetti P, Zimmer-Nechemias L, Daugherty C, Pelli MA, Vaccaro R, Gentili G, Distrutti E, Dozzini G, Morelli A, Clerici C. Oral bile acid treatment and the patient with Zellweger syndrome. Hepatology 1992; 15:198-207.
65. Daugherty CC, Setchell KDR, Heubi JE, Balistreri WF. Resolution of liver biopsy alterations in three siblings with bile acid treatment of an inborn error of bile acid metabolism (D4-3-oxosteroid 5b-reductase deficiency). Hepatology 1993; 18:1096-1101.

Gene Therapy and Liver Diseases

G. Y. Wu, C. H. Wu

INTRODUCTION

We have shown previously that cell-surface receptors have been used as natural internalization sites for targeting genes to hepatocytes (1). This targeting is based on the fact that parenchymal liver cells are the only cells that have large numbers of high affinity receptors that can recognize galactose-terminal (asialo-) glycoproteins. Binding of these glycoproteins by the receptor leads to invagination of the plasma membrane and internalization of the ligand-receptor complex in membrane-bound vesicles.

METHODS AND RESULTS

A carrier system was developed consisting of two components: *a*) an asialoglycoprotein ligand covalently bound to *b*) a polymer containing multiple positive charges, a polycation. The asialoglycoprotein component provided the recognition signal for hepatocyte targeting, while the positively charged polycation served to bind DNA in a strong, non-damaging electrostatic manner to form a soluble protein-DNA complex (2).

To determine whether normal genes could be targeted in vivo to correct metabolic dysfunction in genetically defective animals, the WHHL rabbit model for familial hypercholesterolemia was used. A plasmid carrying a full-length cDNA for the human low density lipoprotein (LDL) receptor was constructed using regulatory elements from the mouse albumin gene inserted upstream to drive the LDL receptor gene. The plasmid was complexed with the carrier and injected intravenously into rabbits. Cellular DNA extracted and analyzed for the presence of human LDL receptor sequences demonstrated approximately 1,000 copies of plasmid per cell, 10 min after injection. These levels declined progressively, and by 48 hours plasmid DNA was less than 0.1 copies/cell. The transcriptional activity of the recombinant gene was analyzed by RNase protection assay for the presence of human LDL receptor transcripts. Exogenous LDL receptor mRNA was detected at 4 hours, reached a peak at 24 hours and decreased to undetectable levels by 72 hours after transfection. Maximal levels of LDL receptor mRNA were found at 24 hours and estimated to be 2-4% of normal endogenous levels. In order to determine the metabolic effects of hepatocyte-directed gene transfer in vivo, WHHL rabbits injected with complexed LDL receptor gene or CAT gene were analyzed for changes in total serum cholesterol. Administration of the LDL receptor gene complex resulted in a rapid, but transient decline in serum cholesterol that lasted 6 days. The drop in cholesterol levels was maximal at 2 days post-injection and was 25% to 30% of pretreatment values (3).

In another model, the Nagase analbuminemic rat model was used. A plasmid containing the structural gene for the human serum albumin under the control of mouse albumin enhancer-rat albumin promoter sequences was constructed and complexed with the targetable conjugate. The soluble complex was injected intravenously into Nagase rats and two-thirds partial hepatectomies were performed in order to stimulate hepatocyte replication and persistence of foreign gene expression. Two weeks after injection, densitometric quantitation revealed an average copy number of 1000 copies of the plasmid/diploid genome with most of the foreign DNA found to be in plasmid form. RNase protection assay estimated the level of human albumin mRNA to be between 0.01 and 0.1% of the normal level of rat albumin in normal rats. Circulating human albumin was determined by Western blot analysis that showed the appearance of human albumin in the serum within 48 hours at a level of 0.05 μg/ml, but increased in concentration to a peak level of 34 μg/ml by 2 weeks post-injection (4). This level remained stable through 4 weeks. No antibodies directed against the human albumin were detected during the 4 weeks of the study.

Based on the recognition that natural infectious agents that have evolved methods of avoiding lysosomal degradation, it was proposed to incorporate these agents into targetable complexes to increase the escape of targeted DNA in a similar manner. In considering this idea, it was noted that adenoviruses are common pathogens in man and animals (5, 6). In susceptible hosts, these viruses have broad tissue specificity (7) normally entering cells by binding to plasma membrane of the host cell via adenovirus fibers that project from the capsid (8). Endocytosis subsequently occurs in which the viral particles are internalized within endosomal vesicles (9). Acidification of endosomes results in a conformational change of the capsid proteins that disrupts the endosomal membrane (10) allowing the viral nucleic acid to enter the cytosolic compartment of the host cell. The endosomolytic property of adenoviruses has been exploited in the past to enhance the introduction of polypeptide molecules (10) and more recently plasmid DNA (11), a method that greatly increased the efficiency of marker gene expression. However, in the latter instance, the DNA complex retained the original infection specificity of the virus. To change the natural infectivity of adenoviruses, chemical coupling of targetable DNA carriers to an adenovirus was attempted. Because the viral fibers govern the infection specificity of adenovirus, chemical coupling of an asialoglycoprotein to these structures could result in a new ability to enter cells by asialoglycoprotein receptors while simultaneously blocking recognition of the cells endogenous receptors for the virus. The strategy was to take advantage of carbohydrate groups that are exclusively located on the fibers (12). Activation of the carbohydrate residues allows modification of the virus by covalent linkage of an asialoglycoprotein-polylysine conjugate to the surface of the virus. Addition of foreign DNA resulted in electrostatic binding to the polylysine of the conjugate and coating of the modified virus by foreign DNA to form a targetable complex. Internalization of the complex is achieved in a cell-specific fashion mediated by receptor recognition of the asialoglycoprotein component of the modified virus.

A wild-type and a replication defective adenovirus, dl312, were modified by coupling an asialoglycoprotein-polylysine conjugate to the virus via carbohydrate residues on the fibers. Wild-type virus modified in this manner had greatly *decreased* infectivity toward normally susceptible HeLa S_3 [asialoglycoprotein receptor (-)] and SK Hep1 [asialoglycoprotein receptor (-)] cells leaving 91 and 86% viable, respectively after 48 hrs. However, with Huh 7 [asialoglycoprotein receptor (+)] cells, *modified* virus *retained* infectivity leaving only 19% of cells viable under identical conditions. Modified virus was complexed to DNA in the form of a plasmid, pSVHBV, containing the gene for hepatitis B surface antigen, as a marker of gene expression. Huh 7, receptor (+), cells treated with modified wild-type, and modified replication-defective dl312 virus complexed to the plasmid increased antigen levels by approximately 13- and 30-fold, respectively, compared to asialoglycoprotein-polylysine DNA complex alone. The enhancement was blocked by more than 95% in the presence of a large molar excess of an asialoglycoprotein. Using a β-galactosidase marker gene, the number of cells transfected by modified virus was found to be 200-fold higher than complex alone (13). Yet, specificity was retained exclusively for asialoglycoprotein receptor-bearing cells. These data indicate that adenovirus can be chemically modified by coupling ligands resulting in targeted gene expression dictated specifically by receptor recognition of the attached ligand.

It was recognized that the carrier system could potentially target single-stranded DNA in the form of antisense oligomers. Because of the remarkable specificity of the action of antisense DNA in the inhibition of the synthesis of specific proteins based on hybridization of antisense to target mRNA, it was hypothesized that receptor-mediated delivery of antisense DNA specific for hepatitis B viral (HBV) mRNA sequences could inhibit viral gene expression in target cells. A 21-mer oligo DNA sequence complementary to the polyadenylation signal for human hepatitis B virus (HBV) was complexed to a soluble DNA-carrier system. A cell line, HepG2 (2.2.15) that possesses asialoglycoprotein receptors (14) and which is permanently transfected with hepatitis B virus (ayw subtype) was exposed to complexed antisense DNA or controls. In the presence of complexed antisense DNA, the concentration of hepatitis B surface antigen in medium was *decreased* by 80% by day 1, and by *more* than 95% through the 6th day compared to untreated cells. There was no significant increase in surface antigen concentration in the presence of complexed antisense DNA after the first day of exposure. This inhibition was blocked by competition with an excess of free asialoglycoprotein. Protein secretion from cells was not affected and could not account for the decrease in HBV surface antigen concentration in the medium after exposure to antisense DNA. Also, total protein synthesis remained unchanged by exposure to complexed antisense sequences under identical conditions. Finally, HBV DNA in the medium and cell layers after 24 hrs exposure to complexed antisense sequences was 80% lower than in controls. Exposure of cells to a random 21-mer oligo DNA sequence under identical conditions failed to alter HBV surface antigen concentration or HBV DNA in medium or cells (15).

The data indicate that antisense oligonucleotides complexed by a soluble DNA-carrier system can be targeted to cells via asialoglycoprotein receptors resulting in specific inhibition of hepatitis B viral gene expression and replication.

CONCLUSIONS

We conclude that a DNA carrier system can target polynucleotides to hepatocytes to provide new gene expression or to inhibit endogenous gene expression in a cell-specific manner and that the effects can be enhanced by the incorporation of natural agents or components that have endosomolytic capabilities.

REFERENCES

1. Wu GY, Wu CH. Receptor-mediated in vitro gene transformation by soluble DNA carrier system. J Biol Chem 1987; 262:4429-4432.
2. Wu GY, Wu CH. Evidence for targeted gene delivery to Hep G2 hepatoma cells *in vitro*. Biochemistry 1988; 27:887-892.
3. Wilson JM, Grossman M, Wu CH, Roy Chowdhury N, Wu GY, Roy Chowdhury J. Hepatocyte-directed gene transfer in vivo leads to transient improvement of hypercholesterolemia in LDL receptor-deficient rabbits. J Biol Chem 1992; 267:963-967.
4. Wu GY, Wilson JM, Shalaby F, Grossman M, Shafritz DA, Wu, CH. Receptor-mediated gene delivery *in vivo*: Partial correction of genetic analbuminemia in Nagase rats. J Biol Chem 1991; 266:14338-14342.
5. Huebner RJ, Rowe WP, Ward TG, Parrott RH, Bell JA. Adenoidal-Pharyngeal-Conjunctival Agents —A newly recognized group of common viruses of the respiratory system. N Engl J Med 1954; 251:1077-1086.
6. Pereira HG, Huebner RJ, Ginsberg HS, Van der Veen J. A short description of the adenovirus group. Virology 1963; 20:613-620.
7. Grayston JT, McCarthy MA, Smith M, Loosli, CG. Adenoviruses II. The sensitivity of different tissue culture strains of cells to adenoviruses. J Infect Dis 1958; 103:86-92.
8. Hennache B, Boulanger P. Biochemical study of KB-cell receptor for adenovirus. Biochem J 1977; 166:237-247.
9. Chardonnet Y, Dales S. Early events in the interaction of adenoviruses with HeLa cells; I. Penetration of Type 5 and, intracellular release of the DNA genome 1. Virology 1970; 40:462-477.
10. Seth P, FitzGerald D, Ginsberg H, Willingham M, Pastan I. Evidence that the Penton base of adenovirus is involved in potentiation of toxicity of pseudomonas exotoxin conjugated to epidermal growth factor. Mol Cell Biol 1984; 4:1528-1533.
11. Curiel DT, Agarwal S, Wagner E, Cotten M. Adenovirus enhancement of transferrin polylysine mediated gene delivery. Proc Natl Acad Sci USA 1991; 88:8850-8854.
12. Ishibashi M, Maizel JV Jr. The polypeptides of adenovirus IV early and late glycopolypeptides. Virology 1974; 58:345-361.

13. Wu GY, Zhan P-L, Sze LL, Rosenberg AR, Wu CH. Incorporation of adenovirus into a ligand-based DNA carrier system results in retention of the original receptor specificity and enhances targeted gene expression. J Biol Chem 1994; 269:11542-11546.
14. Sells MA, Chen ML, Acs G. Production of hepatitis B virus particles in HepG2 cells transfected with cloned hepatitis B virus DNA. Proc Natl Acad Sci USA 1987; 84:1005-1009.
15. Wu GY, and Wu CH. Specific inhibition of hepatitis B viral gene expression *in vitro* by targeted antisense oligonucleotides. J Biol Chem 1992; 267:12436-12439.

Prescribing in Liver Disease

J. Reichen

INTRODUCTION

When prescribing drugs to patients with liver disease, the following questions should be asked:

1. Does the drug need adjustment of loading and/or maintenance dose?
2. Is there altered response of this patient to drug once dosage is adjusted?
3. Is there increased susceptibility of this patient to adverse effects?

In answering these questions, one will answer questions about altered pharmacokinetics, altered pharmacodynamics and altered susceptibility of patients with liver disease.

In the practice of the clinical pharmacologist, all three questions are asked; thus, figure 1 gives the reasons for consultation during a one year period in different departments of our university hospital. In the following, all three questions will be addressed with some thought given to pathogenic background for altered pharmacokinetic and pharmacodynamic behavior of drugs as well as for altered susceptibility of the host with liver disease to drug toxicity.

PHARMACOKINETIC ALTERATIONS IN CHRONIC LIVER DISEASE

The hepatic clearance (Cl_{hep}) of drugs is the product of hepatic blood flow (Q) and the extraction (E) of the drug across the liver:

$$Cl_{hep} = Q \cdot E = Q \cdot f_u \cdot Cl_{int}/(Q + f_u \cdot Cl_{int}) \quad [1]$$

where f_u stands for unbound fraction of drug and Cl_{int} for intrinsic clearance.

$$Cl_{int} = V_{max}/K_m \quad [2]$$

where V_{max} and K_m stand for the maximal velocity and half-saturation constant of the removal process of the drug under study, respectively. This process is usually a metabolic step, but in some instances possibly also an active transport process (1, 2).

This relationship predicts the flow- and enzyme-limited regime of hepatic drug removal: in

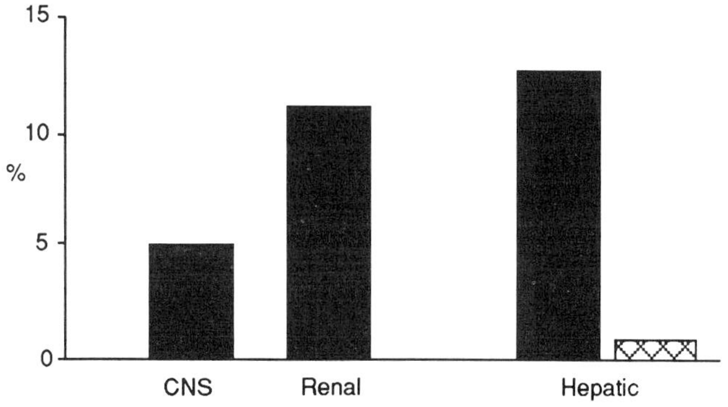

Fig. 1. Reasons for 200 consecutive consultations in patients with chronic liver disease; 5.3% concerned adverse effects of drugs on the central nervous system, most often prolonged action of sedatives and/or induction of porto-systemic encephalopathy; 11.8% concerned renal adverse effects, most often of diuretics, but also of non-steroidal anti-inflammatory drugs. Questions concerning the liver were seen most often, namely clearance to use potentially hepatotoxic drugs in 12.3% (hepatic: solid bar). Only 0.3% of consultations dealt with dosage adjustments in chronic liver disease (hepatic: hatched bar).

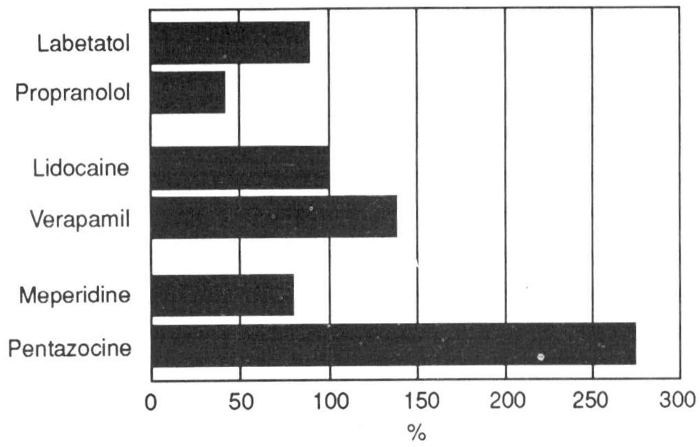

Fig. 2. The increase in bioavailability of selected high-extraction compounds in patients with liver cirrhosis compiled and averaged from different sources. The figure is given to illustrate orders of magnitude and should not be used for dosage adjustment since the variability is high, the coefficient of variation even within studies often exceeding 100%.

the flow-limited regime —when extraction approaches 1— clearance equals flow. Such drugs exhibit a high first pass-effect, i.e., systemic administration requires a much lower dosage than when given orally; the increase in bioavailability of some common compounds with a high hepatic exctraction ratio is shown in figure 2. It is evident that porto-systemic shunting —spontaneous or surgically induced— has a major bearing on the handling of high extraction compounds (3, 4). It is less realized that sinusoidal capillarization also has major impact on the hepatic handling in particular of highly protein bound drugs (5) but is also a major determinant of the elimination of enzyme-limited compounds which are less or not protein bound (6).

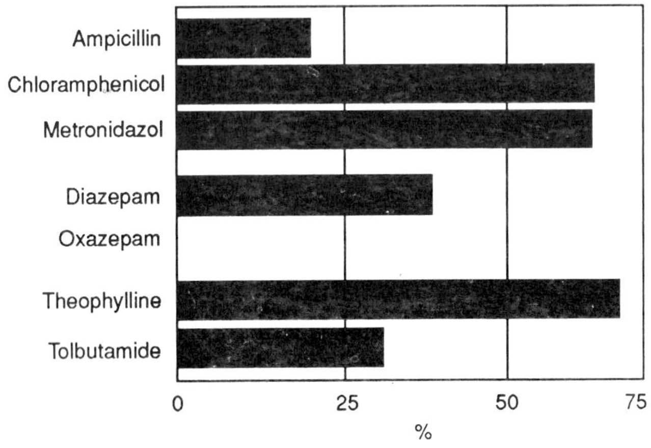

Fig. 3. The decrease in clearance of selected antibiotics, benzodiazepines and other compounds potentially used in patients with chronic liver disease. All drugs have a relatively low hepatic extraction and therefore follow an enzyme-limited regime. The data are compiled and averaged from different sources. The figures given serve to illustrate the orders of magnitude of the alterations seen with low extraction compounds and should not be used for dosage adjustment since the variability is high, the coefficient of variation even within studies often exceeding 100%.

In contrast, drugs subject to the enzyme-limited regime are independent of hepatic perfusion and their clearance is determined by enzymatic or transport activity in the liver as expressed by the intrinsic clearance (equation 2); the hepatic clearance of such drugs is much more dependent on protein binding since in equation 1 intrinsic clearance is adjusted by f_u, the fraction of free drug. It is evident that a lowered albumin level —often encountered in patients with liver disease— will affect the clearance and distribution of drugs bound to albumin; this includes most anionic drugs. It is often less appreciated that basic drugs bind to other serum proteins, in particular α_1-acid glycoprotein which are also reduced in cirrhosis. This has been shown to be germane in particular for antidysrhythmic drugs such as lidocaine (7) and disopyramide (8). The decrease in hepatic clearance of some important drugs, compiled from different sources, is shown in figure 3.

Intuitively, one would predict that the clearance of flow-limited drugs is much more affected in chronic liver disease than that of enzyme-limited compounds due to the profound alterations in hepatic perfusion. However, different investigations have established this not to be the case (9-11), the clearance of both class of compounds being affected to a similar extent (fig. 4). This apparent paradox has been resolved by the "intact cell hypothesis" which states that a reduced number of intrinsically normal hepatocytes is either normally perfused or circumvented by intrahepatic shunting (12). This hypothesis has been proven by morphometric means in experimental animals (6, 13) and recently in man (14). However, not all animal models conform to this model, e.g., rats with bile duct ligation demonstrate decreased activity expressed per hepatocyte, thus obey the "sick cell hypothesis" (15); whether similar instances occur in man remains yet to be formally proven.

Different processes affecting the parameters determining hepatic clearance in cirrhosis —pro-

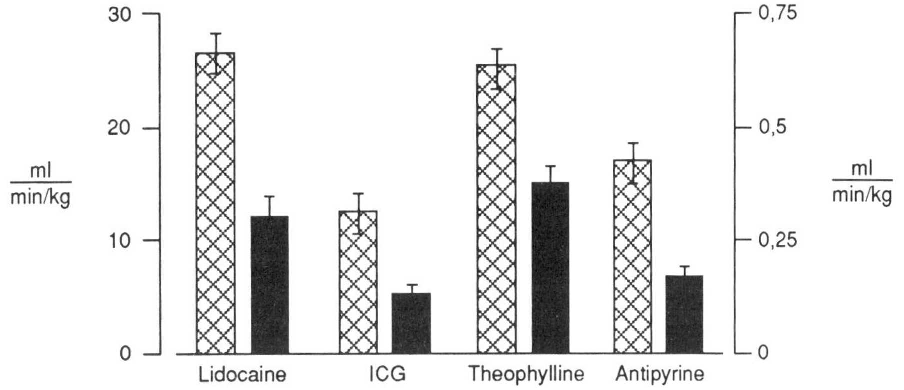

Fig. 4. Hepatic clearance of two model drugs with high hepatic extraction —lidocaine and indocyanine green (ICG)— and of two compounds with low extraction —theophylline and antipyrine— are decreased to a similar extent in patients with cirrhosis of the liver (solid bars) compared with controls (hatched bars). Mean ± SEM are shown. (Drawn from a publication by Colli et al. Clin Pharmacol Ther 1988; 44:642-649, and Kawasaki et al. Am J Gastroenterol 1985; 80:801-806.)

ven and speculative— are listed in table 1. Since apparently both, flow and intrinsic clearance are affected to variable extents in cirrhosis, the concept of hepatic clearance as outlined in equation 1 remains theoretical and cannot be translated directly into practice. In particular, high extraction compounds become enzyme-limited as liver disease progresses (16-18). The factors listed in table 1 have only been partially explored in man. Shunting is highly variable (19); in man, serum bile acid levels have been found to correlate with scintigraphically determined shunt fractions (20). Shunt flow has also been assessed after rectal instillation of different radioisotopes (21, 22) or by determination of azygos vein flow by thermodilution. Application of shunt fractions thus determined to dosage adjustment has not been used in clinical practice and it remains doubtful whether it would add any benefit.

Determination of hepatic flow is a difficult endeavor in cirrhosis since at low extraction fractions the Fick principle by e.g. indocyanine green, for estimation of nutritional hepatic flow becomes difficult if not impossible. Nevertheless, different attempts at improvement have been made, among others clearance of low dose galactose (23) or of sorbitol (24, 25). Again, their utility for dosage adjustement remains to be proven.

A variety of model compounds have been proposed to measure metabolic activity of the liver. Among the most popular are the galactose elimination capacity (26, 27), antipyrine clearance (28, 29), the aminopyrine breath test (30, 31) and more recently the so-called MEGX test (32, 33) which measures the formation of a main metabolite, monoethylglycinexylidide. All of these tests carry some prognostic information; however, it remains unclear what they really do measure with the exception of the metabolism of the substance administered. Thus, aminopyrine N-demethylation as measured by the aminopyrine breath test correlates with liver cell mass in cirrhotic rats (13) but is determined mainly by flow and sinusoidal capillarization (6). Unless we have a battery of tests which unambiguously measures the factors lined out in equation 1 and table 1, an accurate prediction of drug metabolism in a a given patient with cirrhosis will remain a dream.

Table 1. Reasons for altered drug disposition in chronic liver disease due to alterations in hepatic clearance

Perfusion	Intrinsic clearance
Decreased or increased flow	Reduced hepatocyte mass
Porto-systemic shunts	Altered mass or characteristics of responsible enzymes («sick cell»)
Sinusoidal capillarization	Regenerative hepatocytes
	Alterations of hepatic membranes

The formula for hepatic clearance, being determined mainly by perfusion and intrinsic clearance, is given in the text.

Thus, the individual prediction of drug adjustment is difficult; the clinician's task is further complicated by often contradictory reports in the literature. Thus, for the antibiotic metronidazole markedly decreased (34), mildly decreased (35) or unaffected (36) clearance in patients with cirrhosis have been described. This is quite often due to the fact that different populations of cirrhotics are studied. One would always like to know at least the Child classification of the study population. Some investigators try to correlate drug disposition in patients with cirrhosis with different measures of hepatic reserve, so-called quantitative liver function tests *(vide supra)*. While such measures of hepatic perfusion or metabolic capacity often correlate with the clearance of a given drug, these correlations are not tight enough to be used for dosage adjustment. This is due to the extreme heterogeneity of the factors listed in table 1 and the many different iso-enzymes are affected to different extents by chronic liver disease (37-41).

The exception to this observation follows from it: the disposition of a model drug will accurately predict its own clearance and —of more practical use— if the elimination of a model drug depends on chiefly one iso-enzyme it will predict the metabolism of other drugs whose elimination depends on this same iso-enzyme. This is the case for, e.g., the ^{14}C-erythromycin breath test which has been useful to predict cyclosporine disposition in liver transplantation (42, 43).

While most phase I reactions in drug metabolism are affected to varying degrees by chronic liver disease, it was initially thought that phase II reactions, in particular glucuronidation, is spared in cirrhosis. This has been shown to be true among others for morphine (44) and phenprocoumon (45). However, this cannot be generalized to all glucuronidation reactions: glucuronidation of zomepirac is diminished in parallel with the galactose elimination capacity (46) and that of oxazepam in parallel with the clearance of antipyrine (47). Pacifici et al. investigated a variety of phase II enzymes of human liver *in vitro* and found conjugating activity —including sulfotransferase, glutathione transferase, acetyl-transferase and thiomethyl-transferase to be diminished but glucuronidation using two different substrates to be maintained (7).

One should realize that liver disease not always leads to abnormally high drug concentrations and/or accumulation but can also be associated with inadequate drug levels. Nowadays, drugs are very often designed as prodrugs to achieve better bioavailability or even organ- or cell-specific delivery. Such prodrugs require metabolic activation by hepatic enzyme systems which can be impaired in cirrhosis. Such an example is provided by spirapril, a novel ACE inhibitor (48): this compound needs to be activated to spiraprilate, a process which occurs less efficiently in cirrhosis leading to decreased concentrations of the active drug and lesser pharmacological effects. With all these difficulties of individual dosage adjustment in mind, a few rules can nevertheless be deduced from these considerations:

1. For high extraction compounds, the loading dose for peroral administration has always to be adjusted.
2. For both, high and low extraction compounds *with a narrow therapeutic window* the maintenance dose should be adjusted.
3. In such cases, whenever possible, therapeutic drug monitoring should be employed to adjust dosage to the individual requirements.

PHARMACODYNAMIC ALTERATIONS

The pharmacodynamics of many vasoconstrictors are altered —most often blunted— in cirrhosis. Thus, a blunted response to angiotensin II (49-51), β-adrenergic agents (50, 52, 53), atrial natriuretic peptide (53) and endothelin among other mediators has been described. This was initially thought to be due to down-regulation of receptors (54) but this has not held up to closer scrutiny (55). Other authors have implicated altered physical properties of biomembranes to be responsible for this phenomenon (56).

Altered phamacodynamic behavior has also been demonstrated for furosemide: although neither plasma disappearance nor urinary furosemide levels differed between controls, cirrhotics responsive and cirrhotic not responsive to the drug, in both patient groups there was a decreased response in urinary sodium secretion for any given furosemide level (57). A similarly reduced sensitivity has been described to the novel loop diuretic torsemide; in this instance, however, pharmacokinetic changes compensated for the pharmacodynamic alterations (58).

Prescribing sedatives, in particular benzodiazepines, to patients with chronic liver disease is a source of worry for the clinician (see also fig. 1) since they could precipitate hepatic encephalopathy. While pharmacokinetic alterations in benzodiazepine handling are well established (59) it remains unclear whether the response of the brain is altered in cirrhosis. Baktir and colleagues demonstrated quite clearly altered pharmacodynamics in response to the short-acting triazolam (60). A later investigation found no difference albeit using less sensitive tests in either pharmacokinetics or —dynamics in patients of Child Pugh A (61); these authors ascribed this discrepancy to the fact that in the former study the differences were due to the inclusion of patients with surgical porto-systemic shunts.

ALTERED SUSCEPTIBILITY OF THE CIRRHOTIC PATIENT TO ADVERSE EFFECTS

There is often concern to prescribe potentially hepatotoxic drugs to patients with chronic liver disease. Indeed, the Physician's Desk Reference will almost universally indicate that such drugs should not be used in patients with established liver disease. With few exceptions, this is not due to an increased susceptibility of these patients to the hepatotoxic effect but to the concern that if they develop hepatotoxicity their hepatic reserve will be insufficient to survive an episode of drug-induced hepatotoxicity.

A notable exception to this rule is acetaminophen which can lead to severe hepatotoxicity at therapeutic dosage in patients with alcoholic liver disease (62). This is due to the decreased glutathione levels in such patients; glutathione detoxifies the cytochrome P 450-generated hepatotoxic acetaminophen metabolite (63, 64).

Another notable interaction of drug toxicity —in this case directed at the kidney— is the use of aminoglycosides in patients with liver cirrhosis; while the risk of nephrotoxicity was increased six-fold compared to antibiotic regimes not containing an aminoglycoside, the relative risk increased to 32-fold in patients with liver disease (65).

Another practically important altered susceptibility is that to non-steroidal inflammatory agents in patients with ascites (66, 67); earlier claims that sulindac was devoid of this effect (68) could not be substantiated (66, 67). This interaction is due to cyclo-oxygenase inhibition in the kidney leading then to unopposed vasoconstriction by the activated renin-angiotensin-aldosterone system (67, 69).

Recently, three cases of seizures induced by pefloxacin in cirrhotic patients have been ascribed to lower metabolism and increased permeability of the blood-brain barrier to the drug (70). In this instance it remains yet unclear whether this phenomenon is due to increased susceptibility of the cirrhotic patient and/or altered pharmacokinetic behavior since markedly elevated blood levels of the compound in 2/3 patients were also found. Another antibiotic implicated to provoke serious adverse effects in cirrhotic patients are β-lactam antibiotics implicated in neutropenia (71).

CONCLUSIONS

Hepatic clearance is determined by hepatic perfusion and intrinsic clearance; the difference derived from the classic equation between flow- and enzyme-limited regimes gets lost as liver disease progresses. Actually, there is still no reliable predictor of drug handling by the patient with liver disease. Consideration of a few pharmacokinetic principles and close surveillance for untoward effect will nevertheless allow safe use of drugs in patients with cirrhosis of the liver.

ACKNOWLEDGEMENTS

The author gratefully acknowledges the support of his research by the Swiss National Foundation for Scientific Research over the past ten years (last grant no. 32.30168).

REFERENCES

1. Wilkinson G R, Shand DG. A physiologic approach to hepatic drug clearance. Clin Pharmacol Ther 1975; 18:377-390.
2. Rowland M, Benet LZ, Graham GG. Clearance concepts in pharmacokinetics. J Pharmacokinet Biopharm 1973; 1:123-136.
3. Pomier Layrargues G, Huet PM, Villeneuve JP, Marleau D. Effect of portacaval shunt on drug disposition in patients with cirrhosis. Gastroenterology 1986; 91:163-167.
4. Poupon RY, Poupon RE, Lebrec D, LeQuernec L, Darnis F. Mechanisms for reduced hepatic clearance and elevated plasma levels of bile acids in cirrhosis. A study in patients with and end-to-side portacaval shunt. Gastroenterology 1981; 80:1438-1444.
5. Gariépy L, Fenyves D, Kassissia I, Villeneuve JP. Clearance by the Liver in Cirrhosis. 2. Characterization of Propranolol Uptake with the Multiple-Indicator Dilution Technique. Hepatology 1993; 18:823-831.
6. Reichen J, Egger B, Ohara N, Zeltner TB, Zysset T, Zimmermann A. Determinants of hepatic functions in liver cirrhosis in the rat: A multivariate analysis. J Clin Invest 1988; 82:2069-2076.
7. Pacifici GM, Viani A, Franchi M, Santerini S, Temellini A, Giuliani L, Carrai M. Conjugation pathways in liver disease. Br J Clin Pharmacol 1990; 30:427-435.
8. Echizen H, Saima S, Umeda N, Ishizaki T. Protein binding of disopyramide in liver cirrhosis and in nephrotic syndrome. Clin Pharmacol Ther 1986; 40:274-280.
9. Branch RA, James JA, Read AE. The clearance of antipyrine and indocyanine green in normal subjects and in patients with chronic liver disease. Clin Pharmacol Ther 1976; 20:81-89.
10. Kawasaki S, Sugiyama Y, Iga T, Hanano M, Sanjo K, Beppu T, Idezuki Y. Pharmacokinetic study on the hepatic uptake of indocyanine green in cirrhotic patients. Am J Gastroenterol. 1985; 80:801-806.
11. Colli A, Buccino G, Cocciolo M, Parravicini R, Scaltrini G. Disposition of a flow-limited drug (lidocaine) and a metabolic capacity-limited drug (theophylline) in liver cirrhosis. Clin Pharmacol Ther 1988; 44:642-649.
12. Wood AJJ, Villeneuve JP, Branch RA, Rogers LW, Shand DG. Intact hepatocyte theory of impaired drug metabolism in experimental cirrhosis in the rat. Gastroenterology 1979; 76:1358-1362.
13. Reichen J, Arts B, Schafroth U, Zimmermann A, Zeltner TB, Zysset T. Aminopyrine N-demethylation by rats with liver cirrhosis: Evidence for the intact cell hypothesis. A morphometric-functional study. Gastroenterology 1987; 93:719-726.
14. Kawasaki S, Imamura H, Bandai Y, Sanjo K, Idezuki Y. Direct evidence for the intact hepatocyte therory in patients with liver cirrhosis. Gastroenterology 1992; 102:1351-1355.
15. Ohara N, Schaffner T, Reichen J. Structure-function relationship in secondary biliary cirrhosis in the rat: Stereologic and hemodynamic characterization of a model. J Hepatol 1993; 17:155-162.
16. Pessayre D, Lebrec D, Descatoire V, Peignoux M, Benhamou JP. Mechanism for reduced drug clearance in patients with cirrhosis. Gastroenterology 1978; 74:566-571.
17. Huet PM, Villeneuve JP. Determinants of drug disposition in patients with cirrhosis. Hepatology 1983; 3:913-918.
18. Callaghan R, Desmond P, Paull P, Mashford M. Hepatic enzyme activity is the major factor determining elimination rate of high-clearance drugs in cirrhosis. Hepatology 1993; 181:54
19. Huet PM, Marleau D, Lavoie P, Viallet A. Extraction of [125I]-albumin microaggregates from portal blood. An index of functional portal blood supply in cirrhosis. Gastroenterology 1976; 70:74-81.
20. Ohkubo H, Okuda K, Iida S, Ohnishi K, Ikawa S, Makino I. Role of portal and splenic vein shunts and impaired hepatic extraction in the elevated serum bile acids in liver cirrhosis. Gastroenterology 1984; 86:514-520.
21. Kashiwagi T, Azuma M, Ikawa T, Takehara T, Matsuda H, Yoshioka H, Mitsutani N, et al. Portosystemic shunting in portal hypertension: evaluation with portal scintigraphy with transrectally administered I-123 IMP. Radiology 1988; 169:137-140.
22. D'Arienzo A, Celentano L, Scuotto A, DiSiervi P, Lombardi V, Squame G, Mazzacca G. Thallium-201 per rectum for the diagnosis of cirrhosis in patients with asymptomatic chronic hepatitis. Hepatology 1988; 8:785-787.
23. Henderson JM, Hanna SS. Effective liver blood flow: determination by galactose clearance. Can J Surg 1983; 26:129-132.
24. Molino G, Avagnina P, Cavanna A, Ballare M, Torchio M, Bona B, Belforte G. Sorbitol clearance: A parameter reflecting liver plasma flow in the rat. Res Comm Chem Pathol Pharmacol 1986; 52:119-132.
25. Zeeh J, Lange H, Bosch J, Pohl S, Loesgen H, Eggers R, Navasa M et al. Steady-state extrarenal sorbitol clearance as a measure of hepatic plasma flow. Gastroenterology 1988; 95:749-759.
26. Tygstrup N. The galactose elimination capacity in control subjects and in patients with cirrhosis of the liver. Acta Med Scand 1964; 175:281-289.
27. Bircher J, Blankart R, Halpern A, Haecki W, Laissue J, Preisig R. Criteria for assessment of functional impairment in patients with cirrhosis of the liver. Eur J Clin Invest 1973; 3:72-85.
28. Brodie BB, Axelrod J. The fate of antipyrine in man. J Pharmacol Exp Ther 1950; 98:97-104.
29. Andreasen PB, Ranek L, Statland BE, Tygstrup N. Clearance of antipyrine. Dependence of quantitative liver function. Eur J Clin Invest 1974; 4:129-134.
30. Lauterburg BH, Bircher J. Expiratory measurement of maximal aminopyrine demethylation in vivo: Effect of phenobarbital- partial hepatectomy- portacaval shunt and bile duct ligation in the rat. J Pharmacol Exp Ther 1976; 196:501-509.
31. Bircher J, Kuepfer A, Gikalov I, Preisig R. Aminopy-

rine demethylation measured by breath analysis in cirrhosis. Clin Pharmacol Ther 1976; 20:484-492.

32. Oellerich M, Hartmann H, Ringe B, Burdelski M, Lautz H, Pichlmayr R. Assessment of prognosis in transplant candidates by use of the Pugh-MEGX score. Transplant Proc 1993; 25:1116-1119.
33. Schiffman M, Fisher R, Sanyal A, Edinboro L, Luketic, V, Purdum III P, Raymond P et al. Hepatic lidocaine metabolism and complications of cirrhosis. Transplantation 1993; 55:830-834.
34. Farrell GC, Baird-Lambert J, Cvejic M, Buchanan N. Disposition and metabolism of metronidazole in patients with liver failure. Hepatology 1984; 4:722-726.
35. Albani F, Tamè MR, De Palma R, Bernardi M. Kinetics of intravenous metoclopramide in patients with hepatic cirrhosis. Eur J Clin Pharmacol 1991; 40:423-425.
36. Daneshmend TK, Homeida M, Kaye CM, Elamin AA, Roberts CJC. Disposition of metronidazole in hepatic cirrhosis and in hepatosplenic schistosomiasis. Gut 1982; 23:807-813.
37. Murray M, Cantrill E, Mehta I, Farrell GC. Impaired expression of microsomal cytochrome P450 2C11 in choline-deficient rat liver during t6he development of cirrhosis. J Pharmacol Exp Ther 1992; 261:373-380.
38. Babany G, Descatoire V, Corbic M, Gendre S, Degott C, Larrey D, Letteron P et al. Regulation of renal cytochrome p-450. Effects of two-thirds hepatectomy-cholestasis- biliary cirrhosis and postnecrotic cirrhosis on hepatic and renal microsomal enzymes. Biochem Pharmacol 1985; 34:311-320.
39. Buters JTM, Zysset T, Reichen J. Metabolism of antipyrine in vivo in two rat models of liver cirrhosis - its relationship to intrinsic clearance in vitro and microsomal membrane lipid composition. Biochem Pharmacol 1993; 46:983-991.
40. Murray ML, Dannan GA, Guengerich PF, Farrell GC. Altered regulation of cytochrome P-450 enzymes in choline-deficient cirrhotic male rat liver: Impaired regulation and activity of the male-specific androst-4-ene-3-17-dione 16-alpha-hydroxylase-cytochrome P-450 UT-A in hepatic cirrhosis. Mol Pharmacol 1987; 31:117-121.
41. Murray M, Zaluzny L, Farrell GC. Drug metabolism in cirrhosis. Selective changes in cytochrome P-450 isozymes in the choline-deficient rat model. Biochem Pharmacol 1986; 35:1817-1824.
42. Lown K, Kolars J, Turgeon K, Merion R, Wrighton SA, Watkins PB. The erythromycin breath test selectively measures P450IIIA in patients with severe liver disease. Clin Pharmacol Ther 1992; 51:229-238.
43. Watkins PB., Hamilton TA, Annesley TM, Ellis CN, Kolars JC, Voorhees J. The erythromycin breath test as a predictor of cyclosporine blood levels. Clin Pharmacol Ther 1990; 48:120-129.
44. Patwardhan RV, Johnson RF, Hoyumpa A, Sheehan JJ, Desmond PV, Wilkinson GR, Branch RA et al. Normal metabolism of morphine in cirrhosis. Gastroenterology 1981; 81:1006-1011.
45. Kitteringham NR, Büstgens L, Brundert E, Mineshita S, Ohnhaus EE. The effect of liver cirrhosis on the pharmacokinetics of phenprocoumon. Eur J Clin Pharmacol 1984; 26:65-70.
46. Witassek F, Bircher J, Huguenin P, Preisig R. Abnormal glucuronidation of zomepirac in patients with cirrhosis of the liver. Hepatology 1983; 3:415-422.
47. Sonne J, Andreasen PB, Loft S, Dossing M, Andreasen F. Glucuronidation of oxazepam is not spared in patients with hepatic encephalopathy. Hepatology 1990, 11:951.
48. Krähenbühl S, Grass P, Surve A, Kutz K, Reichen J. Pharmacokinetics and hemodynamic effects of a single oral dose or the novel ACE inhibitor spirapril in patients with chronic liver disease. Eur J Clin Pharmacol 1993; 45:247-254.
49. Castro A, Jimenez W, Claria J, Ros J, Martinez JM, Bosch M, Arroyo V et al. Impaired Responsiveness to Angiotensin-II in Experimental Cirrhosis —Role of Nitric Oxide. Hepatology 1993; 18:367-372.
50. Ryan J, Sudhir K, Jennings G, Esler M, Dudley F. Impaired Reactivity of the Peripheral Vasculature to Pressor Agents in Alcoholic Cirrhosis. Gastroenterology 1993; 105:1167-1172.
51. Murray BM, Paller MS. Decreased pressor reactivity to angiotensin II in cirrhotic rats. Evidence for a post-receptor defect in angiotensin action. Circ Res 1985; 57:424-431.
52. Kitano S, Kayanagi N, Sugimachi K, Kobayashi M, Inokuchi K. Mucosal blood flow and modified vascular responses to norepinephrine in the stomach of rats with liver cirrhosis. Eur Surg Res 1982; 14:221-230.
53. Ohsuga M, Moreau R, Hartleb H, Komeichi H, Lebrec D. Blunted Systemic, Splanchnic, and Renal Hemodynamic Responses to Atrial Natriuretic Peptide in Rats with Cirrhosis. J Hepatol 1994; 20:91-96.
54. Gerbes AL, Remien J, Juengst D, Sauerbruch T, Paumgartner G. Evidence for down-regulation of beta-2-adrenoceptors in cirrhotic patients with severe ascites. Lancet 1986; i:1409-1411.
55. Garcia Pagan JC, Navasa M, Rivera F, Bosch J, Rodes J. Lymphocyte beta-1-adrenoceptors and plasma catecholamines in patients with cirrhosis. Gastroenterology 1992; 102:2015-2023.
56. Ma ZH, Meddings JB, Lee SS. Membrane physical properties determine cardiac beta- adrenergic receptor function in cirrhotic rats. Am J Physiol 1994; 267:G87-G93.
57. Villeneuve JP, Verbeeck RK, Wilkinson GR, Branch RA. Furosemide kinetics and dynamics in patients with cirrhosis. Clin Pharmacol Ther 1986; 40:14-20.
58. Schwartz S, Brater DC, Pound D, Green PK, Kramer WG, Rudy D. Bioavailability, Pharmacokinetics, and Pharmacodynamics of Torsemide in Patients with Cirrhosis. Clin Pharmacol Ther 1993; 54:90-97.
59. Klotz U, Avant GR, Hoyumpa A, Schenker S, Wilkinson GR. The effects of age and liver disease on the disposition and elimination of diazepam in adult man. J Clin Invest 1975; 55:347-359.
60. Baktir G, Fisch HU, Karlaganis G, Minder C, Bircher J. Mechanism of the excessive sedative response of

cirrhotics to benzodiazepines: Model experiments with triazolam. Hepatology 1987; 7:629-638.
61. Robin DW, Lee MH, Hasan SS, Wood AJJ. Triazolam in cirrhosis: Pharmacokinetics and pharmacodynamics. Clin Pharmacol Ther 1993; 54:630-637.
62. Seeff LB, Cuccherini BA, Zimmerman HJ, Adler E, Benjamin SB. Acetaminophen hepatotoxicity in alcoholics. A therapeutic misadventure. Ann Intern Med 1986; 104:399-404.
63. Burgunder JM Lauterburg BH. Decreased production of glutathione in patients with cirrhosis. Eur J Clin Invest 1988; 17:408-414.
64. Lauterburg BH Velez ME. Glutathione deficiency in alcoholics: Risk factor for paracetamol hepatotoxicity. Gut 1988; 29:1153-1157.
65. Moore RD, Smith CR, Lietman PS. Increased risk of renal dysfunction due to interaction of liver disease and aminoglycosides. Am J Med 1986; 80:1093-1097.
66. Zambraski EJ, Chremos AN, Dunn M. Comparison of the effects of sulindac with other cyclooxygenase inhibitors on prostaglandin excretion and renal function in normal and chronic bile duct-ligated dogs and swine. J Pharmacol Exp Ther 1984; 228:560-566.
67. Quintero E, Ginès P, Arroyo V, Rimola A, Camps J, Gaya J, Guevara A et al. Sulindac reduces the urinary excretion of prostaglandins and impairs renal function in cirrhosis with ascites. Nephron 1986; 86:298-303.
68. Guarner C, Enriquez J, Guarner F, Quiroga J, Just J, Seres I, Prieto J et al. Effect of sulindac on prostaglandin excretion and renal function in cirrhotic patients with ascites. Scand J Gastroenterol 1986; 21:231-234.
69. Laffi G, Daskalopoulos G, Kronberg I, Hsueh W, Gentilini P, Zipser RD. Effects of sulindac and ibuprofen in patients with cirrhosis and ascites. Gastroenterology 1986; 90:182-187.
70. Chapuis L, Cadranel JF, Nordmann P, Hagege H, Gargot D, Bernard B, Buffet C et al. Grand Mal Seizures as a Complication of Treatment with Pefloxacin in Patients with Cirrhosis —A Report of Three Cases. J Hepatol 1993; 19:383-384.
71. Singh N, Yu VL, Mieles LA, Wagener MM. Beta-lactam antibiotic-induced leukopenia in severe hepatic dysfunction: Risk factors and implications for dosing in patients with liver disease. Am J Med 1993; 94:251-256.